Chapman & Hall/CRC Biostatistics Series

Recently Published Titles

Economic Evaluation of Cancer Drugs: Using Clinical Trial and Real-World Data
Iftekhar Khan, Ralph Crott, Zahid Bashir

Bayesian Analysis with R for Biopharmaceuticals: Concepts, Algorithms, and Case Studies
Harry Yang and Steven J. Novick

Mathematical and Statistical Skills in the Biopharmaceutical Industry: A Pragmatic Approach
Arkadiy Pitman, Oleksandr Sverdlov, L. Bruce Pearce

Bayesian Applications in Pharmaceutical Development
Mani Lakshminarayanan, Fanni Natanegara

Statistics in Regulatory Science
Shein-Chung Chow

Geospatial Health Data: Modeling and Visualization with R-INLA and Shiny
Paula Moraga

Artificial Intelligence for Drug Development, Precision Medicine, and Healthcare
Mark Chang

Bayesian Methods in Pharmaceutical Research
Emmanuel Lesaffre, Gianluca Baio, Bruno Boulanger

For more information about this series, please visit: https://www.crcpress.com/Chapman--HallCRC-Biostatistics-Series/book-series/CHBIOSTATIS

Bayesian Methods in Pharmaceutical Research

Edited by
Emmanuel Lesaffre
Gianluca Baio
Bruno Boulanger

CRC Press
Taylor & Francis Group
Boca Raton London New York

CRC Press is an imprint of the
Taylor & Francis Group, an **informa** business
A CHAPMAN & HALL BOOK

CRC Press
Taylor & Francis Group
6000 Broken Sound Parkway NW, Suite 300
Boca Raton, FL 33487-2742

Printed on acid-free paper

International Standard Book Number-13: 978-1-138-74848-4 (Hardback)

Visit the Taylor & Francis Web site at
http://www.taylorandfrancis.com

and the CRC Press Web site at
http://www.crcpress.com

Aan Hilda en Fons. Altijd bereid te helpen en positief ingesteld.

To Anna and Kobi. If I didn't have you, I would probably be 100 times more productive. But I would ***certainly*** *be a gazillion times less happy!*

A Martine, Eliot, Salomé, Pablo, Nils, Basile, Gaspard, Maxence et .... Que notre projet continue.

Contents

Preface

This edited book finds its origin in a series of Bayesian conferences, the "Bayes2000" meetings, started by the third editor in 2010. The aim of these meetings is to promote the use of applied Bayesian biostatistics in life sciences, pharmaceutical research & development and public health policies. The Bayes2000 meetings have been organized so far primarily in western Europe, namely 2010 (Braine l'Alleud, Belgium), 2011 (Louvain-la-Neuve, Belgium), 2012 (Aachen, Germany), 2013 (Rotterdam, The Netherlands), 2014 (London, UK), 2015 (Basel, Switzerland), 2016 (Leuven, Belgium), 2017 (Albacete, Spain), 2018 (Cambridge, UK) and 2019 (Lyon, France). At all these meetings exchange between industry, regulatory agencies and academics was promoted and established.

At the 2016 meeting, the idea was born to make even more public the possibilities the Bayesian approach can offer for pharmaceutical research. The three editors decided to contact authors active in Bayesian biostatistics coming from industry, regulatory agencies or academia. The purpose of this edited volume is to reflect the different stages of pharmaceutical research. For each of these stages: (1) the reader is introduced to the substantive area; (2) a review is given of the common statistical approaches; (3) the capabilities of the Bayesian approach are discussed and (4) the challenges for the future for the Bayesian approach are presented. Each chapter highlights one or more aspects of pharmaceutical research. The concepts are illustrated with numerous real-life examples.

The volume is divided into four major parts. Part I is the introductory part. In Part II, Bayesian approaches in clinical development are treated. In Part III, Bayesian approaches for post-marketing studies are discussed. In Part IV we look at product development and manufacturing aspects. We close the book with Part V that discusses some additional topics. We now briefly discuss the main aspects of each chapter.

Part I consists of three chapters.

The first chapter introduces the basic Bayesian concepts. To this end primarily clinical examples will be used, with a focus on randomized controlled trials (RCTs). More specifically, after a reflection on the classical frequentist approach, the Bayesian concepts of prior and posterior distribution will be explained. Then follows the posterior summary measures and how to compute the posterior and its summary measures in practice. To this end we explain and illustrate the mechanisms of the Markov chain Monte Carlo techniques. Aspects of the choice of prior will also be discussed. Apart from the standard parametric Bayesian approaches, also non-parametric and semi-parametric Bayesian methods will be discussed, but only briefly. We end the chapter with a brief overview of the popular Bayesian software tools.

The second chapter addresses the status of Bayesian statistics in terms of regulatory acceptance by the U.S. Food and Drug Administration (FDA). The chapter highlights the acceptance of Bayesian statistics in submissions for medical devices in the U.S. for a number of years. This is in contrast to the submission of drugs. The history and the accomplishments of the Bayesian approach for medical devices is reviewed. The chapter also addresses the regulation of pharmaceutical drugs and biologicals and the role of the Bayesian approach in this. While the past has not been favorable for submissions using Bayesian tools, there is hope that things may change in the near future. Finally the challenges and the future of Bayesian statistics in the regulatory environment are tackled.

In Chapter 3 the connection is made between posterior tail probabilities and P-values obtained from frequentist one-sided hypothesis tests. Further, this chapter discusses (1) posterior tail probabilities for decision making and (2) predictive tail probabilities. R code exemplifies the Bayesian calculations.

Part II consists of ten chapters.

Chapter 4 is an introductory chapter to highlight the use and importance of Bayesian ideas in drug development. After an overview of the different stages in drug development, the distinction between classical and Bayesian thinking is pointed out. Four applications of Bayesian methods in drug development illustrate the usefulness of the Bayesian approach.

Chapter 5 consists of a review of different methodologies to elicit prior information from experts. Both elicitation of single as well as multiple parameters is considered. Further, the chapter describes how information from multiple experts needs to be combined. Three examples of eliciting prior information in the context of drug trials are described. The Bayesian approach offers the use of prior information in the analysis of the current data. One possibility is to use prior expert knowledge; another possibility is to incorporate historical data into the analysis. The question is then whether the historical data are suitable for the current analysis, and if so, how much of the historical information should be made use of.

Chapter 6 describes the proposed priors that allow us to incorporate (part of) the historical data into the current analysis, i.e. the power prior, the commensurate prior and the meta-analytic prior. Three applications on non-inferiority studies illustrate the use of these priors and associated topics.

After a potentially potent drug has been discovered, it is important to determine the appropriate dose. In the first part of Chapter 7, dose-response studies are briefly introduced and illustrated in a Bayesian context. In a dose-response or dose ranging study, one seeks to determine the range of doses that determine the therapeutic window. In the second part of this chapter, the Bayesian approach to dose escalation trials in oncology is treated. The goal in such a trial is to find the maximum tolerated dose for the drug. The benefits of the Bayesian approach to the classical frequentist 3+3 design are highlighted. Bayesian dose escalation designs are a special case of adaptive designs. In (Bayesian) adaptive study design modifications of the study design or conduct are prospectively planned and appropriately taken into account at the analysis stage.

Chapter 8 reviews Bayesian adaptive designs, including: (1) adapting the size and/or duration of the study, (2) changing the in- and exclusion criteria of the trial and (3) adapting the probability to be assigned to the treatment arms. Clinical trials are inherently longitudinal, since one has to measure (and compare) the change in disease status of the patients to conclude whether the experimental treatment has an effect and/or is safe. Typically, one records in a longitudinal study either repeatedly the response (repeated measurements) or the timing that it takes to achieve a certain response (survival data).

In Chapter 9, Bayesian methods for repeated measurements obtained in a longitudinal study are discussed. Modeling longitudinal data involves specifying a mean & covariance structure and therefore also their prior distributions. While the prior distributions for the parameters of the mean structure are standard, the prior distributions for the covariance structure need special attention and will be addressed in this chapter. An important part of this chapter is devoted to the Bayesian analysis of longitudinal data in the presence of missing responses and/or covariates. Missing data are present in each study, but in a longitudinal study past responses and covariates can be explicitly used to get an idea what the results would have been if all subjects had complete data.

In Chapter 10, Bayesian methods for the analysis of survival data are treated. Almost invariably survival studies are confronted with censored responses, with right censoring most prevalent. In the frequentist paradigm Cox regression is by far the most popular semi-parametric technique to analyze right-censored event times. In contrast, for a long time the Bayesian survival models were parametric and could not compete with the frequentist semi-parametric methods. With the introduction of Bayesian semi-parametric models the parametric assumptions could be greatly reduced. One could even show that in the limit a particular Bayesian semi-parametric approach leads to a Cox regression model.

Chapter 11 is an illustration of a possible Bayesian approach to study cognitive decline and brain imaging for precision medicine.

Apart from the 'standard' advantages that Bayesian methods have over classical approaches for the analysis of RCT data, in two settings the Bayesian approach is particularly interesting and fruitful, i.e. when dealing with RCTs on orphan products for rare diseases and in pediatric trials. In both cases the trials suffer from small study sizes.

Chapter 12 is devoted to the unique clinical and statistical challenges for the design and analysis of orphan products in rare diseases. The regulatory background for orphan drugs is different from classical drugs, and therefore extensively reviewed in this chapter. The chapter then reviews trial designs for such drugs that can incorporate Bayesian statistics. The methods make use of the various priors for the inclusion of historical data seen in Chapter 6.

Also the Bayesian approaches to analyze trial results from a pediatric population make use of such priors, borrowing information from adult population results. This is seen in Chapter 13.

Part III hosts four chapters that basically all deal with Bayesian methods for explorative analyses.

When several RCTs evaluate the relative performance of an experimental intervention versus a control intervention, one may extend the external validity of the individual studies by combining the results in a meta-analysis. A meta-analysis also increases the power to examine efficacy and safety of the experimental intervention in a subgroup of patients, e.g. elderly patients. Finally, a meta-analysis allows us to examine whether the effect or the safety of an experimental intervention remains constant over different RCTs. All of this is discussed in Chapter 14, but with a focus on a Bayesian analysis. Classical meta-analysis is also called pairwise analysis. But if several interventions are available for the treatment of the same disease or symptoms, one might wonder which of the treatments is 'best'. Such a question can be addressed in a network meta-analysis, which is also discussed and illustrated in this chapter. Network meta-analyses are also the tool to compare the relative efficacy and safety of interventions in case there are no or only a limited number of head-to-head trials.

The availability of efficacious and safe interventions is of primary importance, but when several interventions enjoy these characteristics it is important from a public health point of view to also evaluate their cost-effectiveness ratio. This is done in an economic evaluation. Economic evaluations in healthcare comprise a set of analytical tools to combine all relevant evidence on costs and consequences of intervention(s) compared to a control or status quo. Recently, such evaluations are primarily based on Bayesian decision-theoretic foundations making use of utility functions and evaluating the uncertainty with which evaluations are made. All of this is explained and illustrated in Chapter 15.

Chapter 16 treats the Bayesian modeling for the economic evaluation of the performance of health interventions by making use of real world data. The chapter describes the basic concepts of real world evidence obtained from several types of real world data. The rest of the chapter is basically an illustration of an economic analysis using survival analysis of a particular case study.

Chapter 17 looks at the decision-making process when deciding regulatory approval of new pharmaceutical interventions, from a slightly different perspective than Chapter 15. In this case, the focus is on the immediate comparison between the clinical benefits and risks associated with a given intervention. While there are commonalities between this and the wider economic evaluation discussed in Chapter 15, in this chapter, methods such as Multi-Criteria Decision making are presented and discussed. A recent trend in medicine, is to look for treatments that are subject-specific, called precision medicine. This is an emerging field that aims to improve disease prevention and treatment by accounting for individual variations in genes, lifestyle and environment making use of extensive datasets. The aim is to uncover subpopulations with different biological characteristics and susceptibility to the disease or response to treatment to identify clinical biomarkers that help in predicting the risk of disease or its progression, or estimate treatment effects at the individual level.

Part IV on product development and manufacturing contains seven chapters.

Chapter 18 gives first an overview of the common problems that need to be addressed during the development of new drug products, namely (1) development of robust processes as required by the quality by design regulation, (2) the qualification and the control of the processes, (3) the development, validation and control of the measurements systems used to evaluate the drug products and (4) common quality evaluations of batches of drug products produced such as the stability, the content uniformity and the dissolution. The problem and comparability of two processes and analytical similarity are addressed from a Bayesian perspective.

Chapter 19 shows that the Bayesian approach is very flexible for modeling complex (manufacturing or assay) processes or complex quantifications of a such a process. This chapter reviews two important aspects of process development and validation, namely: (1) the design space and (2) the assessment of assay robustness. In addition, the chapter demonstrates that natural quality criteria may exist in complex quantitative forms.

Chapter 20 aims to show how an analytical method or an assay can be developed following the best practice of the industry — namely, the Analytical Quality by Design — to ensure a high reliability of the results obtained. Then, it illustrates how measurement error (also known as total error) can be used to better predict the impact of the uncertainty during routine use, but also during activities like assay transfer between sites.

Stability studies are facing the emergence of new issues related to quality risk management going from the quantification of the risk of Out-of-Specification products in future production, the determination of a shelf-life that guarantees acceptable risks to both patients and manufacturers, the definition of a robust set of storage conditions under which the labeled shelf-life remains valid, to the validation of a process modification and so on. Statistical modeling plays a prominent role in the design and analysis of stability studies, and in Chapter 21 the benefits of using the Bayesian framework to manage risks and make decisions is demonstrated. Content uniformity is a measure of the amount of active pharmaceutical ingredient in the units of a batch of drug product.

Before a batch of a newly manufactured drug product is released to consumers, content uniformity testing is used to establish that the dosage units of a drug product consistently contain the specified amount of drug (active pharmaceutical ingredient). Content uniformity testing establishes whether a sample of units from a batch of drug product meets specified criteria on the amount of drug present. The foundation for most content uniformity testing stems from USP guidelines, namely USP<905> for solid dosage units, USP<3> for topical and transdermal products, and USP<601> for inhaled products. In Chapter 22, a thorough review of two USP guidelines is provided along with their Bayesian counterparts and extensions.

Chapter 23 gives a brief review of current practice in in-vitro (IV) dissolution. IV dissolution studies replace the in-vivo studies that evaluate in real-life the dissolution of the active pharmaceutical ingredient in the body. Drug molecules must first dissolve in the patient's gastro-intestinal tract and then in a dissolved state be transported into the dedicated sites in the body. This makes the understanding and control of the dissolution rate of a pharmaceutical product a key goal of both pharmaceutical sponsors and regulators.

According to the 2011 U.S. Food and Drug Administration Guidance for Industry Process Validation, biopharmaceutical manufacturing processes are considered in three stages: Process Development and Design (Stage 1), Process Qualification (Stage 2), and Continued Process Verification (Stage 3). The focus of Chapter 24 are Stages 2 and 3 of the commercial manufacturing process. In many cases, simple statistical tools available in off-the-shelf statistical software for Stages 2 and 3 are used to meet these objectives. Often these simple tools are adequate; however, there are limitations to their use and interpretation. The application of Bayesian methods to address these limitations is the subject of this chapter.

The book ends with Part V that contains two chapters.

Chapter 25 reviews the use of Bayesian methods in the medical device industry. In contrast to drug trials, FDA has accepted the Bayesian approach as one of the mainstream statistical approaches that can be used for registration purposes. The Bayesian methods are basically used here in two areas. The first is in the creation of stochastic engineering models (SEM) to analyze the performance of the device during its design stage prior to release to market. A SEM attempts to simulate the performance of a medical device in the intended patient population. In the second area the Bayesian methods address the modeling and analysis of clinical trials to demonstrate the safety and efficacy of the device. These methods include adaptive Bayesian device trials, and augmenting trials with historical data using dynamic borrowing informative prior methods.

Chapter 26 shows that the Bayesian approach is well suited to analyze the factors that determine the drug development costs. An overview is given of the area of quantitative modeling to support drug development decisions at program and portfolio levels. First, classical statistical approaches currently used to manage programs and portfolios are reviewed and their pitfalls are shown. Then, the elegance of the Bayesian approach is demonstrated and it is shown to inform and improve decisions made to promote or abort programs or products in development. The focus lies here on approaches that explicitly model the relationship between trial designs and performance criteria.

The editors wish to thank Pablo Boulanger for the design of the cover page of the book. We also thank Rob Calver and his team to help us in the editorial process.

Editors

Emmanuel Lesaffre studied mathematics at the University of Antwerp and received his PhD in statistics at the University of Leuven, Belgium. He is full professor at L-Biostat, KU Leuven, and part-time professor at University of Hasselt. He had a joint position at Erasmus University in Rotterdam, the Netherlands from 2007 to 2014.

His statistical research is rooted in medical research questions. He has worked in a great variety of medical research areas, but especially in oral health, cardiology, nursing research, ophthalmology and oncology. He also contributed on various statistical topics, i.e. discriminant analysis, hierarchical models, model diagnostics, interval-censored data, misclassification issues, variable selection, various clinical trial topics and diagnostic tests both under the frequentist and Bayesian paradigm. He has taught introductory and advanced courses to medical and statistical researchers. In the last two decades, his research focused on Bayesian techniques resulting in a textbook and courses taught at several universities and governmental organizations. Recently, he co-authored a textbook on interval censoring. In total he (co)-authored nine books and more than 600 papers. He has served as statistical consultant on a great variety of clinical trials in various ways, e.g. as a steering committee and data-monitoring committee member.

He is the founding chair of the Statistical Modelling Society (2002) and was ISCB president (2006–2008). Further, he is ASA and ISI fellow and honorary member of the Society for Clinical Biostatistics and of the Statistical Modelling Society. He has been involved in the organisation of the Bayes 20XX conference since 2013.

Gianluca Baio is a Professor of Statistics and Health Economics in the Department of Statistical Science at University College London. He graduated in Statistics and Economics from the University of Florence (Italy). He then completed a PhD programme in Applied Statistics again at the University of Florence, after a period at the Program on the Pharmaceutical Industry at the MIT Sloan School of Management, Cambridge (USA). He then worked as a Research Fellow and then Lecturer in the Department of Statistical Sciences at University College London (UK). His main interests are in Bayesian statistical modelling for cost effectiveness analysis and decision-making problems in the health systems, hierarchical/multilevel models and causal inference using the decision-theoretic approach. He also leads the Statistics for Health Economic Evaluation research group within the department of Statistical Science, whose activity revolves around the development and application of Bayesian statistical methodology for health economic evaluation, e.g. cost-effectiveness or cost-utility analysis. He also collaborates with the UK National Institute for Health and Care Excellence (NICE) as a Scientific Advisor on Health Technology Appraisal projects and has served as Secretary (2014-2016) and then Programme Chair (2016-2018) in the Section on Biostatistics and Pharmaceutical Statistics of the International Society for Bayesian Analysis. He has been involved in the organisation of the Bayes 20XX conference since 2013.

Bruno Boulanger, PhD
Organization: PharmaLex Belgium
Chief Scientific Officer, PharmaLex Belgium, Belgium
Lecturer, School of Pharmacy, Université de Liège, Belgium

After a post-doctorate at the Université Catholique de Louvain (Belgium) and the University of Minnesota (USA) in Statistics applied to simulation of clinical trials, Bruno joined Eli Lilly in Belgium in 1992. Bruno holds various positions in Europe and in the USA where he gathered experience in several areas of the pharmaceutical industry including discovery, toxicology, CMC and early clinical phases. Bruno joined UCB Pharma in 2007 as Director of Exploratory Statistics, contributing the implementation of Model-Based Drug Development strategy and applied Bayesian statistics. Bruno is also, since 2000, Lecturer at the Université of Liège, in the School of Pharmacy, teaching Design of Experiments and Statistics. Bruno has organized and contributed since 1998 to Non-Clinical Statistics Conference in Europe and set up in 2010 the Applied Bayesian Biostatistics conference. Bruno is also a USP Expert, member of the Committee of Experts in Statistics since 2010. Bruno has authored or co-authored more than 100 publications in applied statistics.

Contributors

Suresh Ankolekar
Maastricht School of Management
Maastricht, Netherlands

Gianluca Baio
University College London
London, UK

Cynthia Basu
Pfizer
San Diego, CA, US

Alun Bedding
Roche Products Ltd
Welwyn Garden City, UK

Nicky Best
GlaxoSmithKline Pharmaceuticals
London, UK

Bruno Boulanger
PharmaLex Belgium
Mont-saint-Guibert, Belgium

Gregory Campbell
GCStat Consulting LLC
Knoxville, TN, US

Bradley P. Carlin
Counterpoint Statistical Consulting
Minneapolis, MN, US

Freda Cooner
Amgen Inc.
Thousand Oaks CA, US

Maria Costa
Novartis Pharmaceuticals Corporation
Basel, Switzerland

Nigel Dallow
GlaxoSmithKline Pharmaceuticals
London, UK

Michael J. Daniels
University of Florida
Gainsville, FL, US

David Dejardin
F. Hoffmann-La Roche
Basel, Switzerland

Nikolaos Demiris
Cambridge Clinical Trials Centre, University of Cambridge
Cambridge, UK

Sofia Dias
University of Bristol
Bristol, UK

Carl Di Casoli
Halozyme Therapeutics
San Diego, CA, US

Katherine Giacoletti
SynoloStat
New York, NY, US

Tarek Haddad
MedTronic
Minneapolis, MN, US

Leonhard Held
University of Zurich
Zurich, Switzerland

Tonakpon Hermane Avohou
University of Liége, Belgium
Liége, Belgium

Buffy Hudson-Curtis
GlaxoSmithKline Pharmaceuticals
Zebulon, NC, US

Masanori Ito
Astellas Pharma Inc.
Tokyo, Japan

Christopher Jackson
MRC Biostatistics Unit
Cambridge, UK

Yannis Jemiai
Cytel Inc
Cambridge, MA, US

Hayley E Jones
University of Bristol
Bristol, UK

Pierre Lebrun
Pharmalex
Mont-saint-Guibert, Belgium

Dave LeBlond
CMC Statistical Studies
Wadsworth, IL, US

Emmanuel Lesaffre
KU Leuven
Leuven, Belgium

Charles Liu
Cytel Inc
Cambridge, MA, US

Linas Mockus
Purdue University
West Lafayette, IN, US

Timothy Montague
GlaxoSmithKline Pharmaceuticals
London, UK

Timothy Mutsvari
Pharmalex, Belgium

Beat Neuenschwander
Novartis Pharma AG
Basel, Switzerland

Steven Novick
AstraZenica
Gaithersburg, MD, US

David Ohlssen
Novartis Pharmaceuticals Corporation
Randolph, NJ, US

Nitin Patel
Cytel Inc
Cambridge, MA, US

John J. Peterson
GlaxoSmithKline Pharmaceuticals
Philadelphia, PA, US

Sylvia Richardson
MRC Biostatistics Unit
Cambridge, UK

Gary L. Rosner
Johns Hopkins University
Baltimore, MD, US

Anaïs Rouanet
MRC Biostatistics Unit
Cambridge, UK

Eric Rozet
Pharmalex
Mont-saint-Guibert, Belgium

Tara Scherder
SynoloStat
New York, NY, US

Heinz Schmidli
Novartis Pharma AG
Basel, Switzerland

Linda D. Sharples
London School of Hygiene and Tropical Medicine
London, UK

Pritibha Singh
Novartis Pharmaceuticals Corporation
Basel, Switzerland

Mark Strong
University of Sheffield
Sheffield, UK

Brian Tom
MRC Biostatistics Unit
Cambridge, UK

Nicky J. Welton
University of Bristol
Bristol, UK

Forrest Williamson
Eli Lilly ad Company
Indianapolis, IN, US

Phil Woodward
Independent Consultant, Suffolk
UK

Dandan Xu
US Food and Drug Administration
Silver Spring, MD, US

Yusuke Yamaguchi
Astellas Pharma Inc.
Japan

Yueqin Zhao
Food and Drug Administration
Silver Spring, MD, US

List of abbreviations

Term	Explanation
AAD	Antiarrhythmic Drug
ACDRS	American Course on Drug Development and Regulatory Science
ACMV	Available Case Missing Value
ACR	American College of Rheumatology
AD	Alzheimer's Disease
ADSWG	Adaptive Design Scientific Working Group
ADNI	Alzheimer's Disease Neuroimaging Initiative
ADAPT-IT	Adaptive Designs Accelerating Promising Trials into Treatments
AE	Adverse Event
AF	Atrial Fibrillation
AI	Artificial Intelligence
AIC	Akaike's Information Criterion
ANCOVA	Analysis of Covariance
ANOVA	Analysis of Variance
AQbD	Analytical Quality by Design
API	Active Pharmaceutical Ingredient
AR	Accept-Reject
ARS	Adaptive Rejection Sampling
ASA	American Statistical Association
ASTIN	Acute Stroke Therapy by Inhibition of Neutrophils
ATP	Analytical Target Profile
AUC	Area Under the Curve
BATTLE	Biomarker Based Approach for Lung cancer Eradication
BART	Bayesian Additive Regression Trees
BCR	Benefit-Cost Ratio
BF	Bayes Factor
BGR	Brooks-Gelman-Rubin
BIC	Bayesian Information Criterion
BLRA	Benefit-Less-Risk Analysis
BMA	Bayesian Model Averaging
BNP	Bayesian NonParametric
BR	Benefit-Risk
BUGS	Bayesian inference Using Gibbs Sampling
CBER	Center for Biologics Evaluation and Research
CDER	Center for Drug Evaluation and Research
CDRH	Center for Devices and Radiological Research
Cdf	Cumulative distribution function
CKD	Chronic Kidney Disease
CMC	Chemistry and Manufacturing Control
CMHT	Community Mental Health Team
CMP	Critical Method Parameter

Term	Explanation
CPO	Conditional Predictive Ordinate
CPP	Critical Process Parameter
CPV	Continued Process Verification
CQA	Critical Quality Attribute
CR	Complete Response
CRHTT	Crisis Resolution Home Treatment Team
CRM	Continual Reassessment Method
CRP	C-Reactive Protein
CUI	Clinical Utility Index
CUDAL	Content Uniformity and Dissolution Acceptance Limits
CYC	Cyclophosphamide
DA	Data Augmentation
DIA	Drug Information Association
DI	Desirability Index
DIC	Deviance Information Criterion
DLT	Dose Limiting Toxicity
DMC	Data Monitoring Committee
DMD	Duchenne Muscular Dystrophy
DoE	Design of Experiments
DP	Dirichlet Process
DPM	Dirichlet Process Mixture
DPMM	Dirichlet Process Mixture Model
DR	Dosing Range
DS	Design Space
DSMB	Data and Safety Monitoring Board
ECMO	Extra-Corporeal Membrane Oxygenation
ECRP	Erythrocyte Sedimentation Rate
EHR	Electronic Health Record
EHSS	Effective Historical Sample Size
EMA	European Medicines Agency
ENBS	Expected Net Benefit of Sampling
ENPV	Expected Net Present Value
ER	Extended Release
ESS	Effective Sample Size
EURORDIS	European Rare Diseases Organisation
EVPI	Expected Value of Perfect Information
EVPPI	Expected Value of Partial Perfect Information
EVSI	Expected Value of Sample Information
EWOC	Escalation With Overdose Control
FDARA	Food and Drug Administration Reauthorization Act
FDC	Fixed-Dose Combination
FMEA	Failure Mode and Effects Analysis
GBR	Global Benefit-Risk
GBS	Guillain-Barré Syndrome
GARP	Generalized AutoRegressive Parameter
GEE	Generalized Estimating Equations
GH	Growth Hormone
GLM	General Linear Model
GLMM	Generalized Linear Mixed Model
GOF	Goodness-Of-Fit

Term	Explanation
GMRF	Gaussian Markov Random Field
GP	Gamma Process
GP	General Practitioner
GP	General Purpose
GPQ	Generalized Pivotal Quantity
HMC	Hamiltonian Monte Carlo
HN	Half-Normal
HPLC	High-Performance Analytical method and assay Liquid Chromatographic
HPD	Highest Posterior Density
HPT	HyperParaThyroidism
HR	Hazard Ratio
HTA	Health Technology Assessment
ICD	Implantable Cardioverter Defibrillator
ICH	International Conference on Harmonisation
IDE	Investigational Device Exemption
IPD	Individual Patient Data
INHB	Incremental Net Health Benefit
INLA	Integrated Nested Laplace Approximation
iPTH	Intact ParaThyroid Hormone
IR	Immediate Release
IV	Innovation Variance
IVF	In Vitro Fertilisation
IVR	In Vitro Release
IVIVC	In Vitro In Vivo Correlation
JAGS	Just Another Gibbs Sampler
LMM	Linear Mixed Model
LOQ	Lower limit Of Quantification
LPML	Log Pseudo-Marginal Likelihood
MABEL	Minimum Anticipated Biological Effect Level
MAC	Meta-Analytic-Combined
MAP	Meta-Analytic-Predictive
MAR	Maximum Attributable Risk
MAR	Missing-At-Random
MCAR	Missing-Completely-At-Random
MCDA	Multi-Criteria Decision Analysis
MCE	Minimum Clinical Efficacy
MCerror	Monte Carlo Error
MCI	Mild Cognitive Impairment
MCP-Mod	Multiple Comparison Procedure Modeling
MC	Monte Carlo
MCS	Monte Carlo Simulation
MCMC	Markov Chain Monte Carlo
MDIC	Medical Device Innovation Consortium
MDP	Markov Decision Process
MF	Mycophenolate Mofetil
MH	Metropolis-Hastings
MIDD	Model-Informed Drug Development
ML	Maximum Likelihood
MLE	Maximum Likelihood Estimate

Term	Explanation
MMLR	Multivariate Multiple Linear Regression
MNAR	Missing-Not-At-Random
MOA	Mechanism Of Action
MR	Magnetic Resonance
MREM	Marginalized Random Effect Model
MRI	Magnetic Resonance Imaging
MSD	Multivariate Statistical Distance
MSOA	Middle Super Output Area
MTD	Maximum Tolerated Dose
MTM	Marginalized Transition Model
mTSS	Modified Total Sharp Score
MVN	Multivariate Normal Model
MVP	Multivariate Probit Model
NCB	Net Clinical Benefit
NDA	New Drug Application
NDLM	Normal Dynamic Linear Model
NFD	Non-Future Dependent
NI	Non-Informative
NI	Non-Inferior
NICE	National Institute for Health and Care Excellence
NIH	National Institutes of Health
NNHM	Normal-Normal Hierarchical Model
NLMM	Non-Linear Mixed Model
NMA	Network Meta Analysis
NNT	Number Need to Treat
NNTH	Number Need to Treat for Harm
NRS	Numeric Rating Scale
NUTS	No-U-Turn Sampler
OAC	Oral AntiCoagulation
OFAT	One Factor At a Time
OINDP	Oral, Inhaled, and Nasal Drug Product
OPG	Objective Performance Goal
OPV	Ongoing Process Verification
OOS	Out-of-Specification
PAM	Partitioning Around Medoids
PAN	PolyArteritis Nodosa
PANSS	Positive And Negative Syndrome Scale
PICO	Population, Interventions and Comparators, and Outcomes
PoC	Proof of Concept
PoS	Probability of Success
pCR	Pathological Complete Response
PDUFA	Prescription Drug User Fee Act
PEP	Predictive Evidence Probability
PET	Predictive Evidence Threshold
PETS	Predictive Evidence Threshold Scaling
PDUFA	Pharmaceutical Drug Users Fee Act
PH	Proportional Hazards
PK	PharmacoKinetic
PKPD	PharmacoKinetic-PharmacoDynamic
PMA	PreMarket Approval

Term	Explanation
PML	Progressive Multifocal Leukoencephalopathy
PMM	Pattern Mixture Model
PP	Process Parameter
PPC	Posterior Predictive Check
PPD	Posterior Predictive Distribution
PPP	Posterior Predictive P-value
PPQ	Process Performance Qualification
PQ	Process Qualification
PROTECT	Pharmacoepidemiological Research on Outcomes of Therapeutics by a European ConsorTium
PSBF	Pseudo Bayes Factor
PSM	Probabilistic Simulation Methods
PSP	Progressive Supranuclear Palsy
PSPRS	PSP-Rating Scale
PT	Polya Tree
PTH	ParaThyroid Hormone
PV	Process Validation
QA	Quality Attributes
QALY	Quality-Adjusted Life Year
QbD	Quality-by-Design
QbT	Quality-by-Testing
QFRBA	Quantitative Framework for Risk and Benefit Assessment
QTPP	Quality Target Product Profile
Q-TWIST	Quality adjusted Time WIthout Symptoms and Toxicity
RBAT	Risk-Benefit Acceptability Threshold
RBC	Risk-Benefit Contour
RBP	Risk-Benefit Plane
REML	Restricted Maximum Likelihood
ROI	Return On Investment
RV	Relative Value
QDM	Quantitative Decision Making
RAND	Research ANd Development
RCT	Randomized Clinical Trial
RIO	Rational Impartial Prior
RMANOVA	Repeated Measures ANOVA
RSD	Relative Standard Deviation
RV-NNT	Relative Value adjusted Number Needed to Treat
RWD	Real World Data
RWE	Real World Evidence
SAE	Serious Adverse Event
SBRAM	Sarac's Benefit-Risk Assessment Method
SD	Standard Deviation
SHELF	SHeffield Elicitation Framework
SM	Selection Model
SMAA	Stochastic Multicriteria Acceptability Analysis
SoC	Standard of Care
SPM	Shared Parameter Model
SSED	Summary of Safety and Effectiveness Data
SEM	Stochastic Engineering Model
SIP	Stochastic Integer Programming

Term	Explanation
SSLWG	Stability Shelf Lives Working Group
SSS	Scandinavian Stroke Scale
SUBA	Subgroup-Based Adaptive
TI	Tolerance Interval
TPP	Target Product Profile
TSD	Technical Support Document
UHPLC	Ultra High Performance Liquid Chromatography
USP	United States Pharmacopeia
VAP	Ventilator-Associated Pneumonia
WAIC	Widely Available Information Criterion

Part I

Introduction

1

Bayesian Background

Emmanuel Lesaffre

I-Biostat, KU Leuven, Belgium

Gianluca Baio

University College London, UK

In this chapter, we review the fundamental concepts of the Bayesian approach to statistical inference. Bayesian statistics was first introduced over 250 years ago, but became only popular when it could address practical problems. For a long time Fisher's theory based on the likelihood function as the fundamental engine of inference and the frequentist approach of Neyman and Pearson have ruled the statistical world. Until three decades ago, the Bayesian approach was looked upon as more of a curiosity rather than providing a tool for solving practical problems. This changed when Markov chain Monte Carlo techniques were introduced.

The chapter starts with reviewing the concepts of the classical approach, also called the *frequentist approach*. Central to the Bayesian approach is Bayes theorem. The origin of the theorem is a simple factorization of the joint probability into the product of a conditional and a marginal probability. The ingenious idea of Thomas Bayes is to apply this principle to the parameters of a statistical model and to assume that the uncertainty underlying their "true" value can be described using a probability model. We illustrate how the posterior distribution arises and can be computed from prior and data information. The characteristics of the posterior distribution are illustrated for binary and Gaussian responses. In addition, the most common posterior summary measures are discussed. Independent and dependent sampling, including Markov chain Monte Carlo techniques, to approximate the posterior distribution and posterior summary measures are discussed and illustrated. A brief and incomplete review of Bayesian software is then given. Most Bayesian analyses are based on parametric assumptions. Especially in the last decade, nonparametric Bayesian developments have seen the light but the theoretical level prevents us going deep here. Bayesian tools for model selection and model checking are also reviewed. Additional topics are treated in the final section as well as suggestions for further reading.

1.1 Introduction

Medical knowledge has expanded tremendously during the last century. This has given a boost to pharmaceutical and drug research. Following the thalidomide disaster (Kim and Scialli, 2011) in the late 1950's, the involvement of statistics and of statisticians has increased exponentially. Initially, acting more as "policemen", protecting medical researchers against over interpreting positive results, gradually statisticians have become involved and pro-active in all stages of medical research and more specifically also in drug research. The impact of statistics and statisticians on medical research truly cannot be overstated, especially in the course of the last five decades. To a large extent, this is due to the ingenious and hard work of so many statisticians such as Armitage, Cochran, Fisher, Neyman and Pearson, to name a few.

Medical knowledge grows by setting up successive experiments to test theoretical conjectures about the mechanisms of action and the resulting effectiveness of healthcare interventions. Each result, whether a failure or a success, gives insight into the medical processes. This is the successful paradigm that pharmaceutical research has followed over many years. For instance, before drugs enter the market they undergo numerous tests from pre-clinical studies, Phase I studies, Phase II studies to Phase III studies. Even when approved and registered by regulatory authorities such as the US Food and Drug Administration (FDA) and the European Medicines Agency (EMA), large scale studies are set up to evaluate the safety of the drugs. Nevertheless, despite this careful process of learning, the current process of accumulating knowledge has been criticized heavily since it turns out that much of the (medical) scientific results cannot be reproduced (Baker, 2011).

The classical statistical approach following the independent and somewhat adversarial developments of Fisher, on one side and Neyman & Pearson, on the other, has brought in much rigor in empirical medical research. However, classical tools such as the P-value are often misunderstood, overused and misused. In addition, while scientific knowledge is built up from successes and failures in the past, i.e. from learning from the past, the classical statistical tools do not allow us to incorporate explicitly past knowledge. The Bayesian approach, for a long time ignored and even opposed by many statisticians, allows us to incorporate in a flexible way historical information into current statistical analyses. Despite this important feature, until about the 1990's, Bayesian analysis was largely considered a curiosity, due to the fact that, because of computational limitations it was not possible to tackle practical problems using Bayesian tools. This changed with the introduction of Markov chain Monte Carlo sampling techniques. Since then, the Bayesian approach has grown tremendously in popularity, certainly among statisticians and increasingly among clinical researchers.

In the next section we briefly review the basic principles of the frequentist statistical approach, based on a combination of Fisher's P-value and the Type I and II error rates as advocated by Neyman & Pearson. In Section 1.3, we present the basic concepts of the Bayesian approach including prior and posterior distribution, posterior summary measures and the posterior predictive distribution. These concepts will be illustrated for a binary and Gaussian outcome. The case of more than one parameter is treated in Section 1.4. Principles to choose the prior distribution are reviewed in Section 1.5. In Section 1.6, numerical techniques to approximate the posterior distribution and its summary measures are reviewed. This section also discusses Markov chain Monte Carlo techniques. Bayesian concepts applied to hierarchical models are reviewed in Section 1.7, as also the data augmentation approach. Statistical models are selected from a pool of models, but must be checked on the data at hand. Bayesian methods for this analysis step can be found in Section 1.8. Most Bayesian models are parametric, but in the last decade Bayesian nonparametric approaches have been advocated, see Section 1.9. Bayesian software is briefly reviewed in Section 1.10. Additional topics and further reading are given in the concluding section.

1.2 The frequentist approach to inference

1.2.1 Classical hypothesis testing

In this section, a brief review of the basic principles of the classical frequentist approach is given. We refer to the 'classical approach' to statistical inference as the combined use of P-value with controlling for the Type I and II error rates. These two procedures are routinely mixed: Neyman & Pearson's approach (based on *hypothesis testing* and Type I and II error rates) is typically used to *design* a study, for instance by fixing the significance level to $\alpha = 0.05$ and the power to $1 - \beta = 0.8$. However, once the data are obtained, the results are reported in terms of *significance testing* and $P-$values, as recommended by Fisher. To focus ideas, we take the randomized clinical trial (RCT) discussed in Lesaffre and Lawson (2012). This multi-center study compared the efficacy of two oral treatments for toenail infection after 12 weeks of treatment. We take here the subgroup of patients for whom the big toenail was selected as target nail. One group of patients received Lamisil (treatment A, $n_A = 131$), while the other group received Itraconazole (treatment B, $n_B = 133$). The two treatment groups were compared for unaffected nail length at the big toenail after 48 weeks of follow up. More specifically, the researchers are interested in knowing whether $\Delta = \mu_A - \mu_B$ is substantially different from zero, with μ_A the true average unaffected nail length under treatment A and μ_B under treatment B. The 'classical' approach to statistical inference is to first specify a 'straw hypothesis', called the null hypothesis (H_0). Here, H_0 is that $\mu_A = \mu_B$ or equivalently, $\Delta = 0$. Then a test statistic, based on the observed data, is computed that evaluates whether $\Delta = 0$ is reasonable. Here, the test statistic is the t-statistic, which is the standardized difference of the two observed means under treatment A and B, respectively and denoted as t_{obs}. If the null hypothesis is true, the t-statistic has a t-distribution with $n_A + n_B - 2$ degrees of freedom. This means that, if the study had been repeated a large number of times under exactly the same conditions and if the null-hypothesis were true, then the standardized difference of (replicated) means has a $t(n_A + n_B - 2)$-distribution. When t_{obs} is relatively large (in absolute value) compared to what is expected under H_0, we reject that hypothesis and claim that $\Delta \neq 0$. The task is to determine what is 'relatively large', which refers to the region of 'extreme' values of the test statistic under the null hypothesis. This is called the *rejection region.* What we consider as extreme is driven by the probability that H_0 is falsely rejected under repeated sampling. That is, when the current study had been repeated and H_0 holds, it is the probability that we (falsely) claim that $\Delta \neq 0$. This probability is called the *Type I error rate* (α), and in practice we wish to keep α relatively low, say $\alpha = 0.05$. In order not to miss a clinically important difference, say $\Delta = \Delta_a$, one determines also the study size such that (under repeated sampling) the probability of rejecting H_0 in favor of the alternative hypothesis $H_a : \Delta \neq 0$ is high. In other words, one wishes to find with high probability that there is a different effect in the two treatments. This probability is called the power of the test, and 1-power $= \beta$ is called the *Type II error rate.* For RCTs, one aims to have a power of at least 80% or $\beta \leq 0.2$. The above strategy was developed by Neyman and Pearson (1928a,b).

Upon completion of the study, one can estimate the true difference in effect between the two treatments and t_{obs}. For the toenail study, one obtained $\widehat{\Delta} = 1.38$ and $t_{obs} = 2.19$, which is in the 0.05-rejection region. Hence, we reject H_0 that $\Delta = 0$. Fisher (1934) proposed to express the extremeness of the observed result in relation to the null hypothesis by means of the *P-value.* This is the probability under H_0 of observing a numerical result that is as extreme as, or even more extreme than the one actually observed. He also suggested that one might take $P < 0.05$ as a possible sign that the null hypothesis does not hold. When the extremeness is defined in the two directions (t_{obs} is too big in absolute value), one computes a *two-sided P-value*. For the toenail study, we obtained as 2-sided $P = 0.03$, smaller than 0.05 and thus we again reject the null-hypothesis.

Fisher proposed 0.05 as a possible threshold, but of course, there is nothing special about this cut-off. An "error rate" of 1 in 20 (i.e. 0.05) is a reasonable target, but nowadays 0.05 has become a magical value in clinical research against with each P-value should be compared. When $P < 0.05$, one classically refers to a *statistically significant result.* Thus in the toenail RCT, one argues that the two treatments are statistically significantly different.

Finally, an alternative way of expressing the results of a statistical test, and nowadays often preferred way, is the $(1-\alpha)100\%$ confidence interval. For $\alpha = 0.05$, this leads to the 95% confidence interval. The technical interpretation of this interval is that, if we repeat our study many times, then in 95% of the times the true, but unknown, value of Δ is located in the interval. The 95% confidence interval for Δ based on the above study results is equal to $[0.14, 2.62]$. Note that the adjective 95% refers to the repeated sampling mechanism. For an individual study, the 95% confidence interval either contains or does not contain the true value of Δ.

1.2.2 Reflections on the classical approach

Fisher and Neyman & Pearson had an enormous impact on all clinical research. Fisher and Neyman & Pearson clashed during their lives in their views on statistical inference. Among many fundamental differences in their two approaches, one common trait is the fact that in both approaches inference depends on the observed result but also on other, possible but never observed, results. This is the *repeated sampling idea.* In the toenail RCT, the conclusion that the two oral treatments have a different effect depends on the difference between the two observed means, but also on what difference could have happened if the null hypothesis applied. The probability calculations are based on (at least conceptually) repeating the study under identical conditions, assuming H_0 holds.

The repeated sampling strategy may lead to confusion in practice. As an example, take the chi-square test and Fisher's Exact test applied to the same 2×2-contingency table. It is well-known that the tests yield different P-values, often not materially different, but still observable. This has to do with the fact the X^2-measure comparing observed with expected frequencies is compared to different reference distributions, yielding possible different conclusions yet based on the same data. Hence, although the two statistical tests are based on the same observed table, the practical conclusion based on the P-value may be different because the sampling spaces (possible tables) are different. While this difference in conclusion can easily be explained, and is acceptable to many statisticians, others may find it difficult to grasp that statistical conclusions are different by just looking differently on what could have happened, but never happened.

The P-value is often misinterpreted. Namely, it is wrong to interpret the P-value as the probability that H_0 is not true. In a frequentist sense, H_0 is either true or false, so it does not make sense to make probabilistic statements about it. Rather, the P-value is more like a surprise index expressing the probability of observing a more extreme result than the observed one given that the null hypothesis is true. In fact, any probability statement of an hypothesis given observed data is a Bayesian probability. In addition, the epidemiological literature is divided when it comes to appreciating the value of a significant result in relation to the size of the study. While some argue that a significant P-value weighs more in a small study than in a big study, others just claim the opposite, see e.g. Royall (1997).

Moreover, classical statistical inference arguably leans too heavily on the P-value. In virtually every clinical paper, numerous P-values are computed. Too often interest lies in discovering 'small P-values' (smaller than 0.05) upon which to attach then strong conclusions. These are called 'data dredging exercises' or 'fishing expeditions' and are possibly the most common misuses of the P-value and probably responsible for much of the unreproducible (clinical) research. Recently, members of the American Statistical Association (ASA) expressed their concern about the large number of clinical studies whose results are unreproducible, which is clearly linked to the predominant role of P-values. In 2016, ASA published a position paper about the (mis)use of P-values, see Wasserstein and Lazar (2016). The paper expresses the consensus viewpoint of many influential statisticians of the limited value of a significant P-value. While, their six conclusions basically reflect what most trained statisticians would claim, the article is important in making it clear that the scientific attitude needs to change. Here are three of their statements:

- "P-values can indicate how incompatible the data are with a specified statistical model."
- "P-values do not measure the probability that the studied hypothesis is true, or the probability that the data were produced by random chance alone."
- "By itself, a P-value does not provide a good measure of evidence regarding a model or hypothesis."

Finally, despite the fact that scientific knowledge builds on past successes and failures, there is nothing in classical statistical inference that allows to take historical information explicitly into account. This is a pity since in pharmaceutical research numerous pre-clinical and clinical studies are done in sequence. It may therefore be more cost effective to explicitly use past data and/or information in current analyses. There is of course always the fear that in this way current conclusions are influenced in a subjective way. While a justified fear, it is equally unwise never to use what we have learned in the analyses of today.

1.3 Bayesian concepts

1.3.1 Bayes Theorem

The Bayesian approach is based on the famous *Bayes Theorem* due to Thomas Bayes. Thomas Bayes was a Presbyterian minister with strong mathematical interests. His friend, Richard Price, submitted in 1763 (two years after Bayes' death), the document "An Essay toward a Problem in the Doctrine of Chances". This document is generally accepted as containing the fundamental ideas of Bayes Theorem. It is a combination of original writings of Thomas Bayes with remarks of Richard Price.

The origin of the theorem lies in a basic property of the joint probability of, say, events A and B: $\Pr(A, B) = \Pr(A \mid B)\Pr(B) = \Pr(B \mid A)\Pr(A)$. This gives

$$\Pr(B \mid A) = \frac{\Pr(A \mid B)\Pr(B)}{\Pr(A)},$$

with a similar result holding for the negations of the events, i.e. A^C and B^C. When A represents the binary outcome of a diagnostic test and B indicates whether an individual suffers from a particular disease or not, the above property leads to an expression of the positive predictive value $\Pr(B \mid A)$ of the diagnostic test as a function of the sensitivity $\Pr(A \mid B)$ and specificity $\Pr(A^C \mid B^C)$ of that test, and the prevalence of the disease, $\Pr(B)$. If the prevalence represents the prior probability of having the disease (without seeing the results of the diagnostic test) and the sensitivity/specificity related to the outcome of the diagnostic test, then the positive predictive value can be interpreted as the posterior probability being diseased after having seen the results of the diagnostic test.

Bayes lived in a period when mathematicians were eager to describe the probability that certain events could happen given that the known distribution of the data and thus assuming its true parameter(s), say θ, were also known. But, Bayes was more intrigued by knowing what the observed data could tell us about the unknown (continuous) parameter θ. The ingenious idea of Bayes was to apply the above formula to the setting where A represents collected data and B stands for an unknown parameter. He realized that to draw conclusions from the collected data to the unknown parameter θ one must be willing to make probability statements about θ. Such statements can be interpreted as follows. We humans will basically never know what the true value is, but we may believe in certain values more than in others. This leads to attaching (prior) probabilities to all possible values of θ. In this way the parameter θ becomes stochastic. In other words, in a Bayesian context, parameters are considered stochastic just because we wish to express our uncertainty about the true value and that using prior probabilities. When the unknown parameter θ is continuous, this leads to a *prior density (or prior)* for θ. Combined with the information about θ in the collected data, Bayes derived how this leads to a *posterior density (or posterior)* for θ. This is the essential idea of Bayes Theorem.

More formally, suppose that the data set $\boldsymbol{y} = \{y_1, \ldots, y_n\}$ is observed where the y_i ($i = 1, \ldots, n$) are independent with distribution $p(y \mid \theta)$. The likelihood function $L(\theta \mid \boldsymbol{y}) = \prod_{i=1}^n p(y_i \mid \theta)$ shows which values of θ can be plausibly supported by, or are consistent with the observed data. Together with the prior $p(\theta)$ the likelihood function gives the posterior $p(\theta \mid \boldsymbol{y})$ as follows:

$$p(\theta \mid \boldsymbol{y}) = \frac{L(\theta \mid \boldsymbol{y})p(\theta)}{\int L(\theta \mid \boldsymbol{y})p(\theta)\, d\theta},$$

whereby the following factorization is used: $p(\theta, \boldsymbol{y}) = L(\theta \mid \boldsymbol{y})p(\theta) = p(\theta \mid \boldsymbol{y})p(\boldsymbol{y})$ with $p(\boldsymbol{y}) = \int L(\theta \mid \boldsymbol{y})p(\theta)\, d\theta$.

Thus, the posterior at each value of θ is obtained by a simple product of the likelihood and the prior at that value, divided by a normalizing constant. Further, values of θ that are most supported by the data (read: likelihood) and the prior will yield θ values for which the posterior is relatively high. The posterior distribution tells everything what we need to know about θ. In contrast to the classical approach, in the Bayesian approach only the current data matter and one does not care what other data could have happened. We say that in the Bayesian approach one conditions on the observed data, i.e. the data are generated from a stochastic mechanism expressed by the likelihood function but once observed, the data $\boldsymbol{y}$ are considered as fixed. That is why, one often sees also the following statement

$$p(\theta \mid \boldsymbol{y}) \propto L(\theta \mid \boldsymbol{y})p(\theta),$$

because $p(\boldsymbol{y})$ is fixed in the Bayesian approach.

Below we illustrate the computation of the posterior distribution via two motivating examples.

1.3.2 The computation of the posterior distribution

We illustrate first the computation of the posterior for a binary outcome, and then repeat (briefly) the computations for a Gaussian outcome.

1.3.2.1 Example: Under-use of oral anticoagulants in atrial fibrillation

Atrial fibrillation (AF) is associated with substantial mortality and morbidity from stroke and thromboembolism. Despite the existence of an efficacious oral anticoagulation (OAC) therapy, namely warfarin, AF patients at high risk for stroke are often under-treated. In Ogilvie et al. (2010) a systematic review of 98 studies was reported on current treatment practices for AF. Evidence was found that high-risk patients are not given AF as much as they should. One clinical researcher (Deplanque, who we abbreviated as D) studied twice the under-use of oral anticoagulants in AF in Europe, first in 1999 and then in 2006. Let us now suppose that D is inclined to use the 1999 results to obtain a better estimate of the OAC use in 2006. In other words, D might wish to incorporate prior information in the analysis of the current data, but wonders how to do that.

From Figure 2 in Ogilvie et al. (2010) one can read off the results of the different studies at the time of the meta-analysis, including the results of the 1999 study and the 2006 study. We now consider three possible actions D can undertake to estimate the true proportion θ of high risk AF patients in Europe to receive OAC in 2006:

1. Do not include prior information;
2. Make use of the reported 1999 odds ratio and its 95% confidence interval to analyze the 2006 data;
3. Transform the likelihood of the 1999 data into a prior for the 2006 data.

In the 2006 study, only 151 patients of the 260 high risk AF patients received OAC yielding the Binomial likelihood function

$$L(\theta \mid y) = \binom{n}{y} \theta^y (1-\theta)^{(n-y)}, \tag{1.1}$$

with $y = 151$ and $n = 260$ and θ being the true proportion of European AF patients receiving OAC treatment. From $L(\theta \mid y)$, one can find the best estimate of θ but also those θ-values that are not supported by the 2006 data. To apply Bayes Theorem, a prior for θ is needed to be combined with the likelihood of the 2006 data. In Figure 1.1 we show four possible prior densities for θ. The Uniform prior on [0,1] in Figure 1.1(a) expresses that all possible values for θ are a priori equally plausible. Such a prior could be labeled as non-informative since one does not prefer one θ value over the other. The flat prior on [0.2, 0.6] in Figure 1.1(b) is derived from looking at the supported θ values in the 1996 likelihood function, showing no support outside the range [0.2, 0.6] for θ values. Several priors can be constructed that are approximately restricted on the same interval, as illustrated in Figure 1.1(c) (extending a bit beyond 0.6). Finally, we can also explicitly use the 1996 likelihood function to yield the Beta prior shown in Figure 1.1(d), see derivations below for details.

The four priors are combined with likelihood (1.1) using Bayes Theorem to yield four posteriors. The four posteriors together with the 2006 (standardized, see below) likelihood are also shown in Figure 1.2. One can observe that in Figure 1.2(a) the (standardized) likelihood coincides with the posterior. Hence the most plausible value of θ based on the posterior is equal to the maximum likelihood estimate (MLE). In the three other cases, the posterior differs from the likelihood and varying the prior will cause the posterior to vary. The interpretation of these results is:

- Figure 1.2(a): the aim is not to make use of the 1999 data. Therefore the Bayesian results will be basically the same as for the classical approach. This prior is called non-informative, but nowadays one prefers the terms vague prior, objective prior, indifferent prior, etc. for reasons explained in Section 1.5;

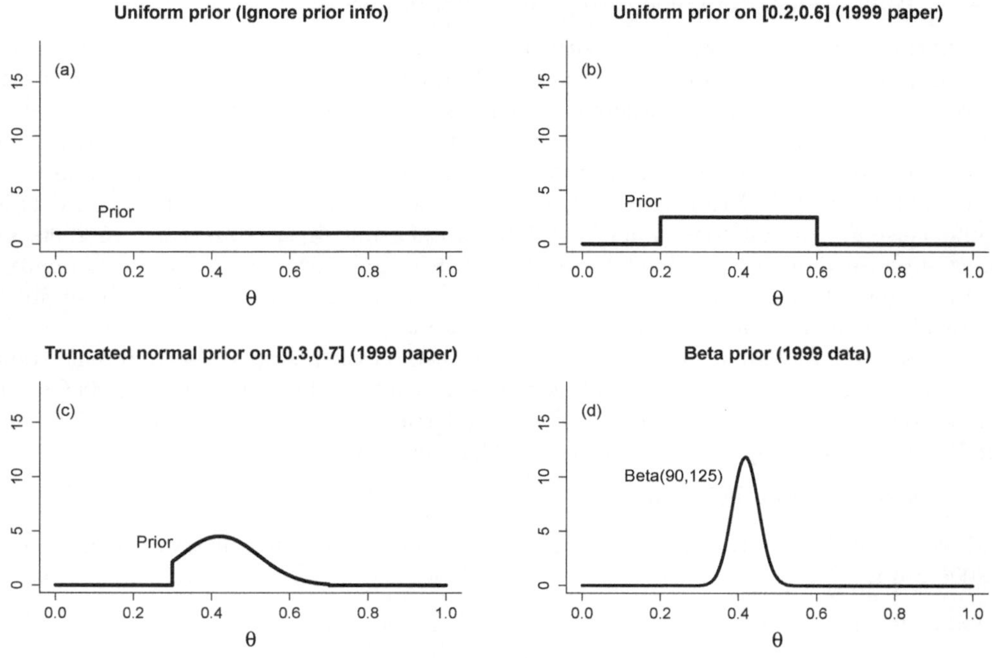

FIGURE 1.1: Under-use of OAC for AF patients: Priors for θ of the 2006 data.

- Figure 1.2(b): since the prior is zero outside [0.2, 0.6], the same is true for the posterior. This is called a subjective prior, since one assumed a priori that θ cannot lie outside this interval;
- Figure 1.2(c): another subjective prior that expresses no belief in values below 0.2;
- Figure 1.2(d): this prior is obtained by standardizing the 1999 likelihood so that area-under-curve is equal to 1.

All four posteriors summarize our information on θ for a given prior in an understandable manner. Namely, for each posterior one can compute probabilities such as $\Pr(\theta > a \mid y), \Pr(\theta < b \mid y), \Pr(a < \theta < b \mid y)$, for any a and b. Such posterior probabilities are much better understood by (clinical) researchers than a P-value. However, in Chapter 3, one shows that one-sided P-values can be interpreted as posterior probabilities. In the same chapter, it is shown that the classical P-value, i.e. when $H_0 : \theta = \theta_0$, is quite different from above probabilities.

We end this example showing how we arrived at the posterior in Figure 1.2(d). In this case, the prior is obtained by standardizing the 1999 Binomial likelihood $L(\theta \mid y_0) = \binom{n_0}{y_0}\theta^{y_0}(1-\theta)^{(n_0-y_0)}$ with $y_0 = 89$ and $n_0 = 213$ by recognizing that the part that depends on θ is the kernel of a Beta density. Then we replace the Binomial coefficient by an appropriate constant (such that "area under the curve", AUC, = 1) and obtain the prior Beta density $\text{Beta}(\alpha_0, \beta_0)$:

$$p(\theta) = \frac{1}{B(\alpha_0, \beta_0)}\,\theta^{\alpha_0-1}(1-\theta)^{\beta_0-1},$$

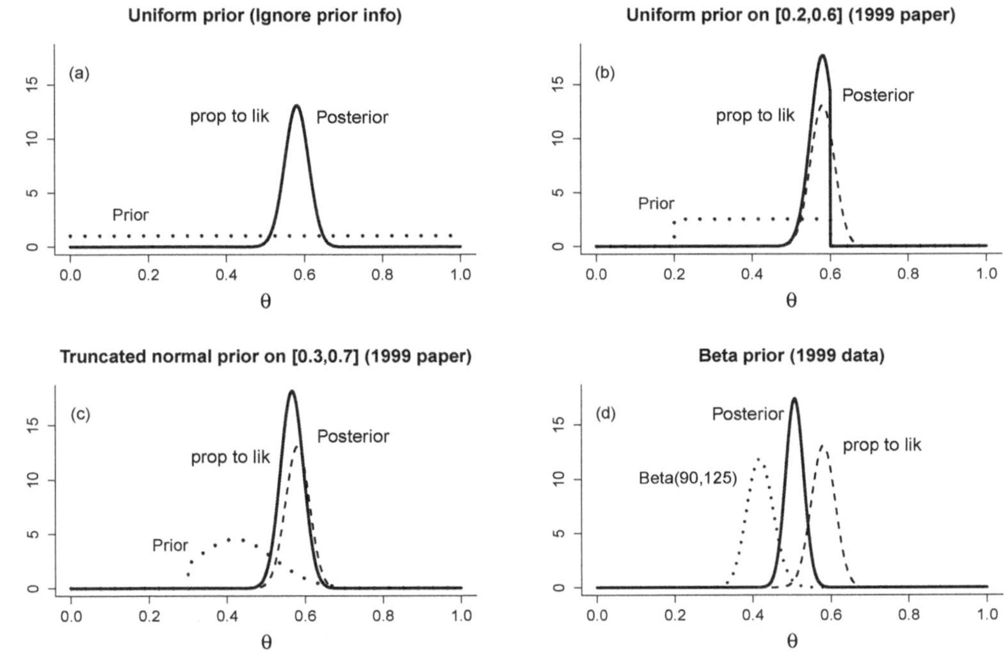

FIGURE 1.2: Under-use of OAC for AF patients: Posteriors for θ (solid line) of the 2006 data based on priors (dotted line) shown in Figure 1.1 combined with likelihood of 2006 data (dashed line).

with $B(\alpha_0, \beta_0)$ the Beta coefficient, $\alpha_0 = y_0 + 1 = 90$ and $\beta_0 = n_0 - y_0 + 1 = 125$. The multiplication of $p(\theta)$ with the 2006 likelihood $L(\theta \mid y) = \binom{n}{y}\theta^y(1-\theta)^{(n-y)}$ yields the posterior of θ based on the 2006 likelihood and the 1999 historical data, i.e.

$$p(\theta \mid y) = \frac{1}{B(\overline{\alpha}, \overline{\beta})}\,\theta^{\overline{\alpha}-1}(1-\theta)^{\overline{\beta}-1},$$

with $\overline{\alpha} = \alpha_0 + y = 90 + 151 = 241$ and $\overline{\beta} = \beta_0 + n - y = 125 + 260 - 151 = 234$, which is again a Beta distribution with parameters $\overline{\alpha}$, $\overline{\beta}$ showing clearly the impact of the prior and data information. For instance, when α_0 and β_0 are small, as in the case of a Uniform prior on [0,1], which is a Beta(1,1), then the impact of the prior when combined with the likelihood of a reasonably sized study is minimal. Finally, because the Beta prior together with the Binomial likelihood yields a Beta posterior, we say that the Beta (distribution) is *conjugate to the Binomial* (likelihood).

The above construction assumes that the information contained in the 1999 data can be simply taken over as information for the 2006 data. This is most often a too strong assumption, and at least some downplaying (also called discounting) of the prior data will be necessary. More details are given in Section 1.5.

1.3.2.2 Example: Comparing efficacy of oral drugs for toenail infection

In Section 1.2 we have used the toenail infection RCT to illustrate the classical statistical approach to inference. Here we illustrate a possible Bayesian analysis of the data. The original outcome has a skewed distribution. Therefore, we have taken the square root of the unaffected nail length as outcome as its distribution is closer to the Normal.

For a better illustration of the concepts, we simplified matters. Firstly, we assume that the standard deviation associated with the observed data σ is common across the two treatment arms and known. Secondly, we assume that for the sake of the comparison of the efficacy of the two treatments it is sufficient to look at the Gaussian likelihood of the difference in observed means, $\widehat{d}$. We thus assume that the likelihood of $\Delta = \mu_A - \mu_B$ (on transformed scale) depends only on $\widehat{d}$ and that, because of the Central Limit Theorem, $\widehat{d}$ has a Normal distribution with mean Δ and standard deviation equal to σ_Δ also assumed known and here set equal to 0.15. When we combine this Gaussian likelihood with a Gaussian prior for Δ, i.e. $\mathrm{N}(\Delta_0, \sigma_0^2)$, we obtain a Normal posterior with mean:

$$\overline{\Delta} = \frac{w_0}{w_0 + w_1}\,\Delta_0 + \frac{w_1}{w_0 + w_1}\,\widehat{d},$$

with

$$w_0 = \frac{1}{\sigma_0^2} \;\&\; w_1 = \frac{1}{\sigma_\Delta^2}.$$

The *posterior precision*, equal to 1/posterior variance, can simply be obtained from

$$\frac{1}{\overline{\sigma}_\Delta^2} = \frac{1}{\sigma_0^2} + \frac{1}{\sigma_\Delta^2}.$$

Therefore it is said that the *Gaussian prior is conjugate to the Gaussian likelihood* (when variance is known). Note that the posterior mean is pulled towards the prior mean with a force that depends on the relative information in the prior and in the data. This phenomenon is called *shrinkage*. It is easy to see that the posterior is dominated by the data when the prior variance is large compared to σ_Δ^2. Shrinkage will be minimal for a *vague (Gaussian) prior*, which is a prior that aims to contribute as little as possible to the posterior.

Figure 1.3 shows the impact of three priors when combined with the toenail likelihood. In Figure 1.3(a) we have used a vague Normal prior with variance 100^2. Inference based on the posterior will then be basically the same as when based on the likelihood alone. When monitoring a RCT, an option is to let the prior represent a skeptical opinion about the difference in efficacy between the two treatments in order not to stop the RCT too early for a possible positive result obtained by chance. In this case it could imply a Normal prior with mean zero and a small variance. This skeptical prior implies a strong shrinkage effect for the estimate of Δ towards zero. This is clearly seen in Figure 1.3(b). By the same token, we could assume in the data monitoring process an enthusiastic prior to avoid stopping too early with a (temporarily) disappointing result, see Figure 1.3(c). See Freedman et al. (1994) for suggesting skeptical and enthusiastic priors in the context of RCTs. For all three posteriors one can compute the posterior evidence that $\Delta > 0$, i.e. that Lamisil shows a better performance than Itraconazole after 48 weeks follow-up. The results are: (a) $\Pr(\Delta > 0 \mid \boldsymbol{y}) = 0.987$; (b) $\Pr(\Delta > 0 \mid \boldsymbol{y}) = 0.895$ and (c) $\Pr(\Delta > 0 \mid \boldsymbol{y}) = 0.998$ for the three posteriors, respectively. As argued above, such summaries of the results are much more intuitive than to give a P-value.

1.3.3 Summarizing the posterior distribution

In a Bayesian context, we only need the posterior distribution to draw conclusions about the parameters of interest. Indeed, we can explore the posterior directly by probabilities $\Pr(a < \theta < b \mid \boldsymbol{y})$ for various a and b. Nevertheless, we can also summarize the posterior with simple measures as what we do to summarize collected data. For estimates of location it is common to use posterior mean, median and mode and variance and standard deviation for variability. In addition, one reports intervals of high posterior belief, in other words Bayesian confidence intervals.

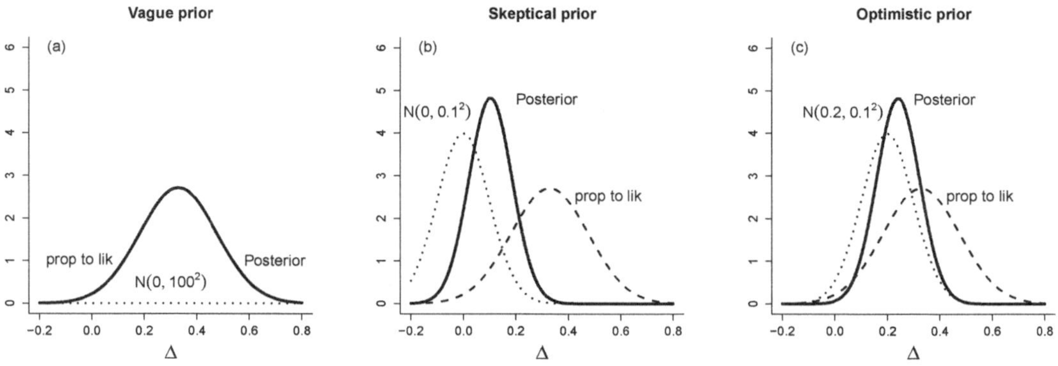

FIGURE 1.3: Toenail RCT: Posteriors for Δ depending on three choices of Gaussian priors.

The two examples we have discussed in the previous section allowed for analytically deriving the posterior. This implies that the denominator of Bayes Theorem, i.e. the integral $\int L(\theta \mid \boldsymbol{y})p(\theta)\,d\theta$ could be analytically determined. In these cases, also the posterior summary measures are most often easy to compute, but this will be in general not the case, as seen in Section 1.6.3.

1.3.3.1 Bayesian measures of location

The usual posterior summary measures that characterize the location of the posterior are the mode, mean and median. The *posterior mode* is the value $\widehat{\theta}_M$, for which the posterior distribution for θ is maximum. In other words, the posterior mode is the value of θ most supported by the posterior. Yet, in practice one most often will compute either (a) *posterior mean* $\overline{\theta}$, defined as $\overline{\theta} = \int \theta\, p(\theta \mid \boldsymbol{y})\,d\theta$, or (b) *posterior median* $\overline{\theta}_M$, computed from $\int_{\overline{\theta}_M}^{max} p(\theta \mid \boldsymbol{y})\,d\theta = 0.5$. Hence $\overline{\theta}_M$ is the value of θ such that the AUC left to it is 0.5. We note that only for the mode, there is no need to compute an integral, since the denominator $p(\boldsymbol{y})$ is a constant in a Bayesian context. The choice between the mean and median depends on the skewness of the posterior, with the mean taken for a symmetric posterior while the median is taken for a skew posterior.

1.3.3.2 Bayesian measures of uncertainty

The location measures indicate our best guess for the parameter θ in a posterior sense, but they do not tell us how uncertain we are about θ. A classical measure of variability is the *posterior variance* $\overline{\sigma}^2_\theta$ and the derived *posterior standard deviation* (SD), defined here as $\overline{\sigma}^2_\theta = \int (\theta - \overline{\theta})^2\, p(\theta \mid \boldsymbol{y})\,d\theta$, and thus $\overline{\sigma}_\theta$ measures the spread of the θ-values around their (posterior) mean.

A *Bayesian confidence interval* also known as *credibility or credible interval* indicates the most plausible values of θ a posteriori. We say that [a,b] is a 95% credible interval (CI) for θ if $\Pr(a \leq \theta \leq b \mid \boldsymbol{y}) = 0.95$. Since this definition is not uniquely defining the 95% CI, one entertains two versions of this interval in practice. With the 95% *equal tail (or equal-tailed) CI* [a, b], the AUC left to a is 0.025 as well as the AUC right to b. The interval [a, b] is called 95% *highest posterior density (HPD) interval* if [a, b] contains the most plausible values of θ, i.e. for all values θ_1 inside [a, b] and all values θ_2 outside that interval: $p(\theta_1 \mid \boldsymbol{y}) \geq p(\theta_2 \mid \boldsymbol{y})$. When the posterior is symmetric as for the toenail study, the two types of credible intervals are the same. In practice, the equal tail CI is more popular since it is often easier to compute, both when analytical calculations are possible or when sampling is involved, see further. Also, the image of the equal tail CI under a monotone transformation $\psi = h(\theta)$ is again an equal tail 95% CI. This is not the case for the HPD interval. In Figure 1.4, the 95% equal tail CI and the 95% HPD interval are shown for a Beta(20,130)-distribution for a proportion θ. In the same figure, we show that the image of θ after log-transformation is not a HPD interval anymore, but the image of a 95% equal tail CI will be again an equal tail interval with the same size on the transformed scale. All such intervals can be obtained in practice (when based on Markov chain Monte Carlo computations) from standard R software such as coda.

Note that in some cases, a Bayesian confidence interval is identical or at least approximately equal to a classical confidence interval. An example of this is the confidence interval of the unknown population mean when the data have a Normal distribution and a flat prior is taken for the mean parameter. In other cases, the Bayesian and classical confidence intervals are often close with weak priors and/or large sample sizes. However, for small sample sizes they tend to differ especially when the classical confidence interval is based on asymptotic arguments, in which case the Bayesian confidence interval often has better coverage properties, see e.g. Lesaffre and Lawson (2012).

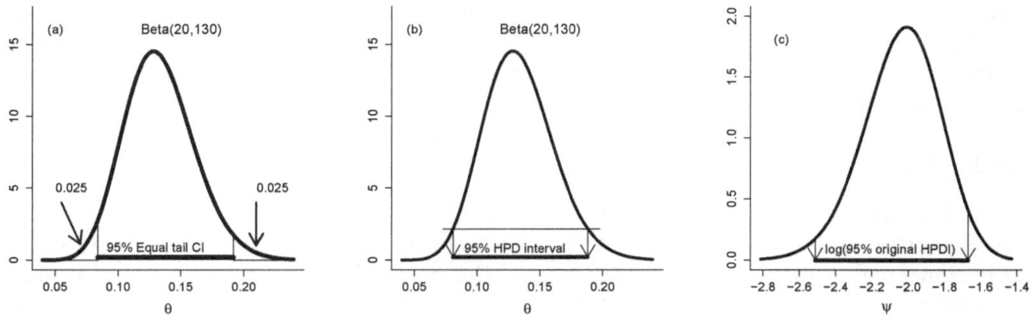

FIGURE 1.4: Bayesian 95% CI: (a) equal tail CI, (b) HPD interval and (c) image of HPD interval for $\psi = \log(\theta)$.

1.3.3.3 Comparison with frequentist summary measures

For a vague prior, the frequentist summary measures for θ will be often close and sometimes identical to the corresponding Bayesian summary measures. For instance, the posterior mode is equal to the MLE for θ when $p(\theta) \propto c$. Another example is when we combine the constant prior $p(\mu) \propto c$ for the mean of a Gaussian distribution (assuming σ known), with a Gaussian likelihood; then, as mentioned above, the estimates and the confidence intervals are the same under the frequentist and Bayesian paradigms. But, of course, their interpretation is different. For instance, the meaning of '95%' in the classical confidence interval refers to the repeated sampling property of that interval, while for a Bayesian confidence interval it can be directly interpreted as 'we are with 95% (posterior) probability sure that θ lies in that interval'. This interpretation is in fact also the interpretation that we attach to the classical confidence interval when discussing our statistical results with (clinical) researchers.

1.3.3.4 Example: OACs in atrial fibrillation: posterior summary measures

The posterior in the OAC example is a Beta(241, 234) distribution, which is a fairly symmetric distribution implying that the measures of location will be practically coinciding. The posterior mode is obtained by maximizing $(\overline{\alpha}-1)\log(\theta)+(\overline{\beta}-1)\log(1-\theta)$ with respect to θ yielding $\widehat{\theta}_M = (\overline{\alpha}-1)/(\overline{\alpha}+\overline{\beta}-2)$ equal to $240/473 = 0.507$. The posterior mean involves the integral $\frac{1}{B(\overline{\alpha},\overline{\beta})}\int_0^1 \theta\,\theta^{\overline{\alpha}-1}(1-\theta)^{\overline{\beta}-1}\,d\theta = B(\overline{\alpha}+1,\overline{\beta})/B(\overline{\alpha},\overline{\beta}) = \overline{\alpha}/(\overline{\alpha}+\overline{\beta})$, which is basically again 0.507. The posterior median one needs to solve $0.5 = \frac{1}{B(\overline{\alpha},\overline{\beta})}\int_{\theta_M}^1 \theta^{\overline{\alpha}-1}(1-\theta)^{\overline{\beta}-1}\,d\theta$ for θ, which can be done with the R function *qbeta* yielding again 0.507.

The variance of the Beta($\overline{\alpha},\overline{\beta}$) distribution is equal to

$$\overline{\alpha}\,\overline{\beta}/\left[(\overline{\alpha}+\overline{\beta})^2(\overline{\alpha}+\overline{\beta}+1)\right].$$

For $\overline{\alpha} = 241$ and $\overline{\beta} = 234$, the posterior standard deviation is therefore equal to $\overline{\sigma} = 0.0229$. Finally, the 95% equal tail interval is [0.46, 0.55], basically the same as the 95% HPD interval.

1.3.4 Prediction

The question arises about what we can expect as future observations if we draw from the same population as that of the current data $\boldsymbol{y}$. This requires us to determine the predictive distribution of a future observation $\widetilde{y}$ after having observed the sample $\boldsymbol{y} = \{y_1, \ldots, y_n\}$. We can only determine this distribution if the future observations are assumed to be associated with the same sampling variability, described by the distribution $p(y \mid \theta)$ as the current observations and that the future observations are independent of the current observations given θ. In fact, we assume that the future observations are *exchangeable* with the current observations.

If we know θ, then the above assumptions imply that we also know that the distribution of $\widetilde{y}$ is $p(\widetilde{y} \mid \theta)$. But, there is uncertainty about the true value of θ expressed by $p(\theta \mid \boldsymbol{y})$. The posterior distribution attaches posterior beliefs to each possible θ-value, which then can be used as weights for $p(y \mid \theta)$. This yields the *posterior predictive distribution* (PPD) given by

$$p(\widetilde{y} \mid \boldsymbol{y}) = \int p(\widetilde{y} \mid \theta)\, p(\theta \mid \boldsymbol{y})\, d\theta. \tag{1.2}$$

Hence, the PPD is not the true distribution of the future data, but represents our estimate of that true distribution given the current uncertainty expressed by the posterior distribution. We note that in the case of a Beta prior combined with a Binomial likelihood this gives a *Beta-Binomial PPD*. For a Gaussian prior combined with a Gaussian likelihood (σ fixed), this gives a *Gaussian PPD* and for a Gamma prior combined with a Poisson likelihood, one obtains a *Negative Binomial PPD*. We will only illustrate the Binomial case here.

Note that the PPD has many practical applications. For instance, it is used to calculate the probability of success of a clinical trial, called *assurance*, see e.g. Chapters 3, 4, 5 and 22. Another application is checking the appropriateness of the chosen statistical model, see Section 1.8.

1.3.4.1 Example: Treating hemophilia A patients

Hemophilia A is a genetic rare disease in which the clotting factor VIII is deficient. Patients with a low level of FVIII have an increased bleeding tendency, which can be life threatening. The incidence of hemophilia A is 1/5000 male births. Patients with that disease are administered factor VIII (FVIII) from donated blood plasma, or DNA recombinant FVIII. With blood donation, there is always the risk of transmission of diseases, while with DNA recombinant FVIII products the body can develop inhibitors (antibody formation) to factor VIII. In Recht et al. (2009) the process is described by which a new drug Refactor® AF was developed in 2005 and registered by the Food and Drug Administration (FDA). The task was to show its safety. Prior to the development on this new compound, 6 out 329 patients (1.8%) treated by 4 other compounds developed an inhibitor.

Refactor® AF is a variation of an existing compound but manufactured in a more sophisticated way. The assessment of inhibitor risk in clinical trials of new or modified recombinant FVIII products is challenging, due to the low frequency of inhibitor occurrence and the generally small size of hemophilia studies because of the rarity of the disease. At that time the FDA stated that, for the compound to successfully pass the test, the upper bound of the two-sided (frequentist) 95% CI for the product inhibitor incidence rate must be below 6.8%. However, this requirement necessitated an unrealistically large study size (based on assumed incidence rates). Therefore a Bayesian approach was worked out.

Lumping together the results found for four existing drugs, it was found that 6 out of 329 patients developed an inhibitor. They considered a Beta(1,1) prior, expressing a belief that before observing any data the probability mass is evenly spread over the interval $[0; 1]$. Combined with the data, this gives a Beta(7,324) posterior for θ, the probability of developing an inhibitor. This gives a posterior mean rate of $7/(7+324)$, corresponding to a 2.1% mean rate and a 99%-ile of 4.4%. FDA accepted the use of a Bayesian approach and to take 4.4% as upper limit for the future 95% equal tail CI based on Refactor® AF data. We could now ask what the probabilities are of future rates when we plan a new study of 100 patients treated with Refactor® AF. For this we assume that the past results obtained from the other compounds are representative for the future results. As seen above, the combination of a Beta prior with a Binomial likelihood leads to a Beta-Binomial PPD.

In Figure 1.5 we show: (a) the Binomial distribution based on 2.1% rate. This is the predictive distribution of future events when we ignore the posterior uncertainty in θ and (b) the Beta-Binomial distribution (BB(100, 7,234)), which takes into account the uncertainty expressed by the Beta(7,324) posterior, is more dispersed than the Binomial distribution.

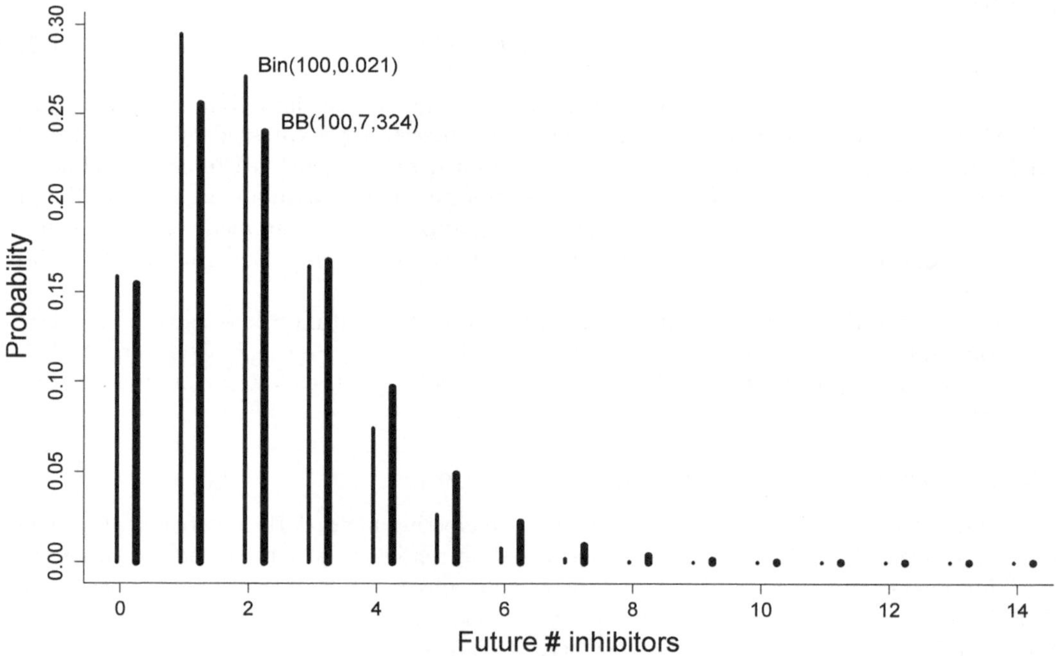

FIGURE 1.5: Hemophilia study: Binomial distribution and PPD (Beta-Binomial distribution) for a future sample of 100 patients.

Note that the prior used for the registration of Refactor® AF, was actually based on the incidence rates from earlier studies with Refactor. We refer to Recht et al. (2009) to see what results and calculations led to the acceptance of Refactor® AF for hemophilia patients by FDA.

1.4 More than one parameter

Most statistical models involve more than one parameter to estimate; examples include the Normal distribution with mean μ and variance σ^2 unknown, linear regression with regression coefficients $\beta_0, \beta_1, \ldots, \beta_d$ and residual variance σ^2, logistic regression with regression coefficients $\beta_0, \beta_1, \ldots, \beta_d$, etc.

To apply the Bayesian approach, we need a (joint) prior for all parameters and to express our prior beliefs on all model parameters. This will turn into a multivariate posterior distribution for all parameters and posterior summary measures, via the *multivariate Bayes Theorem* given by

$$p(\boldsymbol{\theta} \mid \boldsymbol{y}) = \frac{L(\boldsymbol{\theta} \mid \boldsymbol{y})p(\boldsymbol{\theta})}{\int L(\boldsymbol{\theta} \mid \boldsymbol{y})p(\boldsymbol{\theta})\, d\boldsymbol{\theta}}.$$

Hence, the multivariate Bayes Theorem is no different than the univariate version, but now we are dealing with a vector of parameters $\boldsymbol{\theta} = (\theta_1, \theta_2, \ldots, \theta_d)^\top$. The prior $p(\boldsymbol{\theta})$ is also multivariate. One possibility is to specify for each parameter separately a prior distribution and then multiply these univariate priors. Namely, we specify $p(\theta_j)$ independently for each $j = 1, \ldots, d$ and then compute $p(\boldsymbol{\theta}) = p(\theta_1) \times p(\theta_2) \times \ldots \times p(\theta_d)$. This is of course, often, a gross simplification. Other priors can be given, e.g. it is common to give location parameters a joint prior separate from the prior for the variance parameter(s). An example is a multivariate Normal prior for the regression coefficients and an Inverse Gamma prior for the residual variance in a linear regression settings. But, one could also define a prior of one set of parameters conditional on another set of parameters. All of this (and more complex priors) are possible. The posterior $p(\boldsymbol{\theta} \mid \boldsymbol{y})$ is again multivariate, but in general does not factorize into independent components. However, in practice we are most interested in inference for each parameter separately. This implies the determination of the (marginal) posterior distributions $p(\theta_j \mid \boldsymbol{y})$. And, ... again we need for each parameter the posterior mean, median and credible intervals. The problem is that in basically all cases the integral cannot be computed analytically and a numerical solution is desperately needed. We will return to this problem in Section 1.6.3.

1.5 Choosing the prior distribution

Incorporating prior information *formally* into the statistical analysis is a unique feature for the Bayesian approach, but is also often the aspect of criticism by non-Bayesians. We give here a short overview of the different principles of constructing prior distributions.

An important class of priors are those *conjugate to the likelihood*, because they allow for an analytical expression of the posterior and often also of the posterior summary measures. We have seen examples of conjugate priors in previous sections. Namely, the Beta distribution is a conjugate prior for the Binomial likelihood. The Gaussian distribution is a conjugate prior for the Gaussian likelihood, when the variance is known. Also, a Gamma distribution is conjugate to the Poisson likelihood. For multivariate data, popular conjugate priors are the multivariate Normal distribution for the mean vector of Gaussian outcomes and the Dirichlet distribution for the parameters of the Multinomial distribution in case of categorical responses. For the covariance matrix of Gaussian data, the conjugate prior is the Inverse-Wishart distribution. In fact, there exists a simple rule to construct the conjugate prior when the distribution of the data belongs to the exponential family. For a more elaborate list of conjugate priors, we refer to any of the books discussed in Section 1.11. Unfortunately, conjugate priors rarely are available for more complex models, but *conditional conjugate* priors are still possible to construct. Such a prior is conjugate to the conditional likelihood when some (or all other) parameters are fixed. An example is a Gaussian prior for a Normal distribution where its standard deviation is fixed. Another example is the *Inverse Gamma distribution* $IG(\alpha, \beta)$ for the variance of a Gaussian likelihood with the mean fixed. Note that $\sigma^2 \sim IG(\alpha, \beta)$ if and only if $1/\sigma^2 \sim Gamma(\alpha, \beta)$. The product of conditional conjugate priors is called a *semi-conjugate prior.* Conditional conjugate priors are quite useful in combination with Gibbs Sampling as seen in Section 1.6.3, and are therefore much used with standard Bayesian software.

Conjugate, but may be also conditional conjugate, priors are often regarded as too restrictive. One way to relax the prior is to replace the parameter values of the conjugate prior by unknown parameters and to give these parameters also a prior distribution. Such higher level parameters are called *hyperparameters* and their priors are called *hyperpriors.* For example, in Section 1.3.2.1 we can replace the Beta(90, 125) prior, by a Beta(α, β) and give α and β also a prior, for instance each a Gamma prior.

When a prior expresses information obtained in the past, we call it a *subjective prior.* Such priors can be based on historical data, expert knowledge or a combination of both. Examples of such priors in Section 1.3.2.1 are those based on the 1996 data, and the skeptical and enthusiastic priors of Section 1.3.2.2. Clearly, subjective beliefs can be expressed with a variety of priors. The same is true for *objective priors,* i.e. priors that have the aim not to bring subjective information into the Bayesian analysis. Objective priors were often called *non-informative* (NI) priors, but also terms have been used such as *reference priors, vague priors,* etc. One may recall that for the binary outcome in Section 1.3.2.1, we have chosen for θ a flat prior on [0,1] as non-informative prior. However, it turns out that each (NI) prior does bring in some information into the analysis and that a truly non-informative prior does not exist! One could see this by computing the compatible prior for $\psi = \log\{\theta/(1-\theta)\}$ in the OAC example. This prior is obtained by realizing that in a Bayesian context parameters are stochastic. But the distribution of a transformed random variable is obtained from the original distribution multiplied with the Jacobian. This is called the *transformation rule of random variables.* In Figure 1.6, we have given the corresponding prior for ψ. Clearly small values for ψ are now preferred for this prior. The problem is that the original flat prior on [0,1] does not express ignorance, but rather indifference and therefore such a prior is also called an *indifference prior.*

The criticism of non-Bayesians is that always some prior knowledge creeps into any Bayesian analysis, no matter what the prior is. Note that the amount of information that is induced by an (informative) prior is given by the effective sample size (ESS), which is the information in the prior equivalent to the size of a fictive data set. Note that this ESS is different from what is used in Section 1.6.3.4 to assess the information that is present in a MCMC chain. One can find more details on the effective sample size in a prior in Chapter 6 (Section 6.4.6) and Chapter 13 (Section 13.3.1). Since, all priors bring in some information, even vague priors, one recommends performing in practice a *sensitivity analysis* by varying the (vague) priors and showing how much posterior inference varies.

Note that in practice, often *local uniform priors* are taken. A local uniform prior is approximately flat in the region when the likelihood is (approximately) non-zero. For instance, in Figure 1.3 the likelihood for Δ is basically zero outside the interval [-0.2, 0.8]. A Gaussian prior with mean zero and SD=1 will be relatively flat in that interval, and is therefore a locally uniform prior here.

The prior could be quite different from the likelihood based on obtained data. For example, suppose that in the oral anticoagulants example the prior based on the 1999 data would point toward a proportion of AF patients not properly treated with medication is close to zero, while the 2006 data support a proportion close to 1. In that case, we speak of a *prior-data conflict*. It is not immediately clear what to do with such a prior. But, one should definitely have a closer look at the circumstances under which the prior and the data were determined.

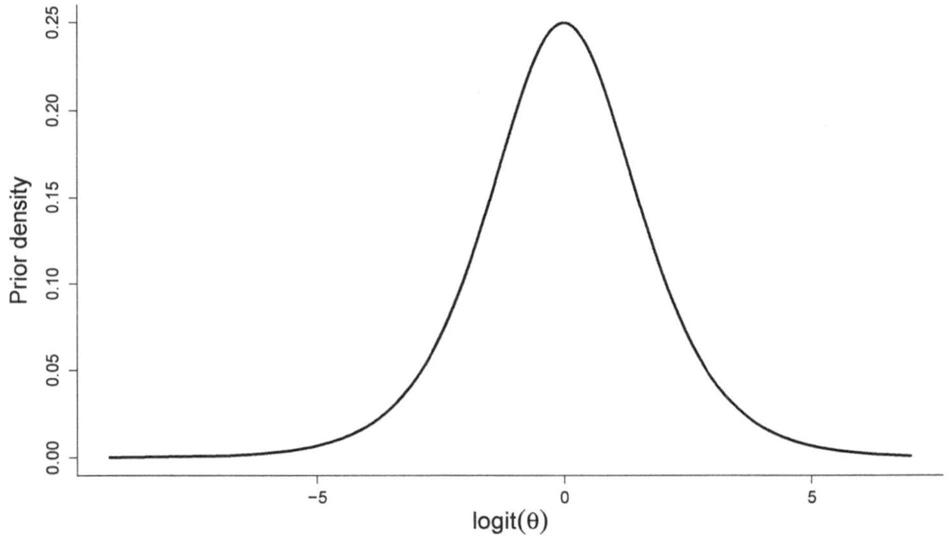

FIGURE 1.6: Prior for logit(θ) when θ has a uniform prior on the unit interval.

Finally, an important class of objective priors is the class of *Jeffreys' priors*. One says that this class is based on the *invariance principle*. This means that it does not matter on what scale (θ or ψ or ...) one applies Jeffreys' construction, the priors will always be compatible. More specifically, Jeffreys suggested the following prior

$$p(\boldsymbol{\theta}) \propto \mathcal{J}^{1/2}(\boldsymbol{\theta}), \tag{1.3}$$

with $\mathcal{J}^{1/2}(\boldsymbol{\theta}) = -E\left(\dfrac{\partial^2 \log\{p(\boldsymbol{y} \mid \boldsymbol{\theta})\}}{\partial \boldsymbol{\theta}\, \partial^\top \boldsymbol{\theta}}\right)$. It can be seen that by this construction $p(\boldsymbol{\psi}) \propto \mathcal{J}^{1/2}(\boldsymbol{\psi}) = \mathcal{J}^{1/2}(\boldsymbol{\theta}) \left|\dfrac{\partial \boldsymbol{\theta}}{\partial \boldsymbol{\psi}}\right| = p(\boldsymbol{\theta}) \left|\dfrac{\partial \boldsymbol{\theta}}{\partial \boldsymbol{\psi}}\right|$, which shows its invariance to whatever scale the principle is applied. Using this principle, Jeffreys also derived on which scale $\boldsymbol{\psi}$ the prior is flat. Finally, for multivariate parameters Jeffreys suggested to apply the principle on location and scale parameters separately. Using this principle, he arrived at a prior for the Gaussian distribution: $p(\mu, \sigma^2) = p(\mu) \times p(\sigma^2) = C \times \sigma^{-2}$. In, e.g. Lesaffre and Lawson (2012), it is shown that with this prior frequentist results are reproduced. But, also in other settings Jeffreys' priors results can exactly or closely reproduce frequentist results.

However, the problem with Jeffreys' priors is that they are often *improper*, which means that their AUC is infinite and therefore may cause the posterior to be improper. The risk with an improper prior is therefore that the posterior summary measures may not exist, and thus that a Bayesian analysis is not possible. That is why BUGS-related software does not allow improper priors (except for the dflat prior), but rather chooses locally uniform priors. For instance, in most `WinBUGS` examples one makes use of a $N(0, 10^6)$ prior for a location parameter and $IG(10^{-3}, 10^{-3})$ for σ^2 (locally uniform prior for σ on log scale).

1.6 Determining the posterior distribution numerically

Most often the posterior cannot be determined analytically, and then we need a numerical way to compute it. Because the numerator is just the product of the likelihood with the prior, computing the posterior boils down to computing the denominator $p(\boldsymbol{y})$, or equivalently determining the integral $\int L(\boldsymbol{\theta} \mid \boldsymbol{y})p(\boldsymbol{y})\, d\boldsymbol{\theta}$.

One may attempt to directly compute the integral and there are, indeed, numerous methods to do so with the Gaussian quadrature methods being the more sophisticated ones. We will return to such methods in Section 1.10. For now, we will concentrate on sampling techniques. First, we consider *independent sampling techniques.*

1.6.1 Monte-Carlo integration

The idea behind *Monte Carlo integration* is to approximate the (posterior) distribution with a histogram of sampled values. The true (posterior) summary measures are then approximated by summary measures based on the Monte Carlo sample. Suppose that we have sampled $\theta^1, \ldots, \theta^K$ from the posterior distribution; then the histogram of $\{\theta^1, \ldots, \theta^K\}$ approximates the underlying posterior distribution. In addition, the mean, standard deviation (SD), etc. of $\{\theta^1, \ldots, \theta^K\}$ can be used to approximate corresponding "true" values. The sampling variability of the sample mean is given by the *Monte Carlo error* (MCE) equal to $s_\theta/\sqrt{K}$, with s_θ the estimated SD of the sampled values of θ. To get an idea of how accurate the sample mean is, or to obtain an estimate of where the true posterior mean could be located, we can compute a frequentist 95% confidence interval based on the Central Limit Theorem given by

$$[\widehat{\overline{\theta}} - 1.96\, s_\theta/\sqrt{K}, \widehat{\overline{\theta}} + 1.96\, s_\theta/\sqrt{K}],$$

with $\widehat{\overline{\theta}}$ the Monte Carlo estimate of the true posterior mean.

It may seem, given that we know the posterior distribution of θ, Monte Carlo sampling has not much extra to offer. However, knowing the posterior distribution does not automatically mean that we can analytically calculate all its posterior summary measures. In addition, suppose that we are interested in the posterior distribution of $\psi = h(\theta)$, with h a monotonic transformation; then we need to apply the transformation rule to obtain the posterior distribution of ψ. Not a big deal you may say. However, it takes you only a few seconds to transform the sampled values of θ, to get (an approximation of) its posterior and posterior summary measures.

1.6.1.1 Example: OACs in atrial fibrillation – sampling from the posterior

The posterior for θ (probability that AF patient is treated with OAC) is Beta(241, 234) and all posterior summary measures can be computed analytically. So we do not really need to sample from the posterior to draw inference about θ, but still ... it can be useful as we will show now. Based on 5,000 sampled values of θ, the Beta(241, 234)-distribution is closely approximated by the sample histogram of the sampled θ's using, for example, the following R commands.

```
# Simulate K=5000 random draws from a Beta(a=241, b=234) distributions
K=5000                # number of Monte Carlo simulations
a=241; b=234          # parameters for the Beta posterior distribution
theta=rbeta(K,a,b)    # simulated Monte Carlo values

# Plots the resulting histogram to approximate the "true" posterior
hist(theta, main="Monte Carlo approximation of the Beta(241, 234)
     posterior distribution",freq=F)
# Superimposes the "true" posterior
points(seq(0,1,.001),dbeta(seq(0,1,.001),a,b),t="l",lwd=2)
```

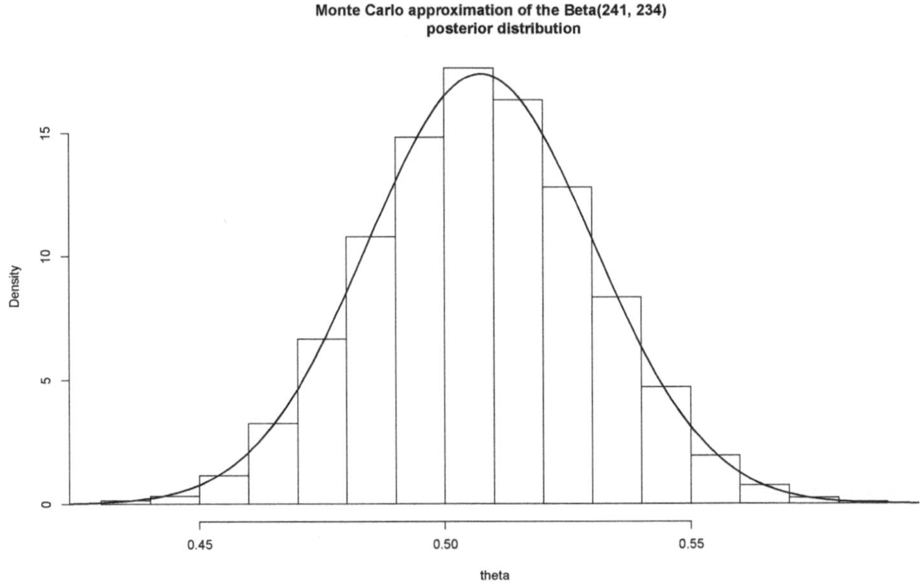

FIGURE 1.7: OAC study: Histogram based on R code that generates Monte Carlo samples from the posterior overlaid with true Beta posterior.

As can be seen in Figure 1.7, the histogram obtained using the Monte Carlo simulations is an extremely good approximation of the true, underlying Beta posterior.

```
# Use the sampled theta's to produce a sample from log(theta)
log.theta=log(theta)
# Produces a histogram to approximate the posterior
# distribution for log(theta)
hist(log.theta)


# Produce summaries to describe the posterior numerically
c("mean"=mean(log.theta),"sd"=sd(log.theta),
      quantile(log.theta,.025),quantile(log.theta,.975))

       mean          sd        2.5%       97.5%
-0.67940181  0.04474143 -0.76856597 -0.59478706
```

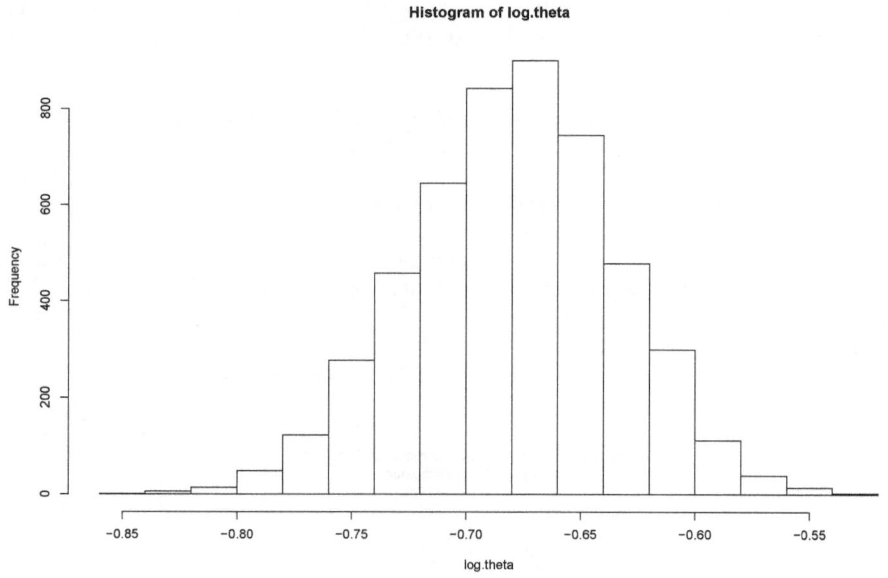

FIGURE 1.8: OAC study: Histogram based on `R` code to obtain Monte Carlo samples from the posterior of transformed parameters.

The same is true for the posterior summaries. The advantage of the sampling approach is immediately seen when we wish to obtain the posterior distribution and the posterior summary measures of $\log(\theta)$. It just involves one extra line in our `R` program, see `R` code and Figure 1.8. For instance, the 95% equal tail CI for $\log(\theta)$ is immediately obtained (and equal approximately to [-0.7686 -0.5948]).

1.6.2 General purpose (univariate) independent sampling algorithms

Many algorithms are available to sample from standard distributions. However, *general purpose* (GP) *sampling algorithms* are required to sample from non-standard distributions. A powerful univariate GP algorithm is the *Accept-reject* (AR) *algorithm* used by e.g. `WinBUGS`. The algorithm assumes that there exists a dominating instrumental distribution $g(\theta) > 0$. This means that there exists a constant $A > 0$ such that $Ag(\theta) \geq p(\theta \mid \boldsymbol{y})$ for all θ. If such an instrumental distribution exists or can be constructed, we sample from $g(\theta)$, and then we reject certain generated values to obtain a sample from the posterior. The advantage of the AR algorithm is that only the product of the likelihood and the prior is needed to sample from the posterior. There are several versions of the AR algorithm implemented in the popular Bayesian algorithms, but also other general purpose algorithms are available, see e.g. Robert and Casella (2004).

1.6.3 Markov chain Monte Carlo techniques

Independent sampling will rarely be available to sample from the posterior. In general, we need more sophisticated sampling tools. Bayesians had to wait until about 1990, when Gelfand and Smith (1990) proposed the use of a general sampling methodology, called *Markov chain Monte Carlo (MCMC) sampling.* MCMC technique(s) were immediately recognized as the solution to many practical issues with Bayesian computations and therefore almost instantaneously caused a revolution in Bayesian statistics, and in statistics on the whole.

We discuss below two popular MCMC techniques: (a) Gibbs Sampling and (b) the Metropolis(-Hastings) algorithm. Next, we will briefly discuss other approaches and Bayesian software. We introduce Gibbs Sampling via the data collected for an oncology study.

1.6.3.1 Example: Trastuzumab RCT – Introduction

Buzdar et al. (2005) describes the results of a Phase II neoadjuvant HER2/neu-positive breast cancer trial to determine whether the addition of trastuzumab to chemotherapy in the neoadjuvant setting could increase pathological complete response (PCR) of the tumor. The plan was that 164 patients would be randomized to chemotherapy with and without trastuzumab. However, the recruitment of patients was slower than expected. At the first interim analysis the Data and Safety Monitoring Board (DSMB) assessed the results when data on 34 patients were available for assessing PCR. Sixteen control patients with four complete responses were observed, together with 12 complete responses for 18 patients under the experimental treatment. Using a Bayesian predictive calculation based on the PPD, they computed the probability to obtain a classical statistical significant result (based on the χ^2-test) at the end of the trial. Since there was about 95% chance to reach significance, the DSMB advised to stop the trial.

Here, we look at the 95% Bayesian CI of the true odds ratio based on the comparison of the results under experimental treatment with probability θ_E and under control treatment with probability θ_C. In case we do not wish to use prior information on the two probabilities, we could give them a uniform prior. Independent sampling then yields easily the posterior distribution of the probabilities and thus also of the odds ratio $\psi = \dfrac{\theta_E/(1-\theta_E)}{\theta_C/(1-\theta_C)}$. We obtained as posterior median (95% CI) for ψ: 5.26 [1.33, 25.22], clearly pointing in the direction of an important effect of adding trastuzumab to chemotherapy.

However, typically the research community is rather skeptical when conclusions are based on small sized studies. We therefore wonder what would be the conclusion of the DSMB if they had combined prior beliefs on the odds ratio with the trial results. Say that a skeptical prior on ψ is used combined with a prior on θ_C based on historical results. What would then be the 95% CI on ψ? Such an analysis is more complicated, but easily solved by applying Gibbs sampling.

1.6.3.2 Gibbs Sampling

The origin of the Gibbs sampling technique can be traced back to a publication of Geman and Geman (1984) in thermodynamics. It was Gelfand and Smith (1990) who saw the importance of this technique for Bayesian computations. In the bivariate case with parameters θ_1, θ_2, Gibbs sampling goes as follows.

Gibbs sampling is based on the following mathematical property that the posterior $p(\theta_1, \theta_2 \mid \boldsymbol{y})$ is completely determined by the two conditional distributions

$$p(\theta_2 \mid \theta_1, \boldsymbol{y}) \qquad \text{and} \qquad p(\theta_1 \mid \theta_2, \boldsymbol{y}).$$

This property yields a simple way to sample from the joint posterior distribution, as follows:

- Select suitable starting values θ_1^0 and θ_2^0, but only one starting value is needed

- Given θ_1^k and θ_2^k at iteration k, generate the $(k+1)$-th value according to iterative scheme:

  1. Sample $\theta_1^{(k+1)}$ from $p(\theta_1 \mid \theta_2^k, \boldsymbol{y})$;
  2. Sample $\theta_2^{(k+1)}$ from $p(\theta_2 \mid \theta_1^{(k+1)}, \boldsymbol{y})$.

The above algorithm is called *Gibbs sampling* and results in a chain of vectors: $\boldsymbol{\theta}^k = (\theta_1^k, \theta_2^k)^\top, k = 1, 2, \ldots$. The elements of the chain are dependent, but they enjoy the Markov property, which means that $p(\boldsymbol{\theta}^{(k+1)} \mid \boldsymbol{\theta}^k, \boldsymbol{\theta}^{(k-1)}, \ldots, \boldsymbol{y}) = p(\boldsymbol{\theta}^{(k+1)} \mid \boldsymbol{\theta}^k, \boldsymbol{y})$. That is why the Gibbs sampler is called a *Markov chain Monte Carlo method.* The chain depends on the starting value and therefore an initial portion of the chain, called the *burn-in part* must be discarded. Under mild regularity conditions, one then obtains a sample from the posterior distribution, also called the target distribution. This means that from a certain iteration k_0 on, we can use the computed summary measures from the chain as an approximation to the true posterior measures. A good approximation of the true posterior summary measures is obtained by running the chain long enough.

The Gibbs sampler can easily be generalized to more than two dimensions. The general case goes as follows. We take a starting position $\boldsymbol{\theta}^0 = (\theta_1^0, \ldots, \theta_d^0)^\top$, and at iteration $(k+1)$ we subsequently sample from the following conditional distributions, also called *full conditionals*:

1. $\theta_1^{(k+1)}$ from $p(\theta_1 \mid \theta_2^k, \ldots, \theta_{(d-1)}^k, \theta_d^k, \boldsymbol{y})$;

2. $\theta_2^{(k+1)}$ from $p(\theta_2 \mid \theta_1^{(k+1)}, \theta_3^k, \ldots, \theta_d^k, \boldsymbol{y})$;

⋮

d. $\theta_d^{(k+1)}$ from $p(\theta_d \mid \theta_1^{(k+1)}, \ldots, \theta_{(d-1)}^{(k+1)}, \boldsymbol{y})$.

The implementation of the Gibbs sampler in practice requires that one can sample from all full conditionals. Often the general purpose algorithms mentioned in Section 1.6.2 are needed to sample from non-standard distributions. As seen, they enjoy the important property that only the product of the likelihood and prior is required to get an idea of the posterior distribution.

1.6.3.3 Example: Trastuzumab RCT – Gibbs sampling the posterior

Suppose that the DSMB is skeptical about the additional effect of trastuzumab. This opinion can be expressed by a skeptical prior on $\psi = \dfrac{\theta_E/(1-\theta_E)}{\theta_C/(1-\theta_C)}$. For instance, a Normal prior on $\log(\psi)$ with mean 0 and SD $= 0.5$, implies that a priori ψ lies in the interval [0.38, 2.66] with 95% probability. Further, suppose that the success rate under the control group is around 33% with 95% prior uncertainty given by the interval [22%, 46%]. The aim is, as before, to determine the odds ratio and its 95% posterior uncertainty.

Now we need Gibbs sampling to determine the posterior $p(\psi, \theta_C \mid \boldsymbol{y})$ and the marginal posteriors $p(\psi \mid \boldsymbol{y})$ and $p(\theta_C \mid \boldsymbol{y})$. The two conditional distributions are determined from the following product:

$$p(\psi, \theta_C \mid \boldsymbol{y}) \propto \theta_C^{r_C}(1-\theta_C)^{n_C - r_C} \times \\ \left(\frac{\psi(1-\theta_C)}{\psi(1-\theta_C)+\theta_C}\right)^{r_E} \left(\frac{\theta_C}{\psi(1-\theta_C)+\theta_C}\right)^{n_E - r_E} \times \\ \frac{1}{\psi} \exp\left\{-\frac{1}{2}\left(\log(\psi)-\mu_0\right)^2/\sigma_0^2\right\} \times \\ \theta_C^{\alpha_C - 1}(1-\theta_C)^{\beta_C - 1},$$

where r_C is the number of control patients that showed PCR among nC treated control patients, and similarly r_E is the number of patients among n_E treated patients in the experimental arm that showed PCR.

From this expression, one determines the conditional $p(\psi \mid \theta_C, \boldsymbol{y})$ by fixing θ_C to a constant. The next step is to look for a sampling technique. The same is done for $p(\theta_C \mid \psi, \boldsymbol{y})$. In Figure 1.9, the two conditional distributions (for two values of the other parameter) are shown up to their normalizing constant. The distributions look smooth but are not (immediately) recognized as standard distributions (from their mathematical expressions). `WinBUGS` takes a version of the AR algorithm to sample ψ from the first conditional, and the *slice sampler* to sample θ_C from the second conditional.

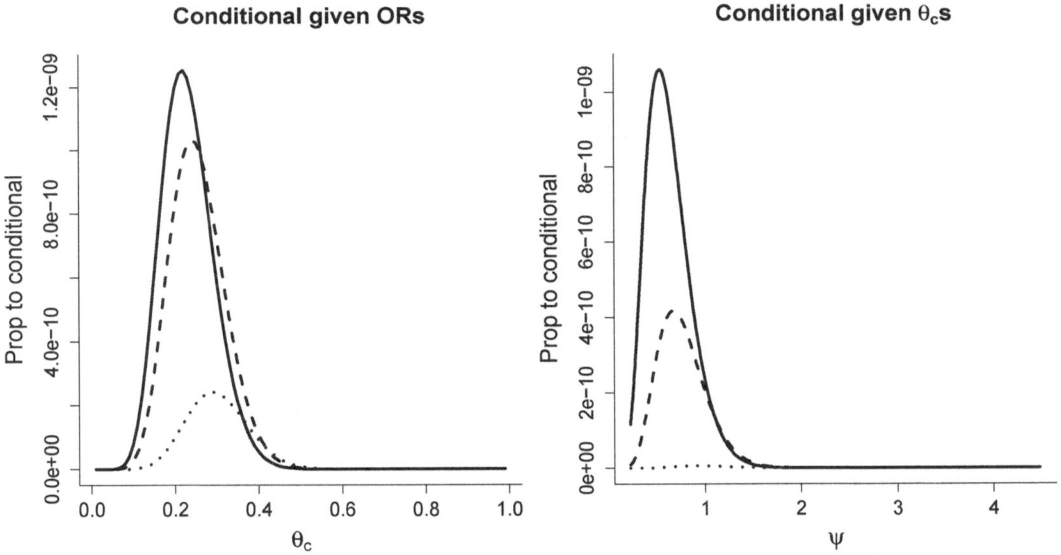

FIGURE 1.9: Trastuzumab RCT: Two (proportional to) conditional distributions of: (1) LHS: θ_C given $\psi = 0.48$ (solid), $\psi = 0.62$ (dashed), $\psi = 1.02$ (dotted) and (2) RHS: ψ given $\theta_C = 0.26$ (solid), $\theta_c = 0.34$ (dashed), $\theta_C = 0.51$ (dotted).

In Figure 1.10(a) the ten first steps (20 substeps) of the Gibbs sampler are shown using the `R` package `R2WinBUGS` in combination with the `R` package `coda`. `R2WinBUGS` has been developed by Sturtz et al. (2005) and runs `WinBUGS` in the background to perform the MCMC simulations. The zig-zag behavior is typical for Gibbs sampling, as the posterior distribution is sampled along the co-ordinate axes. Figure 1.10(b) is based on 500 iterations from a chain of 1,000 sampled values where we have removed the first 500 iterations. Note that we show the behavior of the Gibbs Sampler for $\log(\psi)$ and θ_C only because of graphical reasons. Figure 1.10(c) shows the posterior distribution of the parameters of interest, ψ and θ_C.

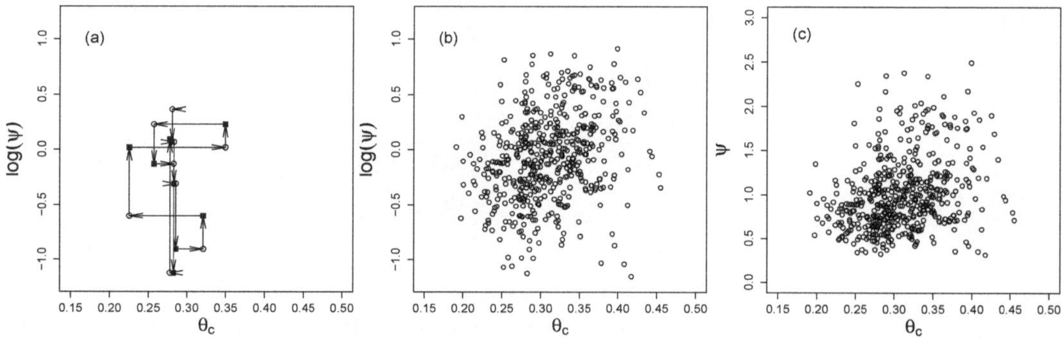

FIGURE 1.10: Trastuzumab RCT: (a) First ten iterations of the Gibbs Sampler, with starting position given by filled circle, (b) 500 sampled values of the joint posterior distribution of $\log(\psi)$ and θ_C, (c) 500 sampled values of the joint posterior distribution of ψ and θ_C.

1.6.3.4 Evaluating the Markov chains

To judge the quality of the sample, or equivalently to know whether we have sampled from the posterior distribution, one should inspect the *trace plots.* A trace plot is a times-series plot with the iteration number on the X axis, and on the Y-axis the corresponding sampled value of the parameter. Convergence to the posterior is characterized by a stationary behavior of the chain. If this is the case, the marginal posterior distributions are estimated. There are also formal convergence procedures. Quite popular is the *Geweke diagnostic*, which compares the early mean (based on first 10% of the chain) and late mean (based on last 50% of the chain). An even more popular diagnostic was suggested by Brooks, Gelman and Rubin, usually referred to as the *BGR diagnostic* or *Potential Scale Reduction*, often indicated as $\widehat{R}$. See Gelman and Rubin (1992) and Brooks and Gelman (1998). They suggested launching multiple chains (say 3) and to evaluate whether these chains are mixing well. The mixing of the chains is evaluated by comparing the overall variability of the chains to the within-chain variability. If the ratio (R-statistic) is close to one (typically < 1.1), then convergence is concluded.

Under mild regularity conditions, MCMC sampling gives eventually the true posterior distribution. We must, however, point out that in practice it can never be proven that convergence to the true posterior distribution has been established, but a similar issue occurs when maximizing the likelihood of a complex model often exhibiting multiple (local) maxima. Further, in practice, one can with a finite number of iterations only approximate the true posterior distribution and its summary measures. That is why we need to sample long enough to guarantee enough precision for, say, the posterior mean. Typically, one requires that the *Monte Carlo error* (MCerror) for the posterior mean is less than 5% of the posterior SD. Note that the MCerror obtained from MCMC is larger than with independent sampling, because the sampled MCMC values are in general not independent. A classical way to express the dependence in the chain goes via the *autocorrelation function*, which expresses the correlation of each parameter at iteration k and $k+\ell$, with ℓ the lag time. These are the correlations of θ^k and $\theta^{k+\ell}$, ℓ for $\ell = 0, 1, 2, \ldots$, respectively. The higher the autocorrelations the less information there is in the chain on the posterior distribution of θ. A useful measure is the *effective sample size* (ESS), which is equal to the size of an independent chain with the same MCerror as for the Markov chain.

1.6.3.5 Example: Trastuzumab RCT – Final steps in establishing the posterior

We started a single chain Gibbs sampler using `WinBUGS` via `R2WinBUGS`. Convergence was easily reached after 1,000 iterations. In Figure 1.11 the traceplots of the two parameters and

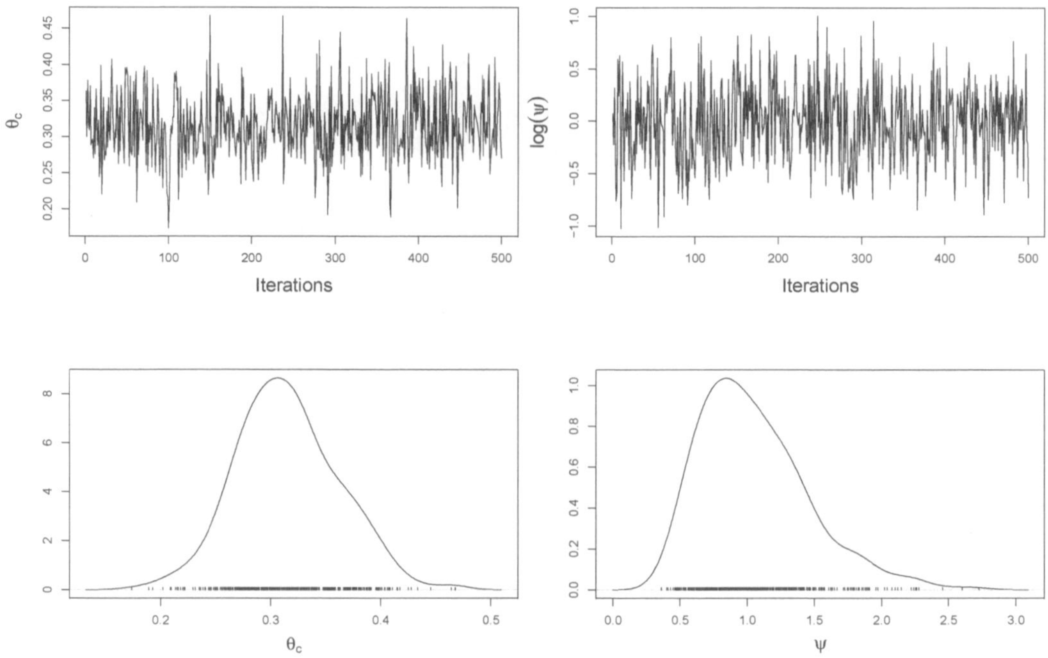

FIGURE 1.11: Trastuzumab RCT: Trace plots of parameters (top), estimated marginal posterior densities (bottom).

estimates of their marginal densities are shown based on the last 500 iterations. Here, the autocorrelations were quite low for both parameters, e.g. for lag 1 they are 0.317 for θ_C and 0.343 for $\log(\psi)$. Further, we obtained for θ_C: ESS=359.51, and for $\log(\psi)$: ESS=244.11. Note that convergence as expressed by the BGR diagnostic (< 1.1) was also easily established when launching 3 chains.

The posterior of $\log(\psi)$ is symmetric, so we report the posterior mean (SD) = -0.07 (0.40), while the posterior for ψ is skewed and so we chose to report the posterior median = 0.92 with 95% equal tail CI = [0.43, 1.97]. Hence our skeptical prior rendered null the evidence obtained from the small study. A Bayesian sensitivity analysis could consist of varying the prior on θ_C. When allowing more uncertainty for this parameter, i.e. 95% prior equal tail CI of [5.3%, 72%] the posterior equal tail 95% CI for ψ is [0.26, 3.06].

1.6.3.6 Metropolis(-Hastings) algorithm

The *Metropolis-Hastings (MH) algorithm* is a general MCMC technique to sample from the posterior distribution without the need for the full conditionals. This algorithm was first proposed by Metropolis (Metropolis et al., 1953), and then extended by Hastings (Hastings, 1970). It can be shown that the Gibbs Sampler is a special case of the MH algorithm, yet the algorithm only became popular after the introduction of Gibbs sampling by Gelfand and Smith in 1990. In practice, though, the two algorithms are treated separately.

The *Metropolis algorithm* makes use of a *proposal density* q that suggests new values for $\boldsymbol{\theta}$. The proposed value will be accepted if it has a higher posterior probability than the existing value, otherwise it will be accepted with a certain probability. More formally, when the chain is at $\boldsymbol{\theta}^k$, then the Metropolis algorithm samples a candidate $\widetilde{\boldsymbol{\theta}}$ from the (symmetric) proposal density $q(\widetilde{\boldsymbol{\theta}} \mid \boldsymbol{\theta})$, with $\boldsymbol{\theta} = \boldsymbol{\theta}^k$. Then $\boldsymbol{\theta}^{(k+1)}$ will be equal to:

- $\widetilde{\boldsymbol{\theta}}$ with probability $\alpha(\boldsymbol{\theta}^k, \widetilde{\boldsymbol{\theta}})$ (accept proposal),
- $\boldsymbol{\theta}^k$ otherwise (reject proposal),

with

$$\alpha(\boldsymbol{\theta}^k, \widetilde{\boldsymbol{\theta}}) = \min\left(r = \frac{p(\widetilde{\boldsymbol{\theta}} \mid \boldsymbol{y})}{p(\boldsymbol{\theta}^k \mid \boldsymbol{y})}, 1\right).$$

This algorithm satisfies again the Markov property, and is therefore again an MCMC algorithm. Note that the adjective 'symmetric' means that $q(\widetilde{\boldsymbol{\theta}} \mid \boldsymbol{\theta}) = q(\boldsymbol{\theta} \mid \widetilde{\boldsymbol{\theta}})$. Often a multivariate Normal or a multivariate t-distribution is chosen. An example of a univariate symmetric proposal density is the Gaussian density with mean that varies with the iteration: $q(\widetilde{\theta} \mid \theta) \propto \exp(-\frac{1}{2\sigma^2}(\widetilde{\theta} - \theta)^2)$. The function $\alpha(\boldsymbol{\theta}^k, \widetilde{\boldsymbol{\theta}})$ is called the *probability of a move.*

The *acceptance rate* is the proportion of times that the proposed value will be accepted. It is not immediately clear what this rate should be here. For a multivariate Normal or t proposal density, taking too small variances corresponds to a high acceptance rate, but will lead to small steps and a slow exploration of the posterior. On the other hand, too large variances correspond to a low acceptance rate due to large explorations outside where the posterior mass is. Roberts, Gelman and Gilks derived that the acceptance rate should be around 0.4 for a univariate posterior, while an acceptance rate of about 0.24 seems optimal for higher dimensions (Roberts et al., 1997).

The above described algorithm is known as the *Random Walk Metropolis* algorithm. Hastings generalized this algorithm by allowing for an asymmetric proposal density, i.e. $q(\widetilde{\boldsymbol{\theta}} \mid \boldsymbol{\theta}) \neq q(\boldsymbol{\theta} \mid \widetilde{\boldsymbol{\theta}})$. An example is the *Independent MH algorithm.* In this case, the proposal density does not move with the locations and one should aim for a high acceptance rate. An example in the univariate case is the Gaussian density with fixed mean: $q(\widetilde{\theta} \mid \theta) \propto \exp\left(-\frac{1}{2\sigma^2}(\widetilde{\theta} - \mu)^2\right)$.

1.6.3.7 Example: Trastuzumab RCT – sampling from the posterior with Metropolis algorithm

To avoid range restrictions, the posterior of logit(θ_C) and log(ψ) was first explored, then back transformed to that of (θ_C, ψ). On this transformed scale, a bivariate Normal proposal density was chosen with correlation zero and variances equal to 0.3 and 0.5, respectively. This choice of proposal density resulted in an acceptance rate of 0.26. We show in Figure 1.12(a) the first fifteen iterations of the algorithm with the accepted and rejected values. In Figures 1.12(b,c) we show the last 4,500 sampled values.

Now the autocorrelations were considerably higher, e.g. for lag 1 they are 0.74 for logit(θ_C) and 0.82 for log(ψ). Therefore the ESS is considerably lower than the chain length (4,500 last values), i.e. 660.26 for logit(θ_C) and 457.23 for log(ψ).

1.6.3.8 Other numerical procedures to estimate the posterior distribution

Hamiltonian Monte Carlo (HMC) is a MCMC method that uses the Hamiltonian dynamics rather than a probability distribution to propose future states (read: values) of the density function being sampled (Neal, 2011). Starting from an initial state, it uses an approximation of the Hamiltonian dynamics to propose a new state and then performs a Metropolis acceptance step. This algorithm is the basis for `Stan`, an increasingly popular Bayesian software.

To sample from the target distribution $p(\boldsymbol{\theta} \mid \boldsymbol{y})$, HMC introduces an auxiliary momentum variable $\boldsymbol{\rho}$ (randomly sampled from a multivariate Normal distribution $N(0, \Sigma)$, with Σ independent of $\boldsymbol{\theta}$) and one draws from the joint distribution $p(\boldsymbol{\rho}, \boldsymbol{\theta} \mid \boldsymbol{y}) = p(\boldsymbol{\rho} \mid \boldsymbol{\theta}, \boldsymbol{y})\, p(\boldsymbol{\theta} \mid \boldsymbol{y})$

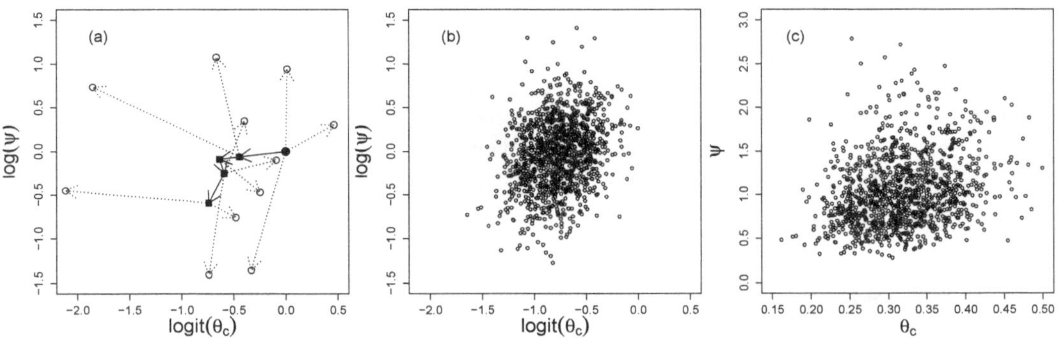

FIGURE 1.12: Trastuzumab RCT: (a) First 15 iterations of Metropolis algorithm, with: starting position (filled circle), accepted values (solid lines) and rejected values (dotted lines), (b) last 4,500 sampled values of the joint posterior distribution of logit(θ_C) and log(ψ), (c) last 4,500 sampled values of the joint posterior distribution of θ_C and ψ.

(Neal, 2011). The joint distribution then defines a Hamiltonian $H(\boldsymbol{\rho}, \boldsymbol{\theta} \mid \boldsymbol{y}) = -\log p(\boldsymbol{\rho}, \boldsymbol{\theta} \mid \boldsymbol{y}) = -\log p(\boldsymbol{\rho} \mid \boldsymbol{\theta}, \boldsymbol{y}) - \log p(\boldsymbol{\theta} \mid \boldsymbol{y})$, which determines the evolution of the point $(\boldsymbol{\rho}, \boldsymbol{\theta} \mid \boldsymbol{y})$ in the parameter space. The trajectory is uniquely defined by the Hamilton's equations of the gradients.

Unfortunately, in many cases, Hamilton's equations can only be solved numerically. `Stan` uses the *leapfrog algorithm* (Carpenter et al., 2017). At the current state at time t, the states at time $t + \varepsilon$, $t + 2\varepsilon$, ..., are approximated (ε is some small time interval called *step size*). After L steps, the state $(\boldsymbol{\rho}^*; \boldsymbol{\theta}^*)$ at time $t + L\varepsilon$ is approximated. To correct for the error introduced by the discrete approximation to the continuous dynamics, a Metropolis step is applied. The probability of accepting the proposal $(\boldsymbol{\rho}^*, \boldsymbol{\theta}^*)$ is

$$\min\left(1, \exp\left(H(\boldsymbol{\rho}, \boldsymbol{\theta}) - H(\boldsymbol{\rho}^*, \boldsymbol{\theta}^*)\right)\right).$$

Three parameters that must to be set are the step size ε, the *mass matrix* Σ^{-1}, and the number of steps L. Sampling efficiency is highly sensitive to these parameters. Fortunately, using the *No-U-Turn sampler* (NUTS) (Hoffman and Gelman, 2014), `Stan` automatically tunes these parameters. It optimizes ε, estimates Σ based on warm-up sample iterations, and is able to dynamically adapt L during the warm-up and sampling.

Integrated nested Laplace approximation (INLA) has been proposed as a computationally convenient alternative for MCMC methods. The classical Laplace approximation is a method to approximate Bayesian parameter estimation, based on a second-order Taylor approximation of the log posterior around the maximum a posteriori estimate. This results in a Gaussian approximation to the posterior, thereby avoiding sampling from the posterior, which can be too time consuming. Note that the Laplace approximation is a special case of *adaptive Gaussian quadrature*, but there is also *non-adaptive Gaussian quadrature*. Gaussian quadrature methods replace the integral by a weighted sum: $\int f(z)\phi(z)dz \approx \sum_{q=1}^{Q} w_q f(z_q)$. Q is the order of the approximation. The higher Q, the more accurate the approximation will be. With non-adaptive Gaussian quadrature, the nodes and weights are fixed, independent of $f(z)\phi(z)$. More specifically the design points are located around zero with dispersion independent of $f(z)\phi(z)$. With adaptive Gaussian quadrature, the nodes and weights are adapted to the 'support' of $f(z)\phi(z)$ with the design points located around the mean of $f(z)\phi(z)$ with appropriate dispersion. Note that the Laplace approximation corresponds to adaptive Gaussian quadrature with $Q = 1$.

To approximate Bayesian inference for latent Gaussian models, a nested version of the classical Laplace approximation is combined with modern numerical techniques for sparse matrices, see e.g. Rue et al. (2017). There are three steps to the approximation. Initially the posterior marginals of the hyperparameters (which are not necessarily Gaussian) are approximated using a Laplace approximation. The Gaussian approximation is then improved by using a Laplace approximation for selected values of the hyperparameters. Finally these two steps are combined using numerical integration. For a more extensive explanation on INLA, we refer to Rue et al. (2009).

1.7 Hierarchical models and data augmentation

Quite often medical data exhibit some hierarchy. Examples can be found in clinical trials conducted at multiple sites, meta-analyses pooling several study results, spatial epidemiology focused e.g. on the estimation of disease intensities in correlated areas or longitudinal studies with repeated measurements over time for the same individual. An appropriate statistical model needs to take into account the hierarchy in the data. Such a model is called an *hierarchical model*. When there are no covariates involved, the model is also called a *variance component model* or a *random effects model*. On the other hand, a *mixed model* is a random effects model that also involves covariates. A *Bayesian hierarchical model* is simply an hierarchical model where all parameters are given a prior distribution.

The following is the description of a *two-level Bayesian Gaussian hierarchical model* when there are n clusters, and in the ith cluster ($i = 1, \ldots, n$) there m_i observed data y_{ij}, ($j = 1, \ldots, m_i$). The true cluster means θ_i, ($i = 1, \ldots, n$), also called *random effects*, are not observed but are assumed to have a common distribution $p(\theta \mid \ldots)$. When the parameters of that distribution are also given a prior, we call it a two-level Bayesian hierarchical model, and it becomes a Gaussian hierarchical model when the random variables Y_{ij}, ($j = 1, \ldots, m_i$) have a Gaussian distribution given θ_i and also the θ_i, ($i = 1, \ldots, n$) have a Gaussian distribution. Formally we assume for a two-level Bayesian Gaussian hierarchical model:

- **Level 1**: $Y_{ij} \mid \theta_i, \sigma^2 \sim \text{N}(\theta_i, \sigma^2) \quad (j = 1, \ldots, m_i;\ i = 1, \ldots, n)$;
- **Level 2**: $\theta_i \mid \mu, \sigma_\theta^2 \sim \text{N}(\mu, \sigma_\theta^2) \quad (i = 1, \ldots, n)$;
- **Priors**: $\sigma^2 \sim p(\sigma^2)$ and $(\mu, \sigma_\theta^2) \sim p(\mu, \sigma_\theta^2)$.

Typically, the hyperparameters μ, σ_θ are given separate independent priors.

The above model is also called a *Bayesian linear model*. The foundations of the Bayesian linear model have been laid down by Lindley and Smith in a series of papers (Lindley, 1971; Lindley and Smith, 1972; Smith, 1973b,a). Some analytical results are available for this model. Namely, there is again *shrinkage* in the estimation of the level-2 means towards the overall posterior mean. If $\overline{y}_i$ is the observed mean of ith cluster, $\overline{\theta}_i$ the estimated mean of ith cluster and $\overline{\mu}$ the posterior mean of μ from a Bayesian analysis, then $\overline{\theta}_i = B_i\,\overline{\mu} + (1 - B_i)\,\overline{y}_i$ with $B_i = \dfrac{\text{prec B}}{\text{prec B} + \text{prec W}_i}$, where $\text{prec B} = \dfrac{1}{\sigma_\theta^2}$, $\text{prec W}_i = \dfrac{1}{\sigma^2/m_i}$. This shows that the estimated means $\overline{\theta}_i$ must show less variability than the original means $\overline{y}_i$, and that the shrinkage is the most for small sized clusters.

The Bayesian linear model can be extended to involve also covariates, and then there are *fixed effects* (regression coefficients) and random effects. A popular model of this type is the *linear mixed model* (LMM) and its extensions, i.e. the *generalized linear mixed model* (GLMM) and the *non-linear mixed model* (NLMM). Although computations are more involved now, we see similar shrinkage of the estimated random effects. Such models are frequently used in longitudinal studies.

Mixed models are also quite popular in a frequentist context. In fact, basically all of the initial developments in mixed models were done under the frequentist paradigm. There is, however, a major difference in estimating the model parameters under the frequentist and the Bayesian paradigm. In the frequentist approach the hyperparameters (in the above example, these are μ and σ_θ) are estimated back from the marginal likelihood. This is called the *empirical Bayesian approach.* In contrast, in the Bayesian approach the hyperparameters are given a prior distribution. Therefore, one argues that (only) the Bayesian approach takes all uncertainty into account and that is why Bayesian credible intervals are usually wider than frequentist confidence intervals. In addition, in Bayesian software one works with the hierarchical specification of the mixed model, while in frequentist software the marginal version of the mixed model (averaged over the random effects) is usually the basis for estimating the parameters.

When fitting the hierarchical model to the data, the random effects are treated as parameters. That is, the original set of model parameters is augmented with the random effects parameters to render the (Bayesian) estimation of the model easier. This technique is called *data augmentation* (DA). Data augmentation is the Bayesian equivalent of the popular Expectation-Maximization algorithm, and is an elegant way to simplify the estimation of model parameters in a Bayesian context. For instance, it can be used to handle missing data in the response and covariates, but it also allows us to deal easily with censored responses.

1.8 Model selection and model checking

A central question in each statistical modeling exercise is: *Which model should we choose for the data at hand?* This question refers to *model selection.* a second important question is: *Does the chosen model fit the data well (enough)?* Or in other words: *Is the chosen model appropriate?*

Model selection and model checking are as important in a Bayesian as in a frequentist context, but now also a prior distribution is involved. Also, as we will see in the next two subsections, these areas are still much under development. However, instead of selecting a 'best' model, one could also opt for letting inference depend on a combination of 'good' models, which leads to model averaging. This will be briefly treated in the third subsection.

1.8.1 Model selection

There are basically two types of model comparisons: nested and non-nested. We speak of a comparison of two nested models, if one model is a simplification of the other model. When this is not the case, we speak of non-nested models. In a frequentist context model comparison (and model selection) is different for nested and non-nested comparisons. For nested comparisons, one makes use of the likelihood ratio statistic, while for non-nested comparisons there is no formal statistical tool. In practice, one most often makes use of *Akaike's Information Criterion* (AIC) or the *Bayesian Information Criterion* (BIC) to select among non-nested models. In a Bayesian context, one does not make the distinction between nested and non-nested comparisons, since one simply does not make use of statistical tests that are based on the repeated sampling idea.

The most popular Bayesian tool for model selection, is the *Deviance Information Criterion* (DIC) suggested by Spiegelhalter et al. (2002). One of the reasons for its popularity is that DIC combines nicely with MCMC computations and has been implemented in `WinBUGS` for many years. DIC can be seen as the Bayesian equivalent of AIC. It measures in a Bayesian way the predictive ability of the model fitted to the data at hand. DIC is formally defined as:

$$\text{DIC} = -2\log p(\boldsymbol{y} \mid \bar{\boldsymbol{\theta}}) + 2p_{DIC}, \tag{1.4}$$

where p_{DIC} corresponds to the effective number of parameters, given by

$$p_{DIC} = -2\ E_{\boldsymbol{\theta}|\boldsymbol{y}}[\log p(\boldsymbol{y} \mid \boldsymbol{\theta})] + 2\log[p(\boldsymbol{y} \mid \bar{\boldsymbol{\theta}})],$$

which quantifies the number of parameters to be estimated after incorporating the prior information into the model. Defining the deviance as $D(\boldsymbol{\theta}) = -2\log\{p(\boldsymbol{y} \mid \boldsymbol{\theta})\}+2\log\{f(\boldsymbol{y})\}$, the effective number of parameters can alternatively be written as $p_D = \overline{D(\boldsymbol{\theta})} - D(\bar{\boldsymbol{\theta}})$ where $\overline{D(\boldsymbol{\theta})}$ is the posterior mean of the deviance.

For practical purposes, we can ignore $f(\boldsymbol{y})$. The mean deviance $\overline{D(\boldsymbol{\theta})}$ can be approximated by $1/K\sum_{k=1}^{K} D(\boldsymbol{\theta}^k)$ and the plug-in deviance $D(\bar{\boldsymbol{\theta}})$ by $D(1/K\sum_{k=1}^{K}\boldsymbol{\theta}^k)$. As can be seen, this criterion is easy to compute given a sampling algorithm is available. Smaller values of DIC indicate better models, but a difference of at least 5 is needed to choose between the two models. However, DIC has been criticized from different angles. For instance, DIC is not invariant to non-linear transformations of $\boldsymbol{\theta}$. Quite disturbing is that negative values for p_{DIC} can occur in which case DIC is not to be used. Note also, that the values of DIC and p_{DIC} are subject to random fluctuations since they depend on the sampled values of the chain. For hierarchical models, p_{DIC}, and thus DIC, depends on the variability of the θ_i, $(i = 1, \ldots, n)$, see e.g. Lesaffre and Lawson (2012).

Recently, the *widely available information criterion* (WAIC) has been suggested as an alternative for DIC because it is invariant to transformations of $\boldsymbol{\theta}$. However, the computation of WAIC needs to be done outside most Bayesian software packages. The same is true for the *pseudo-Bayes factor* (PSBF) derived from the *Bayes factor* (BF). One may argue that the Bayes factor is the ideal Bayesian tool for model selection, and that is true if it were easier to compute and not so dependent on the choice of prior. The Bayes factor can be considered as the Bayesian equivalent of the likelihood ratio test. When we need to choose between two models M_1, M_2 with parameters $\boldsymbol{\theta}_1$ and $\boldsymbol{\theta}_2$, respectively, the Bayes factor is given by $\text{BF}_{1,2} = p(\boldsymbol{y} \mid \text{M}_1)/p(\boldsymbol{y} \mid \text{M}_2)$ where $p(\boldsymbol{y} \mid \text{M}_m) = \int p(\boldsymbol{y} \mid \boldsymbol{\theta}_m, \text{M}_m)p(\boldsymbol{\theta}_m \mid \text{M}_m)d\boldsymbol{\theta}_m$ for $m = \{1, 2\}$. Thus, the BF is the ratio of the marginal likelihoods under the two models. Unfortunately, these marginal likelihoods are often computationally quite involved and (too much) dependent on the choice of the prior distributions. The pseudo-Bayes factor is one way to bypass the dependence on the prior, by partitioning the data set into a learning set $\boldsymbol{y}_L = \{y_i : i \in L\}$ and a testing set $\boldsymbol{y}_T = \{y_i : i \in T\}$. When the testing and learning parts are defined respectively as $T = \{i\}$ and $L = \{1, ..., i-1, i+1, ..., n\}$, the pseudo-Bayes factor in favor of model M_1 with respect to model M_2 is obtained as

$$\text{PSBF}_{1,2} = \frac{\prod_{i=1}^{n} p(y_i \mid \boldsymbol{y}_{(i)}, \text{M}_1)}{\prod_{i=1}^{n} p(y_i \mid \boldsymbol{y}_{(i)}, \text{M}_2)},$$

where $\boldsymbol{y}_{(i)}$ is the sample with all observations except y_i. The logarithm of PSBF is called the *log pseudo-marginal likelihood* (LPML).

As seen in Section 1.7, in a frequentist context the marginal likelihood is used to estimate the parameters of hierarchical models, while in a Bayesian context the random effects with the fixed effects are jointly estimated. The first way produces marginal selection criteria, while the second way leads to conditional (or hierarchical) selection criteria. The conditional criteria measure the predictive ability of the model on future samples from the same subjects as for the data at hand. The marginal criteria, on the other hand, measure the predictive ability of the model on the population of subjects. In practice, the marginal selection criteria are most often relevant. Yet, in a Bayesian analysis almost always the conditional criteria are reported because most Bayesian analyses of hierarchical data make use of the elegant DA algorithm. Recently, this issue has received considerable attention in the literature. We refer to some recent work and references therein that shows the inappropriateness of the hierarchical selection criteria, see e.g. Quintero and Lesaffre (2017); Ariyo et al. (2019); Merkle et al. (2018).

1.8.2 Model checking

The selected model is not necessarily sensible nor does it guarantee a good fit to the data. There is still the need for model evaluation. Some standard activities are (a) checking that inference from the chosen model is reasonable; (b) verifying that the model can reproduce the data well and (c) sensitivity analyses by varying certain aspects of the model. In a sense Bayesian model evaluation is similar to frequentist model evaluation, but now also the prior distribution needs attention. Further, and in contrast to frequentist approaches, most of the Bayesian techniques are based on sampling techniques and do not need any large sample argument.

A popular technique based on sampling is the *posterior predictive check* (PPC). The basic idea is quite simple. One generates replicated data from the assumed model, and compares a statistic based on the replicated data with that computed on the observed data. More formally, let us assume that the data have been generated from distribution $p(y \mid \boldsymbol{\theta})$, which we refer to as model M_0. Given an observed sample $\boldsymbol{y} = \{y_1, \ldots, y_n\}$ we estimate the model parameters $\boldsymbol{\theta}$. Suppose that a large value of the goodness-of-fit test (GOF) statistic $T(\boldsymbol{y})$ or of a discrepancy measure $D(\boldsymbol{y}, \boldsymbol{\theta})$ corresponds to a poor fit. One generates the sample $\widetilde{\boldsymbol{y}} = \{\widetilde{y}_1, \ldots, \widetilde{y}_n\}$ from $p(y \mid \boldsymbol{\theta})$ taking the uncertainty about $\boldsymbol{\theta}$ into account. Thus, one generates in fact samples from the PPD. Then the GOF statistic or the discrepancy measure based on the observed data is compared to that of the replicated data. This gives a proportion of times the statistic of the observed data is more extreme than that of replicated data, producing what is called a *posterior predictive P-value* (PPP-value). Typically PPP-values smaller than 0.05 or 0.10 are an indication that the model fit is not good. However, since the data are used twice (once for estimating the model parameters and once for testing the model) the PPP-value is known to be conservative. Examples of $T(\boldsymbol{y})$ and $D(\boldsymbol{y}, \boldsymbol{\theta})$ are typically GOF statistics such as the X^2-statistic in evaluating discrete models or Normality tests in evaluating the Gaussian distribution of regression residuals.

1.8.3 Model averaging

Finding the true model for the data at hand is a useless exercise. At most one can hope for a reasonable model, either for prediction or for understanding which and why factors determine the response. Instead of focusing on one 'best' model, one might consider the collection of 'good' models and determine overall (posterior) summary measures by averaging these summary measures from this set of models. When applied in a Bayesian context, this is called *Bayesian model averaging* (BMA). Suppose that one is interested in estimating γ, e.g. the response of a future observation. For BMA, one takes the total set of possible models $\{M_1, \ldots, M_K\}$ and uses the model probabilities $p(M_m \mid \boldsymbol{y})$, $(m = 1, \ldots, K)$ to determine the posterior distribution of γ

$$p(\gamma \mid \boldsymbol{y}) = \sum_{m=1}^{K} p(\gamma \mid \boldsymbol{y}, M_m) p(M_m \mid \boldsymbol{y}),$$

with $p(\gamma \mid \boldsymbol{y}, M_m)$ determined from the posterior of the model parameters $p(\boldsymbol{\theta}_m \mid \boldsymbol{y}, M_m)$ by marginalization. The posterior mean and variance of γ are then determined from:

$$\begin{aligned} \mathrm{E}(\gamma \mid \boldsymbol{y}) &= \sum_{m=1}^{K} \widehat{\gamma}_m p(M_m \mid \boldsymbol{y}), \\ \mathrm{Var}(\gamma \mid \boldsymbol{y}) &= \sum_{m=1}^{K} \left[\mathrm{Var}(\gamma \mid \boldsymbol{y}, M_m) + \widehat{\gamma}_m^2\right] p(M_m \mid \boldsymbol{y}) - \mathrm{E}(\gamma \mid \boldsymbol{y})^2, \end{aligned}$$

with $\widehat{\gamma}_m = \mathrm{E}(\gamma \mid \boldsymbol{y}, M_m) = \int \gamma(\boldsymbol{\theta}_m) p(\boldsymbol{\theta}_m \mid \boldsymbol{y}, M_m) d\boldsymbol{\theta}_m$. Further details can be found in Raftery et al. (1997).

1.9 Bayesian nonparametric methods

Parametric inference is still most popular under both the frequentist and the Bayesian paradigm. Largely due to the flexibility of Bayesian software, it is relatively easy to change and relax parametric assumptions. Consequently, most Bayesian analyses and software are still based on (flexible) parametric assumptions. Especially in the last decade, several developments aimed to further relax the distributional assumptions in a Bayesian context leading to *Bayesian nonparametric (BNP) approaches.* When covariates are also involved, they are also called *Bayesian semiparametric (BSP) approaches.* The early BNP approaches aimed for analytical expressions of the posterior. However, this quickly appeared horrendously complicated. Breakthroughs were realized when involving MCMC techniques.

The most successful BNP approach is based on the seminal paper by Ferguson (1973). Ferguson specified a prior on the functional space of cumulative distribution functions, and he called it the *Dirichlet process (DP) prior.* The introduction of the DP prior implied the start of an impressive amount of new statistical developments in BNP analyses. A good overview and further references can be found in Müller et al. (2012).

The Dirichlet process is defined via the Dirichlet distribution. First, choose $c > 0$ and $F^*(x)$, a right-continuous cumulative distribution function (cdf) serving as a kind of template. Then, assume that $P(\cdot)$ is a probability measure on Borel sets of the real axis, i.e. $P([a, b]) = F(b) - F(a)$ with $F(x)$ a cdf, and $P^*(\cdot)$ based on $F^*(x)$ defined in a similar way. Then:

A Dirichlet Process (DP) with parameters $(c, F^*(x))$ *is a random cdf* F*, which for each (measurable) finite partition* $\{B_1, B_2, \ldots, B_k\}$ *of the real axis assigns probabilities* $P(B_j)$ $(j = 1, \ldots, k)$ *such that, the joint distribution of the vector* $(P(B_1), P(B_2), \ldots, P(B_k))$ *is the Dirichlet distribution Dir* $(cP^*(B_1), cP^*(B_2), \ldots, cP^*(B_k))$.

Ferguson (1973) showed that such a process exists. The DP is denoted as $DP(cF^*)$, with c the precision and F^* the centering cdf. In other words, c controls the variation around a template cdf F^*, something like an initial guess of the cdf of the data. The realized F has a discrete nature, with expected value at x equal to $F^*(x)$ and variance $F^*(x)$ $\{1 - F^*(x)\}/(c+1)$. Because of the discrete nature of the realized F, we can write $F(x) = \sum_{h=1}^{\infty} w_h \delta_{m_h}(x)$, with $w_1, w_2, \ldots$ probability weights for the locations m_h and $\delta_{m_h}(x) = 1$ when $x = m_h$ and zero elsewhere. Sethuraman (1994) proposed a sampling procedure to construct the DP, called the *stick breaking construction.* This procedure consists of taking i.i.d. draws m_h from F^*, and with weights in the unit interval, as follows: $w_1 \in [0,1]$, $w_2 \in [0, 1 - w_1]$, $w_3 \in [0, 1 - w_1 - w_2]$, etc.

The discreteness of the DP posterior is considered, though, as a limitation, and various extensions have been proposed just to name a few: *Dirichlet Process Mixture* (DPM), *Mixture of Dirichlet Processes* (MDP) and a *Pólya Tree* (PT). For technical details on all these BNP and BSP approaches, but also for yet other BNP and BSP approaches, we refer to Müller et al. (2012).

Until recently nonparametric Bayesian software was largely lacking, but this changed with the introduction of the `R` package **`DPpackage`** developed by Jara, see Jara et al. (2011). This package allows for a great variety of BNP and BSP analyses based on the Dirichlet process and its variants.

In Chapter 9 such BNP models will be used in a longitudinal context, while in Chapter 10 an alternative BNP model based on Gamma Processes is used in a survival context.

1.10 Bayesian software

1.10.1 BUGS-related software

The introduction of the MCMC techniques combined with the `BUGS` (**B**ayesian inference **U**sing **G**ibbs **S**ampling) software caused a revolution in the Bayesian world. The `BUGS` project started in 1989 in the MRC Biostatistics Unit in Cambridge. First, there was the classical `BUGS` program. The stand alone `WinBUGS` program (Lunn et al., 2000) equipped with GUI capabilities was further developed in cooperation with Imperial College School of Medicine at St. Mary's, London. But the developments have stopped and the successor of `WinBUGS`, `OpenBUGS` is hosted at the University of Helsinki. `OpenBUGS` version 3.2.3 offers more sampling and modeling tools than `WinBUGS`. See Lunn et al. (2009), for the history of the `BUGS` project.

`WinBUGS` and `OpenBUGS` are examples of click-and-point software, and are therefore unhandy and time consuming when data and models change in the process of analyzing the data. Batch processing via `R` is handled using packages `R2OpenBUGS`, `R2WinBUGS`, or `BRugs`. Additional `R` software, such as the packages `coda` and `boa` provide tools for exploring the sampled chains outside the `BUGS` software.

`JAGS` (Just Another Gibbs Sampler) is `BUGS`-like software, with practically the same syntax as `WinBUGS` and `OpenBUGS` but provides some extra functions. `JAGS` (version 4.3.0), written in `C++` by Martyn Plummer, is platform independent. Practice shows that `JAGS` is in general faster than `WinBUGS` and `OpenBUGS`. `JAGS` can be called from `R` via the packages `rjags`, `R2jags` and `runjags`. The package `runjags` allows also for parallel processing using multiple cores on the computer, see Plummer (2003) and the webpage of JAGS.

1.10.2 Stan

`Stan` is an probabilistic programming language based on `C++`. `Stan` is based on HMC sampling seen in Section 1.6.3.8 and uses NUTS as a default sampler. A `Stan` program is composed of separate blocks where the user specifies observed and unobserved quantities. Several interfaces with general statistical software packages have been developed, e.g. with `R` (`RStan`). `Rstan` also provides informal and formal diagnosis for checking convergence. `Shinystan` is a powerful package for exploring the posterior sample.

For small and simple models, there is no practical difference between `Stan` and the `BUGS` software. `Stan` with NUTS performs more efficiently for a high-dimensional target distribution although computation is more intensive at each iteration. However, at the time this book is written Stan cannot deal with discrete parameters because HMC or its variant NUTS requires gradients. In addition, Stan does not allow missing input in the data block; therefore some extra programming is required to deal with missing values.

1.10.3 SAS software

The SAS® package is a vast software package providing the user facilities to set up data bases, general data handling, statistical programming and analysis. SAS offers the user also a broad range of statistical procedures, primarily organized in SAS procedures. Most of the SAS procedures deal with frequentist methods, but the number of Bayesian SAS procedures has been increasing in the last decade. With version 14.0, SAS offers tools for Bayesian analyses of finite mixture models (PROC FMM), generalized linear models (PROC GENMOD), accelerated life failure models (PROC LIFREG), Cox regression models, and piecewise exponential hazard models (PROC PHREG). In each of these procedures, the model is specified as for a frequentist analysis but adding a BAYES statement calls for a Bayesian estimation method. For sampling from the posterior distributions, one makes use of adaptive rejection sampling (ARS), conjugate sampling, Metropolis, and other algorithms. The BCHOICE procedure is a purely Bayesian procedure written specifically for discrete choice models. But, the most advanced SAS procedure for Bayesian modeling is the MCMC procedure. PROC MCMC uses a random walk Metropolis algorithm to obtain posterior samples. The syntax is similar to that of the procedure NLMIXED, i.e. users can freely define their model in combination with a great variety of priors. Recently, SAS launched the BGLIMM procedure for Bayesian generalized linear mixed models.

1.10.4 R-INLA

R-INLA is the interface to INLA from R. Briefly, the R-INLA package fits Bayesian models using Integrated Nested Laplace approximation (INLA), which makes use of latent Gaussian Markov random field (GMRF) models (Rue and Held, 2005).

1.10.5 Further R software

There has been recently an explosion of Bayesian R software. Numerous dedicated R programs have been developed for a great variety of applications. Hence, it is unfeasible trying to give a comprehensive overview of the available packages. The advantage of dedicated software is that the numerical algorithms are optimized for the specific applications at hand.

1.11 Further reading

This chapter serves as a general introduction to Bayesian methods. Further reading is necessary to grasp the technicalities of the material. Apart from the books already mentioned above, general background to Bayesian methods can be found in:

- Box and Tiao (1973): the classical early book on parametric Bayesian methods;
- O'Hagan and Forster (2004): containing many theoretical results presented in a mathematically elegant manner;

- Gelman et al. (2004) and Carlin and Louis (2000): two standard books on Bayesian methods for data analysis that triggered many statistical modelers to start using the Bayesian approach;
- Robert and Casella (2004): a fundamental book on MCMC sampling;
- Ntzoufras (2009) and Kruschke (2015): two books that nicely combine the application of Bayesian methods with Bayesian software.

Bibliography

Ariyo, O., Quintero, L., Muñoz, J., Verbeke, G., and Lesaffre, E. (2019). Bayesian model selection in linear mixed models for longitudinal data. *Journal of Applied Statistics*, in press.

Baker, M. (2011). Is there a reproducibility crisis? *Nature*, 533(7604):452–454.

Box, G. and Tiao, G. (1973). *Bayesian Inference in Statistical Analysis.* Addison-Wesley, Reading, MA.

Brooks, S. and Gelman, A. (1998). General methods for monitoring convergence of iterative simulation. *Journal of Computational and Graphical Statistics*, 7:434–455.

Buzdar, A., Ibrahim, N., Francis, D., Booser, D., Thomas, E., Theriault, R., Pusztai, L., Green, M., Arun, B., Giordano, S., Cristofanilli, M., Frye, D., Smith, T., Hunt, K., Singletary, S., Sahin, A., Ewer, M., Buchholz, T., Berry, D., and Hortobagyi, G. (2005). Significantly higher pathologic complete remission rate after neoadjuvant therapy with trastuzumab, paclitaxel, and epirubicin chemotherapy: results of a randomized trial in human epidermal growth factor receptor 2-positive operable breast cancer. *Journal of Clinical Oncology*, 23(16):3676–3685.

Carlin, B. and Louis, T. (2000). *Bayes and Empirical Bayes Methods for Data Analysis.* Chapman and Hall, Boca Raton, FL, 2nd edition.

Carpenter, B., Gelman, A., Hoffman, M., Lee, D., Goodrich, B., Betancourt, M., Brubaker, M., Guo, J., Li, P., and Riddell, A. (2017). Stan: A probabilistic programming language. *Journal of Statistical Software*, 76(1):1–32.

Ferguson, T. (1973). A Bayesian analysis of some nonparametric problems. *The Annals of Statistics*, 1 (2):209–230.

Fisher, R. A. (1934). *Statistical Methods for Research Workers.* Oliver & Boyd, Edinburgh, UK, 3rd edition.

Freedman, L., Spiegelhalter, D., and Parmar, M. (1994). The what, why and how of Bayesian clinical trials monitoring (with discussion). *Statistics in Medicine*, 13:1371–1389.

Gelfand, A. and Smith, A. (1990). Sampling-based approaches to calculating marginal densities. *Journal of the American Statistical Association*, 85:398–409.

Gelman, A., Carlin, J., H.S., S., and D.B., R. (2004). *Bayesian Data Analysis.* Chapman & Hall/CRC, Florida, USA, 2nd edition.

Gelman, A. and Rubin, D. (1992). Inference from iterative simulation using multiple sequences. *Statistical Science*, 7:457–511.

Geman, S. and Geman, D. (1984). Stochastic relaxation, Gibbs disributions, and the Bayesian restoration of images. *IEEE Transactions on Pattern Analysis and Machine Intelligence*, 6:721–741.

Hastings, W. (1970). Monte Carlo sampling methods using Markov chains and their applications. *Biometrika*, 57:97–109.

Hoffman, M. and Gelman, A. (2014). The No-U-Turn sampler: Adaptively setting path lengths in Hamiltonian Monte Carlo. *Journal of Machine Learning Research*, 15:1593–1623.

Jara, A., Hanson, T., Quintana, F., Müller, P., and Rosner, G. (2011). DP-package: Bayesian semi- and nonparametric modeling using R. *Journal of Statistical Software*, 40(5):1–30.

Kim, J. and Scialli, A. (2011). Thalidomide: The tragedy of birth defects and the effective treatment of disease. *Toxicological Sciences*, 122:1–6.

Kruschke, J. (2015). *Doing Bayesian Data Analysis. A Tutorial with R, and Stan.* London: Academic Press, 2nd edition.

Lesaffre, E. and Lawson, A. (2012). *Bayesian Biostatistics.* Statistics in Practice. John Wiley, New York, NY.

Lindley, D. (1971). The estimation of many parameters. In *V.P. Godambe and D.A. Sprott (eds): Foundations of Statistical Inference*, pages 435–455, Toronto: Holt, Rinehart and Winston.

Lindley, D. and Smith, A. (1972). Bayes estimates for the linear model (with discussion). *Journal of the Royal Statistical Society — Series B*, 34:14–46.

Lunn, D., Spiegelhalter, D., Thomas, A., and Best, N. (2009). The BUGS project: evolution, critique and future directions. *Statistics in Medicine*, 25:3049–3067.

Lunn, D., Thomas, A., Best, N., and Spiegelhalter, D. (2000). WinBUGS - a Bayesian modelling framework: Concepts, structure, and extensibility. *Statistics and Computing*, 10:325–337.

Merkle, E. C., Furr, D., and Rabe-Hesketh, S. (2018). Bayesian model assessment: Use of conditional vs. marginal likelihoods. *arXiv preprint arXiv:1802.04452.*

Metropolis, N., Rosenbluth, A., Rosenbluth, M., Teller, A., and Teller, E. (1953). Equations of state calculations by fast computing machines. *Journal of Chemical Physics*, 21:1087–1092.

Müller, P., Quintana, F., Jara, A., and Hanson, T. (2012). *Bayesian Nonparametric Data Analysis.* Springer-Verlag, New York, NY.

Neal, R. (2011). MCMC using Hamiltonian dynamics. In Brooks, S., Gelman, A., Jones, G., and Meng, X.-L., editors, *Handbook of Markov Chain Monte Carlo*, pages 113–162. Chapman & Hall/CRC Press, New York, NY.

Neyman, J. and Pearson, E. (1928a). On the use and interpretation of certain test criteria for purposes of statistical inference. Part I. *Biometrika*, 20A:175–240.

Neyman, J. and Pearson, E. (1928b). On the use and interpretation of certain test criteria for purposes of statistical inference. Part II. *Biometrika*, 20A:263–294.

Ntzoufras, I. (2009). *Bayesian Modeling using WinBUGS*. John Wiley, New York, NY.

Ogilvie, I., Newton, N., Welner, S., Cowell, W., and Lip, G. (2010). Underuse of oral anticoagulants in atrial fibrillation: A systematic review. *The American Journal of Medicine*, 123:638–645.

O'Hagan, A. and Forster, J. (2004). *Bayesian Inference. In: Kendall's Advanced Theory of Statistics. Volume 2B*. Arnold, London.

Plummer, M. (2003). JAGS: A program for analysis of Bayesian Graphical Models using Gibbs Sampling, *Proceedings of the 3rd International Workshop on Distributed Statistical Computing (DSC 2003)*, March 20–22, Vienna, Austria. ISSN 1609-395X. http://www.ci.tuwien.ac.at/Conferences/DSC-2003/Proceedings/Plummer.pdf

Quintero, A. and Lesaffre, E. (2017). Multilevel covariance regression with correlated random effects in the mean and variance structure. *Biometrical Journal*, 59 (5):1047–1066.

Raftery, A., Madigan, D., and Hoeting, J. (1997). Bayesian model averaging for linear regression models. *Journal of the American Statistical Association*, 92:179–191.

Recht, M., Nemes, L., Matysiak, M., Manco-Johnson, M., Lusher, J., Smith, M., Mannucci, P., Hay, C., Abshire, T., O'Brien, A., Hayward, B., Udata, C., Roth, D., and Arkin, S. (2009). Clinical evaluation of moroctocog alfa (AF-CC), a new generation of B-domain deleted recombinant factor VIII (BDDrFVIII) for treatment of haemophilia A: demonstration of safety, efficacy, and pharmacokinetic equivalence to full-length recombinant factor VIII. *Haemophilia*, 15:869–880.

Robert, C. and Casella, G. (2004). *Monte Carlo Statistical Methods*. Springer Texts in Statistics, New York, NY.

Roberts, G., Gelman, A., and Gilks, W. (1997). Weak convergence and optimal scaling of random walk Metropolis algorithms. *The Annals of Applied Probability*, 7:110–120.

Royall, R. (1997). *Statistical Evidence. A Likelihood Paradigm*. Chapman and Hall.

Rue, H. and Held, L. (2005). *Gaussian Markov Random Fields: Theory and Applications*. Chapman & Hall, Boca Raton, FL.

Rue, H., Martino, S., and Chopin, N. (2009). Approximate Bayesian inference for latent Gaussian models by using integrated nested Laplace approximations (with discussion). *Journal of the Royal Statistical Society — Series B*, 71:319–392.

Rue, H., Riebler, A., Sorbye, S., Illian, J., Simpson, D., and Lindgren, F. (2017). Bayesian computing with INLA: A review. *Annual Review of Statistics and Its Application*, 4:395–421.

Sethuraman, J. (1994). A constructive definition of Dirichlet priors. *Statistica Sinica*, 4:639–650.

Smith, A. (1973a). Bayes estimates in one-way and two-way models. *Biometrika*, 60:319–329.

Smith, A. (1973b). A general Bayesian linear model. *Journal of the Royal Statistical Society — Series B*, 35:67–75.

Spiegelhalter, D., Best, N., Carlin, B., and van der Linde, A. (2002). Bayesian measures of model complexity and fit (with discussion). *Journal of the Royal Statistical Society — Series B*, 64:1–34.

Sturtz, S., Ligges, U., and Gelman, A. (2005). R2WinBUGS: A package for running WinBUGS from R. *Journal of Statistical Software*, 12 (3):1–17.

Wasserstein, R. and Lazar, N. (2016). The ASA's statement on p-values: context, process, and purpose. *The American Statistician*, 70 (2):129–133.

2

FDA Regulatory Acceptance of Bayesian Statistics

Gregory Campbell
GCStat Consulting LLC, US

Regulatory acceptance of the use of Bayesian statistics in clinical studies in the United States is addressed. The U.S. Food and Drug Administration (FDA) has for the past 20 years signaled a willingness to review applications for design and analysis of pivotal clinical studies for medical devices. The state of regulatory acceptance is much less enthusiastic for confirmatory trial submissions to FDA for pharmaceutical drugs and biological products and for submissions to European and Japanese regulatory authorities. Differences between drugs and devices are highlighted in exploring this acceptance gap. There is a natural reluctance by regulators to entertain any new innovative method and Bayesian statistics can signal a major paradigm shift. Companies, especially large ones, can be particularly hesitant to try a new methodology since it may not be as predictable and there can be a fear that the regulatory review staff might be less than enthusiastic. In addition, there are several technical challenges that Bayesian methods pose. Promising opportunities for the use of Bayesian methods in pharmaceutical submissions are explored, including the use of data from control arms in other randomized trials and the planning of Bayesian adaptive trials. The future of Bayesian statistics in the regulatory environment is addressed.

2.1 Introduction

This chapter addresses the status of Bayesian statistics in terms of regulatory acceptance by the U.S. Food and Drug Administration (FDA). In the United States Bayesian statistics has been used in submissions for medical devices for a number of years, which does not seem to be the case for any confirmatory trials in Europe or Japan. The history and the accomplishments for medical devices will be reviewed. Attention is then turned to the regulation of pharmaceutical drugs and biologicals. There are harbingers of change in the wind and these will be reviewed. Finally the challenges and the future of Bayesian statistics in the regulatory environment will be tackled.

2.2 Medical devices

In 1998, FDA's Center for Devices and Radiological Health (CDRH) began an initiative to investigate the extent to which Bayesian statistics could contribute to the design and analysis of medical device clinical trials. The motivation for the initiative stemmed from several factors. There was often a great deal of available information for many medical devices because the device development tended to be iterative and incremental and the mechanism of action is usually well-understood, being physical and local. So rather than ignore all prior information and start a pivotal trial as if one knew nothing, the philosophy was to leverage the prior information and arrive at the same regulatory decision sooner. Second, there has been a revolution in both computing power and in algorithms such as MCMC that facilitated the calculation of a posterior distribution for virtually any set of modeling assumption. In that same year CDRH co-sponsored a meeting in which FDA signaled to industry that Bayesian submissions would be entertained. With the full support to the senior leadership of CDRH, FDA produced a guidance document in draft form in 2005, finalized in 2010 (U.S. Food and Drug Administration, 2010). It laid out a pathway for industry for the use of Bayesian statistics in medical device clinical trials.

The guidance advocated two basic approaches. One used prior quantitative information in the form of previous study or studies; the approach advocated was a Bayesian hierarchical model that used previous studies, evaluated to be exchangeable with each other, and updated with the current study of the investigational device to produce a posterior distribution for the new device. The second was a Bayesian adaptive approach, usually with a non-informative prior, that allowed for the preplanned modifications to the trial based on accumulating data in the trial. The advantage of a Bayesian as opposed to a frequentist adaptive approach is that intermediate endpoints can be used to model the ultimate efficacy endpoint using accumulated data to allow for early stopping and, more importantly, early recruitment curtailment. The guidance noted in both cases that it was important to understand the operating characteristics of the design and to calculate the probability of the Type I error as well as the power for all realistic alternatives. The decision criterion was based on the posterior distribution and not on hypothesis testing significance levels and P-values.

Many *PreMarket Approval* (PMA) applications and a large number of *Investigational Device Exemptions* (IDEs) have been approved by FDA for trials designed and analyzed as Bayesian. Campbell (2010, 2013) provide a list of the publicly available Bayesian designed and analyzed clinical trials submissions that had been submitted to FDA.

Almost all the Bayesian trials were adaptive for the study size. In the case of prior information, the size of the current study could depend on the amount of borrowing that the Bayesian hierarchical model allowed. And in the Bayesian adaptive model the study size would depend on the outcomes observed in the current trial. Computer simulations under various scenarios were essential to understanding the operating characteristics of the trial, as emphasized in Berry et al. (2010). The similarities of Bayesian and adaptive designs was highlighted by Campbell (2013). The Bayesian thinking and experience was instrumental in forming the basis of a guidance document on adaptive designs for a medical device that was finalized in 2016 (U.S. Food and Drug Administration, 2016a). Review experiences for Bayesian submission are discussed by Pennello and Thompson (2008). Yang et al. (2016) reported 250 adaptive submissions to CDRH for the period from 2007 to 2013, of which about 30% were Bayesian.

Another outgrowth of the Bayesian effort was its contribution to the thinking about extrapolating (adult) data for pediatric medical devices, see Chapter 6. This is reflected in the final guidance released in 2016, in which an appendix lays out a Bayesian hierarchical model for the possible borrowing of adult data for pediatric populations in some circumstances (U.S. Food and Drug Administration, 2016d).

2.3 Pharmaceutical products

The question of whether a Bayesian approach could be of use in the regulatory submissions of pharmaceutical drugs and biologics was broached fairly early. The International Conference on Harmonisation (ICH) guideline "Statistical Principles for Clinical Trials" (E9) released by the U.S., Europe and Japan in 1998, allows for Bayesian approaches: ". . .because the predominant approaches to the design and analysis of clinical trials have been based on frequentist statistical methods, the guidance largely refers to the use of frequentist methods when discussing hypothesis testing and/or confidence intervals. This should not be taken to imply that other approaches are not appropriate: the use of Bayesian and other approaches may be considered when the reasons for their use are clear and when the resulting conclusions are sufficiently robust" (U.S. Food and Drug Administration, 1998).

In 2004, FDA and the Department of Biostatistics at Johns Hopkins University co-sponsored a workshop at the National Institutes of Health entitled "Can Bayesian Approaches to Studying New Treatments Improve Regulatory Decision-Making?" It featured presentations by Steve Goodman, Tom Louis, Don Berry, FDA officials from CDRH, Center for Drug Evaluation and Research (CDER) and the Center for Biologics Evaluation and Research (CBER), three case studies and panel discussions. The August, 2005 issue of the journal Clinical Trials was devoted to this workshop. At that time the effort in medical devices was quite well known and deemed successful and the focus was on pharmaceutical drugs and biologics. It is not clear that the workshop accomplished much to change the view of Bayesian statistics in the pharmaceutical world at that time.

The Center for Drug Evaluation and Research has been a leader in the use of Bayesian statistics in the regulation of pharmaceutical drugs in the post-market. CDER led an effort to use Bayesian data mining of safety signals in its post-market data bases and used this information to take action for various concerning safety signals that are detected. The machinery to accomplish this was a Gamma-Poisson model to borrow strength from similar drugs (DuMouchel, 1999). A major application of Bayesian methods in recent years has been the dose-finding effort for modeling a drug's dose response curve. An early Bayesian effort was the report of the ASTIN trial (Grieve and Krams, 2005). There are now a number of examples of Bayesian adaptive designs used in dose-finding for dose establishment for Phase III studies. These studies do not use prior information but rely on accumulating information in the Phase II trial in a treatment response adaptive randomization scheme to well-characterize the dose response curve; this approach illustrates the Bayesian adaptive power of learning and confirming within the trial.

There has been even more evidence of Bayesian movement for premarket Phase III trials. A recent example is the AWARD-5, a successful Bayesian adaptive seamless Phase 2-3 trial for the drug dulaglutide, which was later approved by FDA (Skrivanek et al., 2012). CDER has been researching the use of Bayesian methods for non-inferiority trials for anti-infective drugs (Gamalo et al., 2014) and the extrapolation of adult data in pediatric drug applications (Gamalo-Siebers et al., 2017). A Drug Information Association (DIA) Scientific Working Group consisting of industry and regulatory members has been meeting over the past several years to explore the various uses of Bayesian statistics in the U.S. regulatory environment. A January-February 2014 issue in the journal Pharmaceutical Statistics, edited by Karen Price and CDER Office of Biostatistics Director Lisa LaVange, is devoted to Bayesian methods in drug development and regulatory review by this group. A draft ICH addendum for the clinical study of pediatric populations mentions Bayesian methods as one possible approach (see U.S. Food and Drug Administration, 2016c). In April, 2016, a special workshop "Substantial Evidence on 21st Century Regulatory Science: Borrowing Strength from Accumulating Data" sponsored by American Course on Drug Development and Regulatory Science (ACDRS), was convened in Washington, DC. It featured industry leaders and FDA officials from CDER and CBER, including CDER Director Janet Woodcock and Bob Temple. The U.S. evidentiary standard for pharmaceutical products was reviewed and it was noted that there is a lack of specificity concerning statistical analysis in the regulations and that neither frequentist methods nor Bayesian methods are referenced in U.S. Food Drug & Cosmetic Act or federal regulations.

More recently, the 21st Century Cures Act was passed by the U.S Congress and signed into law on December 13, 2016. While an earlier draft of the bill had mentioned Bayesian statistics explicitly, the final version in Section 3021 mentions "use of novel clinical trial designs for drugs and biological products" and in particular addresses "the use of complex adaptive and other novel trial designs" and "how sponsors may obtain feedback from the Secretary on technical issues related to modeling and simulations" (U.S. Congress, 2016). It also specified a public meeting and a draft guidance document on this topic. Regarding pharmaceutical drug user fees, in a commitment for the Pharmaceutical Drug Users Fee Act (PDUFA) VI "FDA agrees to develop staff capacity to facilitate appropriate use of complex adaptive, Bayesian and other novel clinical trial designs". FDA also agreed to conduct a pilot program for "highly adaptive trial designs for which analytically derived properties (e.g. Type 1 error rate) may not be feasible, and simulations are necessary to determine trial operating characteristics", to convene a public workshop to discuss complex adaptive trial designs and publish draft guidance on complex adaptive trial designs (Federation of American Scientists, 2017).

2.4 Differences between devices and drugs

For a pharmaceutical product, there is often little prior information derived from similar products since a similar pharmaceutical product often may have very different safety and efficacy profiles. The drug action is pharmacological and systemic and in contrast the device mechanism of action is usually physical, well-understood and local.

To some extent it is not surprising that there has been some regulatory hesitation by pharmaceutical firms when it comes to the use of Bayesian methods. The drug industry is relatively risk averse and this is in stark contrast to a more innovative and risk-taking medical device industry. The current drug regulatory system has been highly predictable as the rules of the games, as it were, are well understood; historically, if the primary efficacy analysis results in a statistically significant P-value in a frequentist paradigm, then the trial is termed a success for the drug's efficacy. This frequentist paradigm has been strongly embraced by the entire statistical and medical establishment, even by persons who are unable to explain exactly what a frequentist confidence interval means. When there is little or no apparent perceived advantage and no encouragement from the regulatory authorities, drug companies are reluctant to embrace a new statistical approach.

2.4.1 The challenge of introducing any different paradigm

A challenge for the use of Bayesian methods is that they have not been used extensively and there are those who are unfamiliar with them and perhaps distrustful. The impression is that Bayesian methods can rely upon unrealistic subjective prior information and the view that is that these methods are perceived as inherently unscientific. The scientific and medical communities and their journals pose a hurdle. This is ironic since Bayesian methodological and theoretical articles are not at all controversial and are well-accepted in statistical journals. Many scientists resist the use of Bayesian methods and there are examples of Bayesian trials that are reported in the literature using only frequentist methods. There are examples in `www.clinicaltrials.gov` where trials known to be Bayesian (or adaptive) are not reported as such. (This is also true in some instances in the Summary of Safety and Effectiveness Data (SSED) issued upon FDA's PMA approval, which does not always adequately reflect the Bayesian or adaptive nature of the study.) Some journals have insisted incorrectly on inappropriate frequentist analyses for Bayesian studies; such failure to report accurately the important details of an experiment, in this case a clinical trial, is extremely poor scientific practice. A Bayesian clinical trial report does need to rely on the authors to accurately convey the ideas and a readership that can understand what is written.

2.4.2 The challenge of perceived FDA reviewer resistance

There may be some reluctance in the pharmaceutical industry to approach CDER with a Bayesian proposal because there is a perception that the FDA reviewers would be antagonistic to it. While that may have been true historically, there is evidence that this may be changing.

This same reluctance plays out in the medical and statistical review divisions of CDER and CBER. Several keys to the success that was achieved by CDRH were due to the strong support by the center leadership and the concerted effort to educate the statistical, medical and engineering review staffs of CDRH. Without strong leadership at every level of CDER and a strong educational outreach program, any change will be slow at best.

One educational idea that could help to familiarize reviewers and scientists and statisticians is to take some old clinical trials and apply both a Bayesian and a frequentist approach and see how they agree and how they differ. While this might be of some use in the beginning when first getting started, it is not recommended as a routine practice since data should be analyzed according to the pre-specified statistical analysis plan.

An effort to address the lack of federally funded large confirmatory clinical trials that are adaptive was an NIH-FDA funded project called Adaptive Designs Accelerating Promising Trials into Treatments (ADAPT-IT). One target of ADAPT-IT has been the study sections that evaluate NIH proposals since adaptive proposals have rarely been successful in the NIH evaluation process. The overarching objectives of ADAPT-IT were to identify and quantitatively characterize the adaptive clinical trial methods of greatest potential value in confirmatory clinical trials, and to elicit and understand the enthusiasms and concerns of key stakeholders that influence their willingness to try these innovative strategies. The five pilot projects were all Bayesian adaptive (Meurer et al., 2012).

A practical regulatory consideration is that the statistical review for a Bayesian submission generally tends to be more complicated at both the design as well as the analysis stage. This translates into more review time and the need for additional review resources. An associated concern is that there may not be enough reviewers with the necessary Bayesian experience. Both statistical and medical reviewers may be unfamiliar and uncomfortable with the Bayesian approach. Additionally there appears to be reluctance within some of the statisticians in CDER to rely on simulations to provide information about the operating characteristics of the design. This then becomes a problem for almost all complicated adaptive designs including Bayesian ones. Ironically, the reliance on large-sample asymptotic theory for the operating characteristics of a design may be more unreliable than the simulated results. A valid concern for simulations is the additional review burden they pose. Rather than rely on well-known statistical theory, one must rely on programming skills by the company and its assessment by the FDA reviewer to assure that no programming mistake has jeopardized the calculations. However computer simulations of the operating characteristics of the design can provide accurate estimates of Type I error probabilities and power for both relatively straightforward and very complicated designs. An additional concern for the Type I error probability simulation is that the null space may be very complicated and multiple simulations may be needed to fully characterize the maximum Type I error probability.

2.4.3 Several technical challenges

There are several technical challenges for the use of Bayesian statistics in a regulatory environment. The first has to do with the Bayesian hierarchical modeling. It tends to work well when there are a fair number of previous studies and they are all exchangeable with each other and the new investigational study. It is well recognized that if there is a single prior study, then the study variance is being estimated with only two observations and consequently is very unstable; this is reflected in the sensitivity of the result to the selection of the particular non-informative prior. The power prior allows for the discounting of the prior distribution (Ibrahim and Chen, 2000) but the results can still be sensitive to the particular non-informative prior on the discount exponent. More recent efforts by Hobbs and his colleagues using commensurate priors have shown some promise (Hobbs et al., 2011, 2012; Murray et al., 2014).

It is sometimes the case that exchangeability is not a reasonable assumption. The evaluation of the reasonableness of this assumption is not merely a statistical exercise but can depend appropriately on clinical and for some devices engineering expertise. If, for example, the new investigational product is thought to perform better than the prior studies or the prior studies represent an improving trend over time, then exchangeability is problematic. This can occur in the medical device world where a newer model of a device is thought to have improved and consequently may no longer satisfy study exchangeability with its previous models.

One challenge that requires some further research concerns how to think about the Type I error probability when there is prior information. If one simulates under the null hypothesis of no treatment effect, however unrealistic it is, then the stringent control of the Type I error probability means that the prior information is effectively ignored in its entirety and consequently the Bayesian approach's advantage is nullified. One view is to presuppose that the Type I error probability is stringently controlled before any data have been collected and then to introduce the prior studies and then the current study. In my opinion, more theoretical work needs to be done in this area to clarify that the stringent control of the Type I error probability when there is prior information is not an appropriate way to think about this problem.

2.5 Some promising opportunities in pharmaceutical drugs

One use of Bayesian hierarchical modeling that has been underutilized and would be low-hanging fruit is the use of control data from previous studies. In many drug studies for the same studied populations for the same indication, the control groups from these previous studies could provide valuable prior information for use in a hierarchical manner for the control data in the current drug trial. The data from these controls could be "borrowed" for a new clinical trial so that many fewer control patients would be needed in the current drug study, saving both time and effort (Viele et al., 2014). Some caution needs to be exerted to make sure that a bias is not introduced, either intentionally or unintentionally, by using control data that is extremely non-representative of what might be expected. One area that has been largely ignored in practical situations has been the use of Bayesian methods in non-inferiority studies. If relevant data exist for the comparison of the active control to the placebo, then that data can be directly leveraged in a Bayesian model that would provide assurance of assay sensitivity of the current study of the investigational new drug to the active control.

There are several clinical areas where it appears that the frequentist statistical approaches are inadequate. This could afford a unique opportunity for the use of Bayesian thinking. The outbreak of the Ebola virus in Africa posed one such challenge where a possible vaccine could be studied in a flexible way that uses prior information which may be more realistic and superior to any frequentist alternative. Oncology trials provide another area where the need is great and the stakes are high (life or death) and there is a willingness to innovate. Patients with rare diseases pose a challenge since there may not be enough patients for a large confirmatory frequentist trial and that a smaller, more efficient trial that uses prior information and possibly accumulating information in the study may be the only alternatives. Pediatric patients also pose a challenge as well since there may not be a willingness to randomize children in a trial but use of prior information from adult studies or other children studies may be brought to bear in some clinically appropriate cases. Another opportunity is in the regulation of anti-infective drugs where a real concern is the degradation of antibiotic resistance as well as evidence from the laboratory of the clinical effectiveness of some drugs in eradicating infectious agents.

A promising development has been the accelerated approval program in CDER and the expedited access program in CDRH. Both programs can lend themselves very nicely to a Bayesian adaptive approach, in which a successful intermediate endpoint or posterior predictive probability is the basis for a conditional approval and the final approval is highly confident since the posterior predictive probability is so high that it is simply a matter of time and leaves very little to chance.

2.6 The future

One perceptible trend in the device world has been an increase in the use of Bayesian adaptive trials in the pivotal (confirmatory) setting. At the same time there seems to have been somewhat less activity in leveraging prior information, a trend that may be due to the lack of good prior studies that are exchangeable. In the drug world, there is a definite trend toward more seamless Phase II-III trials that require extensive planning at the outset. There should be more reliance on control data from previous trials of the same agent for the identical population.

One interesting pharmaceutical development has been the use of Bayesian platform trials, including I-SPY-2, BATTLE project and more recently GBM AGILE. All are Bayesian adaptive umbrella trials, each using a master protocol that studies one disease and many pharmaceutical agents in Phase 2. I-SPY-2 is a collaborative effort among academic investigators, the National Cancer Institute, FDA, and the pharmaceutical and biotechnology industries to study oncologic therapies and biomarkers using a Bayesian adaptive Phase 2 clinical trial design in the neoadjuvant setting for women with locally advanced breast cancer (Barker et al., 2009). Biomarker Based Approach for Lung cancer Eradication (BATTLE) studies four treatments with 11 biomarkers in non-small cell lung cancer (Zhou et al., 2008). GBM AGILE is a global platform trial, driven by Bayesian statistics, where agents to treat glioblastoma (GBM) if successful will proceed via an algorithm through two seamless stages that combine Phase II screening and registration trials (Alexander et al., 2018).

An interesting development has been the effort to incorporate a stochastic engineering model using simulated virtual patients as prior information in Bayesian medical device trials. A power prior approach together with a discount function that takes into account the similarity between the modeled and observed data is illustrated in a case study of cardiac lead fracture. Simulated "virtual patients" are generated according to the stochastic engineering model and used to model clinical outcomes, see Haddad et al. (2017) and Chapter 25.

Yet another topic that could well call upon Bayesian methods is the clear effort by FDA to consider the use of real world evidence in regulatory decision making. There is a guidance document for medical devices (U.S. Food and Drug Administration, 2017b). The Bayesian approach could be utilized to combine data across different sources using Bayesian machinery.

A recent initiative is the use of formal decision analysis in a quantitative manner in order to make regulatory benefit-risk decisions. Here risk is couched in terms of public health implications and not monetary ones. FDA has released several guidance documents in regulating medical devices on this topic, one for PMAs (U.S. Food and Drug Administration, 2016b) and one for IDEs (U.S. Food and Drug Administration, 2017a). A Bayesian approach to benefit-risk could result in the future in decision-theoretic clinical trials. A noteworthy historic decision-theoretic trial in emergency medicine trial is reported by Lewis and Berry (1994).

The future is enormous for Bayesian adaptive designs. When no prior information is being used, one obvious advantage is being able to seamlessly model the predictive capability of intermediate endpoints in predicting the primary effectiveness endpoint. This could enable the cessation of recruitment at an earlier stage than without it. A second advantage is that a Bayesian approach allows for the calculation at different stages of the probability of trial success and futility. This can be extremely helpful in trial planning under various scenarios and also in its use by Data Monitoring Committees (DMCs) during the trial. A third advantage is in the analysis of adaptive trials. A frequentist analysis is very challenging since the probability modeling depends on the sample space. However for an adaptive (and/or Bayesian) trial, this is quite difficult to write down since the number of patients is not fixed. This was readily apparent in the famous device trial for extracorporeal membrane oxygenation (ECMO), an adaptive play-the-winner trial which generated substantial statistical controversy (Ware, 1989). The future may lie in Bayesian treatment adaptive response trials not just for dose-finding but for pivotal/confirmatory clinical trials. Such trials may be more ethical and easier to recruit investigators and patients for since the probabilities can be updated in real time to make sure that a person gets the treatment most likely at the time to be optimal, see also Chapter 8.

2.7 Conclusion

It is an exciting time for Bayesian statistics in clinical trials and the future is brighter than ever. In my opinion we are at or nearing a tipping point for the use of Bayesian methods for pharmaceutical drugs and biologics in a regulatory environment. What is needed is to buy-in at all levels of the regulatory agencies, from the top to the bottom, and an educational effort for statisticians and clinicians within the pharmaceutical industry and the regulatory authorities.

Bibliography

Alexander, B., Ba, S., Berger, M., Cavenee, W., Chang, S., Cloughesy, T., T., J., Khasraw, M., Li, W., Mittman, R., Poste, G., Wen, P., W.K.A., Y., Barker, A., and Network, G. A. (2018). Adaptive Global Innovative Learning Environment for Glioblastoma: GBM AGILE. *Clinical Cancer Research*, 24(4):737–743.

Barker, A., Sigman, C., Kelloff, G., Hylton, N., Berry, D., and Esserman, L. (2009). I-SPY2: an adaptive breast cancer trial design in the setting of neoadjuvant chemotherapy. *Clinical Pharmacology and Therapeutics*, 86 (1):97–100.

Berry, S., Carlin, B., Lee, J., and Müller, P. (2010). *Bayesian Adaptive Methods for Clinical Trials*. CRC Press, Boca Raton, FL.

Campbell, G. (2010). Bayesian statistics in medical devices: Innovation sparked by the FDA. *Journal of Biopharmaceutical Statistics*, 21(5):871–887.

Campbell, G. (2013). Similarities and differences of Bayesian designs and adaptive designs for medical devices: A regulatory view. *Statistics in Biopharmaceutical Research*, 5:356–368.

DuMouchel, W. (1999). Bayesian data mining in large frequency tables, with an application to the FDA spontaneous reporting system (with discussion). *The American Statistician*, 53:177–202.

Federation of American Scientists (2017). Prescription Drug User Fee Act (PDUFA): 2017 Reauthorization as PDUFA VI. `"https://fas.org/sgp/crs/misc/R44864.pdf (accessed August 2017)"`.

Gamalo, M., Tiwari, R., and LaVange, L. (2014). Bayesian approach to the design and analysis of non-inferiority trials for anti-infective products. *Pharmaceutical Statistics*, 13(1):25–40.

Gamalo-Siebers, M., Savic, J., Basu, C., Zhao, X., Gopalakrishnan, M., Gao, A., Song, G., Baygani, S., Thompson, L., Xia, H., Price, K., Tiwari, R., and Carlin, B. (2017). Statistical modeling for Bayesian extrapolation of adult clinical trial information in pediatric drug evaluation. *Pharmaceutical Statistics*, 16:232–249.

Grieve, A. and Krams, M. (2005). ASTIN: A Bayesian adaptive dose response trial in acute stroke. *Clinical Trials*, 2(4):340–351.

Haddad, T., Himes, A., Thompson, L., Irony, T., Nair, R., and MDIC Computer Modeling and Simulation Working Group Participants (2017). Incorporation of stochastic engineering models as prior information in Bayesian medical device trials. *Journal of Biopharmaceutical Statistics*, 10:1–15.

Hobbs, B., Carlin, B., Mandrekar, S., and Sargent, D. (2011). Hierarchical commensurate and power prior models for adaptive incorporation of historical information in clinical trials. *Biometrics*, 67(3):1047–1056.

Hobbs, B., Sargent, D., and Carlin, B. (2012). Commensurate priors for incorporating historical information in clinical trials using general and generalized linear model. *Bayesian Analysis*, 7(3):639–674.

Ibrahim, J. and Chen, M. (2000). Power prior distributions for regression models. *Statistical Science*, 15(1):46–60.

Lewis, R. and Berry, D. (1994). Group-sequential clinical trials: A classical evaluation of Bayesian decision-theoretic designs. *Journal of the American Statistical Association*, 89:1528–1534.

Meurer, W., Lewis, R., Tagle, D., Fetters, M., Legocki, L., Berry, S., Connor, J., Durkalski, V., Elm, J., Zhao, W., Frederiksen, S., Silbergleit, R., Palesch, Y., Berry, D., and Barsan, W. (2012). An overview of the adaptive designs accelerating promising trials into treatments (ADAPT-IT) project. *Annals Emergency Medicine*, 60(4):451–457.

Murray, T., Hobbs, B., Lystig, T., and Carlin, B. (2014). Semiparametric commensurate survival model for post-market medical device surveillance with non-exchangeable historical data. *Biometrics*, 70(1):185–191.

Pennello, G. and Thompson, L. (2008). Experience with reviewing Bayesian medical device trials. *Journal of Biopharmaceutical Statistics*, 18(1):81–115.

Skrivanek, Z., Berry, S., Berry, D., Chien, J., Geiger, M., Anderson, J., and Gaydos, B. (2012). Application of adaptive design methodology in development of a long-acting glucagon-like peptide-1 analog (dulaglutide): Statistical design and simulations. *Journal of Diabetes Science and Technology*, 6(6):1305–1318.

U.S. Congress (2016). 21st Century Cures Act. "https://www.govtrack.us/congress/bills/114/hr34/text".

U.S. Food and Drug Administration (1998). Guidance for Industry: E9 Statistical Principles for Clinical Trials. "https://www.fda.gov/downloads/drugs/guidancecomplianceregulatoryinformation/guidances/ucm073137.pdf".

U.S. Food and Drug Administration (2010). The Use of Bayesian Statistics in Medical Device Clinical Trials: Guidance for Industry and Food and Drug Administration Staff. "http://www.fda.gov/MedicalDevices/DeviceRegulationandGuidance/GuidanceDocuments/ucm071072.htm".

U.S. Food and Drug Administration (2016a). Adaptive Designs for Medical Device Clinical Studies: Guidance for Industry and Food and Drug Administration Staff. "https://www.fda.gov/downloads/medicaldevices/deviceregulationandguidance/guidancedocuments/ucm446729.pdf (accessed August, 2017)".

U.S. Food and Drug Administration (2016b). Factors to Consider When Making Benefit-Risk Determinations in Medical Device Premarket Approval and De Novo Classifications. Guidance for Industry and Food and Drug Administration Staff. "https://www.fda.gov/downloads/medicaldevices/deviceregulationandguidance/guidancedocuments/ucm517504.pdf".

U.S. Food and Drug Administration (2016c). ICH Harmonised Draft Guideline Addendum to ICH E11: Clinical Investigation of Medicinal Products in the Pediatric Population. "https://www.fda.gov/downloads/Drugs/GuidanceComplianceRegulatoryInformation/Guidances/UCM530012.pdf".

U.S. Food and Drug Administration (2016d). Leveraging Existing Clinical Data for Extrapolation to Pediatric Uses of Medical Devices: Guidance for Industry and Food and Drug Administration Staff. "http://www.fda.gov/downloads/MedicalDevices/DeviceRegulationandGuidance/GuidanceDocuments/UCM444591.pdf".

U.S. Food and Drug Administration (2017a). Factors to Consider When Making Benefit-Risk Determinations for Medical Device Investigational Device Exemptions. Guidance for Investigational Device Exemption Sponsors, Sponsor Investigators and Food and Drug Administration Staff. "https://www.fda.gov/downloads/MedicalDevices/DeviceRegulationandGuidance/GuidanceDocuments/UCM451440.pdf (accessed August, 2017)".

U.S. Food and Drug Administration (2017b). Use of Real-World Evidence to Support Regulatory Decision-Making for Medical Devices. "https://www.fda.gov/downloads/medicaldevices/deviceregulationandguidance/guidancedocuments/ucm513027.pdf (accessed August, 2017)".

Viele, K., Berry, S., Neuenschwander, B., Amzal, B., Chen, F., Enas, N., Hobbs, B., Ibrahim, J., Kinnersley, N., Lindborg, S. Micallef, S., Roychoudhur, S., and Thompson, L. (2014). Use of historical control data for assessing treatment effects in clinical trials. *Pharmaceutical Statistics*, 13:41–54.

Ware, J. (1989). Investigating therapies of potentially great benefit: ECMO. *Statistical Science*, 4:298–306.

Yang, X., Thompson, L., Chu, J., Liu, S., Lu, H., Zhou, J., Gomatan, S., Tang, R., Zhao, Y., Ge, Y., and Gray, G. (2016). Adaptive design practice at the Center for Devices and Radiological Health (CDRH), January 2007 to May 2013. *Therapeutic Innovation & Regulatory Science*, 50(6):710–717.

Zhou, X., Liu, S., Kim, E., Herbst, R., and Lee, J. (2008). Bayesian adaptive design for targeted therapy development in lung cancer – a step toward personalized medicine. *Clinical Trials*, 5(3):463–467.

3

Bayesian Tail Probabilities for Decision Making

Leonhard Held

University of Zurich, Switzerland

Bayesian tail probabilities are commonly used for decision making in medical and pharmaceutical research. The close correspondence between posterior tail probabilities and one-sided P-values is reviewed with the analysis of 2×2 tables as a prominent example. Application of the methodology is illustrated both for superiority and equivalence trials and allows for the integration of prior knowledge in decision making. I then move on to predictive tail probabilities and their usage in clinical trials. Specifically I discuss the concept of assurance and describe computation of the posterior predictive probability of trial success in sequential and group-sequential trials. Box's P-value is described as a method to assess potential prior-data conflict based on a prior predictive tail probability. I conclude the chapter with a discussion of predictive evidence threshold scaling, an application of predictive tail probabilities to assess the evidential strength of non-confirmatory studies. The computation of posterior or predictive tail probabilities can be done analytically or with Monte Carlo methods and this is illustrated with `R` code.

3.1 Introduction

This chapter gives an introduction to the use of Bayesian tail probabilities in medical and pharmaceutical research. I start in Section 3.2 with the close correspondence of one-sided P-values and *posterior tail probabilities* under non-informative priors, to emphasize important links between frequentist and Bayesian inference for *tests for direction*. This link is investigated further in Section 3.2.1 for 2×2 tables. Monte Carlo computation of posterior tail probabilities is described in Section 3.2.2 and its use in a Bayesian analysis of a clinical trial is outlined in Section 3.2.3. The applicability of Bayesian tail probabilities for decision making is described in greater generality in Section 3.2.4, before I move to *predictive tail probabilities* in Section 3.3. This section revisits the application from Section 3.2.3 from a predictive perspective and outlines the Box (1980) method for the assessment of prior-data conflict based on a Bayesian predictive tail probability in Section 3.3.1. I continue with two more advanced Bayesian predictive methods used in pharmaceutical research, predictive probability of success (Section 3.3.2) and predictive evidence threshold scaling (Section 3.3.3), before I close with some discussion in Section 3.4. In particular, I emphasize that the close correspondence between frequentist and Bayesian methods is lost for significance tests of point null hypothesis, so-called *tests for existence*.

Throughout I try to follow the notation from Held and Sabanés Bové (2020), which is also recommended for a more detailed exposition of the frequentist and Bayesian approach to statistical inference. Similar to Kruschke (2014) I provide R code which I hope will make it easy to understand the material and to apply the methods discussed to other statistical problems. I am using a few functions that I have written myself where the code is given in the Appendix.

```
## source functions detailed in Appendix
source("appendix.R")
```

3.2 Posterior tail probabilities

In classical hypothesis testing, a commonly encountered procedure is the *one-sided hypothesis test* (see for example Cox, 2005) where the evidence against a point null hypothesis $\dot{H}_0$: $\theta = \theta_0$ is quantified using a P-value:

$$P\text{-value } = \Pr(T(X) \geq T(x) \mid \theta = \theta_0), \tag{3.1}$$

where $T(X)$ is a suitable summary of the data $X = x$, for example the mean. For a one-sided test the interest is in departures in a pre-specified direction towards the alternative H_1: $\theta > \theta_0$, say.

The P-value obtained from a one-sided hypothesis test has sometimes a Bayesian interpretation as the posterior probability of the composite null hypothesis H_0: $\theta \leq \theta_0$:

$$\Pr(H_0 \mid x) = \Pr(\theta \leq \theta_0 \mid x). \tag{3.2}$$

The switch from $\dot{H}_0$ to H_0 is important, since both $\Pr(\dot{H}_0)$ and $\Pr(\dot{H}_0 \mid x)$ will be zero if θ is a continuous parameter with absolutely continuous prior distribution. It also constitutes an important shift in interpretation: If θ_0 represents the case of no effect, then the test of $\dot{H}_0$ versus H_1 is a *test for existence* of an effect, whereas the test of H_0 versus H_1 is a *test for direction* of an effect, assuming its existence.

For illustration, consider a random sample $X_{1:n} = (X_1, \ldots, X_n)$ of size n from a Normal sampling distribution $\mathrm{N}(\theta, \sigma^2)$ with unknown mean θ and known variance σ^2. Having observed the data $X_{1:n} = x_{1:n}$ and under the assumption of a flat reference prior $p(\theta) \propto 1$, the posterior distribution is $\theta \mid x_{1:n} \sim \mathrm{N}(\overline{x}, \sigma^2/n)$, here $\overline{x}$ denotes the sample mean. Therefore

$$\Pr(H_0 \mid x_{1:n}) = \Pr(\theta \leq \theta_0 \mid x_{1:n}) = \Phi(\sqrt{n}(\theta_0 - \overline{x})/\sigma), \tag{3.3}$$

where Φ denotes the cumulative distribution function of the standard Normal distribution. The posterior probability (3.3) is the lower tail of the posterior distribution $p(\theta \mid x_{1:n})$ below the threshold θ_0, an example of a posterior tail probability. The P-value (3.1), based on the sample mean $T(X_{1:n}) = \overline{X} \sim \mathrm{N}(\theta, \sigma^2/n)$ as summary statistic, is

$$P\text{-value } = \Pr(\overline{X} \geq \overline{x} \mid \theta = \theta_0) = 1 - \Phi(\sqrt{n}(\overline{x} - \theta_0)/\sigma) = \Phi(\sqrt{n}(\theta_0 - \overline{x})/\sigma). \tag{3.4}$$

Comparison of (3.3) with (3.4) reveals that the one-sided P-value is equal to the posterior probability $\Pr(H_0 \mid x)$.

Use of the improper reference prior $p(\theta) \propto 1$ in the computation of (3.3) gives rise to a so-called objective Bayesian method (Bayarri and Berger, 2004; Berger, 2006). Objective Bayesian methods often give similar results to the corresponding frequentist methods. The posterior probability (3.2) can also be calculated for other (more informative) prior distributions on θ, in which case (3.2) will in general change and the analogy between posterior probabilities and P-values will be lost.

It may also be of interest to relate the posterior probability (3.2) to the corresponding prior probability $\Pr(H_0)$. The reference prior $p(\theta) \propto 1$ could perhaps be said to imply $\Pr(H_0) = 1/2$ for any θ_0, but this argument comes from taking $\infty/(2\infty) = 1/2$, so is not mathematically rigorous (Lee, 2004, Section 4.2). However, a proper prior $p(\theta)$ makes $\Pr(H_0)$ and $\Pr(H_1) = 1 - \Pr(H_0)$ well-defined, and then Bayes theorem gives

$$\frac{\Pr(H_0 \mid x)}{\Pr(H_1 \mid x)} = \frac{p(x \mid H_0)}{p(x \mid H_1)} \times \frac{\Pr(H_0)}{\Pr(H_1)}, \tag{3.5}$$

where the Bayes factor

$$\text{BF} = \frac{p(x \mid H_0)}{p(x \mid H_1)} \tag{3.6}$$

provides a direct quantitative measure how the data x have increased or decreased the odds of H_0 (Kass and Raftery, 1995). If prior and posterior probabilities are available, the Bayes factor can thus be computed as the ratio of posterior to prior odds:

$$\text{BF} = \frac{\Pr(H_0 \mid x)/\Pr(H_1 \mid x)}{\Pr(H_0)/\Pr(H_1)}. \tag{3.7}$$

Another possibility is to specify the prior probability $\Pr(H_0)$ directly together with conditional prior distributions $p(\theta \mid H_0)$ and $p(\theta \mid H_1)$ under the two hypotheses. The latter can then be combined with the likelihood $p(x \mid \theta)$ to compute the *marginal likelihood*

$$p(x \mid H_i) = \int p(x \mid \theta) p(\theta \mid H_i) d\theta \quad i = 0, 2$$

and to obtain the Bayes factor via (3.6). Such a formulation is particularly useful for a point null hypothesis $\dot{H}_0$: $\theta = \theta_0$, where

$$\Pr(\theta \mid \dot{H}_0) = \begin{cases} 1 & \text{for } \theta = \theta_0 \\ 0 & \text{elsewhere} \end{cases}$$

and so $p(x \mid \dot{H}_0) = p(x \mid \theta_0)$. However, the correspondence between frequentist and Bayesian methods will then be lost; see Section 3.4 for more discussion and some references.

3.2.1 Bayesian analysis of 2×2 tables

Does the analogy of one-sided P-values and posterior tail probabilities (for non-informative priors) also hold for non-Normal data? In a very remarkable but largely overlooked contribution, published in 1877, the medical doctor Carl von Liebermeister (1833-1901), Professor of Internal Medicine at the University of Tübingen in southern Germany, proposed a Bayesian approach for the analysis of counts in a 2×2 table.

Liebermeister's (1877) contribution had a clinical focus, and we reproduce here one of the examples of his paper.

> *"Es seien von einer gewissen Zahl von Wechselfieberkranken ohne jede Auswahl 12 mit ausreichenden Dosen Chinin und 12 andere rein exspectativ behandelt worden. Bis zum dritten Tage der Behandlung seien von den mit Chinin behandelten 10 fieberfrei geworden; von den exspectativ behandelten sei nur bei 2 Fällen das Fieber ausgeblieben. Wie gross ist die Wahrscheinlichkeit, dass das Chinin eine das Fieber coupierende Wirkung ausübt?"*

Twelve patients with remittent fever (presumably caused by malaria infections) were treated with quinine, another 12 control patients were followed-up without treatment. After three days, 10 patients in the treatment group, but only 2 patients in the control group, had not had a fever. Liebermeister raises the question of how large the probability, that quinine has an antipyretic effect, is.

To introduce some notation, let n_1 and n_0 be the number of patients in the treatment and control group, respectively, here $n_1 = n_0 = 12$. Let $x_1 = 10$ be the number of patients with a positive clinical outcome in the treatment (quinine) group and $x_0 = 2$ the corresponding number in the control group. The corresponding 2×2 table thus has entries x_1, y_1, x_0 and y_0, where $y_i = n_i - x_i$, $i = 0, 1$, is the number of patients with a negative outcome in each group.

We thus have two independent Binomial samples, the number of positive outcomes

$$\begin{aligned} X_1 &\sim \text{Bin}(n_1, \pi_1) \text{ in the treatment group and} \\ X_0 &\sim \text{Bin}(n_0, \pi_0) \text{ in the control group,} \end{aligned}$$

and we wish to compare the success probability π_1 that a patient in the treatment group has a positive outcome with the corresponding probability π_0 in the control group. Liebermeister proposed to compute the posterior probability

$$\Pr(\pi_1 > \pi_0 \mid \text{Data}) \tag{3.8}$$

in order to quantify the evidence for superiority of the treatment under study. To do so, he followed Laplace (1814) and selected independent uniform prior distributions for the unknown probabilities π_1 and π_0, which ensures clinical equipoise *a priori*, *i. e.* $\Pr(H_1\colon \pi_1 > \pi_0) = \Pr(H_0\colon \pi_1 \leq \pi_0) = 0.5$. Note that in modern clinical trials terminology, (3.8) is the posterior probability that the ***absolute risk reduction*** ARR $= \pi_1 - \pi_0$ is positive, but it can also be interpreted as the posterior probability that the corresponding *risk ratio* or *odds ratio* is greater than one. Note also that the formulation is a test for direction, not a test for existence.

Analytic computation of (3.8) is far from trivial, and it is very remarkable that Liebermeister was able to provide a general formula (Seneta, 1994). Interestingly it turns out that the complementary probability to (3.8), $\Pr(H_0 \mid \text{Data}) = \Pr(\pi_1 \leq \pi_0 \mid \text{Data})$, is closely related to the P-value from Fisher's exact test when testing the null hypothesis $H_0\colon \pi_1 = \pi_0$ against the alternative $H_1\colon \pi_1 > \pi_0$. Specifically, $\Pr(\pi_1 \leq \pi_0 \mid \text{data})$ is exactly equal to the one-sided P-value from Fisher's test applied to the slightly modified table, where the entries x_1 and y_0 on the diagonal are both increased by one count. This result holds in general and has been rediscovered nearly a century later by Altham (1969), without knowledge of the pioneering work by Liebermeister (1877). Note that the increase by one on the diagonal increases the observed absolute risk reduction and hence decreases the P-value.

```
print(quinine.table)

        positive negative
Quinine       10        2
Control        2       10

(fisher.p <- fisher.test(quinine.table, alternative="greater")$p.value)

[1] 0.001664

(quinine.table.modified <- quinine.table + diag(2))

        positive negative
Quinine       11        2
Control        2       11
```

```
(liebermeister.p <- fisher.test(quinine.table.modified, alternative="greater")$p.value)

[1] 0.0006013
```

For Liebermeister's example, Fisher's exact test (without any additions on the diagonal) gives $P = 0.0017$, while $\Pr(\pi_1 \leq \pi_0 \mid \text{Data}) \approx 0.0006$, and Liebermeister's posterior probability (3.8) is $\Pr(\pi_1 > \pi_0 \mid \text{Data}) = 0.9993987$. It is very remarkable that Liebermeister (1877, page 950) correctly reports this probability to the same degree of accuracy, i.e. to seven decimal places.

Note that the Bayes factor (3.7) is equal to the posterior odds $\Pr(H_0 \mid x)/\Pr(H_1 \mid x) = 0.0006013/(1 - 0.0006013) = 1/1662$, since π_1 and π_0 are independent and have the same distribution *a priori*, so the prior odds $\Pr(H_0)/\Pr(H_1)$ is simply $1/1 = 1$. Adopting the categorization of Bayes factors proposed by Held and Ott (2016, Table 1), a Bayes factor of 1/1662 translates into decisive evidence against H_0 (see Kass and Raftery, 1995, Section 3.2 for a similar categorization). Again there is a need to emphasize that H_0 is *not* a point null hypothesis, so the Bayes factor against the point null hypothesis $\dot{H}_0$: $\pi_1 = \pi_0$ would be different.

The close numerical connection to Fisher's test, which was developed more than 50 years later (Fisher, 1934, Section 21.02), has led Seneta (1994) to call the Liebermeister approach a "Bayesian test procedure". Fisher was unaware of the work by Liebermeister, and it took another 25 years until Liebermeister's work was first mentioned in the English-language literature (Winsor, 1948). However, this had virtually no impact in the field of statistics so more recent work on the Bayesian analysis of the 2×2 table (Altham, 1969; Nurminen and Mutanen, 1987; Howard, 1998) all fail to acknowledge Liebermeister's pioneering contribution.

Winsor (1948) appreciates Liebermeister's "recognition of the problem" but concludes that "it is clear that few of us today would use the Liebermeister solution"; instead he favours the decision-theoretic null hypothesis significance testing framework by Neyman and Pearson. However, even if we dichotomize Liebermeister's probability into "significant" and "non-significant" based on some threshold, the frequentist performance of Liebermeister's test is remarkable, in particular less conservative than Fisher's test itself (Seneta and Phipps, 2001). This parallels the superior frequentist behaviour of another famous objective Bayes procedure, Jeffreys' equal-tailed credible interval for a proportion (Brown et al., 2001; Bayarri and Berger, 2004). Moreover, Liebermeister is clear in his paper that he prefers the exact tail probability over a dichotomized categorization into "significant" or "non-significant":

> *"In der That, wenn die Wahrscheinlichkeitsrechnung für die Beurtheilung therapeutischer Resulatate mit Nutzen und in ausgedehnter Weise angewendet werden soll so ist erforderlich: nicht, dass man mittels einer Tabelle oder Formel sich überzeugen könne, es sei für die Ausschliessung des Zufalls ein gewisser willkürlich angenommener Grad von Wahrscheinlichkeit erreicht; sondern vielmehr, dass man für jedes vorliegende Beobachtungsmaterial mit Sicherheit und Genauigkeit berechnen könne, mit w e l c h e m Grade von Wahrscheinlichkeit der Zufall ausgeschlossen ist."*

In this paragraph Liebermeister emphasizes that it is not enough to investigate whether or not the probability that the observed difference is due to chance is smaller than some arbitrary threshold; instead this probability should be calculated and reported for any data at hand. This parallels the call for a quantitative interpretation of the P-value, as originally proposed by Fisher (Goodman, 2016) and recently reiterated in the American Statistical Association Statement on P-values (Wasserstein and Lazar, 2016).

Liebermeister has used independent uniform priors for the two success probabilities π_1 and π_0. Of course, other choices can be made, for example priors from the family of Beta distributions, denoted by Beta(a, b). Informative priors can be used to represent prior knowledge, for example from expert knowledge or previous studies. Lee (2004, Appendix A.22) gives a formula for the posterior probability (3.8) under independent Beta(a, b) and Beta(c, d) priors, where a, b, c and d are integers. Howard (1998, Appendix) gives an analytic formula for the posterior probability (3.8) based on independent Beta(a, a) priors, where a can be even non-integer. However, in practice it will be more common to have prior information for comparative measures such as the risk difference, the risk ratio or the odds ratio. In Section 3.2.3 we will use an informative prior distribution for an odds ratio.

3.2.2 Monte Carlo integration

Many applied Bayesian statisticians will not bother about the exact computation of the tail probability (3.8). Instead they will employ Monte Carlo methods (Robert and Casella, 2010) to simulate from the posterior distribution of π_1 and π_0, independent Beta distributions

$$\begin{aligned} \pi_1 \mid x_1 &\sim \text{Beta}(1 + x_1, 1 + n_1 - x_1) \text{ and} \\ \pi_0 \mid x_0 &\sim \text{Beta}(1 + x_0, 1 + n_0 - x_0) \ , \end{aligned}$$

to obtain samples from the absolute risk reduction ARR as shown in the code below. The tail probability (3.8) can then be estimated directly as the proportion of samples from ARR greater than zero, as implemented in the R function `tailProbMC`; see the Appendix for the code. This estimate will be prone to Monte Carlo error, which can be quantified with the corresponding Monte Carlo standard error (Ripley, 1987).

```
set.seed(12345)
nsim <- 10000
pi1 <- rbeta(nsim, 1+quinine.table[1,1], 1+quinine.table[1,2])
pi0 <- rbeta(nsim, 1+quinine.table[2,1], 1+quinine.table[2,2])
arr <- pi1 - pi0
(pEffective <- tailProbMC(0, arr, lower.tail=FALSE))

        Tail probability Monte Carlo standard error
               0.9993000                  0.0002645
```

The output can be used to compute a 95% Monte Carlo confidence interval for the exact tail probability, using the function `confidenceInterval`:

```
confidenceInterval(mean=pEffective[1], se=pEffective[2])

Lower limit Upper limit
     0.9988      0.9998
```

This is a confidence interval in the frequentist sense that in repeated independent simulations (with identical samples size `nsim`) the interval will cover the exact tail probability about 19 out of 20 (95%) times. From Section 3.2.1 we recall that the exact tail probability is 0.9993987, so is contained in the 95% Monte Carlo confidence interval quoted above for this specific simulation. Note that the Monte Carlo sample size `nsim`=10,000 has been chosen quite large, to achieve a high level of precision with small Monte Carlo standard error.

The Monte Carlo approach gives us great flexibility to compute any tail probability of interest. In particular, it is often of interest to compute the posterior probability for a clinically relevant treatment effect. Suppose the clinically relevant difference for the current problem has been fixed at 20%; then we can also estimate the posterior probability of a clinically relevant effect using `tailProbMC`:

```
(pRelevant <- tailProbMC(0.2, arr, lower.tail=FALSE))

        Tail probability Monte Carlo standard error
                0.986700                   0.001146
```

The posterior probability of clinically relevant effect is only slightly smaller than Liebermeister's probability for any (positive) effect, but the Monte Carlo error has increased somewhat. This example illustrates how easy Monte Carlo computations are, even if analytic formulae are available for this particular problem (Nurminen and Mutanen, 1987). And of course, the whole posterior distribution of the absolute risk reduction may also be of interest and can be easily visualized with a histogram based on the posterior samples, as shown in Figure 3.1.

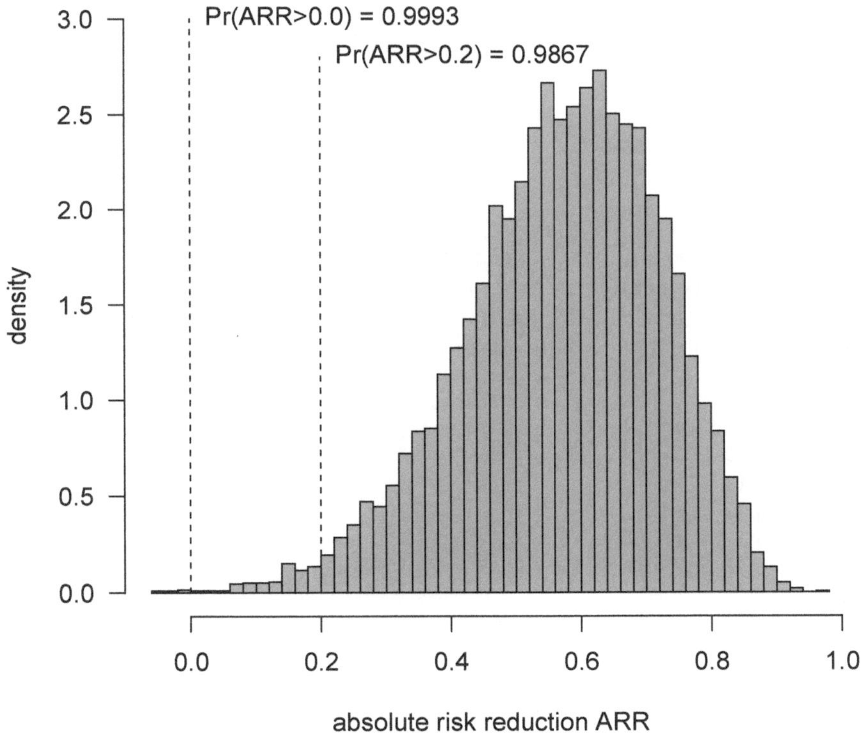

FIGURE 3.1: Histogram of 10,000 samples from the posterior distribution of the absolute risk reduction ARR in Liebermeister's Quinine example. The two thresholds shown are for a positive risk reduction (threshold 0.0) and for a clinical relevant risk reduction (threshold 0.2) with estimated tail probabilities given in the figure.

3.2.3 Posterior tail probabilities today

In their book on Bayesian approaches to clinical trials, Spiegelhalter et al. (2004, Chapter 3) make extensive use of posterior tail probabilities. To avoid Monte Carlo computations, they use the so-called Normal-Normal framework, where the data $X = x$ are represented by a sample from a Normal distribution with unknown mean θ and (usually known) variance σ^2. An informative prior for the mean is used, also assumed to be Normal.

If we model both the data and the prior using Normal distributions, say $X \mid \theta \sim \mathrm{N}(\theta, \sigma^2)$ and $\theta \sim \mathrm{N}(\nu, \tau^2)$, then the posterior is also Normal:

$$\theta \mid x \sim \mathrm{N}\left(\frac{\kappa x + \delta \nu}{\kappa + \delta}, (\kappa + \delta)^{-1}\right), \tag{3.9}$$

here $\kappa = 1/\sigma^2$ and $\delta = 1/\tau^2$ are the corresponding precisions. Tail probabilities based on this posterior distribution can then be computed based on the cumulative distribution function of the Normal distribution, as implemented in the R function `tailProb`.

To illustrate the procedure, we consider Example 3.6 from Spiegelhalter et al. (2004), who report results from the GREAT trial on early thrombolytic therapy after myocardial infarction, given at home by general practitioners. The data x now represent the observed log odds ratio and θ is the underlying true log odds ratio. The 30-day mortality rate was 13/163 in the treatment and 23/148 in the control arm. This corresponds to an observed odds ratio of 0.47 and an absolute risk reduction of 7.6% (number needed to treat: 13.2).

```
print(thrombo.table)

             deaths survivors
Thrombolytics    13       150
Control          23       125
```

Spiegelhalter et al. (2004) elicited a prior distribution for the odds ratio with the help of a senior cardiologist based on empirical evidence from previous trials. The prior is expressed as a Log-Normal distribution with prior median of 0.77 and 95% equal-tailed credible interval from around 0.60 to 1.00. This is equivalent to a $\theta \sim \mathrm{N}(-0.26, 0.13^2)$ distribution for the log odds ratio θ:

```
## prior mean and standard deviation for log odds ratio
thetaPriorMean <- -0.26
thetaPriorSD <- 0.13
## prior median odds ratio
exp(thetaPriorMean)

[1] 0.7711

## 95% prior credible interval for odds ratio
exp(thetaPriorMean + 1.96*c(-1,1)*thetaPriorSD)

[1] 0.5976 0.9948
```

The likelihood can be approximated by a Normal observation equal to the observed log odds ratio `thetaHat` with mean equal to the true log odds ratio θ and standard deviation equal to its standard error `thetaHatSE`:

```
## log odds ratio (thetaHat) and corresponding standard error
(thetaHat <- log(odds.ratio(thrombo.table)))

[1] -0.7529

(thetaHatSE <- sqrt(sum(1/thrombo.table)))

[1] 0.3675
```

Note that Spiegelhalter et al. (2004) use a slightly modified estimate of the log odds ratio and the associated standard error, where 1/2 has to be added to all entries of the 2×2-table `thrombo.table`. This modified estimate has been shown to reduce bias (Haldane, 1956) and is often used to approximate the likelihood with a Normal distribution (Lee, 2004).

Combining the above prior with the Normal likelihood for the log odds ratio thus gives the posterior distribution (3.9), as implemented in the function `posteriorNormal`.

```
(thetaHatPost <- posteriorNormal(thetaPriorMean, thetaPriorSD, thetaHat, thetaHatSE))

Posterior mean   Posterior SD
       -0.3148         0.1226

(probEffectivePost <- tailProb(0, pnorm, mean=thetaHatPost[1], sd=thetaHatPost[2]))

Tail probability
          0.9949
```

The posterior distribution of the log odds ratio is $\theta \mid \text{Data} \sim \text{N}(-0.31, 0.12)$ with posterior probability $\Pr(\theta < 0 \mid \text{data}) = 0.9949$ for a treatment effect. For comparison, Liebermeister's tail probability is slightly smaller, since it is based on a different prior distribution:

```
(thrombo.table.modified <- thrombo.table + diag(2))

              deaths survivors
Thrombolytics     14       150
Control           23       126

(liebermeister.p <- fisher.test(thrombo.table.modified, alternative="greater")$p.value)

[1] 0.9807
```

Also in this example it may be of interest to calculate the posterior probability of a clinically relevant effect (or the corresponding Bayes factor). In the present example, Spiegelhalter et al. (2004) consider odds ratios smaller than 0.5 as clinically relevant. The corresponding posterior probability can now be calculated analytically based on the cumulative probability function `pnorm` of the Normal distribution:

```
(probRelevantPost <- tailProb(log(0.5), pnorm, mean=thetaHatPost[1], sd=thetaHatPost[2]))

Tail probability
        0.001011
```

This tail probability turns out to be very small. However, the corresponding prior probability for an OR smaller than 0.5 is even smaller, so the corresponding Bayes factor (see the `R` function `bayesFactor` in the Appendix for details) is greater than one:

```
(probRelevantPrior <- tailProb(log(0.5), pnorm, mean=thetaPriorMean, sd=thetaPriorSD))

Tail probability
       0.0004313

(bayesFactorRelevant <- bayesFactor(probRelevantPrior, probRelevantPost))

Bayes factor
       2.346
```

We can also compute this posterior probability and the corresponding Bayes factor under the Liebermeister prior using Monte Carlo simulation:

```
## posterior simulation
pi1 <- rbeta(nsim, 1+thrombo.table[1,1], 1+thrombo.table[1,2])
pi0 <- rbeta(nsim, 1+thrombo.table[2,1], 1+thrombo.table[2,2])

odds1 <- odds(pi1)
odds0 <- odds(pi0)
oddsRatioPost <- odds1/odds0

(probRelevantLieberPost <- tailProbMC(0.5, oddsRatioPost))

          Tail probability Monte Carlo standard error
                  0.536700                   0.004987

## prior simulation
pi1Prior <- rbeta(nsim, 1, 1)
pi0Prior <- rbeta(nsim, 1, 1)

odds1Prior <- odds(pi1Prior)
odds0Prior <- odds(pi0Prior)
oddsRatioPrior <- odds1Prior/odds0Prior

(probRelevantLieberPrior <- tailProbMC(0.5, oddsRatioPrior))

          Tail probability Monte Carlo standard error
                  0.384600                   0.004865

(bayesFactorRelevantLieber <- bayesFactor(probRelevantLieberPrior[1],
                                          probRelevantLieberPost[1]))

Bayes factor
       1.854
```

The posterior probability for a clinically relevant effect (0.54) is much larger now, due to Liebermeister's uninformative prior distribution. However, the corresponding Bayes factor is still not much greater than one, illustrating that the data have increased the odds for a clinically relevant effect only by a factor of 1.85. This is similiar to the result reported by Spiegelhalter et al. (2004), where the corresponding Bayes factor is 2.35. Note that the two Bayes factors are not identical because the prior distributions on θ are not exactly compatible.

3.2.4 Using posterior tail probabilities for decision making

Frequentist confidence intervals are the established tool to conclude superiority of a new treatment in a clinical study. Specifically, if the lower limit of a 95% confidence interval for the treatment effect is positive, then superiority can be concluded at one-sided Type I error rate of 2.5%. Likewise, if the limits of the 95% confidence interval are within a pre-specified equivalence margin $[-\Delta, \Delta]$, say, then equivalence has been established, again controlling the Type I error rate at approximately 2.5% (Matthews, 2006).

The analogy between frequentist confidence intervals and Bayesian credible intervals under non-informative reference priors makes it natural to use (equal-tailed) Bayesian credible intervals for decision making. Specifically, this suggests to conclude superiority if the 2.5%

quantile of the posterior distribution is greater than zero or a pre-specified clinically relevant difference δ, say. If both the 2.5% and the 97.5% quantile of the posterior distribution are within the equivalence margin $[-\Delta, \Delta]$, then equivalence of the two treatments can be established. However, if the credible intervals are based on informative priors, then these decision rules may have different operating characteristics compared to their frequentist counterparts. Slightly different results are also to be expected if highest posterior density (HPD) rather than equal-tailed credible intervals are used, see Held and Sabanés Bové (2020, Section 6.2) for a general introduction to different types of credible intervals. Type I and II error rates then have to be established for the specific problems considered (Grieve, 2016).

3.3 Predictive tail probabilities

Various statistical researchers have emphasized the importance of modeling and reporting uncertainty in terms of *observables*, as opposed to inference about (unobservable) parameters. In medical research we are often interested in predictive probabilities, such as the probability of success of a future trial or the probability that a patient will respond to treatment. The more traditional approach to inference based on unobservable parameters can be seen as a limiting form of *predictive* inference about observables (Bernardo and Smith, 1994, Appendix B.4.3). Parametric inference is therefore an intermediate structural step in the predictive process.

A predictive model for observables, for example future outcomes of a clinical trial, can be constructed easily within the Bayesian framework (Held and Sabanés Bové, 2020, Chapter 9). As we will see in this section, the prior predictive distribution also plays a key role in Bayesian clinical trial methodology.

Suppose we want to predict future data x^{new}, say, which are assumed to arise from the same sampling distribution as the original data x. Bayesian prediction is based on the simple identity

$$p(x^{\text{new}} \mid x) = \int p(x^{\text{new}} \mid \theta) \times p(\theta \mid x)\, d\theta, \tag{3.10}$$

so the *predictive distribution* of x^{new} given x is the integral over the product of the sampling distribution of x^{new} and the posterior distribution $p(\theta \mid x)$ with respect to θ.

For example, consider the Normal-Normal framework with posterior distribution (3.9), abbreviated as

$$\theta \mid x \sim \mathrm{N}(\tilde{\nu}, \tilde{\tau}^2).$$

Further assume that the future observation x^{new} comes from a Normal distribution with unknown mean θ and known variance $\tilde{\sigma}^2$, say. It is then easy to show that the predictive distribution (3.10) of x^{new} takes the form

$$x^{\text{new}} \mid x \sim \mathrm{N}(\tilde{\nu}, \tilde{\tau}^2 + \tilde{\sigma}^2). \tag{3.11}$$

The assumption of a known variance $\tilde{\sigma}^2$ in (3.11) is less restrictive than it seems. For example, for rare binary outcomes where θ represents a log odds ratio, $\tilde{\sigma}^2 \approx 4/m^{\text{new}}$ where m^{new} is the number of events in the new study (Spiegelhalter et al., 2004, Section 2.4.1). A similar approximation exists for the log hazard ratio.

Spiegelhalter et al. (2004, Example 3.11) reconsider the GREAT trial where x represents the observed log odds ratio. The goal is to predict the log odds ratio x^{new} in a hypothetical new trial with 100 patients in each arm. Assuming a mortality rate of around 10%, the variance of x^{new} can thus be fixed at $\tilde{\sigma}^2 = 4/(0.1 \cdot 200) = 1/5$. Combining this with the results from Section 3.2.3 thus gives the predictive distribution (3.11), which can easily be computed with the R function `predictiveNormal`, from which we obtain the posterior tail probabilities of interest:

```
thetaHatNewSD <- 1/sqrt(5)
(thetaHatPred <- predictiveNormal(thetaHatPost[1], thetaHatPost[2], thetaHatNewSD))

Predictive mean   Predictive SD
        -0.3148          0.4637

(predProbEffective <- tailProb(0, pnorm, mean=thetaHatPred[1], sd=thetaHatPred[2]))

Tail probability
          0.7514

(predProbRelevant <- tailProb(log(0.5), pnorm, mean=thetaHatPred[1], sd=thetaHatPred[2]))

Tail probability
          0.2073
```

Assuming Normality of the log odds ratio, the posterior probability that the observed OR in the new trial is less than 1, turns out to be 0.75 while the posterior probability that the observed OR in the new trial is less than 0.5, turns out to be 0.21.

We repeat this calculation with Monte Carlo, avoiding the Normality assumption for the distribution of the log odds ratio in the new trial. Specifically, we use an initial $\text{Beta}(1+23, 1+125)$ distribution for the probability of survival in the control arm, based on an initial $\text{Beta}(1,1)$ prior and the observed mortality rate (23/148) in the GREAT control arm. Using samples from the Normal posterior distribution `thetaHatPost` for the log odds ratio, we can generate Binomial samples in both groups and finally samples from the odds ratio `oddsRatioPred` in the new study.

```
## simulate posterior distribution of pi0 and pi1
orPost <- exp(rnorm(nsim, mean=thetaHatPost[1], sd=thetaHatPost[2]))
odds1 <- orPost*odds(pi0)
pi1 <- prob(odds1)
pi0 <- rbeta(nsim, 1 + thrombo.table[2,1], 1 + thrombo.table[2,2])

## simulate new trial data
nNew <- 100
XNew1 <- rbinom(nsim, size=nNew, prob=pi1)
XNew0 <- rbinom(nsim, size=nNew, prob=pi0)

oddsRatioPred <- pValues <- numeric()
newData <- matrix(rep(NA, 4), ncol=2, nrow=2)
for(i in 1:nsim){
    ## number of successes in both groups
    newData[,1] <- c(XNew1[i], XNew0[i])
    ## number of failures
    newData[,2] <- nNew-newData[,1]
    oddsRatioPred[i] <- odds.ratio(newData)
    pValues[i] <- fisher.test(newData, alternative="less")$p.value
}

(pred2ProbEffective <- tailProbMC(1.0, oddsRatioPred))

          Tail probability Monte Carlo standard error
                  0.752300                   0.004317
```

```
(pred2ProbRelevant <- tailProbMC(0.5, oddsRatioPred))

        Tail probability Monte Carlo standard error
                0.250700                   0.004334

(prob.significant <- tailProbMC(0.025, pValues))

        Tail probability Monte Carlo standard error
                0.142700                   0.003498
```

Figure 3.2 displays a line plot of 10,000 samples from the posterior predictive distribution of the odds ratio. Note that the observed odds ratio can only take a finite number of values, so it is not unlikely that the hypothetical trial produces an odds ratio of exactly one (with probability around 5%). The histogram of the total number of events has its median at 28, more than the 20 cases that have been expected by Spiegelhalter et al. (2004, Example 3.11).

The cumulative distribution function is well approximated by the Normal distribution based on the moments calculated above. The probabilities that the new trial will give an effect (OR $<$ 1) or a clinically relevant result (OR $<$ 0.5) are only slightly smaller than under Normality. The plot also shows the P-values obtained from the one-sided exact test by Fisher. Those have an interesting pattern, reflecting the discreteness of the data. The probability of a significant result in this hypothetical trial, also known as assurance (O'Hagan et al., 2005), is only 0.14 at one-sided significance level of 2.5%.

3.3.1 Prior-data conflict

The predictive distribution (3.10) is sometimes called *posterior predictive distribution*, since it is conditional on the observed data x. In contrast, the *prior predictive distribution*

$$p(x) = \int p(x \mid \theta) \times p(\theta)\, d\theta \tag{3.12}$$

is derived from the sampling and the prior distribution alone. The prior predictive distribution plays a key role in Bayesian model selection, since the Bayes factor (3.5) compares (3.12) under the two hypotheses. Note that (3.12) is well defined only for proper priors $p(\theta)$.

Box (1980) has suggested an approach to assess a potential conflict between a prior and some data. The method is based on a Bayesian tail probability ("Box's P-value") obtained from the prior predictive distribution and the actually observed datum. Small P-values indicate a *prior-data conflict*, *i. e.* incompatibility of prior assumptions and the actual observations.

Box's P-value is defined as the probability of obtaining a result with prior predictive ordinate $p(X)$ equal to or lower than at the actual observation x:

$$\Pr\left(p(X) \leq p(x)\right).$$

If both data and prior are Normal, $X \mid \theta \sim \mathrm{N}(\theta, \sigma^2)$ and $\theta \sim \mathrm{N}(\nu, \tau^2)$, then the prior predictive distribution is $X \sim \mathrm{N}(\nu, \sigma^2 + \tau^2)$. It can be shown that Box's P-value is then the upper tail probability of a χ^2 distribution with 1 degree of freedom evaluated at

$$t^2 = \frac{(x - \nu)^2}{\sigma^2 + \tau^2}.$$

Here we compute Box's P-value for the prior used in Spiegelhalter et al. (2004) and the results from the GREAT study:

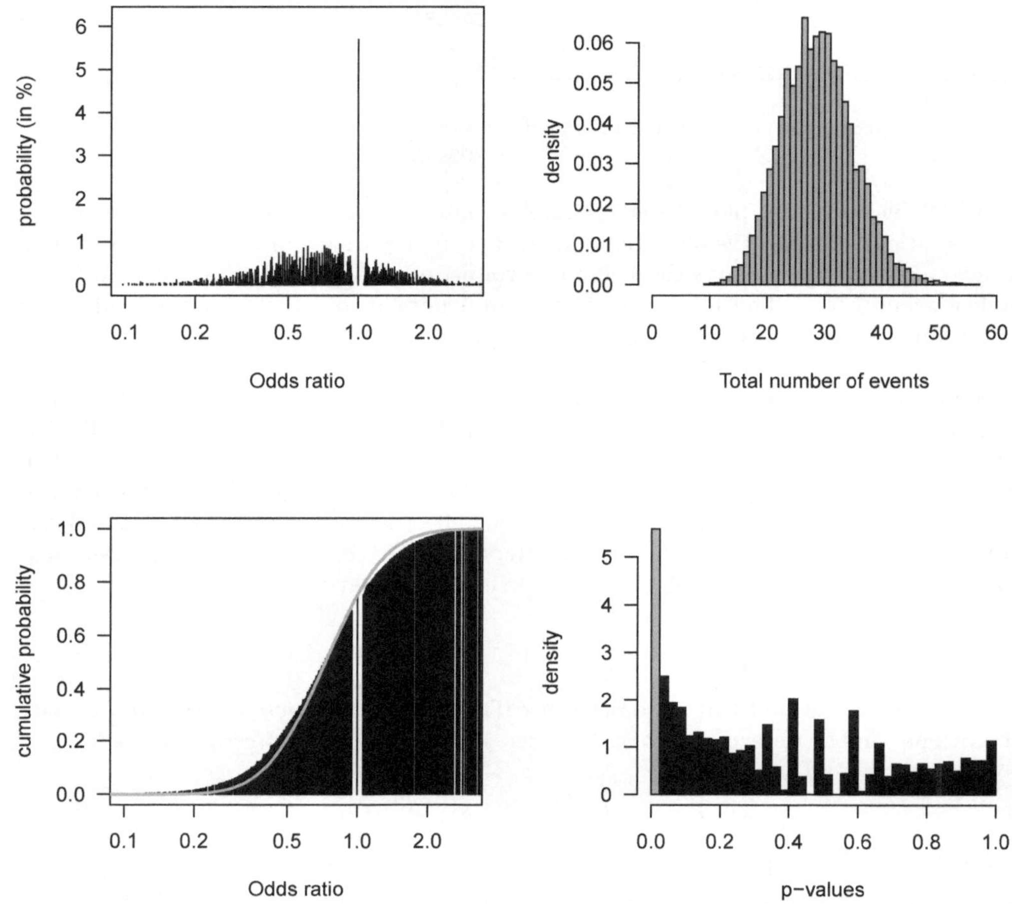

FIGURE 3.2: Top left: Line plot of 10,000 samples from the posterior predictive distribution of the odds ratio in a hypothetical trial with 100 patients in each arm. Top right: Histogram of the total number of events. Bottom left: The corresponding cumulative probability of the odds ratio. Superimposed is a Normal cumulative distribution function with first and second moments calculated under a Normality assumption. Bottom right: The distribution of the P-values obtained from Fisher's one-sided exact test. The grey rectangle marks significant trial results at significance level 2.5%.

```
(t2 <- (thetaHat-thetaPriorMean)^2/(thetaPriorSD^2+thetaHatSE^2))

[1] 1.598

(box.p <- tailProb(t2, pchisq, lower.tail=FALSE, df=1))

Tail probability
          0.2061
```

The resulting tail probability is relatively large and gives no evidence for prior-data conflict. This is the same result as obtained by Spiegelhalter et al. (2004, Example 5.5).

3.3.2 Predictive probability of trial success

In the previous example we calculated already the predictive probability of trial success based on application of Fisher's exact test. An alternative approach is to base the decision of trial success on a Bayesian tail probability, as alluded to in Section 3.2.4. Here we reproduce a conjugate example from Berry et al. (2010, Section 4.2) for a Binomial response rate as outcome, with a Beta(16.6, 7.4) prior. This prior stems from the 16 originally observed responses in 23 patients combined with an initial Beta(0.6, 0.4) prior. Trial success was declared if the posterior probability for a response rate greater than 60% (`probRelevantResponse` in the `R` code chunk below) is greater than than 90%.

```
p <- rbeta(nsim, 16.6, 7.4)
## m: number of patients in future trial
m <- 17
Y <- rbinom(nsim, size=m, prob=p)
## Pr(response rate > 0.60)
probRelevantResponse <- pbeta(0.6, 16.6+Y, 7.4+m-Y, lower.tail=FALSE)
## pps: Predictive probability of success Pr(probRelevantResponse > 0.60) > 0.9
(pps <- tailProbMC(0.9, probRelevantResponse, lower.tail=FALSE))

          Tail probability Monte Carlo standard error
                  0.559200                   0.004965
```

Assuming there are 17 patients in a future trial, the predictive probability of success is 55.9%.

Using a Bayesian test for decision making is important for sequential and group-sequential trials. Berry et al. (2010, Section 4.3) discuss the applicability of Bayesian methods to sequential stopping for futility and efficacy. Specifically, the probability for a response rate greater than 60% is updated after each patient or each group of patients and is used to decide whether or not the trial is being stopped. Stopping can be done based on two different thresholds, one for stopping for futility, one for stopping for efficacy. See Chapter 8 on Adaptive Designs for more details on sequential stopping.

3.3.3 Predictive evidence threshold scaling

Neuenschwander et al. (2018) propose predictive evidence threshold scaling (PETS), an approach to assess the evidential strength of non-confirmatory studies relative to a hypothetical confirmatory standard based on Bayesian tail probabilities. Specifically, they consider the predictive evidence threshold

$$\text{PET} = \Pr(\theta_P > 0 \mid \text{hypothetical confirmatory evidence}), \tag{3.13}$$

i. e. the predictive tail probability of a positive effect θ_P in a new (confirmatory) trial based on hypothetical confirmatory evidence. Confirmatory data usually requires one or two significant trials, with one-sided P-values equal to 0.025 or smaller. Neuenschwander et al. (2018) assume that the hypothetical confirmatory evidence in (3.13) is based on one-sided P-values exactly equal to 0.025.

PET is compared to the predictive evidence probability (PEP)

$$\text{PEP} = \Pr(\theta_P > 0 \mid \text{non-confirmatory evidence}), \tag{3.14}$$

the predictive tail probability of a positive effect θ_P in a new (confirmatory) trial based on the observed non-confirmatory evidence. Computation of (3.13) and (3.14) is based on a meta-analytic model $X_i \mid \theta_i \overset{iid}{\sim} \mathrm{N}(\theta_i, \sigma_i^2)$ and $\theta_i \overset{iid}{\sim} \mathrm{N}(\theta, \tau^2)$ where X_i is the observed treatment effect in study i, θ_i is the true study-specific treatment effect, σ_i is the study-specific standard error, and τ is a heterogeneity parameter. If PEP $\geq$ PET, the non-confirmatory evidence is sufficient for an efficacy claim. Assumptions about the heterogeneity of effects for non-confirmatory (τ_E) and confirmatory (τ_C) studies have to be made. They can be varied in a sensitivity analysis.

To illustrate the approach we revisit the analysis reported in Neuenschwander et al. (2018). Data from a Phase I and Phase II (single arm) study reports promising progression-free-survival of patients with non-small-cell lung cancer treated with Crizotinib. Specifically, the log median survival time in the two studies was estimated to be $\widehat{\theta}_1 = 2.272$ (standard error: 0.13) and $\widehat{\theta}_2 = 2.092$ (0.091) log months, respectively. The confirmatory heterogeneity standard deviation has been fixed at $\tau_C = 1/16$, whereas the non-confirmatory heterogeneity standard deviation τ_E is varied in the range of 0.0 to 0.5.

A hypothetical confirmatory study with 225 patients and one-sided P-value $P = 0.025$ for the null hypothesis of 4.5 months median survival time corresponds to a log median survival time of 1.635 (0.067) log months.

```
## evidential trials
thetaHatEvidential <- c(2.272, 2.092)
thetaHatSeEvidential <- c(0.130, 0.091)

## hypothetical confirmatory trial
nConfirmatory <- 225
(thetaHatSeConfirmatory <- 1/sqrt(nConfirmatory))

[1] 0.06667

## null hypothesis threshold
thetaNull <- log(4.5)
## P-value
pValue <- 0.025
(thetaHatConfirmatory <- qnorm(1-pValue, mean=thetaNull, sd=thetaHatSeConfirmatory))

[1] 1.635

## confirmatory heterogeneity
tauConfirmatory <- 1/16

## predictive confirmatory distribution for one confirmatory study
(pred1Study <- predictiveMetaNormal(thetaHatConfirmatory,
                                    thetaHatSeConfirmatory,
                                    tauConfirmatory))

Predictive Mean   Predictive SD
         1.6347          0.1107

## PET for one confirmatory study
(PET1 <- tailProb(thetaNull, pnorm, mean=pred1Study[1], sd=pred1Study[2],
                  lower.tail=FALSE))

Tail probability
           0.881

## predictive confirmatory distribution for two identical confirmatory studies
(pred2Studies <- predictiveMetaNormal(rep(thetaHatConfirmatory, 2),
                                      rep(thetaHatSeConfirmatory, 2),
                                      tauConfirmatory))
```

```
Predictive Mean   Predictive SD
         1.6347          0.0899

## PET for two identical confirmatory studies
(PET2 <- tailProb(thetaNull, pnorm, mean=pred2Studies[1], sd=pred2Studies[2],
                           lower.tail=FALSE))

Tail probability
           0.927

## predictive evidence probability
## evidential heterogeneity
tauEvidential <- seq(0.0, 0.5, 0.1)
PEP <- numeric()

for(i in 1:length(tauEvidential)){
    predEvidential <- predictiveMetaNormal(thetaHatEvidential, thetaHatSeEvidential,
                                          tauEvidential[i], tauConfirmatory)
    PEP[i] <- tailProb(thetaNull, pnorm, mean=predEvidential[1], sd=predEvidential[2],
                               lower.tail=FALSE)
}

print(PEP)

[1] 1.0000 1.0000 0.9999 0.9980 0.9878 0.9671
```

Even for large values of evidential heterogeneity ($\tau_E = 0.5$), the predictive evidence probability of the non-confirmatory data (PEP=0.967) exceeds the predictive evidence threshold based on one (PET=0.881) or even two (PET=0.927) hypothetical (just) significant studies. Thus, the non-confirmatory evidence can be viewed as sufficient for an efficacy claim.

3.4 Discussion

The chapter has illustrated a number of ways in which Bayesian tail probabilities are used for decision making in clinical trials. Bayesian tail probabilities are based on the posterior or predictive distribution and quantify the probability that the parameter of interest is above a certain threshold.

The close correspondence of one-sided P-values to Bayesian tail probabilities under non-informative reference priors makes the methodology attractive to scientists and regulatory authorities who are trained within the frequentist paradigm. Although Bayesian methods do not rely on the frequentist paradigm of repeated testing, it is still useful to investigate the frequentist operating characteristics of Bayesian methods (Rubin, 1984; Bayarri and Berger, 2004; Grieve, 2016) such as the Type I error rate and the power to detect a clinically relevant difference.

We have also seen that Bayesian tail probabilities can be used to assess the evidence of the data against a null hypothesis H_0. If those tail probabilities are small and the prior odds is 1/1, the posterior probability of H_0 is then approximately equal to the one-sided P-value. However, we have emphasized that this is only true for a test for direction, where we consider a composite null hypothesis of the form H_0: $\theta \leq \theta_0$ versus the alternative H_1: $\theta > \theta_0$. For a point null hypothesis H_0: $\theta = \theta_0$, where we test for the existence of a treatment effect, the analogy between P-values and Bayes factors is lost. Both one-sided and two-sided P-values are then considerably smaller than the corresponding Bayes factors, *i. e.* P-values overstate the evidence against point null hypotheses. This has recently caused a huge amount of discussion in the scientific literature (Johnson, 2013; Wasserstein and Lazar, 2016; Benjamin et al., 2018). We refer the interested reader to the pioneering work by Berger and Sellke (1987); Edwards et al. (1963); Sellke et al. (2001) and to the recent review in Held and Ott (2018).

Acknowledgments

I am grateful to Isaac Gravestock and Goscha Roos for proof-reading a first version of this chapter and to the editors for valuable additional comments.

Appendix: R functions

```
## Two functions to transform probabilities to odds and vice versa
odds <- function(prob)
    return(prob/(1-prob))

prob <- function(odds)
    return(odds/(1+odds))

## function to compute odds ratio from 2x2 table
odds.ratio <- function(table){
    res <- table[1,1]*table[2,2]/table[1,2]/table[2,1]
    return(res)
}

## function to compute tail probability based on Monte Carlo samples
tailProbMC <- function(threshold, samples, lower.tail=TRUE){
    below <- (samples <= threshold)
    p <- mean(below)
    if(lower.tail==FALSE)
        p <- 1-p
    nsim <- length(samples)
    ## Note: Monte Carlo standard error is the same whether or not (lower.tail==TRUE)
    p.se <- sqrt(var(below)/nsim)
    res <- c(p, p.se)
    names(res) <- c("Tail probability", "Monte Carlo standard error")
    return(res)
}

## Computes Wald confidence interval based on estimate and standard error
confidenceInterval <- function(mean, se, level=0.95){
    z <- qnorm((1+level)/2)
    lower <- mean - z*se
    upper <- mean + z*se
    res <- c(lower, upper)
    names(res) <- c("Lower limit", "Upper limit")
    return(res)
}

## function posterior computes mean and standard deviation of posterior distribution
## in Normal-Normal model
```

```
posteriorNormal <- function(prior.mean, prior.sd, estimate, estimate.se){
    prior.var <- prior.sd^2
    estimate.var <- estimate.se^2
    post.var <- 1/(1/prior.var+1/estimate.var)
    post.mean <- (prior.mean/prior.var + estimate/estimate.var)*post.var
    res <- c(post.mean, sqrt(post.var))
    names(res) <- c("Posterior mean", "Posterior SD")
    return(res)
}

## function predictive computes mean and standard deviation of predictive distribution
## in Normal-Normal model
predictiveNormal <- function(prior.mean, prior.sd, data.sd){
    prior.var <- prior.sd^2
    data.var <- data.sd^2
    pred.mean <- prior.mean
    pred.var <- prior.var+data.var
    res <- c(pred.mean, sqrt(pred.var))
    names(res) <- c("Predictive mean", "Predictive SD")
    return(res)
}

## function to compute tail probability based on cumulative probability function
## specified in argument "fn"
tailProb <- function(threshold, fn, lower.tail=TRUE, ...){
    fn1 <- function(par) fn(par, lower.tail=lower.tail, ...)
    res <- fn1(threshold)
    names(res) <- "Tail probability"
    return(res)
}

## calculates Bayes factor based on prior and post probability
bayesFactor <- function(prob.prior, prob.post){
    odds.prior <- odds(prob.prior)
    odds.post <- odds(prob.post)
    res <- odds.post/odds.prior
    names(res) <- "Bayes factor"
    return(res)
}

## function pred
## computes mean and std of predictive distribution
## x and s: means and stds of trial(s)
## tau: heterogeneity of trial(s)
## data.sd: predictive standard deviation
predictiveMetaNormal <- function(x, s, tau, data.sd=tau){
    w <- 1/(s^2+tau^2)
    mean <- sum(w*x)/sum(w)
    std <- sqrt(1/sum(w)+data.sd^2)
    res <- c(mean, std)
    names(res) <- c("Predictive Mean", "Predictive SD")
    return(res)
}
```

Bibliography

Altham, P. M. E. (1969). Exact Bayesian analysis of a 2×2 contingency table and Fisher's "exact" significance test. *Journal of the Royal Statistical Society — Series B*, 31:261–269.

Bayarri, M. J. and Berger, J. O. (2004). The interplay of Bayesian and frequentist analysis. *Statistical Science*, 19(1):58–80.

Benjamin, D. J., Berger, J. O., Johannesson, M., Nosek, B. A., Wagenmakers, E.-J., Berk, R., Bollen, K. A., Brembs, B., Brown, L., Camerer, C., Cesarini, D., Chambers, C. D., Clyde, M., Cook, T. D., De Boeck, P., Dienes, Z., Dreber, A., Easwaran, K., Efferson, C., Fehr, E., Fidler, F., Field, A. P., Forster, M., George, E. I., Gonzalez, R., Goodman, S., Green, E., Green, D. P., Greenwald, A., Hadfield, J. D., Hedges, L. V., Held, L., Ho, T.-H., Hoijtink, H., Jones, J. H., Hruschka, D. J., Imai, K., Imbens, G., Ioannidis, J. P. A., Jeon, M., Kirchler, M., Laibson, D., List, J., Little, R., Lupia, A., Machery, E., Maxwell, S. E., McCarthy, M., Moore, D., Morgan, S. L., Munafò, M., Nakagawa, S., Nyhan, B., Parker, T. H., Pericchi, L., Perugini, M., Rouder, J., Rousseau, J., Savalei, V., Schönbrodt, F. D., Sellke, T., Sinclair, B., Tingley, D., Van Zandt, T., Vazire, S., Watts, D. J., Winship, C., Wolpert, R. L., Xie, Y., Young, C., Zinman, J., and Johnson, V. E. (2018). Redefine Statistical Significance. *Nature Human Behaviour*, 2:6–10.

Berger, J. (2006). The case for objective Bayesian analysis. *Bayesian Analysis*, 1(3):385–402.

Berger, J. and Sellke, T. (1987). Testing a point null hypothesis: Irreconcilability of P values and evidence (with discussion). *Journal of the American Statistical Association*, 82:112–139.

Bernardo, J. M. and Smith, A. F. M. (1994). *Bayesian Theory*. Wiley, Chichester, UK.

Berry, S., Carlin, B., Lee, J., and Müller, P. (2010). *Bayesian Adaptive Methods for Clinical Trials*. CRC Press, Boca Raton, FL.

Box, G. E. P. (1980). Sampling and Bayes' inference in scientific modelling and robustness (with discussion). *Journal of the Royal Statistical Society — Series A*, 143:383–430.

Brown, L., Cai, T., and DasGupta, A. (2001). Interval estimation for a binomial proportion. *Statistical Science*, 16(2):101–133.

Cox, D. R. (2005). *Principles of Statistical Inference*. Cambridge University Press, Cambridge, UK.

Edwards, W., Lindman, H., and Savage, L. J. (1963). Bayesian statistical inference for psychological research. *Psychological Review*, 70(3):193–242.

Fisher, R. A. (1934). *Statistical Methods for Research Workers*. Oliver & Boyd, Edinburgh, UK, 3rd edition.

Goodman, S. N. (2016). Aligning statistical and scientific reasoning. *Science*, 352:1180–1181.

Grieve, A. P. (2016). Idle thoughts of a 'well-calibrated' Bayesian in clinical drug development. *Pharmaceutical Statistics*, 15(2):96–108.

Haldane, J. B. S. (1956). The estimation and significance of the logarithm of a ratio of frequencies. *The Annals of Human Genetics*, 20(4):309–311.

Held, L. and Ott, M. (2016). How the maximal evidence of P values against point null hypotheses depends on sample size. *The American Statistician*, 70(4):335–341.

Held, L. and Ott, M. (2018). On p-values and Bayes factors. *Annual Review of Statistics and Its Application*, 5(1):393–419.

Held, L. and Sabanés Bové, D. (2020). *Likelihood and Bayesian Inference - With Applications in Biology and Medicine.* Springer, Berlin.

Howard, J. V. (1998). The 2×2 table: A discussion from the Bayesian viewpoint. *Statistical Science*, 4:351–367.

Johnson, V. E. (2013). Revised standards for statistical evidence. *Proceedings of the National Academy of Sciences of the United States of America*, 110(48):19313–19317.

Kass, R. E. and Raftery, A. E. (1995). Bayes factors. *Journal of the American Statistical Association*, 90(430):773–795.

Kruschke, J. (2014). *Doing Bayesian Data Analysis: A Tutorial with R, JAGS, and Stan.* Elsevier, 2nd edition.

Laplace, P. S. (1814). *Essai philosophique sur les probabilités.* Courcier, Paris.

Lee, P. (2004). *Bayesian Statistics: An Introduction.* Wiley, third edition.

Liebermeister, C. (1877). Über Wahrscheinlichkeitsrechnung in Anwendung auf therapeutische Statistik. *Sammlung klinischer Vorträge* (Innere Medicin No. 31-64), 110:935–962.

Matthews, J. N. (2006). *Introduction to Randomized Controlled Clinical Trials.* Chapman & Hall/CRC, second edition.

Neuenschwander, B., Roychoudhury, S., and Branson, M. (2018). Predictive evidence threshold scaling: does the evidence meet a confirmatory standard? *Statistics in Biopharmaceutical Research*, 10(2):76–84.

Nurminen, M. and Mutanen, P. (1987). Exact Bayesian analysis of two proportions. *Scandinavian Journal of Statistics*, 14:67–77.

O'Hagan, A., Stevens, J. W., and Campbell, M. J. (2005). Assurance in clinical trial design. *Pharmaceutical Statistics*, 4(3):187–201.

Ripley, B. D. (1987). *Stochastic Simulation.* John Wiley & Sons, Inc., New York, NY.

Robert, C. and Casella, G. (2010). *Introducing Monte Carlo Methods with R.* Springer, Berlin.

Rubin, D. B. (1984). Bayesianly justifiable and relevant frequency calculations for the applied statistician. *The Annals of Statistics*, 12(4):1151–1172.

Sellke, T., Bayarri, M. J., and Berger, J. O. (2001). Calibration of P values for testing precise null hypotheses. *The American Statistician*, 55:62–71.

Seneta, E. (1994). Carl Liebermeister's hypergeometric tails. *Historia Mathematica*, 21:453–462.

Seneta, E. and Phipps, M. C. (2001). On the comparison of two observed frequencies. *Biometrical Journal*, 43:23–43.

Spiegelhalter, D., Abrams, K., and Myles, J. (2004). *Bayesian Approaches to Clinical Trials and Health-Care Evaluation.* Wiley, New York, NY.

Wasserstein, R. L. and Lazar, N. A. (2016). The ASA's statement on p-values: context, process, and purpose. *The American Statistician*, 70(2):129–133.

Winsor, C. P. (1948). Probablity and listerism. *Human Biology*, 20:161–169.

Part II

Clinical development

4

Clinical Development in the Light of Bayesian Statistics

David Ohlssen

Novartis Pharmaceuticals Corporation, US

This chapter focuses on a non-technical introduction to Bayes in drug development where emphasis is placed on the challenges to applying Bayesian thinking. A short introduction to drug development is first provided. Next, the role of quantitative decision making in drug development is discussed in greater detail. In this context, classical thinking and Bayesian thinking is introduced and contrasted. This is followed by several areas of application. While some of these areas are covered in greater detail in other chapters, here we focus on the thought process and critical assumptions. The chapter concludes with a brief discussion of the key challenges and opportunities for Bayesian statistics.

4.1 Introduction

Spiegelhalter et al. (2004) define Bayesian thinking, in the context of health technology assessment, as "The explicit quantitative use of external evidence in the design, monitoring, analysis, interpretation and reporting of a health-care evaluation". In his thought provoking paper on learning versus confirming in drug development, Sheiner (1997) described the Bayesian view as being particularly suited to the learning phases of drug development. He notes: "The Bayesian view is well suited to this task because it provides a theoretical basis for learning from experience; that is, for updating prior beliefs in the light of new evidence". The work goes on to emphasize the term Bayesian is adopted to describe a point of view or a thought process, where prior knowledge (i.e. validated scientific theory) is to be incorporated into the analysis of current data. A clear distinction is made between this thought process and formal Bayesian inference (i.e. a statistical method involving the use of a prior probability distribution when analyzing data), with the former being considered the key concept behind Bayes and the latter more the technical details.

With this background in mind, the remainder of this chapter will focus on a non-technical introduction to Bayes in drug development where emphasis shall be placed on the challenges to applying Bayesian thinking. To begin, a short introduction to drug development will be provided. Next, the role of quantitative decision making in drug development will be discussed in greater detail. In this context, classical thinking and Bayesian thinking will be introduced and contrasted. This will be followed by several areas of application. While some of these areas will be covered in greater detail in other chapters, here we shall focus on the thought process and critical assumptions. Finally, the chapter will conclude with a brief discussion of the key challenges and opportunities for Bayesian statistics.

4.2 Introduction to drug development

Following the discovery of a candidate molecule in the laboratory, a typical drug development process could involve:

- Preclinical safety testing followed by first in human trials to assess safety and tolerability (Phase I);
- Randomized *proof of concept studies* where a basic formulation of the drug is first tested in a patient population (Phase IIA);
- Dose and regimen finding trials to identify the best dose or doses (Phase IIB);
- Confirmatory testing of those doses to demonstrate safety and efficacy for regulatory approval (Phase III);
- Post-approval trials (Phase IIIB & Phase IV), which might investigate the uses of a drug in a different patient population or compare the drug head-to-head with an alternative therapy.

The approach can change substantially in more severe diseases with high unmet medical need (i.e. no treatment options). For example, in the oncology setting, Phase I will typically involve patients (as opposed to healthy volunteers) and emphasis on finding a dose with acceptable toxicity, while Phase II could be based on a series of single arm studies in a number of different populations. In fatal conditions with no treatment options, a successful Phase II study could lead to conditional approval of the therapy by regulatory agencies.

Drug development projects are typically run by groups of experts from a variety of disciplines such as medicine, biostatistics, clinical pharmacology, safety and epidemiology, chemistry and formulation, quality assurance, commercial, health economics, data management, and project management. The teams look to define the product profile of the proposed candidate drug and form a development strategy to support the profile.

In the early phases of drug development (Phases I-II), which are regarded as learning phases and tend to be more exploratory in nature, many changes to the development program can be made. Examples include changes to the target population; formulation and method of administration; and key outcomes of interest. As a result, the drug development team must make many decisions. Ideally, decision-making should be as quantitative as possible, providing substantial opportunity for Bayesian thinking and inference.

The confirmatory stage (Phase III) tends to involve a greater degree of regulation. In the US, the Food and Drug administration (FDA) suggest that the clearest way to establish substantial evidence of effectiveness is from at least two adequate and well-controlled studies each convincing on its own to establish effectiveness (U.S. Food and Drug Administration, 1998). Although quantitative thresholds and the use of a classical approach are not stated in the guidelines, in practice this translates to a minimum requirement of achieving statistical significance (at the 5% level of a two-sided test) in the pre-specified primary analysis that is associated with each of the studies. In some cases, the requirement of two successful studies can be relaxed. This can occur when wider relevant evidence is taken into consideration or in cases with very high unmet need. Bayesian approaches have increasingly been used in these situations, although no systematic approach or guideline has been established.

In addition to decision making within a project, large pharmaceutical companies will manage a portfolio of several hundred drug development projects for different experimental medicines, resulting in a large number of clinical trials conducted simultaneously across all phases of development. A key aspect for senior management is decision making at the portfolio level. Again, this setting provides substantial opportunity for Bayes.

4.3 Quantitative decision making in drug development

Classical hypothesis testing and P-values have provided the cornerstone of *quantitative decision making* (QDM) in drug development. A positive signal, based on a primary analysis resulting in a low P-value, implies that the result seen in a trial would have had low probability under the null model (e.g. a statistical model with a zero treatment effect). Outside the pre-specified primary and key secondary analysis, extreme care must be taken when interpreting P-values. A common mistake is to falsely treat such exploratory analysis with the same type of interpretation as the pre-specified inferential analyses. Such a strategy fails to account for multiplicity and random high bias.

Properly adjusted P-values resulting from pre-specified analyses can be a highly valuable tool in QDM. However, the strength of conclusions that can be drawn from P-values alone, even when associated with the primary analysis, are limited. Unfortunately, there is often a desire to make stronger conclusions and sometimes inadvertently they are made. It has been argued that one of the main reasons for the so-called replication crisis is the misinterpretation of P-values (Wasserstein and Lazar, 2016).

For instance, following a positive signal in the primary analysis of a Phase II study, we ideally would like to make a solid conclusion, such as:

- the statistically significant result is likely to be achieved again if we repeat the same trial (Replication);
- there is a good chance the treatment is efficacious (inversion of the hypothesis testing definition);
- there is a high probability of a successful Phase III study (Prediction).

Replication will depend in part on the strength of the signal observed in the study. For example, it could be argued that when a trial just achieves the significance threshold, an identical replicate study would only have a 50% chance of achieving significance. This is based on the judgment that the most likely treatment effect in the replicate study would be exactly the observed value required to just achieve significance. However, this approach does not account for the broader range of evidence associated with the question of interest. This point will be examined further in the discussion on Bayesian and classical thinking.

As subsequent Phase III studies do not tend to be identical to Phase II studies, the question of replication tends to be of less practical interest than inversion or prediction. Prediction of later phase success depends largely on the definition of success and the relevance of the Phase II study to Phase III.

4.4 Bayesian thinking

The idea of inverting the definition of a hypothesis has links with Bayesian statistics. It is well known that for simple models where so called non-informative or weak priors are applied, the posterior probability of a treatment effect greater than 0 would be equivalent to 1 – the one-sided P-value (Greenland and Poole, 2013), see also Chapter 3. This relationship will also hold even when more complex models are applied, as long as the likelihood dominates the prior.

So does Bayesian inference with weak priors provide a simple way to much stronger conclusions? Well unsurprisingly, there is no free lunch. The big danger with such an approach is that a crucial piece of evidence or context is missed by assuming a weak prior. It is particularly common to overlook evidence associated with the background rate or prevalence of a particular outcome.

A situation might occur where many previous attempts at forming a drug for the disease had failed, with many showing no treatment effect in the clinical outcome of interest. In this case, it could be much more reasonable to put a large prior probability on a zero treatment effect and then smear the rest of the prior over a reasonable range of positive treatment effects.This is referred to as both "lump and smear" and "spike and slab" prior (Madigan and Raftery, 1994). Such a prior is quite informative and the evidence from a typical Phase II study would be unlikely to overwhelm the strong prior evidence of a zero treatment effect. Further, completely different conclusions would be made depending on whether a weak prior or the more informative prior incorporating information about the background success rates was assumed.

The previous discussion highlights that, to put a positive result into context, the wider evidence must be considered. This is where I personally draw one of the main distinctions between classical thinking and Bayesian thinking. While classical thinking tries to bring in other evidence in a more qualitative and descriptive way, Bayesian thinking will try to formally synthesize the broader body of evidence in a quantitative model. In practice, even when Bayesian thinking is used, only some of the wider evidence can be synthesized. This could be due to a subjective judgment on the rigor and relevance of the wider evidence, where evidence not reaching an acceptable standard is not formally incorporated. A further complication occurs when different forms of evidence are difficult to link together and model. For example, it might be difficult to synthesize evidence on the mechanism of action from animal studies with a treatment effect observed in the target population in Phase II. However, positive evidence from the former would imply a greater degree of confidence in biological plausibility and therefore make a successful clinical study more likely.

4.5 Applications of Bayesian methods in drug development

4.5.1 Using historical data in a proof of concept study

Early phase proof of concept studies can provide an opportunity to incorporate historical information from previous studies of the same disease. Often the control treatment or placebo group will be the same in multiple historical studies. This allows the development of an informative prior for the control arm based on synthesis of the control group data from the series of relevant previous trials. As a result, the control group in the new trial can be reduced by the number of virtual patients represented by the historical prior.

One of the main complications involves the careful selection of relevant historical studies. If this is done badly it would basically lead to a poor quantitative evaluation of the new study (e.g. incorrect treatment effect estimation and a lack of a proper understanding of uncertainty). A good selection of relevant previous research requires expert clinical knowledge combined with a systematic approach. However, regardless of the care taken to form the pool of historical trials, there is still a certain level of subjectivity.

Once the historical evidence has been selected, a further challenge is the synthesis of the information to form a prior. Ideally, the historical evidence should be down weighted in some way. Otherwise the historical evidence would dominate the assessment of the control group in the new study. Fortunately, there have been many methodological developments in this area. One of the key ideas involves using a hierarchical model, similar to those used in meta-analysis, to predict the effect of a control group in a new study. This predictive distribution is then used as a prior in the new study (see Figure 4.1). The approach is known as the *meta-analytic predictive* (MAP) *prior* (Neuenschwander et al., 2005); see more about this prior in Chapter 6.

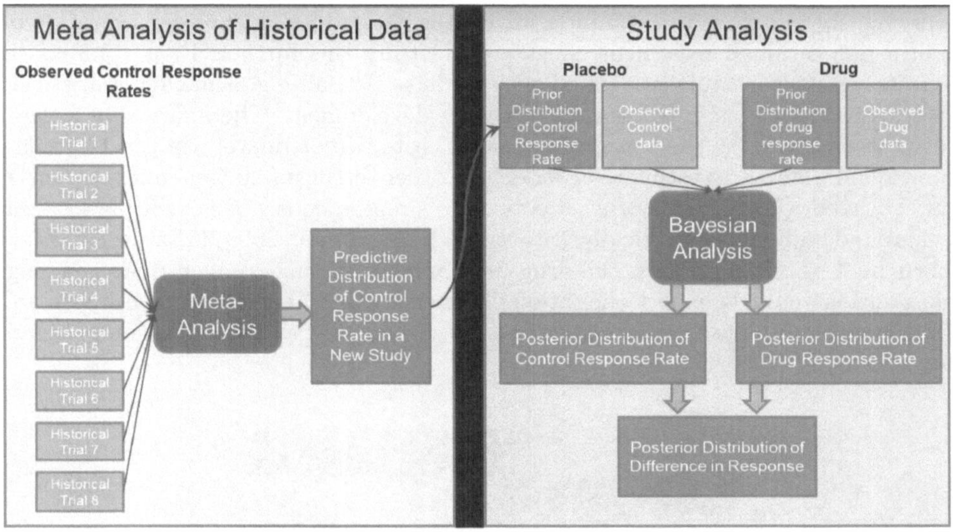

FIGURE 4.1: Using historical control data to form a prior in a proof of concept study. The left side of the figure depicts a hierarchical model of the form used in meta-analysis to predict the effect of a control group in a new study. The right side shows how this predictive distribution is then used as a prior in the new study.

Recent developments have included forming the prior as a mixture distribution and adding an extra weakly informative component to create more flexible borrowing in the case of prior-data conflict (Schmidli et al., 2014). This approach is attractive as the *commensurability* between the observed data and the prior affects the amount of borrowing. However, the concept of flexible borrowing also has a downside as it can lead to a carefully considered assumption (e.g. exchangeability) to be quickly ignored if a small amount of observed data is in conflict with the prior. As the consequences of falsely downweighing important prior evidence can be as serious as prior misspecification, using simulation to understand the characteristics of flexible borrowing procedure (when applied to particular design) is recommended. See also Chapter 6 for an extensive treatment of using historical data in current studies.

4.5.2 Assessing probability of success for portfolio review

At the end of Phase II, there is interest in assessing the probability of a successful Phase III program. The Bayesian framework provides an ideal setup for assessing this, as it provides the tools to synthesize the available evidence, predict the outcome in Phase III and then assess the chance of achieving certain goals on the probability scale (O'Hagan et al., 2005). Even if the modeling required is complex, Markov chain Monte Carlo (MCMC) provides a well-established technique for implementation.

Typically, a model-based approach would be applied to predict the primary outcome of a Phase III trial using Phase II data. This would allow an assessment of the probability of achieving a basic level of success, such as achieving statistical significance in the primary analysis of Phase III. It is easy to change the definition of success to incorporate achieving a clinically meaningful treatment effect estimate and achieving success in two Phase III trials, which form the Phase III program. Furthermore, in many cases, it is possible to incorporate key secondary end points, perhaps key to product labeling, into the definition of success.

As previously mentioned, a common mistake is the failure to consider the prior probability of a null or small treatment effect. To illustrate this further, Figure 4.2 considers the quantitative decision rule associated with a Phase II trial (e.g. achieving statistical significance) to be a diagnostic test for further drug development. The figure shows the false discovery rate is driven by the background success rate. Unfortunately, in practice this rate is unknown and difficult to estimate or model. In other settings (e.g. genomics), where hundreds of thousands of candidate drugs are assessed simultaneously, it is possible to estimate the background null rate empirically (Storey and Tibshirani, 2003). However, without a large clear pool of relevant cases, the drug development setting is much more challenging. Possible solutions include expert elicitation (Kinnersley and Day, 2013) or using historical data from the same disease to form the prior. In either case, subjective assumptions must be made.

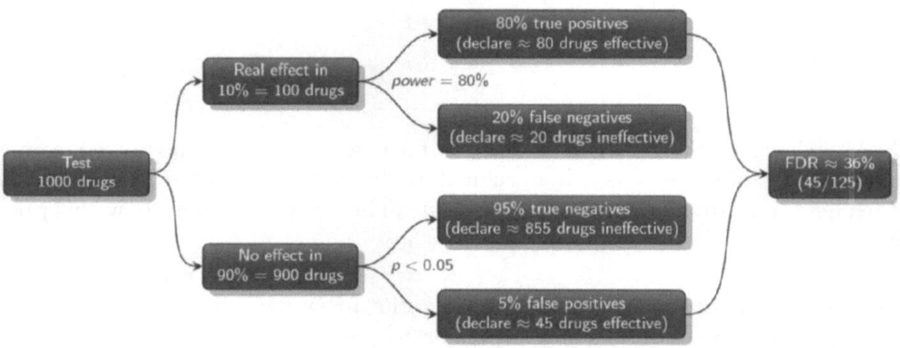

FIGURE 4.2: Considering Phase II clinical trials as a diagnostic test for further drug development. The figure displays 1000 candidate drugs each assessed by a Phase II clinical trial. Classical hypothesis testing is used as a crude diagnostic test for further development of the drug. While the design and analysis will control power and Type I error, the figure illustrates that the false discovery rate is driven by the prevalence of drugs with a real treatment effect.

Further complications occur when the Phase II differs significantly from the proposed Phase III program. Key differences could include changes to the population, changes to the primary outcome of interest; changes to the dose and or regimen. In each situation, the Bayesian paradigm or other model based approaches can help to adjust for these differences (see e.g. Kirby et al., 2012). However, to make progress with these challenges, fairly strong assumptions will often be required and the ability of diagnostics to check the modeling can be limited. For instance, in the development of multiple sclerosis drugs, surrogate outcome meta-analysis of a large number of historical studies can be used to bridge between Phase II outcomes based on MRI and Phase III outcomes based on clinical relapses (Pozzi et al., 2016). A further example could involve the use of model averaging (see Chapter 1) to adjust and shrink effects observed in a sub-population, particularly when the population was found in an exploratory analysis (Bornkamp et al., 2017).

The definition of success is a further area requiring careful attention and is often a cause of confusion. In particular, the drug development team might be focused on a different definition of success (e.g. marketing authorization or commercial viability) to the one that the statistician can realistically assess (e.g. statistical significance in the primary outcome of a planned Phase III study) using data from the drug development program. Therefore, when probability of success metrics are discussed and used to make drug development decisions, clarity on the definition of success is essential.

While a significant primary analysis is necessary for marketing authorization by the regulatory agencies, assessing the probability of achieving this will not directly provide a probability of achieving product approval or commercial viability. The latter two quantities are much harder to assess as they involve many factors or risks that cannot be easily assessed using earlier phase data from a drug development program. Mechanisms of failure of a program could include rare adverse events leading to a safety signal, which only show up during the Phase III program. Further, commercial viability could be determined by the success of competitors. Some data might be available to help assess this. For example, databases of program success rates by broad disease areas are available (DiMasi et al., 2010) and competitive intelligence on rival therapies will be routinely collected. In the case of the former, such data provide a way to get a crude overall estimate of program failure incorporating many mechanisms of failure. However, it is not easy to combine this with the early phase data collected in a drug development program. Therefore, it is difficult to come up with an assessment that is tailored to a specific program.

4.5.3 Extrapolation and partial extrapolation in pediatrics

Once a drug is approved in an adult diseased population, attention often turns to studying the corresponding pediatric population. In some cases, scientific arguments can be made so that no further well controlled clinical trials are required. To achieve this, a sponsor must provide other information to support pediatric use, and the regulator must conclude that the course of the disease and the effects of the drug, i.e. the pharmacokinetic-pharmacodynamic (PK-PD) relationship of the drug, are sufficiently similar in the pediatric and adult populations to permit extrapolation from adult efficacy data to pediatric patients. This approach is sometimes referred to as *full extrapolation* (U.S. Food and Drug Administration, 1998). The European Medical Agency produced a paper addressing extrapolation in the context of pediatrics (European Medicine Agency, 2016). They propose a systematic approach to characterize differences between the source and target population on medicine disposition and effects, disease manifestation and progression, and clinical response to treatment.

In other circumstances, although there might be some case to support full extrapolation, the scientific arguments are not strong enough for the regulatory agencies to accept and therefore there is pressure to conduct a full clinical trial program in the pediatric population. These trials can be very difficult to conduct, as pediatric studies are typically much harder to recruit and often the disease is much less common in the pediatric population.

More recently this type of situation has proved a fertile ground for Bayesian thinking and Bayesian methods. One possibility is to follow similar lines to the historical data example. For instance, the adult data could be used to form a prior either for the treatment effect or background control effect. In the case of the former, it is unlikely that there would be enough adult studies to fit a meta-analytic predictive model. Therefore, a more subjective approach must be taken to discount the adult data.

4.5.4 Big data machine learning and artificial intelligence: Future challenges for Bayesian methods

The hype and excitement surrounding big data, machine learning and *artificial intelligence* (AI) have recently spread to drug development. Areas of interest include: combining clinical data with genetic or proteomic data to create more personalized treatments; using digital devices, such as accelerometers to measure movement, in clinical studies and modeling large observational cohorts, such as UK biobank, to better understand disease progression and build disease models that will help simulate future clinical trials.

Machine learning techniques are well established in situations with big data and where prediction is the main question of interest. The ability to computationally scale machine learning methods has been a key factor in achieving success. Such approaches have had noted success in complex classification problems such as image recognition and natural language processing (both text and speech). A common theme in these areas is a large supply of cheaply available labeled data, where the correct classification or gold standard is known and can be used to train a predictive algorithm. This is in contrast to the clinical research setting, where data from subjects is relatively expensive to collect and the classification of patients into well-defined groups, based on their outcomes, is complex. To expand on the latter point, intra-patient variability and the multi-dimensional nature of measuring how well a patient is doing on a treatment make ranking and classifying patients particularly difficult.

In drug development, the inherent uncertainty surrounding clinical outcomes makes a Bayesian approach an attractive alternative to more traditional machine learning approaches. Bayesian Machine learning approaches based on the Box loop (Blei, 2014) could be particularly well suited to this setting. However, a major challenge is how to appropriately computationally scale. Methods for full Bayesian inference such as Markov chain Monte Carlo and Hamiltonian Monte Carlo (Hoffman and Gelman, 2014, see also Chapter 1) are not well suited to dealing with genuine big data. If Bayesian inference is to succeed in these developing areas, reliable approaches to computationally scale (Li et al., 2017) or robust approximations (e.g. Blei et al., 2017) will be essential. Currently, this has not been established in a clinical development setting and as such provides an opportunity for further research.

4.6 Conclusion

This chapter has provided a non-technical introduction to the current state of Bayesian methods in a drug development setting. Rather than technical details and mathematical formulae, the Bayesian thought process was highlighted. A common theme throughout was the need to make scientifically rational assumptions that allow different information sources to be synthesized through modeling. This is in direct contrast to classical thinking, where emphasis is typically placed on a single data source and one or two key analyses.

Implementing Bayesian thinking in practice is easier said than done. In each of the applications, a critical aspect involves deciding upon the rigor and relevance of different sources of information. As this step is subjective and requires the engagement of domain area scientists, much greater resources are required. Systematic frameworks and guidelines like those produced in device development (U.S. Food and Drug Administration, 2010) could help considerably help with the quality and efficiency of this step.

While the technical solutions required to synthesize different sources of information have been largely solved (e.g. by using MCMC), there are still challenges in terms of having a critical mass of quantitative scientists to implement them. Education of clinicians and statisticians remains a key issue (Natanegara et al., 2005).

To conclude on a positive note, within the pharmaceutical industry, Bayesian thinking is an integral and established part of quantitative decision making (Grieve, 2007). It seems in this setting, Bayesian statistics is here to stay and flourish for the foreseeable future. Following successes in devices (Campbell, 2010), recent experience suggests increasing use of Bayes in regulatory decision making.

Bibliography

Blei, D. (2014). Build, compute, critique, repeat: data analysis with latent variable models. *Annual Review of Statistics and Its Application*, 1:203–232.

Blei, D., Kucukelbir, A., and McAuliffe, J. (2017). Variational inference: A review for statisticians. *Journal of the American Statistical Association*, 112:859–877.

Bornkamp, B., Ohlssen, D., Magnusson, B., and Schmidli, H. (2017). Model averaging for treatment effect estimation in subgroups. *Pharmaceutical Statistics*, 16:133–142.

Campbell, G. (2010). Bayesian statistics in medical devices: Innovation sparked by the FDA. *Journal of Biopharmaceutical Statistics*, 21(5):871–887.

DiMasi, J., Feldman, L., Seckler, A., and Wilson, A. (2010). Trends in risks associated with new drug development: success rates for investigational drugs. *Clinical Pharmacology and Therapeutics*, 8:272–277.

European Medicine Agency (2016). Reflection paper on extrapolation of efficacy and safety in pediatric medicine development. `http://www.ema.europa.eu/docs/en_GB/document_library/Regulatory_and_procedural_guideline/2016/04/WC500204187.pdf`.

Greenland, S. and Poole, C. (2013). Living with p values: resurrecting a Bayesian perspective on frequentist statistics. *Epidemiology*, 24(1):62–68.

Grieve, A. (2007). 25 years of Bayesian methods in the pharmaceutical industry: a personal, statistical bummel. *Pharmaceutical Statistics*, 6:261–281.

Hoffman, M. and Gelman, A. (2014). The No-U-Turn sampler: Adaptively setting path lengths in Hamiltonian Monte Carlo. *Journal of Machine Learning Research*, 15:1593–1623.

Kinnersley, N. and Day, S. (2013). Structured approach to the elicitation of expert beliefs for a Bayesian-designed clinical trial: a case study. *Pharmaceutical Statistics*, 12:104–113.

Kirby, S., Burke, J., Chuang-Stein, C., and Sin, C. (2012). Discounting phase 2 results when planning phase 3 clinical trials. *Pharmaceutical Statistics*, 11:373–385.

Li, C., Srivastava, S., and Dunson, D. (2017). Simple, scalable and accurate posterior interval estimation. *Biometrika*, 104:665–680.

Madigan, D. and Raftery, A. (1994). Model selection and accounting for model uncertainty in graphical models using Occam's window. *Journal of the American Statistical Association*, 89:1535–1546.

Natanegara, F., Neuenschwander, B., Seaman, J., Kinnersley, N., Heilmann, C., Ohlssen, D., and Rochester, G. (2005). The current state of Bayesian methods in medical product development: Survey results and recommendations from the DIA Bayesian Scientific Working Group. *Pharmaceutical Statistics*, 13:3–12.

Neuenschwander, B., Capkun-Niggli, G., Branson, M., and Spiegelhalter, D. (2005). Summarizing historical information on controls in clinical trials. *Clinical Trials*, 7:5–18.

O'Hagan, A., Stevens, J., and Campbell, M. (2005). Assurance in clinical trial design. *Pharmaceutical Statistics*, 4(3):187–201.

Pozzi, L., Schmidli, H., and Ohlssen, D. (2016). A Bayesian hierarchical surrogate outcome model for multiple sclerosis. *Pharmaceutical Statistics*, 15:341–348.

Schmidli, H., Gsteiger, S., Roychoudhury, S., O'Hagan, A., Spiegelhalter, D., and Neuenschwander, B. (2014). Robust meta-analytic-predictive priors in clinical trials with historical control information. *Biometrics*, 70:1023–1032.

Sheiner, L. (1997). Learning versus confirming in clinical drug development. *Clinical Pharmacology and Therapeutics*, 61:275–291.

Spiegelhalter, D., Abrams, K., and Myles, J. (2004). *Bayesian Approaches to Clinical Trials and Health-Care Evaluation*. Wiley, New York, NY.

Storey, J. and Tibshirani, R. (2003). Statistical significance for genomewide studies. In *Proceedings of the National Academy of Sciences*, volume 100, pages 9440–9445.

U.S. Food and Drug Administration (1998). Guidance for Industry: E9 Statistical Principles for Clinical Trials. "https://www.fda.gov/downloads/drugs/guidancecomplianceregulatoryinformation/guidances/ucm073137.pdf".

U.S. Food and Drug Administration (2010). The Use of Bayesian Statistics in Medical Device Clinical Trials: Guidance for Industry and Food and Drug Administration Staff. "http://www.fda.gov/MedicalDevices/DeviceRegulationandGuidance/GuidanceDocuments/ucm071072.htm".

Wasserstein, R. and Lazar, N. (2016). The ASA's statement on p-values: context, process, and purpose. *The American Statistician*, 70 (2):129–133.

5

Prior Elicitation

Nicky Best
GlaxoSmithKline, UK

Nigel Dallow
GlaxoSmithKline, UK

Timothy Montague
GlaxoSmithKline, US

Expert knowledge is a valuable source of information to augment available data or when interpretation/synthesis of data requires expert judgment. Prior elicitation is a key tool for translating this expert knowledge and judgment into a quantitative probability distribution that can then be used in the design, analysis and/or interpretation of clinical studies. This chapter reviews the different approaches to elicit information from experts and summarize it in a probabilistic language, more specifically into prior distributions. We then focus on how expert knowledge from multiple experts can be summarized. Software to achieve such summaries are reviewed too. The concepts and approaches are illustrated using three real-life examples relating to different aspects of pharmaceutical product development.

5.1 Introduction

Consider the following scenarios:

- A Phase II *proof of concept* (PoC) *study* has been recently completed and provides sufficient evidence of efficacy to warrant further clinical development. To plan the next study, we need an estimate of the expected treatment effect to inform sample size calculations and other design considerations. However, the primary measure of efficacy in the next clinical study will not be the same measure that was utilized in the PoC study. Additionally, the quantitative relationship between the efficacy measure in the PoC study and the efficacy measure of the proposed study is unknown, such that the expected treatment difference in the next study cannot be predicted directly from the PoC data.

- An alternative treatment for a rare disease is being developed for pediatric use. Studies in adults in a different indication provide evidence of similar efficacy and a lower toxicity profile than the currently available *standard of care* (SoC), but no clinical trials have been previously conducted in children with this disease. A randomized trial to assess non-inferiority of the new, less toxic treatment and SoC is currently being planned, but conventional sample size calculations require a sample size that is an order of magnitude larger than is feasible to recruit given the rarity of the disease.

TABLE 5.1: Factors in favor or against use of prior elicitation.

Factors favoring use of prior elicitation
∘ Inadequate empirical data (of suitable quality and relevance) are available to inform a decision
∘ Multiple sources of empirical data are available of differing levels of relevance, with a need to bridge the gap between the historical setting(s) and the current setting
∘ Lack of scientific consensus, or when reliable evidence or legitimate models are in conflict, with a need to quantify the uncertainty due to disagreement
∘ Need to characterize uncertainty
∘ Appropriate experts (and financial resources) are available and elicitation can be completed within the required time frame
Factors suggesting against use of prior elicitation
∘ A large body of empirical data (of suitable quality and relevance) exists with a high degree of consensus
∘ The information that an expert elicitation could provide is not critical to the assessment or decision
∘ Available expertise and/or financial resources are insufficient to conduct a robust and defensible elicitation

In drug development, there are many situations where sponsors, researchers, regulators, clinicians and patients are being asked to make decisions about the clinical development or use of a new medicine with very limited empirical evidence. As in the first example above, data from clinical studies, animal and in vitro studies or other data sources may exist, but cannot be used statistically to predict the treatment effect in the next clinical study due to a lack of direct relevance, high levels of variability or lack of scientific consensus about the appropriate model. Or, as in the second scenario, there may not be any hard data or only very limited data that exist. In such situations, expert knowledge is a valuable source of information to augment available data or when interpretation/synthesis of data requires expert judgment. Prior elicitation is a key tool for translating this expert knowledge and judgment into a quantitative probability distribution that can then be used in the design, analysis and/or interpretation of clinical studies. For example, an elicited prior for the treatment effect of a novel medicine could be used to calculate the probability of success of the next study; this is often termed *assurance* (O'Hagan et al., 2005) and is computed by averaging the conditional probability of study success (e.g. power) for fixed effect sizes over a prior distribution for the true value of the treatment effect of interest. Or the elicited prior may be used as part of the formal data analysis of a clinical study, by combining it with the observed data from the clinical study via Bayesian methods.

Table 5.1 summarizes some of the circumstances where it might or might not be worthwhile to consider use of prior elicitation.

5.2 Methods for prior elicitation

Typically, the desired output of an elicitation is a probability distribution that represents the expert's prior belief about a quantity of interest, such as a treatment difference, denoted here by θ. However, most experts are unfamiliar with expressing their beliefs in the form of a probability distribution, and even when an expert is familiar with this concept, it is very difficult for him or her to produce a distribution directly. A variety of methods and tools are available to help experts to encode their beliefs in a way that can then be represented by a probability distribution. The most commonly used methods are summarized below — see Chapters 5 and 6 of O'Hagan et al. (2006) for more detailed descriptions.

5.2.1 Methodologies for eliciting a prior for a single uncertain quantity

Rather than asking experts directly for statistical quantities like means and standard deviations of a probability distribution, most elicitation techniques involve first asking the expert to provide values of the cumulative distribution function for θ at a small number of points, and then fitting a probability distribution to the values elicited. Expert judgments about values of the cumulative distribution can be obtained in several ways.

5.2.1.1 Fixed interval ("probability") method

Here the expert is asked to consider a fixed value or interval for θ and to provide its corresponding probability. Typical questions may be:

"What is your probability that θ is less than or equal to -1?"

"What is your probability that θ lies between 0 and 1.5?"

The main limitation of this method is that by pre-specifying a particular interval or fixed value for θ, we may sub-consciously draw the expert's attention to particular values for the quantity being elicited, which can introduce 'anchoring bias' in the expert's judgments (see Section 5.2.5). Methods that avoid pre-specifying values for θ are therefore recommended.

5.2.1.2 Variable interval methods

Here the expert is asked about the values of θ that are associated with particular probabilities - typically tertiles or quartiles of the cumulative distribution function. The expert is first asked to state what he/she judges to be the plausible range of values for θ, and to then split this range into three or four intervals of equal probability. For example, to determine the median, the expert is asked to choose a value a such that the true value of θ has the same probability of being above or below a. To determine the lower (upper) quartiles, the expert is asked to condition on the true value being below (above) the value provided for the median, and is then asked to choose a value b_L (b_U) such that the true value of θ has the same probability of being below (above) b_L (b_U) as being between b_L (b_U) and the median.

5.2.1.3 "Roulette" or "Chips in Bins"

Here, the expert is given a certain number of gaming chips/counters and asked to distribute them among the bins of a histogram (see Figure 5.1). The proportion of chips allocated to a particular bin gives the expert's probability that the true value of θ lies in that bin (subject to rounding error). As with the variable interval method, the expert is first asked to state what (s)he judges to be the plausible range of values for θ, and this range is to be split equally into the required number of histogram bins. A small number of bins and/or chips simplifies the elicitation task for the expert (in terms of level of precision required) at the expense of accuracy in representing the expert's "true belief". However, more chips or bins do not necessarily guarantee more accuracy – for example, assigning probability of 0.005 to each chip (i.e. if 200 chips were used) may result in a resolution level beyond the expert's capabilities to conceptualize. A pragmatic choice that appears to work well in practice is to give the expert 20 chips (each corresponding to 5% probability) and split their plausible range into about 8 to 12 bins.

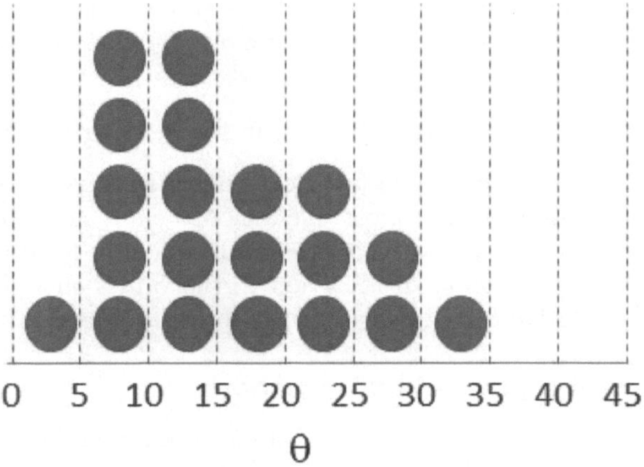

FIGURE 5.1: Example of a 'chips in bins' (roulette) elicitation method.

Practical experience suggests that experts find the roulette method more intuitive than the quartile or tertile methods. However, there is a danger that they can just focus on making the histogram a 'nice' shape rather than thinking carefully about the probabilities they are specifying. Training of the experts is important (see Section 5.2.5) to make them aware that their histogram need not be symmetrical or bell-shaped, and providing them with feedback to check that the histogram truly represents their beliefs, e.g. for the histogram in Figure 5.1, check with the experts that they believe there is a 30% probability that the true value of θ is below 10 and 15% probability it is above 25.

5.2.2 Fitting distributions to the elicited values

Once a number of summary values have been elicited from the expert using one of the methods above, the elicitation task is completed by converting these into a probability distribution. Any convenient distribution can be used so long as it fits the elicited summary values adequately. This could be a simple histogram, but more commonly standard parametric families of distributions are used since these are mathematically convenient to use in subsequent analyses involving the elicited prior. Several standard methods exist for fitting parametric distributions to empirical quantiles, including maximum likelihood, moment matching (suitable if empirical means and standard deviations have been elicited or can be derived), or least squares (which selects the distribution that minimizes the sum of squared differences between the elicited and fitted quantiles). Methods do exist for eliciting non-parametric distributions (e.g. Gosling et al., 2007) but these tend to be more complex and the resulting fitted distributions are often more cumbersome to use in practice. What is important is to ensure that the expert agrees that the fitted distribution is an adequate representation of their beliefs, and to check that the resulting use to which the prior is put is not sensitive to the choice.

5.2.2.1 Bimodal distributions

Most commonly used elicitation approaches fit unimodal parametric distributions to an expert's judgments. However, sometimes such distributions are not flexible enough. For example, judgments of the form "if X occurs then I expect θ to be small, but if Y occurs I expect θ to be large" typically imply a bimodal prior distribution (for example, X and Y might be different potential mechanisms of action for a new drug). Such a bimodal prior distribution could be captured using the roulette method, and either using the roulette histogram directly as the expert's prior or fitting a parametric or non-parametric mixture model to the roulette summaries. However, it is unlikely that the expert will be able to accurately capture the marginal summary of a set of conditional beliefs such as the above. A better approach in this case is to re-structure the elicitation process to elicit conditional distributions – for example:

(i) The distribution of θ conditional on X occurring;

(ii) The distribution of θ conditional on Y occurring;

(iii) The probability that X rather than Y occurs.

The resulting fitted prior is then a mixture of the fitted distributions for (i) and (ii) with mixture weights given by (iii). Dallow et al. (2018) discuss the use of this bimodal elicitation technique to address potential problems of over-optimism when eliciting expert beliefs about the true treatment effect for new medicine. In the early phases of drug development, there is often a reasonable probability that the drug being tested will demonstrate no efficacy in the planned endpoint of interest, but it may be scientifically implausible that it will have a true negative effect. Such beliefs can be hard to capture via a single unimodal prior distribution, so Dallow et al. provide an example where they first elicit the expert's probability, w, that the drug has a true positive/favorable effect, and then elicit the distribution of this effect size conditional on the assumption that the drug does have a favorable effect. They then construct a bimodal prior for the drug response as a weighted mixture of the prior for the placebo or control response (which had been elicited separately), with weight $(1 - w)$, and the conditional distribution for the drug effect given that the drug works, with weight w (see Figure 5.2).

5.2.3 Methodologies for eliciting priors for multiple uncertain quantities

We often want experts to provide judgments about more than one uncertain quantity — for example, treatment effects of both a control therapy and an investigational product, or response rates for several different doses of a drug. With multiple quantities, it is necessary to think about dependence: does the probability that X takes some value depend on what the value of Y is? Independent quantities can just be elicited separately, but if quantities are not independent we must elicit the nature and magnitude of dependence between them, which is generally much harder for experts to think about than eliciting a single quantity. There is no clear understanding among elicitation practitioners on how to elicit dependence, although there has been some work in the literature on methods for eliciting correlated quantities in specific situations (see, for example, Daneshkhah and Oakley, 2010, for an overview) Given the challenges and complexity of eliciting multivariate summaries,

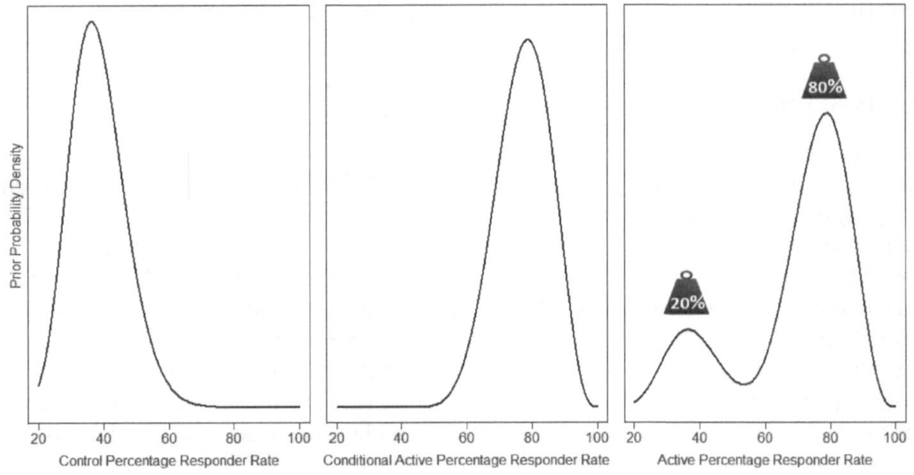

FIGURE 5.2: Example of bimodal prior elicitation.

it is generally recommended to try and address elicitation of dependent quantities by re-defining the quantities of interest in such a way that they can reasonably be assumed to be independent — this is called *elaboration* or *structuring*. Standard methods for eliciting a single quantity can then be used.

5.2.3.1 Structuring

Suppose we are eliciting an expert's belief about both control and active responses. While what an expert believes about the response on treatment will often depend on what he/she believes about the control response, the expert may be willing to assume that the difference between active and control is independent of the value of the control response. We could then first elicit an independent prior for the control response, and then elicit the beliefs about the active response conditional on assuming a particular value for the control response (typically, the mean or mode of the elicited control prior). This conditional distribution can then be converted into a prior for either the relative or absolute treatment difference between active and control (by simply subtracting or dividing by the fixed control value), and then combined (e.g. by Monte Carlo simulation) with the prior for the control response to derive an unconditional (but correlated) prior for the active response. Alternatively, we often elicit the experts' beliefs about the absolute or relative treatment difference directly. The choice of absolute or relative difference will depend on which measure of treatment effect the experts think is most independent of the control response, as well as the type of endpoint (e.g. for mean responses the absolute difference is often used, whereas for rates or risks the relative difference is more often used), and this should be discussed and agreed with the experts at the start of the elicitation.

Another scenario involving correlated quantities is elicitation of parameters for dose-response modeling. For example, we may require prior distributions for the E_{max}, E_0 and ED_{50} parameters of the three-parameter E_{max} model (see Seber and Wild, 2003, and Chapter 7), which are known to be highly correlated. Additionally, experts may be unfamiliar and uncomfortable providing beliefs about these parameters. Rather than directly eliciting expert beliefs about each of these parameters and their dependencies, Huson and Kinnersley (2009) recommend to elicit expert beliefs about the true response for each of a pre-specified set of doses of interest. We then map these beliefs onto the dose-response model parameters by treating the elicited prior for each dose as if it was the sampling distribution for the response at that dose, and fitting an appropriate Bayesian dose-response model with vague priors. The resulting joint 'posterior' distribution for the model parameters represents the implied expert belief distribution for those parameters (see Example 2 in Section 5.3). Note that this approach is similar to earlier methods proposed by Kadane et al. (1980) for eliciting parameters of a Normal linear regression model by asking experts to provide their opinion about quantiles of the response variable at various design points (specific values of the covariates). Even when we are only interested in eliciting beliefs about a single quantity, it can often be helpful to consider breaking the elicitation problem down into a series of components that can be thought about individually. Separate priors can be elicited for each component and then combined to form an overall prior for the quantity of interest.

5.2.4 Combining judgments from multiple experts

When elicitation is used to provide expert input to a decision problem with substantial consequences, we generally want to use the skill of several experts to ensure that range of available knowledge, perspectives and interpretations is represented. There are many legitimate reasons as to why expert opinions will differ and understanding the source of differences between experts can often be as, or more, valuable than any aggregate finding. Nevertheless, it is usually desirable, where possible, to obtain a single distribution that encapsulates the beliefs of several experts and which can be used for decision making and/or analysis.

There is extensive literature on strategies to combine experts' probabilistic judgments – good overviews can be found in Clemen and Winkler (1999), O'Hagan et al. (2006) and European Food Safety Authority (2014). These strategies fall into one of two main classes. The first is to mathematically combine the experts' individual prior distributions into a single distribution. This approach is referred to as *mathematical aggregation* (and the resulting prior is sometimes called a *community prior* (see Lesaffre and Lawson, 2012, p. 123). The second is to create an interaction between the experts, through which a single distribution is elicited from the group as a whole — either directly or, more usually, following an initial stage where prior distributions are elicited individually for each expert and then shared and debated with the group. This is referred to as *behavioral aggregation*, leading to a *consensus prior* (Lesaffre and Lawson, 2012, p. 123). See below for further details of each approach.

Both approaches have pros and cons, and although several attempts have been made to empirically compare different aggregation methods, these have been conducted in an experimental setting as opposed to occurring in the context of a real-world decision analysis and conclusions are hard to generalize (Clemen and Winkler, 2007). The process of behavioral aggregation can help to provide insights and resolve differences of opinion and build commitment to the eventual decision/analysis for which the prior is being elicited. On the other hand, there is a danger that minority or extreme opinions may be lost in building a common group view. Behavioral aggregation requires a trained facilitator to manage the elicitation process and the interactions between the experts to ensure that the process is not dominated by only one or two experts. For a planning or a regulatory decision with a wide variety of stakeholders, mathematical aggregation can be an advantage, both because it is explicit, auditable and, in a sense, objective; and also, because it leaves all opinions and eventualities in the analysis. However, when individual priors are very diverse, then mathematical pooling may create an average set of judgments that lacks any substantive meaning. Ultimately, the choice of aggregation method should be guided by the purpose to which the prior will be used, together with practical considerations such as the feasibility of convening all the experts together (either face-to-face or virtually) weighed against the perceived desirability of exchanging information by enabling interaction between the experts.

5.2.4.1 Behavioral aggregation

Several frameworks have been developed for conducting an expert elicitation using behavioral aggregation. Two of the most popular approaches are the *SHeffield ELicitation Framework* (SHELF) and the *Delphi method*.

SHELF (SHeffield ELicitation Framework)

The *SHeffield ELicitation Framework* (Oakley and O'Hagan, 2016) is a package of documents, templates and software that allows the user to carry out elicitation of probability distributions for uncertain quantities from a group of experts. The SHELF approach is a formal protocol for elicitation, and requires the experts to meet face-to-face (or via video conference) to enable verbal interaction between them. SHELF also requires a facilitator who has expertise in the process of elicitation. The facilitator guides the experts, manages the process and at the end delivers the elicited probability distribution. SHELF provides not only the tools for a facilitator, but advice on their use.

The SHELF protocol involves initially eliciting each individual expert's prior independently and then seeking what is called a 'consensus' or *Rational Impartial Observer* (RIO) *prior.* The RIO consensus prior is intended to represent what it would be reasonable for an independent, impartial observer to think based on the collective views expressed by the group of experts. Importantly, it does not have to be a consensus in the sense that all the experts accept it as a representation of their individual beliefs. A key feature of the SHELF protocol for obtaining a consensus prior is the opportunity for each expert to provide a verbal justification for their individual prior, and for other experts to challenge and debate these views. Careful facilitation is required to manage this debate, and to guide the experts to determine their final consensus prior.

The accompanying `SHELF` software is an `R` package (Oakley, 2018) that provides graphical tools to support elicitation and recording of individual priors and consensus distributions. The software supports use of tertiles, quartiles or roulette for eliciting individual judgments; any of these methods can also be used to aid elicitation of the RIO consensus prior (although roulette is generally not recommended as it can be cumbersome to use with a group). The software also supports use of the probability method for this stage. Note that the SHELF authors do not recommend using probability method for individual judgments due to the potential for anchoring bias, as noted above. At the group stage, there is less risk of anchoring bias because the experts have already provided their initial beliefs about the likely value of the quantity of interest, and so the facilitator can select appropriate values based on the individual judgments, and ask the experts to collectively agree on the probability that the quantity of interest is higher or lower than each chosen value. The `SHELF R` package also implements methods to select and graphically display the parametric distribution (Normal, Student-t, Scaled Beta, LogNormal, LogStudent-t or Gamma) that provides the best fit to each expert's values. An option is also available to mathematically aggregate several individual priors using the linear pool method (see below) and display this alongside all the individual priors.

The most recent version of `SHELF (version 3.0)` has also been extended to include two multivariate elicitation methods that can be used for eliciting individual priors for two or more correlated quantities when it is not possible to remove the dependence through structuring:

- The *Dirichlet method* can be used to elicit a multivariate prior for a set of proportions that must sum to 1; for example, the proportion of subjects scoring in each category of a patient-reported outcome scale. The method works by eliciting independent marginal Beta prior distributions for the proportion in each category, and then adjusting these to find the closest set of Beta marginals that are compatible with a Dirichlet joint distribution.

- The *Gaussian copula method* is more flexible, and can be used to construct a general multivariate distribution for two or more correlated quantities. Marginal distributions (of any functional form) are first elicited for each quantity; one extra judgment is then required for each pair of quantities. This is the concordance probability, which is the probability that the true values of the two quantities will both be on the same side of their elicited medians (i.e. both above their medians or both below). The functional form of the resulting joint distribution is complex but it is straightforward to simulate from.

See the `SHELF R` package documentation (Oakley, 2018) for more details.

Delphi method

The *Delphi method* was originally developed by the RAND corporation in the 1950s for use in classified studies conducted for the US Air Force on bombing requirements (Dalkey and Helmer, 1972). The Delphi framework is an iterative, questionnaire-based approach whereby experts initially independently produce a prior using a survey type tool, together with a brief written justification for their beliefs. Then, through a process of controlled interaction, each expert is given the opportunity to review the anonymized opinions from their peers and to update their prior distribution(s). This process continues iteratively until a consensus prior emerges or the facilitator decides to stop and mathematically aggregate the individual priors. Anonymity of experts is a specific feature of the Delphi protocol, as the technique is intended to reduce the social and political pressures to accept judgments that can arise in interacting groups. By removing identifying information from feedback, it is supposed that experts can/will concentrate on the merits of the feedback information itself without being influenced by potentially irrelevant cues.

The original Delphi method was developed to capture point estimates only and not the uncertainty around these, and there are several online tools available to facilitate use of the Delphi approach in this context. However, the approach can be extended to elicit uncertainty as well, called probabilistic Delphi (see European Food Safety Authority, 2014, Section 6.3). An advantage of the Delphi method is that experts do not have to come together for a face-to-face or video conference meeting, and it eliminates the psychological issues of group discussion. However, there is a risk that experts do not fully engage in the process and careful training and feedback are required to ensure that each expert understands the process and the questions being asked. The limited interaction between experts also loses a principle benefit of the behavioral aggregation approach. Our experience of using prior elicitation to support internal decision-making in a large drug development organization suggests that the process of negotiation among experts and exchange of rationale for the individual priors during the group stage of the elicitation is of value in its own right, allowing stakeholders to see the diversity of opinions that experts hold about a potential drug effect and to uncover the reasons for heterogeneity, and potential resolution of these differences, in a totally transparent way.

Mathematical pooling

Mathematical pooling uses a suitable mathematical formula to combine the individual expert's probability distributions without providing experts with any feedback about the other experts' judgments or justifications. There are two main approaches to mathematical aggregation: opinion pooling and so-called supra-Bayesian methods. We summarize some of the most widely used methods below; see Clemen and Winkler (2007) and European Food Safety Authority (2014) for detailed reviews.

Two commonly-used formulae for opinion pooling are the *linear pool* and the *logarithmic (or multiplicative) pool*. Using the linear pool, a consensus distribution $f(\theta)$ is obtained as a weighted arithmetic mean of the individual distributions $\{f_1(\theta),\ldots,f_n(\theta)\}$ with weights w_i $(i=1,\ldots,n)$ summing to 1:

$$f(\theta)=\sum_{i=1}^{n} w_i f_i(\theta).$$

Alternatively, the logarithmic pool takes a weighted geometric mean of the individual distributions:

$$f(\theta)=k\prod_{i=1}^{n} f_i(\theta)^{w_i},$$

where k is a normalizing constant that ensures $f(\theta)$ integrates to 1. These two methods can lead to very different consensus prior distributions, as illustrated in Figure 5.3: the logarithmic opinion pool is based on the intersection of individual beliefs (which can be thought of as finding a compromise distribution) whereas the linear pool covers the range of the individual beliefs (and so perhaps better reflects a consensus distribution).

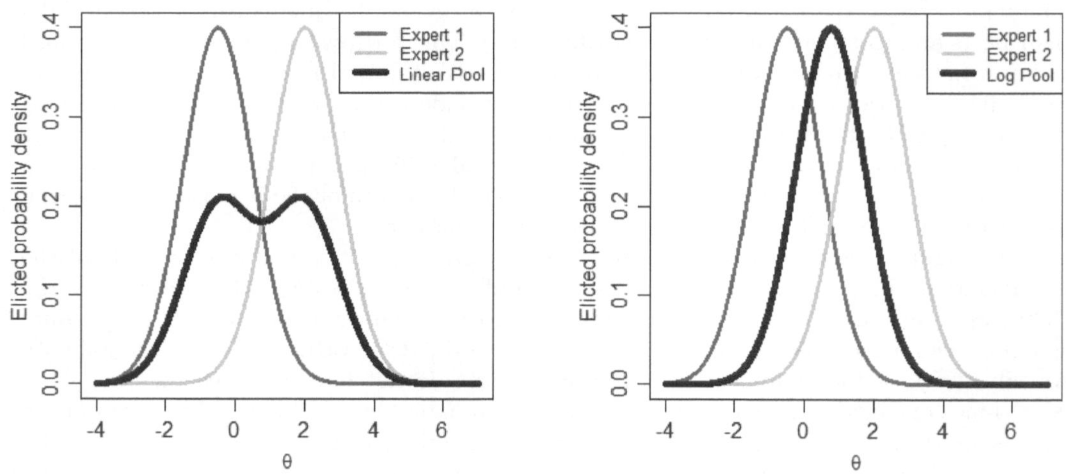

FIGURE 5.3: Example of linear pool (left) and logarithmic pool (right) of individual priors from two experts.

Another challenge is how to weight each expert in the opinion pool. The decision-maker may choose to weight each expert equally, or may assign higher weight to those experts who he/she considers to have greatest expertise. One attempt to assign objective weights to each expert is due to Cooke (1991). Cooke's method uses 'seed questions' in which experts provide probability assessments on quantities for which the decision-maker knows the answer, in order to calculate a measure of the extent to which the experts are calibrated. This calibration measure is then used to assign a weight to each expert. However, it can be difficult to identify relevant seed questions within the experts' general domain for which the true value is available but unlikely to be known with certainty by the experts themselves.

As an alternative to averaging and pooling individual priors to provide a mathematical consensus, *supra-Bayesian methods* can be used. Supra-Bayesian methods are philosophically appealing since they allow the decision-maker to formulate a prior using the elicited information from the experts as data that may be combined with his/her own initial prior distributions via Bayes' rule. Several supra-Bayesian models have been proposed (for example, see Albert et al., 2012, and references therein), and while it has been argued that a Bayesian updating scheme is the most appropriate method to combine information provided by a group of experts for a decision-maker (e.g. Genest and Zidek, 1986), this approach can be complex and difficult to implement in practice. In addition to requiring the decision-maker to conduct an elicitation exercise of their own beliefs, the major feature that makes supra-Bayesian aggregation difficult is the high correlation that typically occurs among the experts' opinions, which needs to be reflected in the likelihood function representing the experts' probability distributions.

5.2.5 Challenges of conducting a prior elicitation

There are many technical and statistical challenges, which can lead to bias in prior elicitation sessions. It is important to be aware and proactively address these when running the elicitation process. O'Hagan (2018) summarizes the keys to a good elicitation as follows:

1. Pay attention to the literature on psychology of elicitation. How you ask a question influences the answer;
2. Ask about the right things: things that experts are likely to assess most accurately;
3. Prepare thoroughly and provide help and training for experts.

There is diverse literature on the heuristics, or rules of thumb, that most people (including experts) employ to make judgments under uncertainty. Several common biases can be attributed to the use of these judgment heuristics. For example, when people are asked to estimate a certain quantity, they often start with an initial estimate (an 'anchor') and then adjust up or down. This is known as the *anchor-and-adjustment heuristic*. Unfortunately, people tend to stick too closely to the initial anchor and do not adjust sufficiently, leading to anchoring bias in their judgments. See Chapter 3 of O'Hagan et al. (2006) and Kynn (2008) for further details of the main heuristics and biases that affect human judgments. Morgan (2014) observes that "because experts are human, there is simply no way to eliminate cognitive bias and overconfidence. The best one can hope to do is to work diligently to minimize its influence".

The potential for introducing bias into an expert elicitation can be reduced by training experts and making them aware of the common pitfalls that people encounter when making judgments under uncertainty, and by following a rigorous protocol for conducting the elicitation, such as those outlined in above. O'Hagan has developed an online training course that can be taken by experts before taking part in an elicitation session conducted using the SHELF framework (`http://www.tonyohagan.co.uk/shelf/ecourse.html`). Most importantly, the facilitator needs to be aware of the key heuristics and biases, which affect human judgments and decision making and understand how he/she can reduce or avoid these. Dallow et al. (2018) provide some further commentary on typical challenges they encountered when conducting prior elicitation within a large drug development organization, and propose some strategies to minimize or overcome these.

5.3 Examples

There is a growing number of examples of use of prior elicitation in drug development. Kinnersley (2015, Table 3) conducted a systematic review of the clinical trial literature on use of expert elicitation, and summarizes 22 clinical trial examples in which expert elicitation was used as a prospective part of the trial design. Dallow et al. (2018) and Crisp et al. (2018) discuss several examples of how prior elicitation has been used within one pharmaceutical company to support clinical trial design and decision making, primarily to inform Bayesian calculations of probability of success (assurance) of different study designs. There has also been some limited application of prior elicitation in areas such as model-based health technology assessment (Soares and Bojke, 2018).

5.3.1 Example 1: Elicitation to support calculation of assurance (probability of success) of a planned clinical trial design within a large pharmaceutical company

Here we take one of the examples from Dallow et al. (2018) to illustrate several features of prior elicitation methodologies discussed in the previous section. This elicitation focused on a fixed-dose combination (FDC) of two different drugs with different mechanisms of action. Positive data were reported in a Phase II PoC study in an allergen challenge model in which rhinitis patients were exposed to controlled amounts of allergen and the effect of the FDC was assessed using symptom scores. The next planned study was to assess the FDC in a Phase III study assessing rhinitic patients in a real-world environmental setting. In addition to the PoC study, data were also available from other similar in-house molecules assessed both in the challenge model as well as an environmental setting, plus summary results from a similar FDC in a series of Phase III trials. This set of data allowed the degree of association between Phase III response and PoC response to be assessed.

The team developing the Phase III study was required to provide an estimate of the study's probability of success (termed assurance) to seek agreement with internal governance boards to commit to Phase III and then to optimize the Phase III trial based on levels of assurance. It was decided that although there was a wealth of available data, there were still uncertainties around what the effect of the FDC would be in the setting of Phase III (i.e. environmental setting), so a prior elicitation session was conducted. A group of six experts attended a three hour elicitation workshop. Their expertise spanned knowledge of the disease area, expertise of the mechanisms of action, knowledge of previous development programs relating to the monotherapies, and statistical expertise within the disease area. It was felt that these six experts provided a balance between those who were or were not directly involved in the project (all were internal to the company) and had a wide enough coverage of relevant backgrounds and specific areas of expertise for a successful elicitation.

When planning the elicitation, one consideration was how to structure the quantities to be elicited. A key uncertainty was how the observed treatment difference between FDC and monotherapy in the PoC challenge model would translate to the environmental setting in Phase III. One option was to break down the elicitation question into two parts: (i) elicit beliefs about the true treatment effect for the FDC in the challenge model in the Phase III target population; (ii) elicit beliefs about the relationship between the allergen challenge model treatment effect and the environmental treatment effect. However, after discussing different structuring options with the experts, they expressed a preference for directly eliciting the Phase III environmental treatment effect, rather than separate elicitation of the different components.

The SHELF protocol was used for the elicitation, using the quartile method to elicit each expert's plausible range, median and upper and lower quartiles for the true mean treatment difference between FDC and monotherapy in the Phase III setting. Figure 5.4a illustrates one expert's quartile judgments together with several alternative fitted parametric distributions. Figure 5.4b shows the fitted prior distributions for all six experts, together with the final consensus prior which was obtained using the SHELF behavioral aggregation approach.

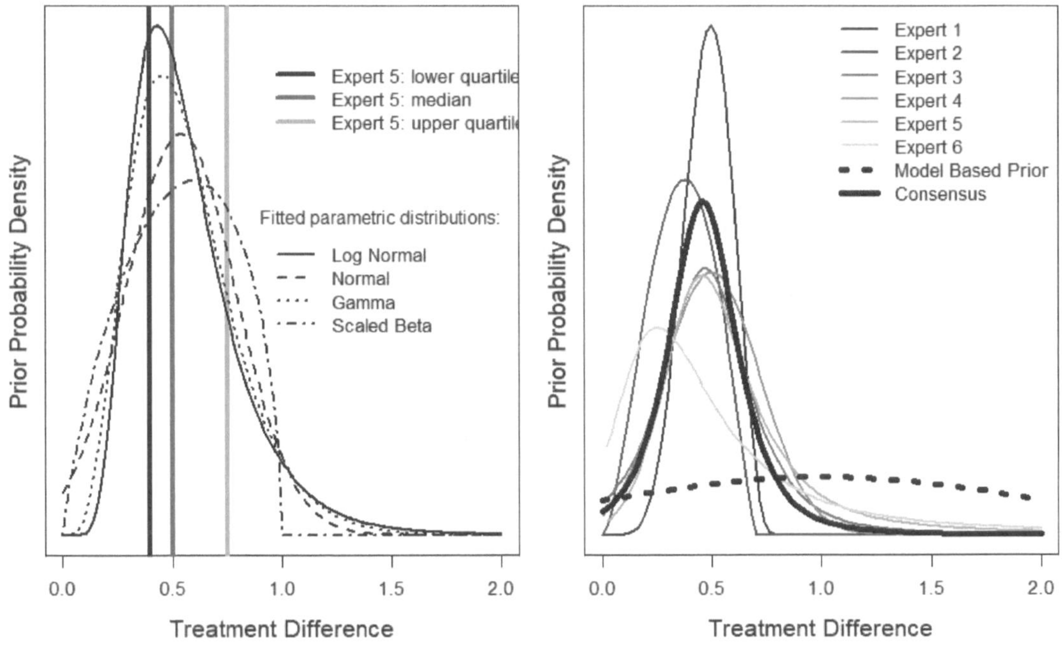

FIGURE 5.4: Rhinitis example from Dallow et al. (2018): (a) Quartile judgments for one expert and fitted parametric prior distributions; (b) Best-fitting individual priors, consensus prior and model-based prior.

In parallel with the expert elicitation, a model-based prior was derived for comparison purposes. For the model-based prior, a logic similar to the 2-step structuring discussed above was used: a linear relationship was assumed between the true treatment differences in the challenge model and environmental settings. A Bayesian hierarchical model was specified for the intercept and slope parameters and fitted to all available PoC (allergen challenge model) and Phase III (environmental) study results from other compounds. The predicted Phase III treatment difference based on the PoC data for the investigational product was then used as the model-based prior. This model-based prior is also shown in Figure 5.4b (bold dotted curve). It is noticeable that this has considerably more uncertainty than the experts' elicited priors. The elicited priors have negligible probability that the treatment effect is less than zero (for the mechanisms of action in this setting, it was considered to be scientifically implausible for the combination to be worse than monotherapy), while the model-based approach suggests this is plausible. Conversely, the model-based prior also has considerable probability of a treatment difference above 1.0, in contrast with the elicited priors. A benefit of the elicited priors is the fact that the experts are able to bring in the broader knowledge of the FDC mechanisms and published data on other molecules leading to belief that the effect would be very unlikely to be negative, while clinical expertise of the disease informed a maximal plausible efficacy threshold. The elicited consensus prior was subsequently used to determine estimates for assurance (approximately 55%), which in turn informed the sample size of the Phase III studies as well as the overall development strategy. As a result of quantifying the risk of failure, the development team favored a staggered approach to the two Phase III studies to mitigate the cost and risk of a parallel Phase III approach. The model-based assurance (approximately 80%) was higher than that based on the elicited prior, and would have led to a less appropriate development plan. See Crisp et al. (2018) for further discussion of the assurance calculations for this case study.

5.3.2 Example 2: Elicitation of dose-response curves

Phase II dose-ranging trials aim to establish the efficacy of a drug and to identify the dosing regime(s) with favorable benefit-risk profile to take forward into confirmatory trials. Dose ranging clinical trial designs have evolved from traditional pairwise comparisons to the more recent focus on model-based approaches involving (typically non-linear) regression modeling of the dose-response relationship. Prior information in the form of data-based or elicited priors for the dose-response curve can be helpful to aid both trial design (e.g. to estimate assurance for designs with different doses, randomization ratios/sample size per dose, trial adaptations, etc.) and/or to increase power and precision of the estimated dose-response curve in the analysis of the trial data.

Kinnersley (2015, Chapter 5) gives a detailed description of an elicitation carried out using the SHELF protocol to elicit parameters of a logistic dose-response model for an academic trial of kisspeptin as a potential treatment for in vitro fertilization (IVF). The aim of the elicitation was to generate prior information to help inform recommendations of alternative study designs that could provide similar information with fewer patients or provide answers to additional questions that would improve the design of subsequent Phase II or III trials. The logistic dose-response model for a binary response variable Y_i given dose x_i $(i = 1, \ldots, n)$ is given by

$$\Pr(Y_i = 1 \mid x_i) = \frac{e^{\beta_0 + \beta_1 x_i}}{1 + e^{\beta_0 + \beta_1 x_i}}.$$

Since eliciting priors for regression coefficients is not straightforward, Kinnersley uses an alternative formulation. He re-expresses the regression coefficients in terms of parameters that reflect observable quantities that are more intuitive to experts to think about: ρ_0 (the probability of response on the lowest dose, denoted x_{min}) and γ (the dose giving the target response rate, θ):

$$\beta_0 = \frac{1}{\gamma - x_{min}} \{\gamma \operatorname{logit}(\rho_0) - x_{min} \operatorname{logit}(\theta)\},$$

$$\beta_1 = \frac{1}{\gamma - x_{min}} \{\operatorname{logit}(\theta) - \operatorname{logit}(\rho_0)\}.$$

Kinnersley notes that the experts were most comfortable with the elicitation of γ using the question "By assuming that a dose-response curve has a plateau at the 90% response rate then where does that plateau start?"; ρ_0 was elicited by asking experts to consider the expected proportion of patients responding in the lowest dose to be used in the trial.

Crisp et al. (2018) also present an example of eliciting dose-response curves, but adopt a slightly different approach to structuring the elicitation. They focus on eliciting priors for the parameters of the three-parameter E_{max} model (Seber and Wild, 2003). However, rather than directly eliciting the model parameters (E_{max}, E_0 and ED_{50}), experts were asked for their beliefs about the true response rate for specific doses. These beliefs are then mapped onto the dose-response model parameters by treating the elicited prior for each dose as if it was the sampling distribution for the response at that dose, and fitting an appropriate Bayesian dose-response model assuming a *functional uniform prior* — that is, a prior that is uniform over the space of potential shapes for the dose-response curve (Bornkamp, 2014). The resulting joint 'posterior' distribution for the model parameters represents the implied expert belief distribution for those parameters.

Both of these dose-response examples illustrate an important aspect of structuring an elicitation exercise, which is that the quantities that the experts were asked to elicit were framed in a language that was familiar to the experts (observable quantities rather than model parameters). One advantage of the Crisp et al. (2018) approach of eliciting beliefs about specific doses is that this also allows for uncertainty about the functional form of the dose-response model. This is illustrated by one of the case studies in Dallow et al. (2018). As with the example in Crisp et al. (2018), expert beliefs were elicited about the true response for each of several doses. A range of standard dose-response models, including linear, log-linear, quadratic, exponential and three-parameter E_{max}, were then fitted to these elicited response distributions for each dose and the experts were shown fitted dose-response profiles and associated uncertainty bands for each model. Experts were then asked to collectively agree which of the fitted curves most appropriately reflected their beliefs about the likely dose-response profile for the drug of interest. Figure 5.5 shows the consensus prior for the response at each of the three doses considered, together with the fitted dose response curves for a selection of different models.

5.3.3 Example 3: Elicitation of treatment response rates for a trial of a very rare disease

Childhood polyarteritis nodosa (PAN) is a serious inflammatory blood vessel disease affecting around one per million children. Untreated, mortality is close to 100%, but with aggressive immunosuppression mortality is around 4%. Cyclophosphamide (CYC) has been the standard treatment for over 35 years, but a research trial (MYPAN) is underway to assess non-inferiority versus CYC of another immunosuppressant, Mycophenolate mofetil (MMF) which is thought to have a lower risk of toxicity. No randomized trials have previously been carried out in children with PAN, and Hampson et al. (2015) report that, due to the rarity of the disease in children, a conventionally-powered non-inferiority trial to compare MMF and CYC would require over 500 patients per arm and take over 30 years to recruit. Regulatory guidance on trials in small populations (European Medicines Agency, 2006) advises that alternative approaches to the design and analysis of such trials might be suitable if they can improve the interpretability of trial results. Hampson et al. (2014, 2015) propose a Bayesian framework for the MYPAN trial, using an expert-elicited informative prior distribution which will then be updated with the data collected from a pragmatically-sized trial (planned to recruit $n = 20$ subjects per arm). They argue that the posterior distribution of the treatment effect would represent the current state of knowledge after the trial had been conducted and may be useful for assessing treatment options even when the limited data available do not allow definitive conclusions to be drawn.

Full details of the MYPAN elicitation can be found in Hampson et al. (2014). Broadly speaking, Hampson et al. (2015) follow an approach similar to the SHELF framework. Individual priors were first elicited from each of 15 expert pediatric consultants from across Europe and Turkey who attended a 2-day face-to-face prior elicitation meeting, before using behavioral aggregation to reach consensus prior distributions. As with all the examples in this chapter, a key feature of the elicitation is how to structure the questions posed to the experts in a way that is familiar to them, and that also appropriately captures correlation when multiple quantities are being elicited. The primary endpoint for MYPAN is probability

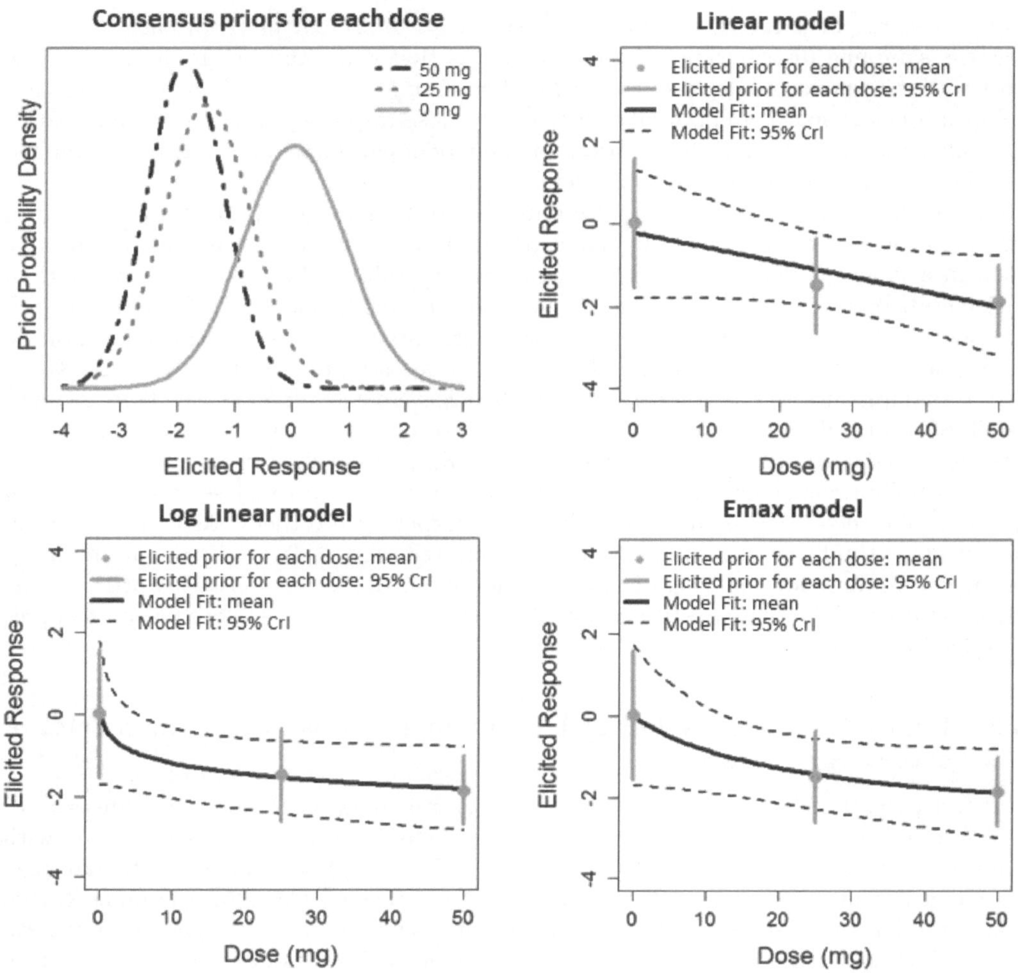

FIGURE 5.5: Consensus prior for the response at each of the three doses and fitted dose response curves for three alternative dose-response models.

of remission within six months, and hence prior distributions were required for p_c and p_e (the probabilities of remission on CYC and MMF, respectively). The authors chose to elicit independent distributions for p_c and θ (the log odds ratio, $\log[p_e(1-p_c)/p_c(1-p_e)]$, since opinions about these two quantities are less likely to be correlated than opinions about p_c and p_e will be. The functional forms of the prior distributions for p_c and θ were then chosen to be Beta(a, b) and N(μ, σ^2), respectively. The authors acknowledge that these functional forms may not accommodate all expert opinion, but argue that it is unlikely that prior knowledge is so detailed that they will not provide an adequate approximation. They also acknowledge that it would be more direct to ask experts about the treatment difference $\Delta = (p_e - p_c)$ rather than the log odds ratio, but argue that assuming a Normal prior for a bounded quantity such as Δ may not be reasonable. Note that an alternative could have been to assume a scaled Beta distribution as the prior for Δ. A mix of variable and fixed interval methods was then used to determine the parameter values of these two priors for each expert. Experts were asked directly for their beliefs about p_c (most likely value and the lower quartile, which were then used to solve for a and b), but - recognizing that log odds ratios can be challenging to interpret — beliefs about θ were elicited indirectly by asking the following questions:

Q1: What is the chance that the 6-month remission rate on MMF is higher than that on CYC?

Q2: What is the chance that the 6-month remission rate on CYC exceeds that on MMF by more than 10%?

The answer to Q1 equates to the prior probability that $p_e > p_c$, which is $\Phi(\mu/\sigma)$ where Φ is the standard Normal distribution function. The answer to Q2 can be expressed as the following integral and solved for σ given values already elicited for a, b and μ/σ:

$$\int_0^1 \int_0^{max(p_c-0.1,0)} g_0(p_c, p_e;\, a, b, \mu/\sigma, \sigma)\, dp_e dp_c,$$

where $g_0(.)$ is the joint prior density of p_e and p_c. See Hampson et al. (2014) for further details.

Each expert was then provided with feedback showing graphical and numerical summaries of their fitted prior distributions, including the implied prior distribution for the remission rate on MMF assuming the remission rate on CYC was equal to the expert's prior mode. The latter distribution was compared to each expert's answers to two additional questions asking for their beliefs about p_e. This is a useful technique to assess goodness of fit of the fitted priors and to detect inconsistencies in experts' opinions. Experts were also provided with the *effective sample size* (ESS; see Chapter 1) of their priors, and Hampson et al. (2014) comment that experts found this very helpful as a measure of the strength of opinion that their distributions represented and was influential on the group's eventual consensus priors (achieved using behavioral aggregation). The ESS for the consensus prior for p_c was five patients, whereas the consensus prior for θ was 'worth' 39 patients on each treatment, reflecting much greater confidence about the relative efficacies of the two treatments than about the absolute remission rates in the pediatric population (see Figure 5.6 for the elicited priors).

5.4 Impact and outlook

In pharmaceutical research and development, we are regularly required to make decisions (e.g. whether to progress a new molecular entity or new biologic to the next phase of development, what doses of a compound to test, how many subjects to study, whether a medicine approved for use in adults is safe and efficacious for use in children, etc.) in the face of imperfect evidence. While the cornerstone of pharmaceutical research and development remains the requirement for valid and substantial evidence of efficacy and safety from well-controlled investigations, there are many situations, both in pre- and post-marketing development, where limitations in data and/or our understanding mean that a definitive body of empirical evidence is not available to support inference and decision making. We have discussed several such examples in this chapter, which can be broadly split into two types of scenario:

1. Settings where the available data are only indirectly relevant to the current setting (e.g. different populations, endpoints, or durations, with limited or no empirical data on how these relate to the previously studied setting).

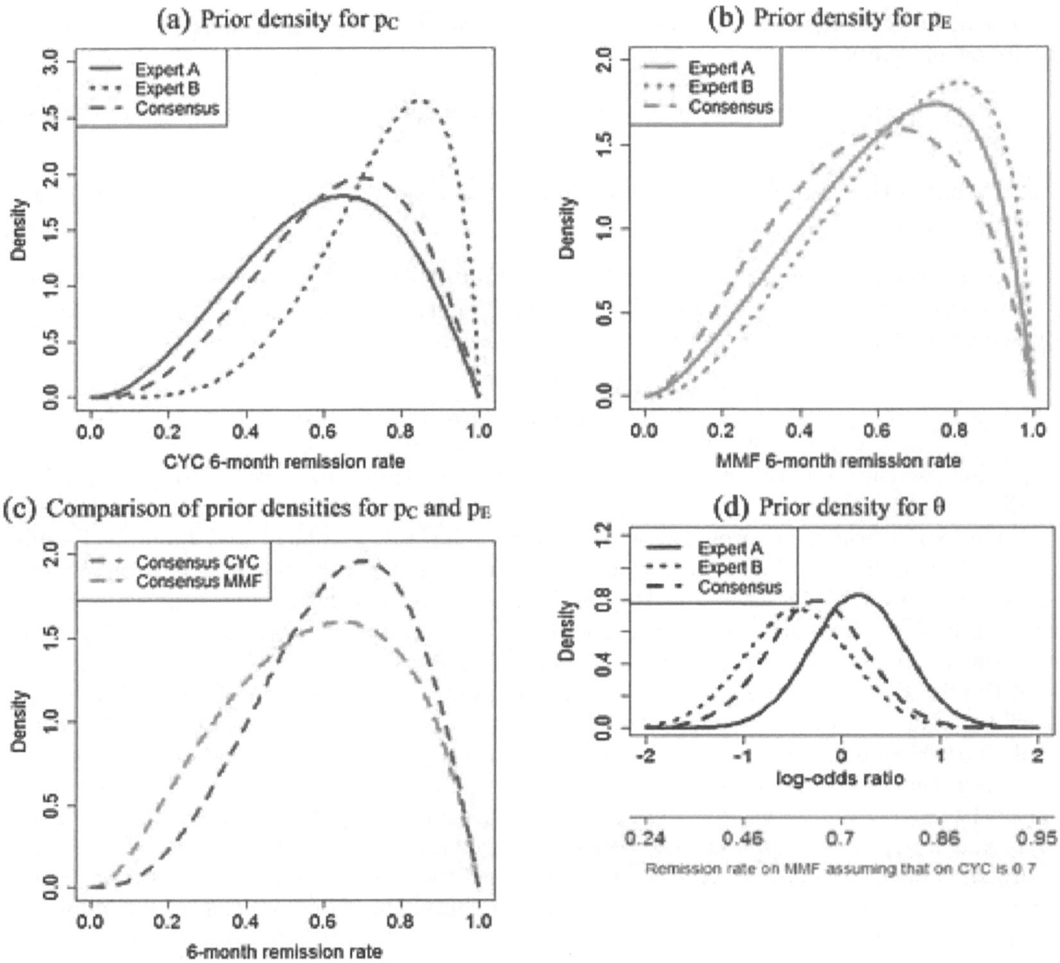

FIGURE 5.6: Prior densities for p_c, p_e and θ elicited from two individuals (labeled experts A and B) and the densities of the consensus prior distributions agreed by the 15 participating experts as representing their collective opinion. Source: Hampson et al. (2014), Figure 2, p. 4191.

2. Settings where little or no relevant data exist, either because the setting is novel (e.g. new mechanism of action or new indication) or because there are ethical and/or logistical constraints on collecting relevant empirical data (e.g. rare diseases, pediatric populations).

In these settings, expert knowledge is a valuable source of information to augment available data or when interpretation or synthesis of data requires expert judgment, and prior elicitation is a key tool that allows for capturing expert beliefs plus appropriate uncertainty in a rigorous and repeatable way.

According to the National Research Council (US) Committee on Estimating the Health-Risk-Reduction Beneffts of Proposed Air Pollution Regulations (2002), the rigorous use of expert elicitation for the analyses of risks is considered to be quality science, and the present authors' experience of using expert elicitation at a major pharmaceutical company endorses the value of this process. During 2015-2018 we have conducted over 40 formal prior elicitation sessions across a variety of therapeutic areas and all phases of drug development using the SHELF approach (see Dallow et al., 2018, for further details). The majority of these elicitations have been used to formulate prior distributions to support clinical trial simulations and assurance calculations to inform scientific and investment board decisions about trial design and probability of success of alternative development strategies. Some of the key benefits we have experienced from the routine use of prior elicitation include that it:

- provides a rigorous way to tap into the wealth of knowledge and experience of medical researchers and drug development scientists in a form that can directly inform decision making;
- is particularly useful when there is an absence of directly relevant data, when there is a translational gap between the completed study(ies) and planned study(ies), where there is a lack of scientific consensus, or when reliable evidence or legitimate models are in conflict;
- provides transparency about the beliefs in the effect(s) of a potential medicine not only by producing a prior probability distribution, but through the process itself, in which all relevant data are summarized and reviewed and expert opinions are discussed, debated and documented.

Both in Dallow et al. (2018) and Crisp et al. (2018) several case studies are discussed where use of prior elicitation has proved impactful. The elicitation process enables the degree of agreement/divergence among experts, and the rationale for this - to be clearly established, enabling project teams to have balanced and transparent discussions at governance boards. Where relevant, assurance calculations based on multiple priors might be presented, e.g. from individual expert opinions, a data-driven prior, and consensus prior, allowing for a better understanding of the risks. In some cases, this may simply provide confidence that the proposed study design is reasonable, and that there are no obvious concerns in terms of re-visiting the fundamental value–proposition of the project. In other cases, this has prompted teams to make critical changes to trial design, e.g. to include a futility interim or make changes to inclusion/exclusion criteria — in order to mitigate risks highlighted by different expert beliefs and the associated assurance calculations (see Case Study 2 in Dallow et al., 2018, for an example).

Experience of using expert elicited priors for Bayesian analysis of clinical trial data is more limited. Use of informative priors based directly on data from other studies is becoming increasingly common in pharmaceutical development, particularly in early phase drug trials (Novick et al., 2018), in pediatric trials (Gamalo-Siebers et al., 2017), and in some medical device trials (Campbell and Yue, 2016). However, to our knowledge, there are no publicly available examples of medicinal product submissions using elicited priors for analysis, which we suspect is largely due to regulatory nervousness at the thought of officially making use of subjective inputs, see Campbell (2016).

The ongoing MYPAN trial discussed above is a potential exception. Here, use of elicited priors for the analysis is proposed as a strategy to enhance interpretability of new trial data in a situation where the feasible sample size is too sparse to allow conclusive inferences to be drawn. A similar approach could be used to support decision making for regulatory or public health purposes in other very rare disease or pediatric settings that lack a good evidence base for treatment decisions, although Hampson et al. (2014) are careful to emphasize that this should only be contemplated when satisfactory sample sizes cannot be accumulated within a reasonable period, and not when a conventional, high-powered trial can (perhaps with some effort, cooperation and adequate funding) be undertaken.

In early phase drug-development, there may be more appetite by sponsors to use elicited prior opinion in a broader range of contexts to inform the analysis of the next study, in order to increase trial efficiency and enable internal decision making based on all available prior knowledge and data, (see Walley et al., 2015, for an example). In all cases, when using informative priors (whether elicited or data-based) for analysis with small anticipated sample sizes, it is important to demonstrate that new trial data has an appropriate chance of shifting prior opinion to avoid trivial and potentially erroneous conclusions (Weber et al., 2018). This can be done by calculation of the posterior under a range of hypothetical future data scenarios, or a formal Bayesian decision theoretic approach could be applied — for example using the elicited priors to calculate the expected value of sample information to determine whether the proposed trial is worthwhile (Welton et al., 2012; Heath and Baio, 2018; Strong et al., 2015).

Another area where use of expert elicited priors has potential value for pharmaceutical research and development is to provide formal judgments about non-identifiable parameters in model-based analyses of trial data. For example, Mason et al. (2017) elicited expert opinion about how missing data on a quality of life endpoint depended on unobserved patient characteristics in a trial comparing two treatment strategies for patients with ruptured abdominal aortic aneurysm. The elicited priors were used to perform sensitivity analysis to alternative assumptions about the missing data. In the MYPAN example, in addition to eliciting expert opinion about the likely remission rate in children, Hampson et al. (2014, 2015) also elicited opinion about the similarity of response rates on each treatment in adults and children. This was used to define informative priors for parameters representing the relevance of data from a trial comparing CYC and MMF in adults; the original elicited priors for the pediatric response rates were then updated to incorporate the adult data down-weighted by the relevance priors.

Done well, expert elicitation can make a valuable contribution to informed decision making. It is not a substitute for rigorous empirical evidence, and should be undertaken only when the state of knowledge given the best available research and analysis will remain insufficient to support timely informed assessment and decision making. However, as discussed in this chapter, there are many situations in pharmaceutical research and development where this is the case, and where the prior elicitation process can provide a formal bridge to a missing link between scientific beliefs and how clinical trials are designed, interpreted and acted upon.

Bibliography

Albert, I., Donnet, S., Guihenneuc-Jouyaux, C., Low-Choy, S., Mengersen, K., and Rousseau, J. (2012). Combining expert opinions in prior elicitation. *Bayesian Analysis*, 7:503–532.

Bornkamp, B. (2014). Practical considerations for using functional uniform prior distributions for dose-response estimation in clinical trials. *Biometrical Journal*, 56(6):947–962.

Campbell, G. (2016). Bayesian submissions to FDA and the evidentiary standard for effectiveness: the CDRH experience. `https://pharm.ucsf.edu/sites/pharm.ucsf.edu/files/campbell.pdf`.

Campbell, G. and Yue, L. (2016). Statistical innovations in the medical device world sparked by the FDA. *Journal of Biopharmaceutical Statistics*, 26(1):3–16.

Clemen, R. and Winkler, R. (1999). Combining probability distributions from experts in risk analysis. *Risk Analysis*, 19(2):187–203.

Clemen, R. and Winkler, R. (2007). Aggregating probability distributions. In Edwards, W., Miles, R., and von Winterfeldt, D., editors, *Advances in Decision Analysis: From Foundations to Applications*, pages 154–176. Cambridge University Press.

Cooke, R. (1991). *Experts in Uncertainty: Opinion and Subjective Probability in Science.* Oxford University Press, New York, NY.

Crisp, A., Miller, S., Thompson, D., and Best, N. (2018). Practical experiences of adopting assurance as a quantitative framework to support decision making in drug development. *Pharmaceutical Statistics*, 17(4):317–328.

Dalkey, N. and Helmer, O. (1972). An experimental application of the Delphi Method to the use of experts. *RAND Corporation, Santa Monica, CA Report RM-727/1.*

Dallow, N., Best, N., and Montague, T. (2018). Better decision making in drug development through adoption of formal prior elicitation. *Pharmaceutical Statistics*, 17(4):301–316.

Daneshkhah, A. and Oakley, J. (2010). Eliciting multivariate probability distributions. In Böcker, K., editor, *Rethinking Risk Measurement and Reporting*, volume I, page 23. Risk Books, London.

European Food Safety Authority (2014). Guidance on expert knowledge elicitation in food and feed safety risk assessment. *EFSA Journal*, 12(6):3734.

European Medicines Agency (2006). Guideline on Clinical Trials in Small Populations. "http://www.ema.europa.eu/docs/en_GB/document_library/Scientific_guideline/2009/09/WC500003615.pdf".

Gamalo-Siebers, M., Savic, J., Basu, C., Zhao, X., Gopalakrishnan, M., Gao, A., Song, G., Baygani, S., Thompson, L., Xia, H., Price, K., Tiwari, R., and Carlin, B. (2017). Statistical modeling for Bayesian extrapolation of adult clinical trial information in pediatric drug evaluation. *Pharmaceutical Statistics*, 16(4):232–249.

Genest, C. and Zidek, J. (1986). Combining probability distributions: a critique and an annotated bibliography. *Statistical Science*, 1(1):114–135.

Gosling, J., Oakley, J., and O'Hagan, A. (2007). Nonparametric elicitation for heavy-tailed prior distributions. *Bayesian Analysis*, 2(4):693–718.

Hampson, L., Whitehead, J., Eleftheriou, D., and Brogan, P. (2014). Bayesian methods for the design and interpretation of clinical trials in very rare diseases. *Statistics in Medicine*, 33(24):4186–4201.

Hampson, L., Whitehead, J., Eleftheriou, D., Tudur-Smith, C., Jones, R., Jayne, D., Hickey, H., Beresford, M., Bracaglia, C., Caldas, A., Cimaz, R., Dehoorne, J., Dolezalova, P., Friswell, M., Jelusic, M.and Marks, S., Martin, N., McMahon, A.-M., Peitz, J., Royen-Kerkhof, A. v., Soylemezoglu, O., and Brogan, P. (2015). Elicitation of expert prior opinion: Application to the MYPAN trial in childhood polyarteritis nodosa. *PLOS One*, 10(3):e0120981.

Heath, A. and Baio, G. (2018). Calculating the expected value of sample information using efficient nested Monte Carlo: A tutorial. *Value in Health*, 21(11):1299–1304.

Huson, L. W. and Kinnersley, N. (2009). Bayesian fitting of a logistic dose-response curve with numerically derived priors. *Pharmaceutical Statistics*, 8(4):279–286.

Kadane, J., Dickey, J., Winkler, R., Smith, W., and Peters, S. (1980). Interactive elicitation of opinion for a normal linear model. *Journal of the American Statistical Association*, 75:845–854.

Kinnersley, N. (2015). Incorporation of expert beliefs in the two-parameter Bayesian logistic dose response model. PhD Thesis. "http://spiral.imperial.ac.uk/handle/10044/1/26228".

Kynn, M. (2008). The 'heuristics and biases' bias in expert elicitation. *Journal of the Royal Statistical Society — Series A*, 171(1):239–264.

Lesaffre, E. and Lawson, A. (2012). *Bayesian Biostatistics*. Statistics in Practice. Wiley.

Mason, A., Gomes, M., Grieve, R., Ulug, P., Powell, J., and Carpenter, J. (2017). Development of a practical approach to expert elicitation for randomised controlled trials with missing health outcomes: Application to the IMPROVE trial. *Clinical Trials*, 14(4):357–367.

Morgan, M. (2014). Use (and abuse) of expert elicitation in support of decision making for public policy. *Proceedings of the National Academy of Sciences of the United States of America*, 111(20):7176–7184.

National Research Council (US) Committee on Estimating the Health-Risk-Reduction Beneffts of Proposed Air Pollution Regulations (2002). Estimating the Public Health Beneffts of Proposed Air Pollution Regulations. "http://www.ncbi.nlm.nih.gov/books/NBK221030/".

Novick, S., Ho, S., and Best, N. (2018). Data-driven prior distributions for a Bayesian phase-2 COPD dose-finding clinical trial. *Statistics in Biopharmaceutical Research*, 10(3):166–175.

Oakley, J. (2018). SHELF. R Package version 1.4.0. "https://CRAN.R-project.org/package=SHELF".

Oakley, J. and O'Hagan, A. (2016). SHELF: the Sheffield Elicitation Framework (version 3.0). "http://tonyohagan.co.uk/shelf".

O'Hagan, A. (2018). Elicitation with SHELF. Course book. "http://tonyohagan.co.uk/shelf".

O'Hagan, A., Buck, C., Daneshkhah, A., Eiser, J., Garthwaite, P., Jenkinson, D., Oakley, J., and Rakow, T. (2006). *Uncertain Judgements: Eliciting Experts' Probabilities*. Statistics in Practice. Wiley.

O'Hagan, A., Stevens, J., and Campbell, M. (2005). Assurance in clinical trial design. *Pharmaceutical Statistics*, 4(3):187–201.

Seber, G. and Wild, C. (2003). *Nonlinear Regression*. Wiley Series in Probability and Statistics. Wiley.

Soares, M. and Bojke, L. (2018). Expert elicitation to inform health technology assessment. In Dias, L., Morton, A., and O'Quigley, J., editors, *Elicitation: The Science and Art of Structuring Judgement*, International Series in Operations Research & Management Science, pages 479–494. Springer International Publishing.

Strong, M., Oakley, J., Brennan, A., and Breeze, P. (2015). Estimating the expected value of sample information using the probabilistic sensitivity analysis sample: A fast, nonparametric regression-based method. *Medical Decision Making*, 35(5):570–583.

Walley, R., Smith, C., Gale, J., and Woodward, P. (2015). Advantages of a wholly Bayesian approach to assessing efficacy in early drug development: a case study. *Pharmaceutical Statistics*, 14(3):205–215.

Weber, K., Hemmings, R., and Koch, A. (2018). How to use prior knowledge and still give new data a chance? *Pharmaceutical Statistics*, 17(4):329–341.

Welton, N., Sutton, A., Cooper, N., Abrams, K., and Ades, A. (2012). *Evidence Synthesis for Decision Making in Healthcare*. Statistics in Practice. Wiley.

6

Use of Historical Data

Beat Neuenschwander
Novartis Pharma AG, Switzerland

Heinz Schmidli
Novartis Pharma AG, Switzerland

The use of historical data has gained growing interest and acceptance in recent years. This is not surprising since the call for making better use of all relevant evidence, for adopting adaptive designs, and for embracing Bayesian approaches has been loud and clear. Appropriately implemented, they help speed up and improve drug development for the benefit of patients. The chapter provides an overview of current approaches to using historical data and a more detailed presentation of the hierarchical meta-analytic-predictive approach. It emphasizes the importance of between-trial heterogeneity as the key quantity to discount historical data relative to the data in the actual trial. As a motivating example, the use of historical data on children with Guillain-Barré syndrome, a rare neurologic disease, is discussed. In addition, non-inferiority trials, which compare a test to an active control treatment, are discussed since they rely on historical trials comparing the active control treatment to placebo. Over the past decades, the topic of historical data has evolved considerably, which is reflected in the recent R-package `RBesT` (`https://CRAN.R-project.org/package=RBesT`) and an extensive list of references covering contributions from industry, academia, and health authorities.

6.1 Introduction

Modern drug development and health-technology assessments are complex activities, for which statistical contributions play a key role. They help inform decisions about risks and benefits of compounds, using well-understood inferential methods. Inference is usually of two kinds: either for a single clinical trial, for example when testing for superiority in a randomized clinical trial; or, for multiple trials, carefully selected based on established systematic-review criteria. Both are pillars of modern medical research.

The use of historical data as additional information sits between such single-trial and multiple-trials analyses. The focus is on the actual trial, yet meta-analytic methods combine its data with the historical information. Importantly, the methods discount the historical data and thus respect between-trial heterogeneity, a consequence of the hierarchical data structure.

Such use of historical data has only recently gained wider acceptance, with the exception of pre-clinical research (Kramer and Font, 2017; Spiegelhalter et al., 2004). For clinical trials, the first proposal has been made 40 years ago, putting forward not only selection criteria for historical data but also a solid methodological foundation (Pocock, 1976), which has strongly influenced further developments; for an overview see Spiegelhalter et al., 2004; Viele et al., 2014.

The recent rise in the use of historical data and other extrapolation activities is reflected in encouragements by health authorities (European Medicines Agency, 2006a, 2001; U.S. Food and Drug Administration, 2010, 2015, 2013; Japan's Pharmaceuticals and Medical Devices Agency (PMDA), 2007), inspired by the urge for innovation (European Commission, 2014; U.S. Food and Drug Administration, 2004, 2013; U.S. House of Representatives, 2015). The pressure to innovate drug development is driven by many factors, including costs (Adams and Brantner, 2010; DiMasi et al., 2003) and the obvious goal to get treatments to the patients faster. Recent trials with innovative historical data designs are Baeten et al., 2013; Boonen et al., 2012; Galeva et al., 2013; Inamdar et al., 2014; Schmidli et al., 2019.

In this overview, we discuss the main aspects to be considered when using historical data in clinical trials. After introducing the topic, we go through various methodological aspects in Section 6.4 and provide a concrete implementation based on the familiar and basic hierarchical model for approximately normal data, illustrated by an example for which code is available in Section 6.7. Section 6.5 about non-inferiority trials shows an important application of historical placebo and active-control data. A discussion and extensive list of references, which reflects the many contributions to this field, concludes the overview.

6.2 Identifying historical or co-data

As a first step, it is important to identify relevant data from previous or ongoing studies. These historical — or, more generally, co-data (Neuenschwander et al., 2016) — must be selected carefully in the presence of data from other ongoing trials. This requires subject-matter expertise, interactions and a consensus among all stakeholders.

In his seminal paper, Pocock put forward six conditions that should ideally be fulfilled if one wants to use historical control data in a future randomized controlled trial (Pocock, 1976):

1. Such a group must have received a precisely defined standard treatment which must be the same as the treatment for the randomized controls;
2. The group must have been part of a recent clinical study which contained the same requirements for patient eligibility;
3. The methods of treatment evaluation must be the same;
4. The distributions of important patient characteristics in the group should be comparable with those in the new trial;
5. The previous study must have been performed in the same organization with largely the same clinical investigators;
6. There must be no other indications leading one to expect differing results between the randomized and historical controls. For instance, more rapid accrual on the new study might lead one to suspect less enthusiastic participation of investigators in the previous study so that the process of patient selection may have been different.

If not all conditions are fully met, one should take this into account when addressing between-trial heterogeneity and potential systematic biases in the methods of Sections 6.4.3, 6.4.7, and 6.4.8. In addition to Pocock's conditions, techniques from systematic reviews should be applied, as discussed for example in Egger et al. (1995) and Higgins and Green (2008).

6.3 An example: Guillain-Barré syndrome in children

For illustration, we will use data on Guillain-Barré syndrome (GBS), a rare neurologic disease that affects all age groups but is more common in children. We will only consider the control data for children, for whom summary statistics (mean, median, SD) for time to independent walking (in days) have been identified from the original publications; see Goodman and Sladky (2005) for the totality of evidence for children and adults. As can be seen in Table 6.1, not all statistics were reported for all trials; for example, the fourth trial has only the median and sample size.

TABLE 6.1: Guillain-Barré syndrome data for untreated children from five historical studies: mean, median, and standard deviation (SD) for time to independent walking, in days (Goodman and Sladky, 2005).

Study	n	Median	Mean	SD
1. Korinthenberg (1996)	56	40	45.4	24.7
2. Paradiso (1999)	37		58.7	44.0
3. Epstein (1990)	14		60.2	43.6
4. Lamont (1991)	18	43		
5. Graf (1999)	9		50.0	29.0

6.4 Methods

6.4.1 Hierarchical data and between-trial heterogeneity

We assume that relevant historical or co-data $\boldsymbol{Y}_{\mathcal{J}}$ have been identified from J trials

$$\boldsymbol{Y}_{\mathcal{J}} = \{Y_1, \ldots, Y_J\}.$$

The data structure is hierarchical, with respective trial-specific parameters $\theta_1, \ldots, \theta_J$. For simplicity, we will ignore potential nuisance parameters; that is, the θ parameters will only be the parameters of interest (e.g. response rates for a one-group or odds-ratios for a two-group problem). We are interested in learning from historical data about the parameter in a new trial $\theta_\star$, for which the data are (or will be) $Y_\star$.

How much we can learn about $\theta_\star$ depends on the direct evidence $Y_\star$ and the indirect evidence $\boldsymbol{Y}_{\mathcal{J}}$. For the latter, this is determined by the between-trial heterogeneity of the parameters: the more heterogeneous these parameters are, the less relevant the historical data $\boldsymbol{Y}_{\mathcal{J}}$ will be.

6.4.2 Prospective and retrospective views

Before turning to a concrete implementation, it is important to distinguish between two views. Prospectively, at the design stage of the trial, the information about $\theta_\star$ comes entirely from the historical data: probabilistically, it is the conditional distribution

$$p(\theta_\star \mid \boldsymbol{Y}_{\mathcal{J}}). \tag{6.1}$$

We will refer to this as the *meta-analytic-predictive* prior. It requires a Bayesian analysis of the historical data, which must include the prediction of the new parameter $\theta_\star$. Non-Bayesian quantifications of $\theta_\star$ would typically comprise a point estimate, standard error, and confidence interval.

After the data (interim or final) in the new trial have been observed, this direct evidence is then combined to infer $\theta_\star$ This can be done in two ways:

(i) The *meta-analytic-predictive* (MAP) approach combines the MAP prior (6.1) with the new data $Y_\star$ in a standard Bayesian way.

(ii) The *meta-analytic-combined* (MAC) approach takes the retrospective view: it infers $\theta_\star$ by a single analysis that incorporates the historical and new data, leading to

$$p(\theta_\star \mid \boldsymbol{Y}_{\mathcal{J}}, Y_\star).$$

The MAC approach is an equivalent alternative to the two-step MAP approach, which follows from the sequential updating property of Bayes theorem; for a proof see Schmidli et al. (2014). MAC is convenient for interim analyses with concurrent co-data, because re-deriving the prior with the new co-data is not necessary; an example are Phase I dose-escalation trials with co-data from trials running in parallel (Neuenschwander et al., 2015).

6.4.3 The basic normal-normal hierarchical model (NNHM)

We now turn to the basic hierarchical model, which will be extended in subsequent sections. It assumes source-specific data Y_j ($j = 1, \ldots, J$) as approximately normally distributed point estimates with standard errors s_j, possibly after a suitable transformation

$$Y_j \mid \theta_j \sim \mathrm{N}(\theta_j, s_j^2).$$

We will refer to this as the *data model.* In addition, a hierarchical model requires a relationship between parameters, the *parameter model.* The simplest one is

$$\theta_j = \mu + \epsilon_j, \quad \epsilon_j \sim \mathrm{N}(0, \tau^2), \tag{6.2}$$

or, $\theta_j \mid \mu, \tau \sim \mathrm{N}(\mu, \tau^2)$, the familiar random-effects (exchangeability) model.

For the GBS example of Section 6.3, a one-parameter approximation based on exponential data appears unjustified because the mean is consistently larger than the standard deviation (SD). We therefore consider log-normal distributions for the data in Table 6.1, using moment matching for the mean (or median) and SD. For a log-normal distribution with parameters μ and σ, the median, mean, and variance are

$$\exp(\mu), \quad \exp(\mu)\exp(\sigma^2/2), \quad \exp(2\mu)\exp(\sigma^2)(\exp(\sigma^2) - 1),$$

respectively. From these, taking the mean (for studies 1,2,3,5) or median (study 4) and SD will give an estimate of the parameters μ and σ of the respective log-normal distribution. Note that for study 1, taking the median rather than the mean leads to numerically very similar values. Moreover, for study 4 the maximum SD (44) from the other studies has been used for the missing SD; alternatively, the study could have been excluded, if poor reporting had been suspected. From μ and σ, the point estimate and standard error for the log-median of time to independent walking in Table 6.2 are then $y = \mu$ and $s = \sigma/\sqrt{n}$.

TABLE 6.2: Log-normal approximations for the Guillain-Barré data of Table 6.1, with point estimate (y) and standard error (s) of the log-median of time to independent walking (in days).

Study	log-N(μ, σ)	y	s
1. Korinthenberg (1996)	(3.69, 0.509)	3.69	0.068
2. Paradiso (1999)	(3.85, 0.668)	3.85	0.110
3. Epstein (1990)	(3.89, 0.649)	3.89	0.173
4. Lamont (1991)	(3.76, 0.703)	3.76	0.166
5. Graf (1999)	(3.77, 0.538)	3.77	0.179

6.4.3.1 Inference under known heterogeneity

For the inference of the above normal-normal hierarchical model (NNHM), we first consider classical results under the assumption that τ is known. Results for the overall mean μ, trial-specific parameters θ_j, and the new parameter $\theta_\star$ depend on the trial-specific precisions (inverse-variance weights) and total precision

$$w_j = (s_j^2 + \tau^2)^{-1}, \quad w_+ = \sum_{j=1}^{J} w_j. \tag{6.3}$$

They are called precisions because the marginal distributions of Y_j are

$$Y_j \mid \mu, \tau \sim \mathrm{N}(\mu, s_j^2 + \tau^2), \quad j = 1, \ldots, J,$$

and the estimate of μ

$$\widehat{\mu} = \sum_j w_j Y_j / w_+$$

has variance

$$\mathrm{var}(\widehat{\mu}) = 1/w_+.$$

Using the shrinkage factors

$$B_j = \frac{s_j^2}{s_j^2 + \tau^2} = s_j^2 w_j, \quad j = 1, \ldots, J,$$

the results for the trial-specific parameters θ_j (shrinkage estimates) are

$$\widehat{\theta}_j = (1 - B_j)Y_j + B_j\widehat{\mu}, \quad \mathrm{var}(\widehat{\theta}_j) = B_j(\tau^2 + B_j/w_+).$$

For the new parameter $\theta_\star$, for which no data are available when designing the trial ($s_\star = \infty, B_\star = 1$), the corresponding result is

$$\widehat{\theta}_\star = \widehat{\mu}, \quad \mathrm{var}(\widehat{\theta}_\star) = 1/w_+ + \tau^2.$$

This would be the prior information for $\theta_\star$ if τ were known. The formula shows that increasing amounts of historical data (larger J, smaller s_j) only help reduce the variance of

$\widehat{\mu}$ $(1/w_+)$. However, if between-trial heterogeneity is large, uncertainty about $\theta_\star$ remains large due to the second variance term τ^2.

Under the assumption of known heterogeneity τ, the Bayesian results are numerically equivalent to the classical ones:

$$\mu \mid \boldsymbol{Y_{\mathcal{J}}} \sim \mathrm{N}(\widehat{\mu}, 1/w_+),$$

$$\theta_j \mid \boldsymbol{Y_{\mathcal{J}}} \sim \mathrm{N}\left((1-B_j)Y_j + B_j\widehat{\mu}, B_j(\tau^2 + B_j/w_+)\right),$$

$$\theta_\star \mid \boldsymbol{Y_{\mathcal{J}}} \sim \mathrm{N}(\widehat{\mu}, 1/w_+ + \tau^2).$$

6.4.3.2 Inference under uncertain heterogeneity

While the results of Section 6.4.3.1 are suitable for heterogeneity sensitivity analyses, a principled approach should account for the uncertain τ. It turns out that this complicates inference considerably (Veroniki et al., 2016).

Many non-Bayesian two-step proposals have been made: first choose one of the many available estimates for τ (DerSimonian and Kacker, 2007), and then use this point estimate to infer the main parameter μ, with various suggestions (such as t distributions instead of normal approximations) to account for the uncertainty of the τ estimate. Importantly, the parameter of interest is $\theta_\star$ (not μ), for which recommendations are sparse; an ad-hoc proposal is a t distribution with $J-2$ degrees of freedom (Higgins et al., 2009), which obviously only works for at least three trials.

Another difficulty arises because the number of historical studies is usually small. This may often lead to the too optimistic conclusion of no heterogeneity ($\widehat{\tau}=0$). For example, for two studies, it has been shown that some τ estimators (e.g. the DerSimonian-Laird and MLE) coincide (Rukhin, 2012) and are equal to

$$\widehat{\tau}^2 = \max\left(0, \frac{(Y_1 - Y_2)^2 - (s_1^2 + s_2^2)}{2}\right).$$

This estimate will often be zero for large studies; for an investigation of the difficulties to infer μ arising from few studies, see Friede et al. (2017). These difficulties are most likely aggravated when inferring $\theta_\star$.

The Bayesian approach to the uncertain τ is more promising, but it requires care when specifying its prior (Gelman, 2006; Lunn et al., 2012; Polson and Scott, 2012; Spiegelhalter et al., 2004). This means that one needs to understand the relationship between heterogeneity and τ. In the following, we suggest an approach that may help set up a sensible prior for τ, illustrated for exponential, binary, and normal endpoints.

1) *Heterogeneity scale.* The amount of heterogeneity depends on the scale of the parameter model. Assuming normally distributed θ parameters, we consider the log, logit (log-odds), and identity links for the three endpoints, respectively.

2) *Unit-information standard deviation.* On these scales, we then determine the approximate unit-information standard deviation $\sigma = \sqrt{\mathrm{var}(Y)}$. For an exponential endpoint, $\sigma = 1$ (for one event). For a binary endpoint with response rate $\pi = 0.5$, $\sigma = 2$; more generally $\sigma^2 = \left(\pi(1-\pi)\right)^{-1}$, for example, $\sigma = 2.5$ for $\pi = 0.2$ and $\sigma = 3.33$ for $\pi = 0.1$, respectively.

3) *Degrees of heterogeneity* can then be expressed as values of τ relative to σ. The proposals in Table 6.3 may be convenient defaults, but they may need to be adapted to the specific application (Turner et al., 2012, 2015).

TABLE 6.3: Degrees of heterogeneity for one-group (log-hazard, log-odds, mean) and two-group (log-hazard-ratio, log-odds-ratio, mean difference) parameters θ as a function of the unit-information standard deviation σ.

	One-group θ	Two-group θ
Heterogeneity	τ	τ
Large	$\sigma/2$	$\sigma/4$
Substantial	$\sigma/4$	$\sigma/8$
Moderate	$\sigma/8$	$\sigma/16$
Small	$\sigma/16$	$\sigma/32$

For the one-group case, Table 6.4 shows τ values for the three endpoints. For the exponential and binary distribution ($\pi = 0.5$), the respective population 97.5%-to-median ratio are also shown. For a normal endpoint, the respective difference of quantiles is shown for $\sigma = 8$, which is the approximate standard deviation of a single blood pressure measurement.

For the two-group case, the heterogeneity of contrast parameters is usually smaller than the one for the respective group parameters. Therefore, we suggest to classify heterogeneity using the τ parameters of Table 6.3 and to assess (similar to Table 6.4) the plausibility of the respective population 97.5%-to-median ratio (or difference in the normal case) of trial parameters.

4) *Prior distributions.* Based on these τ values, the prior distribution for τ can then be specified. For weak prior information, we will use a half-normal (HN) or exponential prior with most of their probability mass on small to large heterogeneity (Table 6.5); the latter has maximum entropy for a given mean. For both examples, the second pair of priors is rather conservative: its median lies between substantial and large heterogeneity, in contrast to the first pair of priors (with median between moderate and substantial heterogeneity), which will often be a more sensible representation.

   It should be noted that these one-parameter distributions should not be used when small heterogeneity is unlikely; in such cases, two-parameter distributions that allow moving the bulk of the probability mass away from zero (e.g. Gamma or log-normal) may be used.

   Finally, uniform priors are not recommended (Gelman, 2006; Lunn et al., 2012; Spiegelhalter et al., 2004) for meta-analyses, in particular if the number of trials is small.

For the GBS data of Table 6.2, the results for $\theta_\star$ are summarized in Table 6.6, using the four priors of Table 6.5. The results are very similar for the respective half-normal and exponential priors. However, the very conservative second pair of priors leads to more uncertainty for the new parameter $\theta_\star$.

For the first prior, the results of the MAP analysis are displayed in Figure 6.1 (left panel). It shows the estimates and 95% intervals for stratified trial-specific estimates and the MAP result for the parameter of interest $\theta_\star$. The right panel shows a density plot (solid line) for the Markov Chain Monte Carlo (MCMC) sample of the MAP prior; see Section 6.7 for the `RBesT` code (Weber, 2017).

Table 6.6 also shows the posterior results for τ, which clearly exclude large between-trial heterogeneity. The posterior 95% intervals are shrunk towards zero in comparison to the prior ones, which are $(0.01, 0.36)$, $(0.01, 0.59)$, $(0.01, 0.72)$, and $(0.01, 1.18)$ — from Table 6.5.

TABLE 6.4: Degrees of heterogeneity and respective between-trial standard deviations τ for exponential, binary, and normal one-group data, with population 97.5%-to-median hazard ratio (exponential), odds ratio (binary), and 97.5%-to-median difference (normal); σ is the unit-information standard deviation for the data under the respective log, logit, and identity link.

	Exponential θ: log-hazard $\sigma = 1$	Binary ($\pi = 0.5$) θ: log-odds $\sigma = 2$	Binary ($\pi = 0.1$) θ: log-odds $\sigma = 3.33$	Normal θ: mean $\sigma = 8$
Heterogeneity:				
large	$\tau = 0.5$	$\tau = 1$	$\tau = 1.667$	$\tau = 4$
	ratio = 2.66	ratio = 7.10	ratio = 26.2	diff = 7.84
substantial	$\tau = 0.25$	$\tau = 0.5$	$\tau = 0.833$	$\tau = 2$
	ratio = 1.63	ratio = 2.66	ratio = 5.12	diff = 3.92
moderate	$\tau = 0.125$	$\tau = 0.25$	$\tau = 0.417$	$\tau = 1$
	ratio = 1.28	ratio = 1.63	ratio = 2.26	diff = 1.96
small	$\tau = 0.0625$	$\tau = 0.125$	$\tau = 0.208$	$\tau = 0.5$
	ratio = 1.13	ratio = 1.28	ratio = 1.50	diff = 0.98

TABLE 6.5: Four prior distributions for the between-trial standard deviation τ; σ is the unit-information standard deviation of the outcome Y.

Prior distribution	Median	95% CI
$\tau \sim$ HN(scale=$\sigma/4$)	0.17σ	$(0.01\sigma, 0.56\sigma)$
$\tau \sim$ Exponential(mean=$\sigma/4$)	0.17σ	$(0.01\sigma, 0.92\sigma)$
$\tau \sim$ HN(scale=$\sigma/2$)	0.34σ	$(0.02\sigma, 1.12\sigma)$
$\tau \sim$ Exponential(mean=$\sigma/2$)	0.35σ	$(0.01\sigma, 1.84\sigma)$

However, even though the posterior medians are roughly one tenth of σ, suggesting small to moderate heterogeneity, uncertainty remains large. This can be explained by the small number of trials, a problem that would be aggravated for fewer trials. For the extreme case of one historical trial, the posterior will be equal to the prior, showing that sensible prior specifications become even more important. For example, using the conservative priors 3 or 4 of Table 6.5 would borrow very little information from the historical trial.

TABLE 6.6: Guillain-Barré Syndrome example: Meta-analytic-predictive results for $\theta_\star$ and posterior results for τ, for the two half-normal and exponential priors of Table 6.5; unit-information $\sigma = 0.64$.

	New parameter $\theta_\star$			Between-trial SD τ	
	Mean	SD	95% CI	Median	95% CI
HN(scale=0.16)	3.77	0.122	(3.52, 4.05)	0.064	(0.003, 0.23)
Exponential(mean=0.16)	3.77	0.117	(3.54, 4.02)	0.055	(0.003, 0.23)
HN(scale=0.32)	3.77	0.151	(3.48, 4.09)	0.075	(0.004, 0.31)
Exponential(mean=0.32)	3.77	0.140	(3.50, 4.06)	0.067	(0.003, 0.29)

6.4.3.3 Bayesian Computations

Bayesian computations for the NNHM and its extensions (see following sections) can be done with standard MCMC software (Carpenter et al., 2017; SAS Institute, 2014; Lunn et al., 2012, 2000) or specialized software such as `RBesT` (Weber, 2017). For the basic NNHM,

FIGURE 6.1: Meta-analytic-predictive analysis for Guillain-Barré data: stratified estimates and 95% intervals for trial-specific parameters, and MAP estimate for $\theta_\star$ in left panel, and density estimate of MCMC sample (solid line) with two-component mixture approximation (dotted line) in right panel.

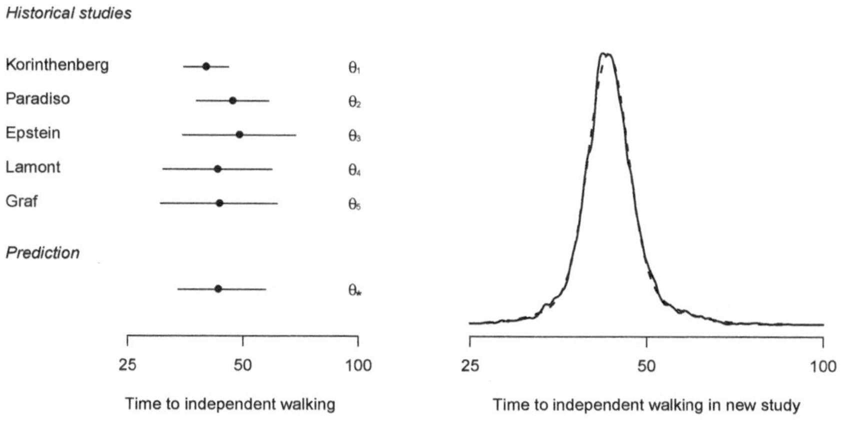

explained above, a non-MCMC approach based on numerical integration can be used as well (Röver, 2015).

6.4.4 Parametric representation of a MAP prior

As MCMC is used for Bayesian evidence synthesis and prediction, no analytical form of the MAP prior is available. Instead, a large sample from the MAP prior is obtained, which is inconvenient for clinical study protocols, medical journals, and reviewers such as health authorities and ethics committees. Moreover, while prior summaries can easily be obtained, combining such a MAP prior with the new data is not straightforward. However, every prior can be well approximated by a mixture of conjugate priors (Dallal and Hall, 1983; Diaconis and Ylvisaker, 1984). For normal endpoints, the MAP prior can be approximated by a mixture of normal distributions,

$$p(\theta_\star \mid \mathbf{Y}_{\mathcal{J}}) = \sum_{k=1}^{K} w_k N(m_k, v_k).$$

The parameters w_k, m_k and v_k can be determined such that the mixture is close to the MAP prior with respect to the Kullback-Leibler divergence (Schmidli et al., 2014). Both numerical criteria and graphical tools can be used to choose an appropriate K. Typically, two or three mixture components provide an acceptable approximation. We used `RBesT` for the mixture approximation in the GBS example. A good approximation of the MAP prior is obtained by the following two-component mixture

$$0.735 \times \mathrm{N}(3.76, 0.076^2) + 0.265 \times \mathrm{N}(3.78, 0.199^2), \tag{6.4}$$

which is shown in the right panel of Figure 6.1 (dotted line).

Mixture representations of MAP priors have two advantages: the prior can be easily communicated, and the posterior distribution from data in a new trial can be evaluated analytically (Schmidli et al., 2014). The latter considerably facilitates evaluation of operating characteristics (Section 6.4.12).

6.4.5 Robustness

If one is concerned about prior-data conflict, that is, the possibility that the historical and new data $\boldsymbol{Y}_{\mathcal{J}}$ and $Y_\star$ contradict each other, a robust version of the original prior should be considered (Box, 1980; O'Hagan and Forster, 2004; O'Hagan and Pericchi, 2012). Such a prior is heavy-tailed, which decreases its influence with increasing prior-data conflict. It can be obtained by a mixture prior of the following form

$$p^R_{MAP}(\theta_\star) = (1 - w_R) \times p_{MAP}(\theta_\star) + w_R \times p_R(\theta_\star). \tag{6.5}$$

Here, $p_{MAP}(\theta_\star)$ is the original MAP prior, for example the two-component mixture (6.4) in the GBS example, and $p_R(\theta_\star)$ is a vague prior. It should be noted that the latter must be proper, and we recommend a unit-information prior (Kass and Wasserman, 1995). The mixture weight w_R should be chosen based on judgment about the relevance of the historical data or based on operating characteristics (see Section 6.4.12, in particular control of type I error). For recent investigations of robust priors in clinical trials, see Li et al., 2016; Mutsvari et al., 2016; Schmidli et al., 2014.

Since priors like (6.5) become less influential under increasing prior-data conflict, this takes for granted that one has stronger beliefs in the data than in the prior. For clinical trials, this will usually be the right thing to do. However, one should always carefully assess the reasons of prior-data conflict. For example, there may be cases where in the actual trial something went wrong or was not as expected, which should be understood when deciding on next steps in the development of a compound.

6.4.6 Effective sample sizes

When using historical data in a new trial, the question about how much these data contribute to the analysis may arise. This can be answered by the *effective sample size* (ESS). If one knows the ESS of the MAP prior $p(\theta_\star \mid \boldsymbol{Y}_{\mathcal{J}})$ (say $ESS_\star$), one may then want to reduce the size of the control group in an upcoming randomized trial by $ESS_\star$.

The influence of the prior via ESS is well understood for members of the one-parameter exponential family. For example, a binary response parameter with prior Beta(a, b) has $ESS = a + b$. For more general situations, various approaches have been proposed. Even though all relate ESS to precisions of $\theta_\star$, they can give fairly different results.

The first, simple idea uses a two-precisions approach (Malec, 2001; Neuenschwander et al., 2010; Pennello and Thompson, 2008). It requires precisions from two analyses: the precision for the analysis of interest, $prec(\theta_\star)$; and, the precision ($prec_0$) of a simpler analysis for which the ESS is known (ESS_0). Assuming that sample sizes are proportional to precisions, it then follows that the ESS of interest is

$$ESS_\star = ESS_0 \times \frac{prec_\star}{prec_0}.$$

Obviously, this does not define a unique ESS because there may be more than one "simple" analysis. However, complete pooling is the obvious analysis. It assumes $\tau = 0$ in the model of Section 6.4.3, for which the precision of $\theta_\star$ is $prec_0 = w_+ = \sum s_j^{-2}$, and $ESS_0 = \sum n_j$, the number of subjects from all trials.

For the example of Section 6.3, the total precision (6.3) and sample size are $prec_0 = 399.8$ and $ESS_0 = 134$. Using the first prior of Table 6.5 and the result of the MAP analysis, the respective ESS is

$$ESS_\star = 134 \times 0.122^{-2}/399.8 \approx 23.$$

For the three other priors, the ESS would be 24, 15, and 17.

A second, technically more involved approximation has been suggested by Morita et al., 2008, 2012; Thall et al., 2014. Unfortunately, for heavy-tailed distributions, the ESS can be quite different. For the two-component mixture of the GBS example, the ESS for the second approach is 52, considerably larger than the one from the first approach (23).

In practice, the various approaches provide a useful range of ESS. From a methodological standpoint, however, an entirely convincing approach to ESS is missing and further research is needed (Neuenschwander et al., in press).

6.4.7 Differential heterogeneity

The heterogeneity across trials, expressed by the single parameter τ in (6.2), assumes the same relevance for all trials, which may not always be reasonable. For example, one may want to account for differential heterogeneity in cases with data from randomized and observational trials, data from company-internal and external studies, or data from children and adult trials.

To account for groups defined by differential heterogeneity, the parameter model needs to be extended. This can be done as follows: for G groups, let the respective between-trial heterogeneity parameters be $\tau_1, \ldots, \tau_G$. Further, let $g(j)$ be the group indicator, which assigns trial j to one of the G groups. Thus, the parameter model under differential heterogeneity is

$$\theta_j = \mu + \epsilon_j, \quad \epsilon_j \sim \mathrm{N}(0, \tau^2_{g(j)}).$$

If the G between-trial standard deviations are known, results similar to the ones in Section 6.4.3.1 are obtained: the Bayesian ones are

$$\mu \mid \mathbf{Y}_{\mathcal{J}} \sim \mathrm{N}(\widehat{\mu}, 1/w_+),$$

$$\theta_j \mid \mathbf{Y}_{\mathcal{J}} \sim \mathrm{N}\left((1-B_j)Y_j + B_j\widehat{\mu}, B_j(\tau^2_{g(j)} + B_j/w_+)\right),$$

$$\theta_\star \mid \mathbf{Y}_{\mathcal{J}} \sim \mathrm{N}\left(\widehat{\mu}, 1/w_+ + \tau^2_{g(\star)}\right),$$

where

$$w_j = (s_j^2 + \tau^2_{g(j)})^{-1}, \quad w_+ = \sum_{j=1}^{J} w_j, \quad \widehat{\mu} = \sum_j w_j Y_j / w_+.$$

What has been said in Section 6.4.3.2 applies here as well. As between-trial standard deviations are not known, priors for the G between-trial parameters will be needed, and they must be chosen sensibly. For example, in a situation with two heterogeneity groups, representing data from observational and randomized trials, a more conservative prior for the former would seem appropriate. Under differential heterogeneity, inferring between-trial heterogeneity becomes even harder since fewer trials contribute to the estimation of each τ.

6.4.8 Systematic biases

So far the parameter model (6.2) assumed all trial parameters centered around the parameter μ. The deviations allow for non-systematic biases, which will be reasonable if criteria for historical data selection have been applied rigorously.

If one wants to include additional data, for which a systematic bias is suspected, it should be accounted for in the model. The idea goes back to Pocock (1976); see Section 6.4.11.1 for the original model formulation. In the NNHM, trial-specific bias parameters δ_j can be added as follows

$$\theta_j = \mu + \delta_j + \epsilon_j, \quad \epsilon_j \sim \mathrm{N}(0, \tau^2).$$

Analyses with systematic biases can be performed in two ways. First, one can assume fixed parameter scenarios for δ_j. These may help sensitivity analyses when taking the retrospective view, that is, when checking conclusions for $p(\theta_\star \mid \boldsymbol{Y}_{\mathcal{J}}, Y_\star)$. This is also simple because the original model can be used with transformed data $Y_j' = Y_j - \delta_j$.

Since the bias parameters are of course not known, one may want to express the uncertainty by prior distributions for δ_j

$$\delta_j \sim \mathrm{N}(m_{\delta_j}, s_{\delta_j}^2).$$

While potentially more data can be incorporated if one allows for systematic biases, the extension of the model becomes clearly more subjective for both approaches. This may, however, be unavoidable in special situations (e.g. for some small populations, rare diseases, and extrapolation problems), where decision making without historical or co-data becomes infeasible.

6.4.9 Covariates

The inclusion of covariates is another extension of the base model. Relevant trial-specific covariates may help to reduce between-trial heterogeneity or even remove systematic biases. If such covariates have been identified (e.g. van Rosmalen et al., 2017), the parameter model can be extended as follows for covariate vectors $\boldsymbol{x_j}$ ($j = 1, \ldots, J$) and regression vector $\boldsymbol{\beta}$

$$\theta_j \mid \mu, \tau, \boldsymbol{\beta} \sim \mathrm{N}(\mu + \boldsymbol{x}_j^\top \boldsymbol{\beta}, \tau^2).$$

The Bayesian implementation requires a prior for $\boldsymbol{\beta}$. This does not pose a serious problem because (as for μ) an uninformative prior can be used, although informative prior distributions may be an option if solid prior information is available.

Finally, it should be noted that a difficulty arises in the prospective setting: to derive the MAP prior $p(\theta_\star \mid \boldsymbol{Y}_{\mathcal{J}})$, the covariates for the new trial $\boldsymbol{x}_\star$ are needed. Retrospectively, $\boldsymbol{x}_\star$ will be known and $\theta_\star$ can be inferred easily.

6.4.10 Further extensions

So far, we only looked at extensions of the parameter model for the main parameters θ_j and $\theta_\star$. Depending on the problem at hand, other extensions may be needed. Here, we briefly mention a few of these extensions.

For the data model, we assumed normal (or approximately normal) parameter estimates. If the original endpoint is not normal, the respective model rather than the normal approximation may be used of course. For example, the model for a binary endpoint would be binomial

$$r_j \mid \pi_j \sim \mathrm{Bin}(\pi_j, n_j), \quad j = 1, \ldots, J.$$

The parameter model would remain the same, using the log-odds transformation $\theta_j = \log(\pi_j/(1 - \pi_j))$. For reasonably large sample sizes, results will usually be similar for the binomial data model and its normal approximation.

More involved data models have been discussed, such as overdispersed count data (Gsteiger et al., 2013), recurrent events (Holzhauer et al., 2018), variance data (Schmidli et al., 2017), and non-parametric survival data (Van Ryzin, 1980). Another extension of the base model allows for individual patient data (IPD) rather than aggregate data, as discussed for example in Higgins et al. (2001); Stewart and Clarke (1995). For an example of IPD and aggregate data, see Gsteiger et al. (2013).

Finally, in the discussion of the previous sections we considered models without nuisance parameters. In the presence of nuisance parameters, various assumptions are possible: unrelated parameters, equal parameters, or related parameters (e.g. exchangeable, as for the θ_j parameters of the base model). For example, unrelated parameters are typically assumed for the control rates (nuisance parameters) in a meta-analysis of randomized controlled trials comparing control to a new treatment (with log-odds-ratio as the main parameter); equal parameters have been assumed for the overdispersion parameter in Gsteiger et al. (2013); for examples of related (modeled) nuisance parameter, see Schmidli et al. (2017, 2013).

6.4.11 Other approaches

In this section, we briefly discuss alternative proposals to incorporating historical data, which are commonly referred to as Pocock's bias model, commensurate priors, power priors, and test-then-pool.

It turns out that the first two are essentially equivalent to the NNHM, of Section 6.4.3. The third is mathematically equivalent to the NNHM for normal data and conceptually similar otherwise. The fourth is completely different in that it only allows for the extremes of complete pooling or stratification.

6.4.11.1 Pocock's bias model

In his seminal paper, Pocock (1976) proposed the following model for the case of no systematic bias for all studies $j = 1, \ldots, J$:

$$\theta_j = \theta_\star + \epsilon_j, \quad \epsilon_j \sim \mathrm{N}(0, \tau_\epsilon^2).$$

This centers all historical parameters at $\theta_\star$ and is equivalent to

$$\theta_j \mid \theta_\star, \tau_\epsilon \sim \mathrm{N}(\theta_\star, \tau_\epsilon^2). \tag{6.6}$$

This conditional distribution is obtained from the standard NNHM, as

$$\theta_j \mid \theta_\star, \tau \sim \mathrm{N}(\theta_\star, 2\tau^2).$$

This shows that the relationship between the variances τ_ϵ^2 in Pocock's model and τ^2 in the NNHM, is

$$\tau_\epsilon^2 = 2\tau^2.$$

The equivalence still holds when allowing for systematic biases, simply by using a non-zero mean (equal to δ_j in Section 6.4.8) of ϵ_j.

6.4.11.2 Commensurate priors

Reversing the conditioning in (6.6) leads to the commensurate priors formulations (Hobbs et al., 2011, 2012; Murray et al., 2014). For one trial, this means

$$\theta_\star \mid \theta_1, \tau_c \sim \mathrm{N}(\theta_1, \tau_c^2).$$

Again, the respective NNHM result is

$$\theta_\star \mid \theta_1, \tau \sim \mathrm{N}(\theta_1, 2\tau^2),$$

which leads to the relationship

$$\tau_c^2 = 2\tau^2.$$

For more than one trial, it has been suggested to use $\theta_1 = \ldots = \theta_J = \mu$ and

$$\theta_\star \mid \mu, \tau_c \sim \mathrm{N}(\mu, \tau_c^2).$$

However, the strong assumption of no between-heterogeneity across historical studies is unrealistic and not really necessary. A more general commensurate prior model is

$$\theta_\star \mid \theta_1, \ldots, \theta_J, \tau_c \sim \mathrm{N}(\overline{\theta}, \tau_c^2).$$

Assuming the same between-trial variance τ^2 for all trials, the corresponding NNHM result is

$$\theta_\star \mid \theta_1, \ldots, \theta_J, \tau \sim \mathrm{N}(\bar{\theta}, \tau^2(J+1)/J).$$

Thus, the NNHM and commensurate prior model are equivalent if

$$\frac{J+1}{J}\tau_c^2 = \tau^2.$$

6.4.11.3 Power priors

In contrast to the approaches discussed so far, power priors (Ibrahim and Chen, 2000; Chen and Ibrahim, 2006; Gravestock and Held, 2017; Held and Sauter, 2017) do not explicitly model the relationship among the new and historical parameters. They express the relevance of the historical data directly via fixed power parameters $0 \leq \alpha_j \leq 1$, with the power prior for $\theta_\star$ defined as the product of the weighted historical data likelihoods

$$\pi(\theta_\star \mid \boldsymbol{Y_{\mathcal{J}}}, \alpha_1, \ldots, \alpha_J) \propto \prod_j L(y_j; \theta_j)^{\alpha_j} \times \pi_0(\theta_\star).$$

Here, the normalizing constant does not depend on $\theta_\star$, and $\pi_0(\theta_\star)$ will usually be noninformative. The idea is appealing because of the interpretation of the power parameters; the fraction of information from historical study j is α_j.

Yet there are difficulties if one wants to incorporate uncertainty via prior distributions $\pi_j(\alpha_j)$. For this case, the original power prior formulation is flawed (Duan et al., 2006; Neelon and O'Malley, 2010; Neuenschwander et al., 2009) and is commonly rectified by the *modified power prior*

$$\pi(\theta_\star \mid \boldsymbol{Y_{\mathcal{J}}}, \boldsymbol{\alpha}) = C(\boldsymbol{\alpha}) \times \prod_j [L(y_j; \theta_j)^{\alpha_j} \pi_j(\alpha_j)] \times \pi_0(\theta_\star).$$

These priors imply technical complications due to the normalizing constant, which now depends on the power parameters $\boldsymbol{\alpha} = (\alpha_1, \ldots, \alpha_J)^\top$; in the above version, they were fixed. Since $C(\alpha)$ can usually not be calculated analytically, power priors with unknown α_j can be computationally challenging.

Interestingly, for normal data there is a one-to-one relationship between power priors and the NNHM. For a single historical trial (i.e. when $\boldsymbol{\alpha} = \alpha$) and outcome standard deviation σ, equivalence is achieved when

$$\alpha = (1 + 2n\tau^2/\sigma^2)^{-1}.$$

This shows two things. First, the often used uniform prior for α has different implications for between-trial heterogeneity, depending on the size of the trial (n): the larger the trial, the smaller the implied heterogeneity. For example, for trials of size 25, 100, and 400, the respective 95% intervals for τ are: $(0.02\sigma, 0.88\sigma)$, $(0.01\sigma, 0.44\sigma)$, and $(0.01\sigma, 0.22\sigma)$. Using the classification in Table 6.3, for a large trial the presumably non-informative prior for α is quite informative on the heterogeneity scale, which drives the amount of borrowing from historical data. Second, the equal relevance case for all trials (common τ) cannot be mapped easily into a single power parameter.

The similarity between hierarchical models and power priors, and the additional technical challenges of the latter, may explain why hierarchical model formulations have been increasingly used recently. Irrespective of the chosen approach, understanding both scales (between-trial heterogeneity and amount of borrowing from historical data) is important.

6.4.11.4 Test-then-pool

So far, we have looked at models that consider intermediate cases between complete pooling and complete stratification, with parameters $\tau > 0$ for all models with between-trial heterogeneities and $0 < \alpha < 1$ for power priors.

The completely opposite approach to these *averaging-between-extremes* approaches is the *select-of-extremes* approach: depending on the data, the historical data will be either simply ignored or fully pooled with the new data. Viele et al. (2014) mention (but do not recommend) this "test-then-pool" approach, calibrating the level of the test of homogeneity with Type I error rate control. However, good operating characteristics, although necessary, are not always sufficient. In a concrete trial, it would be hard to justify full pooling, making no difference between historical and concurrent data.

A slightly improved version of "test-then-pool" is *averaging-of-extremes*. This is model averaging for the model with $\tau = 0$ or $\tau = \infty$ ($\alpha = 0$ or $\alpha = 1$ for power priors). For the NNHM, this could be implemented by a point mass prior on the two parameters. But the question remains: why use a model with extreme parameters when the context tells us that the parameters are between the extremes?

6.4.12 Historical trial designs: Operating characteristics

In the previous sections, we were mainly concerned with the quantification of the parameter $\theta_\star$ based on historical data. In most cases, this information will be used as additional information in a new trial. The most frequent application is the use of historical control data in a randomized trial. The design of such a historical-data trial needs careful considerations (Cuffe, 2011; Galwey, 2017; van Rosmalen et al., 2017). How influential are the historical data? How do the historical data affect the operating characteristics of the design?

For the operating characteristics of most designs, the effect on Type I error is relevant. In particular, the amount of potential Type I error inflation should be known. If deemed too high, a more robust prior (see Section 6.4.5) may be used. However, while Type I error inflation should be controlled, it is important to realize that Type I error deflation is also possible; in particular, the expected Type I error under the prior is controlled (Neuenschwander, 2011).

Depending on the complexity of the design, which will often have at least one interim analysis, assessing operating characteristics may be resource intensive and require simulations. Publicly available tools to address some standard designs with historical data priors have been developed recently (Gerber and Gsponer, 2016; Gsponer et al., 2014; Weber, 2017).

6.5 Application: Non-inferiority trials

6.5.1 Motivation

A new treatment should be better than placebo. For regulatory approval of a test treatment, evidence for this minimal efficacy requirement has to be provided. A clinical trial where patients are randomized to test treatment or placebo allows us to directly evaluate whether the test treatment is superior to placebo. However, if the test treatment is intended for patients with a serious disease, and an approved treatment is already available, using placebo may not be ethical, and a non-inferiority (NI) trial may be the only option (Rothmann et al., 2016).

In NI trials, the test treatment is compared to an active-control (an approved treatment) rather than to placebo. Obviously, NI trials cannot provide direct evidence on whether the test treatment is superior to placebo. However, this question can be addressed indirectly based on historical and active-control data, as emphasized in the FDA guidance on NI trials: "In the absence of a placebo arm, knowing whether the trial had assay sensitivity relies heavily on external (not within-study) information, giving NI studies some of the characteristics of a historically controlled trial." (U.S. Food and Drug Administration, 2016).

6.5.2 The OASIS II trial

Patients with acute coronary syndrome (ACS), e.g. a heart attack, are in a serious condition. In the OASIS II trial, $n_\star^T = 5045$ patients with ACS were randomized to the test treatment *Hirudin* (T) and $n_\star^C = 5033$ to the active-control *Heparin* (C). All patients also received standard of care, including aspirin. The primary endpoint was cardiovascular death or new myocardial infarction by day 7. The proportion of patients with such an event was 3.5% for test ($y_\star^T = 178$) and 4.2% for control ($y_\star^C = 211$). The statistical model is

$$y_\star^T \mid \pi_\star^T \sim \text{Bin}(\pi_\star^T, n_\star^T), \quad y_\star^C \mid \pi_\star^C \sim \text{Bin}(\pi_\star^C, n_\star^C).$$

The minimal efficacy requirement is that *Hirudin* is better than placebo (actually standard of care), which also requires trial-external information for evaluation. In this case, six randomized trials comparing the active-control (C) with placebo (P) were identified (Oler et al., 1996). The number of events and patients in historical trial $j = 1, \ldots, 6$ are denoted by y_j^C and n_j^C for active-control, and y_j^P and n_j^P for placebo. The statistical model for the historical data is

$$y_j^C \mid \pi_j^C \sim \text{Bin}(\pi_j^C, n_j^C), \quad y_j^P \mid \pi_j^P \sim \text{Bin}(\pi_j^P, n_j^P).$$

The log-odds $\theta = \log\{\pi/(1-\pi)\}$ rather than the response rates π are used in the following. The minimal efficacy requirement can be stated as $\theta_\star^T - \theta_\star^P > 0$ (Simon, 1999), which can be re-written as

$$\theta_\star^T - \theta_\star^P = (\theta_\star^T - \theta_\star^C) + (\theta_\star^C - \theta_\star^P) > 0.$$

The OASIS II trial directly provides information on the first term $(\theta_\star^T - \theta_\star^C)$. Information on the second term $(\theta_\star^C - \theta_\star^P)$ can be extracted from the six historical trials by the meta-analytic-predictive (MAP) approach (Schmidli et al., 2013). More precisely, for $\delta_j^{CP} = \theta_j^C - \theta_j^P$ the MAP parameter model is

$$\delta_\star^{CP}, \delta_1^{CP}, \ldots, \delta_6^{CP} \mid \mu^{CP}, \tau \sim \text{N}(\mu^{CP}, \tau^2).$$

The between-trial standard deviation τ quantifies the heterogeneity of treatment effects (C vs. P) across trials. For rare events, the unit-information standard deviation σ for log-odds-ratios is approximately 2 (for one event), so that a half-normal prior with scale 0.5 covering small to very large heterogeneities is rather conservative (see Tables 6.3 and 6.5). For μ, a vague normal prior $\mathrm{N}(0, 100^2)$ can be used as this parameter is well informed by the data.

A sample from the posterior distribution of the parameters can be generated with `WinBUGS` (Schmidli et al., 2013). The posterior for the odds ratio $\exp(\delta_\star^{CP})$ has median (95% interval) 0.61 (0.21,1.42) and is more uncertain than for the odds ratio $\exp(\mu^{CP})$, 0.60 (0.31, 1.02). This is due to between-trial heterogeneity: the posterior median (95% interval) for τ is 0.25 (0.01,0.84).

Figure 6.2 (upper part) summarizes these results. The MAP prediction shows that it seems quite uncertain whether *Heparin (C)* would have been superior to placebo (P) in OASIS II, had placebo been included. The middle part of Figure 6.2 shows that the OASIS II NI trial provides some evidence that *Hirudin* (T) is superior to the active-control *Heparin* (C).

For the result shown in the lower part of Figure 6.2, information from the historical trials and the OASIS II trial have been combined. The posterior median (95% interval) for the odds ratio $\exp(\delta_\star^{TP})$ is 0.51 (0.17,1.23), with $p(\delta_\star^{TP} < 0) = 0.93$. Based on standard regulatory criteria, this does not provide sufficient evidence that *Hirudin* is superior to placebo. Further issues with both the trial (e.g. switching from superiority to non-inferiority) and the historical data were discussed at the FDA advisory committee meeting; see Fleming (2008) and references therein.

6.5.3 Outlook and extensions

In current practice, NI trials are typically designed and analyzed using a non-inferiority margin approach rather than the evidence synthesis approach described above. However, regulators show interest in the latter. For example, the EMA guideline (European Medicines Agency, 2006b) states: "In a submission the applicant should present both the direct confidence interval T minus R and the indirect interval T minus P." (R corresponds to C in our notation). And, the recent FDA guidance (U.S. Food and Drug Administration, 2016) seems to go even a step further: "Use of the synthesis method [..] would also be acceptable and may be recommended for determining whether a loss of effect greater than M2 has been ruled out [..]"; here, M2 refers to the preservation of a fraction of the effect C vs. P.

For the OASIS II NI trial, historical data consists of relevant clinical trials where patients have been randomized to active-control or placebo. This is a common setting, and several examples using a Bayesian evidence synthesis approach have been described (Gamalo-Siebers et al., 2016; Schmidli et al., 2020; Simon, 1999).

However, the approach can be applied more broadly. For example, historical trials comparing C or P with other treatments may provide valuable information. In such a case, a network meta-analytic-predictive approach can synthesize the evidence and predict the C vs. P effect in the NI trial (Schmidli et al., 2013). Usually, summary baseline information is available as well, which may allow a refined prediction of the C vs. P effect using meta-regression; see Section 6.4.9 and Witte et al., 2011. In oncology, some historical trials may be single-arm with just the active-control C, which also can be integrated using a MAP approach (Wandel et al., 2015).

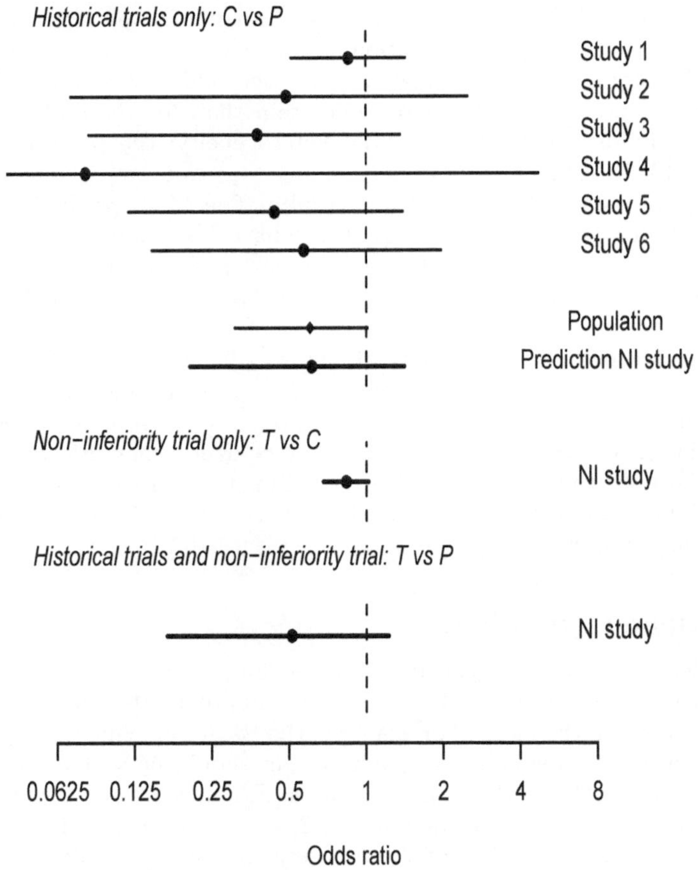

FIGURE 6.2: Results for cardiovascular death or new myocardial infarction by day 7 (median and 95% interval): Historical information from six trials comparing active-control *Heparin (C)* with placebo (*P*), with MAP prediction (upper panel); result from OASIS II non-inferiority trial (middle panel); and, indirect comparison of placebo and *Hidurin (T)* (lower panel).

6.6 Discussion

With increasing amounts of and easier access to data, making better use of these data is mandatory. Statistical analyses are meta-analytic and account for various sources of heterogeneity and potential biases. Such precautions are important if one wants to make use of real world evidence (Eichler et al., 2016; Neuenschwander et al., 2018).

We have discussed the basic statistical framework (with extensions) and an implementation based on the standard normal-normal hierarchical model. The field is rapidly evolving and adapting to the needs of modern drug development (Boonstra et al., 2016; Bhuyan et al., 2016; Chuang-Stein and Kirby, 2017; Desai et al., 2013; Di Scala et al., 2013; Efthimiou et al., 2017; Kelsh et al., 2015; Marringwa et al., 2007; Pozzi et al., 2016; Quan et al., 2017; Takeda and Morita, 2015; van de Wiel et al., 2016; Walley et al., 2015; Wandel and Roychoudhury, 2016; Weaver et al., 2016).

The statistical approach to most applications with co-data is usually Bayesian, which is not strictly necessary. As we have shown, a meta-analytic-combined analysis, a meta-analysis of all the data, can be done in a non-Bayesian way, because a prior distribution is not needed. However, classical inference is challenging with few trials.

We confined our discussion to simple meta-analytic models. Often, however, a network of trials will be available and appropriate methods should be applied to address heterogeneities and biases (Dias et al., 2011; Lu and Ades, 2004; Salanti et al., 2008; Lumley, 2002; Ohlssen et al., 2014). The non-inferiority trial of Section 6.5 illustrates the use of historical data for a simple network of three treatments.

The aspects arising in the historical data setting resemble the ones of other co-data approaches, for example when taking advantage of additional data in the investigation of small populations (Dunne et al., 2011; European Medicines Agency, 2006a, 2001; U.S. Food and Drug Administration, 2015; Gamalo-Siebers et al., 2017; Hampson et al., 2014; Neelon and O'Malley, 2010; Unkel et al., 2016).

The use of historical or other co-data in medical product development is growing, scientifically sound and practically feasible. Yet it is ambitious and requires careful considerations regarding trial design, data analysis, and decision making. If appropriately done, making better use of relevant data will improve drug development, for the benefit of patients in need of better treatments.

6.7 Code

```
# RBesT MAP analysis for GBS example: prior 1 HN(scale=0.16)

# load package
library(RBesT)

# data
dat = data.frame(study=c(1:5),
                 study.labels=c("Korinthenberg","Paradiso",
                 "Epstein","Lamont","Graf"),
                 n=c(56,37,14,18,9),
                 y=c(3.69,3.85,3.89,3.76,3.77),
                 y.se=c(0.068,0.110,0.173,0.166,0.179))
print(dat)

# MAP analysis
set.seed(1)
map = gMAP(cbind(y, y.se) ~ 1 | study, weights=n,data=dat,
           family=gaussian,beta.prior=cbind(3.8,10),
           tau.dist="Half-Normal",tau.prior=cbind(0,0.16))
print(map)
pl = plot(map)
```

```
print(pl$forest_model)

# Approximating the MAP prior by a mixture of conjugate priors
map.approx2 = mixfit(map, Nc=2)
plot(map.approx2)$mixdens

# Effective sample sizes
ess(map.approx2)
ess(map.approx2, method="morita")
```

Bibliography

Adams, C. and Brantner, V. (2010). Spending on new drug development. *Health Economics*, 19(2):130–141.

Baeten, D., Baraliakos, X., Braun, J., Sieper, J., Emery, P., van der Heijde, D., McInnes, I., van Laar, J., Landewé, R., Wordsworth, P., Wollenhaupt, J., Kellner, H., Paramarta, J., Wei, J., Brachat, A., Bek, S., Laurent, D., Li, Y., Wang, Y., Bertolino, A., Gsteiger, S., Wright, A., and Hueber, W. (2013). Anti-interleukin-17A monoclonal antibody secukinumab in treatment of ankylosing spondylitis: a randomised, double-blind, placebo-controlled trial. *The Lancet*, 382(9906):1705–1713.

Bhuyan, P., Desai, J., St Louis, M., Carlsson, M., Bowen, E., Danielson, M., and Cantor, M. (2016). Repurposing historical control clinical trial data to provide safety context. *Drug Discovery Today*, 21(2):212–216.

Boonen, S., Reginster, J., Kaufman, J., Lippuner, K., Zanchetta, J., Langdahl, B., Rizzoli, R., Lipschitz, S., Dimai, H., Witvrouw, R., Eriksen, E., Brixen, K., Russo, L., Claessens, F., Papanastasiou, P., Antunez, O., Su, G., Bucci-Rechtweg, C., Hruska, J., Incera, E., Vanderschueren, D., and Orwoll, E. (2012). Fracture risk and zoledronic acid therapy in men with osteoporosis. *New England Journal of Medicine*, 367(18):1714–1723.

Boonstra, P., Taylor, J., and Mukherjee, B. (2016). Increasing efficiency for estimating treatment-biomarker interactions with historical data. *Statistical Methods in Medical Research*, 25(6):2959–2971.

Box, G. (1980). Sampling and Bayes inference in scientific modeling and robustness. *Journal of the Royal Statistical Society — Series A*, 143:383–430.

Carpenter, B., Gelman, A., Hoffman, M., Lee, D., Goodrich, B., Betancourt, M., Brubaker, M., Guo, J., Li, P., and Riddell, A. (2017). Stan: A probabilistic programming language. *Journal of Statistical Software*, 76(1):1–32.

Chen, M. and Ibrahim, J. (2006). The relationship between the power prior and hierarchical models. *Bayesian Analysis*, 1(3):551–574.

Chuang-Stein, C. and Kirby, S. (2017). Incorporating information from completed trials in future trial planning. In *Quantitative Decisions in Drug Development*, pages 53–67. Springer.

Cuffe, R. (2011). The inclusion of historical control data may reduce the power of a confirmatory study. *Statistics in Medicine*, 30(12):1329–1338.

Dallal, S. and Hall, W. (1983). Approximating priors by mixtures of natural conjugate priors. *Journal of the Royal Statistical Society — Series B*, 45:278–286.

DerSimonian, R. and Kacker, R. (2007). Random-effects model for meta-analysis of clinical trials: an update. *Contemporary Clinical Trials*, 28:105–114.

Desai, J., Bowen, E., Danielson, M., Allam, R., and Cantor, M. (2013). Creation and implementation of a historical controls database from randomized clinical trials. *Journal of the American Medical Informatics Association*, 20(E1):162–168.

Di Scala, L., Kerman, J., and Neuenschwander, B. (2013). Collection, synthesis, and interpretation of evidence: a proof-of-concept study in COPD. *Statistics in Medicine*, 32(10):1621–1634.

Diaconis, P. and Ylvisaker, D. (1984). Quantifying prior opinion. *Bayesian Statistics (Proceedings of the Second Valencia International Meeting)*, 2:133–148.

Dias, S., Welton, N., Sutton, A., and Ades, A. (2011). NICE DSU Technical Support Document 2: A Generalised Linear Modelling Framework for Pairwise and Network Meta-Analysis of Randomised Controlled Trials. "http://www.nicedsu.org.uk".

DiMasi, J., Hansen, R., and Grabowski, H. (2003). The price of innovation: new estimates of drug development costs. *Journal of Health Economics*, 22(2):151–185.

Duan, Y., Ye, K., and Smith, E. (2006). Evaluating water quality using power priors to incorporate historical information. *Environmetrics*, 17(1):95 – 106.

Dunne, J., Rodriguez, W., Murphy, M., Beasley, B., Burckart, G., Filie, J., Lewis, L., Sachs, H., Sheridan, P., Starke, P., and Yao, L. (2011). Extrapolation of adult data and other data in pediatric drug-development programs. *Pediatrics*, 128(5):1242–1249.

Efthimiou, O., Mavridis, D., Debray, T., Samara, M. Belger, M., Siontis, G., Leucht, S., Salanti, G., and GetReal Work Package 4. (2017). Combining randomized and nonrandomized evidence in network meta-analysis. *Statistics in Medicine*, 36(8):1210–1226.

Egger, M., Smith, G., and Altman, D. (1995). *Systematic Reviews in Health Care: Meta-Analysis in Context*. British Medical Journal Publishing Group.

Eichler, H., Bloechl-Daum, B., Bauer, P., Bretz, F., Brown, J., Hampson, L., Honig, P., Krams, M., Leufkens, H., Lim, R., Lumpkin, M., Murphy, M., Pignatti, F., Posch, M., Schneeweiss, S., Trusheim, M., and Koenig, F. (2016). "Threshold-crossing": a useful way to establish the counterfactual in clinical trials? *Clinical Pharmacology and Therapeutics*, 100(6):699–712.

European Commission (2014). Innovative Medicines Initiative 2: Europe's fast track to better medicines. "http://www.imi.europa.eu/sites/default/files/uploads/documents/Horizon2020/EC_factsheet_imi2.pdf".

European Medicines Agency (2001). Note for Guidance on Clinical Investigation of Medicinal Products in the Paediatric Population. Committee for Proprietary Medicinal Products (CPMP). http://www.ema.europa.eu/docs/en_GB/document_library/Scientific_guideline/2009/09/WC500002926.pdf.

European Medicines Agency (2006a). Guideline on Clinical Trials in Small Populations. `"http://www.ema.europa.eu/docs/en_GB/document_library/Scientific_guideline/2009/09/WC500003615.pdf"`.

European Medicines Agency (2006b). Guideline on Clinical Trials in Small Populations. `"http://www.ema.europa.eu/docs/en_GB/document_library/Scientific_guideline/2009/09/WC500003615.pdf"`.

Fleming, T. (2008). Current issues in non-inferiority trials. *Statistics in Medicine*, 27(3):317–332.

Friede, T., Röver, C., Wandel, S., and Neuenschwander, B. (2017). Meta-analysis of two studies in the presence of heterogeneity with applications in rare diseases. *Biometrical Journal*, 59(4):658–671.

Galeva, I., Konstan, M., Higgins, M., Angyalosi, G., Brockhaus, F., Piggott, S., Thomas, K., and Chuchalin, A. (2013). Tobramycin inhalation powder manufactured by improved process in cystic fibrosis: the randomized EDIT trial. *Current Medical Research and Opinion*, 29(8):947–956.

Galwey, N. (2017). Supplementation of a clinical trial by historical control data: is the prospect of dynamic borrowing an illusion? *Statistics in Medicine*, 36(6):899–916.

Gamalo-Siebers, M., Gao, A., Lakshminarayanan, M., Liu, G., Natanegara, F., Railkar, R., Schmidli, H., and Song, G. (2016). Bayesian methods for the design and analysis of noninferiority trials. *Journal of Biopharmaceutical Statistics*, 26(5):823–841.

Gamalo-Siebers, M., Savic, J., Basu, C., Zhao, X., Gopalakrishnan, M., Gao, A., Song, G., Baygani, S., Thompson, L., Xia, A., Price, K., Tiwari, R., and Carlin, B. (2017). Statistical modeling for Bayesian extrapolation of adult clinical trial information in pediatric drug evaluation. *Pharmaceutical Statistics*, 16(4):232–249.

Gelman, A. (2006). Prior distributions for variance parameters in hierarchical models. *Bayesian Analysis*, 1(3):515–534.

Gerber, F. and Gsponer, T. (2016). gsbDesign: an R package for evaluating the operating characteristics of a group sequential Bayesian design. *Journal of Statistical Software*, 69(11).

Goodman, S. and Sladky, J. (2005). A Bayesian approach to randomized controlled trials in children utilizing information from adults: the case of Guillain-Barre syndrome. *Clinical Trials*, 2(10):305–310.

Gravestock, I. and Held, L. (2017). Adaptive power priors with empirical Bayes for clinical trials. *Pharmaceutical Statistics*, 16(5):349–360.

Gsponer, T., Gerber, F., Bornkamp, B., Ohlssen, D., Vandemeulebroecke, M., and Schmidli, H. (2014). A practical guide to Bayesian group sequential designs. *Pharmaceutical Statistics*, 13(1):71–80.

Gsteiger, S., Neuenschwander, B., Mercier, F., and Schmidli, H. (2013). Using historical control information for the design and analysis of clinical trials with overdispersed count data. *Statistics in Medicine*, 32(21):3609–3622.

Hampson, L., Whitehead, J., Eleftheriou, D., and Brogan, P. (2014). Bayesian methods for the design and interpretation of clinical trials in very rare diseases. *Statistics in Medicine*, 33(24):4186–4201.

Held, L. and Sauter, R. (2017). Adaptive prior weighting in generalized regression. *Biometrics*, 73(1):242–251.

Higgins, J. and Green, S. (2008). *Cochrane Handbook for Systematic Reviews of Interventions*. Wiley.

Higgins, J., Thompson, S., and Spiegelhalter, D. (2009). A re-evaluation of random-effects meta-analysis. *Journal of the Royal Statistical Society — Series A*, 172:137–159.

Higgins, J., Whitehead, A., Turner, R., Omar, R., and Thompson, S. (2001). Meta-analysis of continuous outcome data from individual patients. *Statistics in Medicine*, 20(15):2219–2241.

Hobbs, B., Carlin, B., Mandrekar, S., and Sargent, D. (2011). Hierarchical commensurate and power prior models for adaptive incorporation of historical information in clinical trials. *Biometrics*, 67(3):1047–1056.

Hobbs, B., Sargent, D., and Carlin, B. (2012). Commensurate priors for incorporating historical information in clinical trials using general and generalized linear models. *Bayesian Analysis*, 7(3):639–674.

Holzhauer, B., Wang, C., and Schmidli, H. (2018). Evidence synthesis from aggregate recurrent event data for clinical trial design and analysis. *Statistics in Medicine*, 15;37(6): 867–882.

Ibrahim, J. and Chen, M. (2000). Power prior distributions for regression models. *Statistical Science*, 15(1):46–60.

Inamdar, A., Merlo-Pich, E., Gee, M., Makumi, C., Mistry, P., Robertson, J., Steinberg, E., Zamuner, S., Learned, S., Alexander, R., and Ratti, E. (2014). Evaluation of antidepressant properties of the p38 MAP kinase inhibitor losmapimod (GW856553) in Major Depressive Disorder: Results from two randomised, placebo-controlled, double-blind, multicentre studies using a Bayesian approach. *Journal of Psychopharmacology*, 28(6):570–581.

Japan's Pharmaceuticals and Medical Devices Agency (PMDA) (2007). Basic Principles on Global Clinical Trials. `"http://www.pmda.go.jp/kijunsakusei/file/guideline/new_drug/GlobalClinicalTrials_en.pdf"`.

Kass, R. and Wasserman, L. (1995). A reference Bayesian test for nested hypotheses and its relationship to the Schwarz criterion. *Journal of the American Statistical Association*, 90:928–934.

Kelsh, M., Ko, C., Chia, V., Przepiorka, D., and Suissa, S. (2015). Historical comparator studies: strengths, limitations, and analytical considerations in using historical pooled clinical data for evaluating efficacy and safety of new therapies. *Pharmacoepidemiology and Drug Safety*, 24(1):240.

Kramer, M. and Font, E. (2017). Reducing sample size in experiments with animals: historical controls and related strategies. *Biological Reviews*, 92(1):431–445.

Li, J., Chen, W., and Scott, J. (2016). Addressing prior-data conflict with empirical meta-analytic-predictive priors in clinical studies with historical information. *Journal of Biopharmaceutical Statistics*, 26(6, SI):1056–1066.

Lu, G. and Ades, A. (2004). Combination of direct and indirect evidence in mixed treatment comparisons. *Statistics in Medicine*, 23(20):3105–3124.

Lumley, T. (2002). Network meta-analysis for indirect treatment comparisons. *Statistics in Medicine*, 21(16):2313–2324.

Lunn, D., Jackson, C., Best, N., Thomas, A., and Spiegelhalter, D. (2012). *The BUGS Book: A Practical Introduction to Bayesian Analysis*. Chapman & Hall/CRC Texts in Statistical Science.

Lunn, D., Thomas, A., Best, N., and Spiegelhalter, D. (2000). WinBUGS - a Bayesian modelling framework: Concepts, structure, and extensibility. *Statistics and Computing*, 10:325–337.

Malec, D. (2001). A closer look at combining data among a small number of binomial experiments. *Statistics in Medicine*, 20(12):1811–1824.

Marringwa, J., Faes, C., Aerts, M., Geys, H., Teuns, G., Van Den Poel, B., and Bijnens, L. (2007). On the use of historical control data in pre-clinical safety studies. *Journal of Biopharmaceutical Statistics*, 17(3):493–509.

Morita, S., Thall, P., and Müller, P. (2008). Determining the effective sample size of a parametric prior. *Biometrics*, 64(2):595–602.

Morita, S., Thall, P., and Müller, P. (2012). Prior effective sample size in conditionally independent hierarchical models. *Bayesian Analysis*, 7(3):561–614.

Murray, T., Hobbs, B., Lystig, T., and Carlin, B. (2014). Semiparametric Bayesian commensurate survival model for post-market medical device surveillance with non-exchangeable historical data. *Biometrics*, 70(1):185–191.

Mutsvari, T., Tytgat, D., and Walley, R. (2016). Addressing potential prior-data conflict when using informative priors in proof-of-concept studies. *Pharmaceutical Statistics*, 15(1):28–36.

Neelon, B. and O'Malley, A. (2010). Bayesian analysis using power priors with application to pediatric quality of care. *Journal of Biometrics & Biostatistics*, 1:103.

Neuenschwander, B. (2011). From historical data to priors. *ASA Proceedings, Biometrics Section*, pages 3466–3474.

Neuenschwander, B., Branson, M., and Spiegelhalter, D. (2009). A note on the power prior. *Statistics in Medicine*, 28:3562–3566.

Neuenschwander, B., Capkun-Niggli, G., Branson, M., and Spiegehalter, D. (2010). Summarizing historical information on controls in clinical trials. *Clinical Trials*, 7(1):5–18.

Neuenschwander, B., Matano, A., Tang, Z., Roychoudhury, S., Wandel, S., and Bailey, S. (2015). A Bayesian industry approach to phase I combination trials in oncology. In *Statistical Methods in Drug Combination Studies (Eds. W. Zhao and H. Yang)*. Chapman & Hall/CRC Biostatistics Series.

Neuenschwander, B., Roychoudhury, S., and Branson, M. (2018). Predictive evidence threshold scaling: does the evidence meet a confirmatory standard? *Statistics in Biopharmaceutical Research*, 10(2):76–84.

Neuenschwander, B., Roychoudhury, S., and Schmidli, H. (2016). On the use of co-data in clinical trials. *Statistics in Biopharmaceutical Research*, 8(3):345–354.

Neuenschwander, B., Weber, S., Schmidli, H., and O'Hagan, A. Predictively consistent prior effective sample sizes (with discussion). *Biometrics.* doi: 10.1111/biom.13252.

O'Hagan, A. and Forster, J. (2004). *Kendall's Advanced Theory of Statistics Vol 2B Bayesian Inference.* Arnold.

O'Hagan, A. and Pericchi, L. (2012). Bayesian heavy-tailed models and conflict resolution: A review. *Brazilian Journal of Probability and Statistics*, 26(4):372–401.

Ohlssen, D., Price, K., Xia, H., Hong, H., Kerman, J., Fu, H., Quartey, G., Heilmann, C., Ma, H., and Carlin, B. (2014). Guidance on the implementation and reporting of a drug safety Bayesian network meta-analysis. *Pharmaceutical Statistics*, 13(1):55–70.

Oler, A., Whooley, M., Oler, J., and Grady, D. (1996). Adding heparin to aspirin reduces the incidence of myocardial infarction and death in patients with unstable angina: A meta-analysis. *Journal of the American Medical Association*, 276(10):811–815.

Pennello, G. and Thompson, L. (2008). Experience with reviewing Bayesian medical device trials. *Journal of Biopharmaceutical Statistics*, 18(1):81–115.

Pocock, S. (1976). The combination of randomized and historical controls in clinical trials. *Journal of Chronic Diseases*, 29(3):175–188.

Polson, N. and Scott, J. (2012). On the half-Cauchy prior for a global scale parameter. *Bayesian Analysis*, 7(4):887–902.

Pozzi, L., Schmidli, H., and Ohlssen, D. (2016). A Bayesian hierarchical surrogate outcome model for multiple sclerosis. *Pharmaceutical Statistics*, 15(4, SI):341–348.

Quan, H., Zhang, B., Chuang-Stein, C., Jones, B., and Anal, E. I. D. (2017). Integrated data analysis for assessing treatment effect through combining information from all sources. *Statistics in Biopharmaceutical Research*, 9(1):52–64.

Rothmann, M., Wiens, B., and Chan, I. (2016). *Design and Analysis of Non-Inferiority Trials.* Chapman & Hall/CRC Biostatistics Series. CRC Press.

Röver, C. (2015). *bayesmeta: Bayesian Random-effects Meta Analysis.* http://cran.r-project.org/package=bayesmeta.

Rukhin, A. (2012). Estimating common mean and heterogeneity variance in two study case meta-analysis. *Statistics & Probability Letters*, 82:1318–1325.

Salanti, G., Higgins, J., Ades, A., and Ioannidis, J. (2008). Evaluation of networks of randomized trials. *Statistical Methods in Medical Research*, 17(3):279–301.

SAS Institute (2014). SAS User Guide: Statistics. The MCMC procedure.

Schmidli H, Häring DA, Thomas M, Cassidy A, Weber S, Bretz F. (2019). Beyond randomized clinical trials: Use of external controls. *Clinical Pharmacology and Therapeutics.* doi: 10.1002/cpt.1723.

Schmidli, H., Gsteiger, S., and Neuenschwander, B. (2020). Incorporating historical data into randomized clinical trials. In *Handbook of Statistical Methods for Randomized Controlled Trials (Eds. K Kim, F Bretz, YK Cheung, LV Hampson)*, Boca Raton, FL. CRC Press.

Schmidli, H., Gsteiger, S., Roychoudhury, S., O'Hagan, A., Spiegelhalter, D., and Neuenschwander, B. (2014). Robust meta-analytic-predictive priors in clinical trials with historical control information. *Biometrics*, 70(4):1023–32.

Schmidli, H., Neuenschwander, B., and Friede, T. (2017). Meta-analytic-predictive use of historical variance data for the design and analysis of clinical trials. *Computational Statistics and Data Analysis*, 113:100–110.

Schmidli, H., Wandel, S., and Neuenschwander, B. (2013). The network meta-analytic-predictive approach to non-inferiority trials. *Statistical Methods in Medical Research*, 22(2):219–240.

Simon, R. (1999). Bayesian design and analysis of active control clinical trials. *Biometrics*, 55(2):484–487.

Spiegelhalter, D., Abrams, K., and Myles, J. (2004). *Bayesian Approaches to Clinical Trials and Health-Care Evaluation*. Wiley, New York, NY.

Stewart, L. and Clarke, M. (1995). Practical methodology of meta-analyses (overviews) using updated individual patient data. *Statistics in Medicine*, 14(19):2057–2079.

Takeda, K. and Morita, S. (2015). Incorporating historical data in Bayesian phase I trial design: the Caucasian-to-Asian toxicity tolerability problem. *Therapeutic Innovation & Regulatory Science*, 49(1):93–99.

Thall, P., Herrick, R., Nguyen, H., Venier, J., and Norris, J. (2014). Effective sample size for computing prior hyperparameters in Bayesian phase I-II dose-finding. *Clinical Trials*, 11(6):657–666.

Turner, R., Davey, J., Clarke, M., Thompson, S., and Higgins, J. (2012). Predicting the extent of heterogeneity in meta-analysis, using empirical data from the Cochrane Database of Systematic Reviews. *International Journal of Epidemiology*, 41:818–827.

Turner, R., Jackson, D., Wei, Y., Thompson, S., and Higgins, P. (2015). Predictive distributions for between-study heterogeneity and simple methods for their application in bayesian meta-analysis. *Statistics in Medicine*, 34:984–998.

Unkel, S., Röver, C., Stallard, N., Benda, N., Posch, M., Zohar, S., and Friede, T. (2016). Systematic reviews in paediatric multiple sclerosis and Creutzfeldt-Jakob disease exemplify shortcomings in methods used to evaluate therapies in rare conditions. *Orphanet Journal of Rare Diseases*, 11, http://doi.org//10.1186/s13023-016-0402-6.

U.S. Food and Drug Administration (2004). Innovation/Stagnation–Challenge and Opportunity on the Critical Path to New Medical Products. `"http://www.fda.gov/downloads/ScienceResearch/SpecialTopics/CriticalPathInitiative/CriticalPathOpportunitiesReports/ucm113411.pdf"`.

U.S. Food and Drug Administration (2010). Guidance for the Use of Bayesian Statistics in Medical Device Clinical Trials. `"http://www.fda.gov/downloads/MedicalDevices/DeviceRegulationandGuidance/GuidanceDocuments/ucm071121.pdf"`.

U.S. Food and Drug Administration (2013). Paving the Way for Personalized Medicine: FDA's Role in a New Era of Medical Product Development. `"http://www.fda.gov/downloads/ScienceResearch/SpecialTopics/PersonalizedMedicine/UCM372421.pdf"`.

U.S. Food and Drug Administration (2015). Leveraging existing clinical data for extrapolation to pediatric uses of medical devices. Draft Guidance for Industry and Food and Drug Administration Staff. `"http://www.fda.gov/downloads/MedicalDevices/DeviceRegulationandGuidance/GuidanceDocuments/UCM444591.pdf"`.

U.S. Food and Drug Administration (2016). Guidance for industry: Non-inferiority clinical trials to establish effectiveness. `"https://www.fda.gov/downloads/Drugs/Guidances/UCM202140.pdf"`.

U.S. House of Representatives. (2015). 21st Century Cures Act. `"https://www.fas.org/sgp/crs/misc/R44071.pdf"`.

van de Wiel, M., Lien, T., Verlaat, W., van Wieringen, W., and Wilting, S. (2016). Better prediction by use of co-data: adaptive group-regularized ridge regression. *Statistics in Medicine*, 35(3):368–381.

van Rosmalen, J., Dejardin, D., van Norden, Y., Löwenberg, B., and Lesaffre, E. (2017). Including historical data in the analysis of clinical trials: Is it worth the effort? *Statistical Methods in Medical Research*, 11:16, http://doi.org//10.1177/0962280217694506.

Van Ryzin, J. (1980). Designing for nonparametric Bayesian survival analysis using historical controls. *Cancer Treatment Reports*, 64(2-3):503–506.

Veroniki, A., Jackson, D., Viechtbauer, W., Bender, R., Bowden, J., Knapp, G., Kuss, O., Higgins, J., Langan, D., and Salanti, G. (2016). Methods to estimate the between-study variance and its uncertainty in meta-analysis. *Research Synthesis Methods*, 7:55–79.

Viele, K., Berry, S., Neuenschwander, B., Amzal, B., Chen, F., Enas, N., Hobbs, B., Ibrahim, J., Kinnersley, N., Lindborg, S., Micallef, S., Roychoudhury, S., and Thompson, L. (2014). Use of historical control data for assessing treatment effects in clinical trials. *Pharmaceutical Statistics*, 13(1):41–54.

Walley, R., Smith, C., Gale, J., and Woodward, P. (2015). Advantages of a wholly Bayesian approach to assessing efficacy in early drug development: a case study. *Pharmaceutical Statistics*, 14(3):205–215.

Wandel, S. and Roychoudhury, S. (2016). Designing and analysing clinical trials in mental health: an evidence synthesis approach. *Evidence-based Mental Health*, 19(4):114–117.

Wandel, S., Schmidli, H., and Neuenschwander, B. (2015). Use of historical data. In *Cancer Clinical Trials: Current and Controversial Issues in Design and Analysis (Ed. S.George)*. CRC Press.

Weaver, J., Ohlssen, D., and Li, J. (2016). Strategies on using prior information when assessing adverse events. *Statistics in Biopharmaceutical Research*, 8(1):106–115.

Weber, S. (2017). *RBesT: R Bayesian Evidence Synthesis Tools.* http://CRAN.R-project.org/package-RBesT.

Witte, S., Schmidli, H., O'Hagan, A., and Racine, A. (2011). Designing a non-inferiority study in kidney transplantation: a case study. *Pharmaceutical Statistics*, 10(5):427–432.

7

Dose Ranging Studies and Dose Determination

Phil Woodward

Independent Consultant, UK

Alun Bedding

Roche Products Ltd, UK

David Dejardin

F. Hoffmann-La Roche, Switzerland

Dose ranging studies are a critical part of drug development to determine the range of doses that determine the therapeutic window, defined as the difference between the minimal dose providing benefit and the maximum safe dose. The therapeutic window is determined in dose response studies. These studies will ideally model the dose response relationship to determine not only the therapeutic window but also the optimal dose for a future study. In oncology, the dose to be investigated in later phases of drug development is typically determined in dose escalation trials. These trials investigate the safety of different doses of the drug or combination of drug under investigation. The literature describes a variety of Bayesian approaches for dose ranging and dose escalation studies. In this chapter we review the Bayesian approaches for dose ranging and dose escalation trials and discuss their benefits, as well as considerations around these Bayesian methods.

7.1 Introduction

Dose ranging studies are a critical part of drug development to determine the range of doses that determine the therapeutic window, defined as the difference between the minimal dose providing benefit and the maximum safe dose. In order to correctly determine the therapeutic window, dose response studies are carried out. These studies will ideally model the dose response relationship to determine not only the therapeutic window but also the optimal dose for a future study. The dose response is also critical if, at a later stage of development, a dose adjustment is needed. Generally, the determination of dose, and thus a dose ranging study, is carried out differently in oncology than in other therapeutic areas. In oncology, dose determination is carried out in a Phase I dose escalation trial, which will determine the dose to take into Phase III, thus obviating the need for Phase II. However, outside oncology the dose determination is done in a Phase II dose response study. In the next two sections, we will detail first dose finding studies in non-oncology situations and then in oncology studies. Since generic dose ranging methods apply more broadly to all therapeutic areas we cover the non-oncology studies first. We then go on to describe methods specific to dose escalation designs in oncology.

7.2 Dose-response studies

In this section we will describe Bayesian methods used in dose finding studies, mainly conducted outside oncology. Dose-response studies are an important facet of drug development as they provide information needed such as: identifying a target dose for future study, determining which starting dose to give to a patient, helping to decide how to adjust dosage, identifying the minimal dose at which there is benefit and identifying the highest dose beyond which no additional benefit will be gained or unacceptable side effects will occur. The statistical analysis of any data requires some assumptions that relate the observations to the process or system that we are trying to understand. Typically we use statistical models to formalize this relationship and make inference on the unobservable parameters of these models, or quantities derived from them, in order to better understand the process or system, as well as to make more reliable decisions. There is a tension between specifying models which are *assumption-rich* which, if the assumptions are appropriate, will enable us to extract more information from the data, and models which are *assumption-weak* which are more robust to model misspecification, but typically result in weaker inference. This is the classic issue of balancing bias and precision. The analysis of clinical dose ranging studies is no different.

ICH E4 (EMA, 2014) advises that studies "should emphasize elucidation of the dose-response function, not individual pairwise comparisons", providing support for the assumption-rich approach. However, elsewhere it more ambiguously states that "the lowest dose(s) tested, if these are to be recommended, [must] have a statistically significant and clinically meaningful effect." This latter quote suggests that demonstrating that a monotonic dose-response function is statistically significant, when compared to the null hypothesis of no effect at any dose, is not sufficient to be able to claim that all doses have a statistically significant effect, even though this does logically follow under the assumption that the monotonic dose-response function is appropriate. In the vast majority of cases, the dose-response study is not considered pivotal, so a confirmatory Phase III study is run to address this issue. It is in these cases where Bayesian methods can be applied with least controversy. The issue of applying Bayesian methods when strict Type I error rate control is mandated is not specific to dose-response studies and so we will not discuss it any detail here.

The structure of this section is as follows. First we describe the Bayesian methods used for models that are assumption-weak; then we look at the assumption-rich approaches, where a functional relationship is imposed on the dose response relationship. With both of these methods we illustrate how to formulate prior distributions for the Bayesian analysis. Finally, we describe a non-Bayesian method for dose finding, *MCP-Mod*, that has received much attention recently, and briefly discuss this from a Bayesian perspective.

7.2.1 Dose-response in human trial based on pre-clinical data: Background

Woodward (2016, Chapter 7) discusses two experiments, one pre-clinical and the other in human, in which proof of mechanism was being assessed by characterizing the exposure and dose-response of a compound using a pharmacology biomarker. The pre-clinical experiment involved taking human blood and adding (referred to as "spiking") a challenge agent that is known to induce an inflammatory response. A concentration-response relationship between a pharmacology biomarker of inflammation and a novel compound was assessed by spiking separate blood samples of this challenged blood with different amounts of the compound. The response used was derived from counting the number of cells affected by the compound, measured on a multiplicative scale and referred to as the N-fold change relative to an aliquot without any spiked compound. An increase implies the compound affects the pharmacology as hypothesized. This experiment provided sufficient confidence in the pharmacological activity of the compound as a function of the concentration to progress into the clinic. However, this experiment was undertaken under ideal conditions while in practice the compound will be delivered to the patient orally and the actual concentration in the blood will be determined by the pharmacokinetic properties, as well as tablet to tablet and patient to patient variations.

An ex-vivo experiment is used in order to determine the concentration-response for a particular compound. The human PK study determines the dose-concentration model. Combined together the models give the dose-response model, with which it is planned to leverage the pre-clinical information. The amount of a compound that can be administered to humans is limited by the compound's maximum tolerated dose, i.e. only doses below which tolerable adverse events occur can be used. A clinical study was undertaken to assess the pharmacological activity with these practical constraints. The desired outcome of the study was to provide guidance on the dose to be chosen for the subsequent larger study.

In this study 34 subjects were randomly assigned to one of six dose levels of the compound. After sufficient time had elapsed for the compound to have reached its maximum concentration in the blood, a sample was taken and, as before, it was spiked with the challenge agent known to induce an inflammatory response. The actual compound's concentration in the blood, plus the N-fold change in inflammatory response from the pre-treatment baseline was measured for each sample. Figure 7.1 shows a scatter plot of the data.

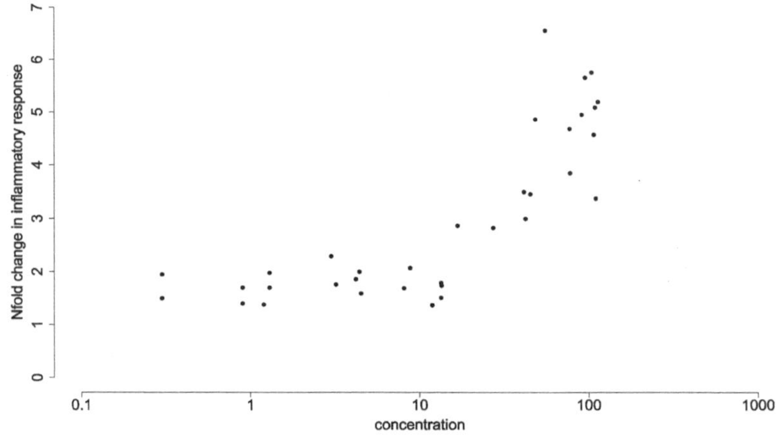

FIGURE 7.1: Clinical pharmacology study: Illustrative scatter plot of the N-fold change in the inflammatory response from baseline to log(concentration).

7.2.2 Assumption-weak models

It is probably still true to say that nowadays most often clinical dose response studies are analyzed with models that assume no relationship between the true mean responses at each dose level. When this happens, we call the statistical model assumption-weak. Of course, such models can still be based on strong parametric assumptions, but with respect to the impact of the dose on the response, they are based on minimal statistical assumptions. For continuous endpoints models such as analysis of variance (ANOVA) or covariance (ANCOVA) or mixed models are common, and when outcomes are binary, logistic regression is often used.

The Bayesian approach to fitting such models is covered in more general Bayesian textbooks, for example Gelman et al. (2013). Software used for implementing these include `WinBugs`, `OpenBugs`, `SAS Proc MCMC`, `Stan` and `JAGS`. For these common cases and when weak prior knowledge is reflected in the choice of priors, the Bayesian credible intervals obtained will be almost identical to the confidence intervals obtained using classical methods, see Chapter 1, Section 1.3. When stronger prior information exists it is necessary to identify the parameter(s), or function of parameters, that need to be assigned informative priors. In some cases this might require the model to be reparameterized. But the most common situation is when we can justify an informative prior for the placebo response based on historical data; refer back to Chapter 6. In the simple case when ANOVA is being used the model can be represented algebraically:

$$Y_{ij} = \mu + \alpha_i + \epsilon_{ij} \quad (i = 1, \ldots, k \quad \text{and} \quad j = 1, \ldots, n_i),$$

where Y_{ij} is the response of the j-th subject receiving the $i-$th treatment, μ is a constant whose meaning depends upon how the treatment factor is parameterized, α_i represents the effects of the treatments, ϵ_{ij} is the residual random error associated with the $j-$th subject receiving the $i-$th treatment with $\epsilon_{ij} \sim \mathrm{N}(0, \sigma^2)$, k is the number of treatment arms and n_i is the number of subjects receiving the $i-$th treatment.

If (in order to make the parameters estimable) the usual convention of constraining one of the α_i to zero is followed then μ and α_i represent the true mean response for the constrained dose level and the true mean differences from that level respectively. It is possible to choose the zero constraint such that μ represents the placebo true mean response, and hence it is a simple matter to incorporate an informative prior that represents knowledge obtained from historical studies. More typically a baseline covariate, as well as possibly other covariates, is included in an ANCOVA model. In that case it is important to realize that μ represents the placebo response when all the covariates equal zero. For an informative prior based on historical data to be credible, not only should the covariates be centered but the variance of the prior distribution should be large enough to accommodate any variation due to differences between the covariates' means in the current study and those in the historical studies. When the prior is based on many historical studies and the between-study heterogeneity is appropriately accommodated for, e.g. using the meta-analytic predictive approach (Schmidli et al., 2017) then, provided the current study is not targeting a niche population, we should not be too concerned. In cases of only a few historical studies then more care is needed and we may wish to inflate the prior variance to address this issue. There may also be concerns around exchangeability when using historical data. For more in depth reference to the use of historical data please refer to Chapter 6. If we knew the covariates' summary statistics in each of the historical studies, or better still had all the individual patient data, then it would be possible to define the placebo prior distribution as a function of the covariates which would then dynamically adjust the prior based on the actual covariate data in the current study.

In studies where there is a positive control, such as a standard of care compound, as well as the placebo arm it is simple to add an informative prior for this arm also. One of the α_i will represent the difference between the positive control and placebo, i.e. the effect of the positive control, which is more stable between studies than the response and hence a better quantity on which to derive an informative prior. In principle it would be possible to define a multivariate prior for the positive control effect and the placebo response, but in practice it is likely to be rare that there will be enough historical studies with which to estimate the correlation parameter with enough precision to make this worthwhile.

7.2.3 Assumption-rich models

It must be true that there exists a difference between two dose levels that is so small that the difference between the mean responses is close to zero. This implies that the dose-response relationship must be smoothly changing. The science of pharmacology has found that a particular shape of dose or exposure-response is ubiquitous: *the sigmoidal curve*, i.e. initially the response changes very slowly as the dose increases, then a stronger dose-response relationship occurs and finally this slows again as some sort of plateau is reached. Thomas et al. (2014) and Thomas and Roy (2017) have shown that, at least for small molecules that show any efficacy, this relationship held for virtually all of the dose-response studies they analyzed. The initial work was based on all such studies undertaken by Pfizer between 1998 and 2009. This was followed up by reviewing all the drugs approved by the FDA between 2009 and 2014. A similar review of large molecules ("biological products") developed by Pfizer (Wu et al., 2018), also showed that this sigmoidal assumption held for the vast majority of cases.

The most commonly used model to describe a sigmoidal relationship is the "$\mathrm{E}_{\max}$ model" (see Chapter 5). This model has four parameters: the response when the dose is zero, E_0, the maximum possible effect, $\mathrm{E}_{\max}$, the dose which produces 50% of this maximum effect, ED_{50}, and a shape parameter (also referred to as *hill parameter*), γ, which determines the steepness of the dose-response. The $\mathrm{E}_{\max}$ model formula is:

$$Y_i = \mathrm{E}_0 + \frac{\mathrm{E}_{\max} X_i^{\gamma}}{\mathrm{ED}_{50}^{\gamma} + X_i^{\gamma}}, \tag{7.1}$$

where X_i is the dose and Y_i is the response (percentage or proportion) of the $i-$th subject. This is a non-linear model since the formula given above implies that the mean response is not a weighted linear combination of the unknown parameters. Figure 7.2 shows the shape of the $\mathrm{E}_{\max}$ model, and how it is affected by the γ parameter. The E_0 and $\mathrm{E}_{\max}$ parameters simply shift and stretch the curves vertically respectively, while the ED_{50} parameter stretches the curves horizontally, in an obvious manner. Although the curves plotted all show an increasing response with increasing dose, a decreasing response can be modeled by a negative $\mathrm{E}_{\max}$ parameter, keeping the γ parameter positive in both cases. Note that between the doses that give 20% and 80% of the effect, the relationship is very close to being linear on the log-dose scale. For this reason, it is usually much easier to interpret plots of the data using the log-scale for the dose. When a zero dose, such as a placebo arm, is included some judgment is needed where to display these data on the log-dose axis to facilitate visual inspection. Also, if it is known, or subsequently discovered, that the active doses are all in this central "log-linear" region, a much simpler linear model, with log-dose as the covariate, should be adequate when modeling the active doses. In this case an indicator function is required to model the response for the placebo arm separately, e.g.

$$Y_i = \alpha + \mathbb{I}(X_i > 0)\left[\beta_0 + \beta \log(X_i)\right]$$

where $\mathbb{I}(X_i > 0)$ is an indicator function equaling 1 if true and 0 if false.

Inspection of the curves on the natural scale suggests that an even simpler linear model could sometimes be adequate. When the hill slope ($= \gamma$) $= 1$, a common assumption supported by the work of Thomas et al. (2014) and Thomas and Roy (2017), and, the compound is only being dosed up to about 60% of its maximum efficacy, the $\mathrm{E}_{\max}$ curve is

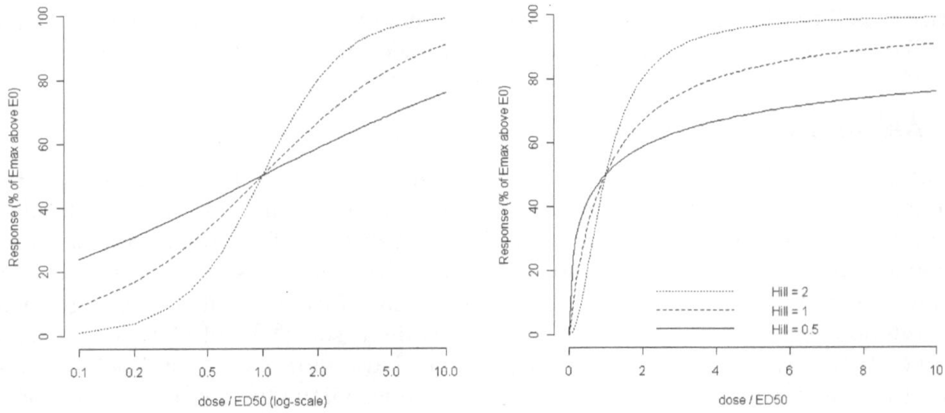

FIGURE 7.2: Percentage of E_{max} above E_0 as a function of a covariate, dose/ED_{50} log scale (left hand panel) and dose/ED_{50} (right hand panel), under different forms of the E_{max} model with varying hill parameter.

approximately linear. When the slope is steeper, i.e. larger γ, the linear range is wider still. Of course, the degree to which a simple linear relationship is adequate will also depend upon the relative size of the variation about the mean response. Since most clinical endpoints used in Phase IIb and III studies tend to have high variance relative to the size of the efficacy signal, and the upper limit of the dose range is often restricted due to safety concerns, possibility of using a simpler linear or log-linear model should be considered.

Finally, before discussing explicitly the Bayesian aspects of dose-response modeling, one should note that in order to cover the majority of the dose-response curve, say between the 10% and 90% maximal effects, the ratio of highest to lowest active dose must be at least 80 for the typical γ of 1. This also assumes we have chosen doses that are centered about the true ED_{50}. Typically doses are chosen on a multiplicative scale, with a 3-fold separation between consecutive doses being common. In this case one would need at least five active doses in order to cover the majority of the dose-response curve. Most dose response studies run in practice (Thomas and Roy, 2017) include fewer active doses than this, and so in most cases it is quite likely that the data in the study alone will be insufficient to provide precise estimates of all of the parameters of the E_{max} model. In particular, it is highly unlikely that such a study will provide enough information to precisely estimate the γ parameter. In fact it is quite common for classical methods of fitting E_{max} models to fail to converge (Thomas and Roy, 2017), which requires an iterative approach to the analysis of the data via the use of ad-hoc constraints or alternative simpler models.

7.2.4 Bayesian modeling

While adaptive designs (see Chapter 8) can help to center the doses, it is still likely that the dose range will not cover the whole dose-response curve suggesting that informative priors could prove valuable. As part of the review undertaken in Thomas et al. (2014) and Thomas and Roy (2017), these authors determined weakly informative priors for the parameters of the E_{max} when used to model small molecule dose-response data in Phase IIb or III studies. Table 7.1 shows priors based on their work. Their work also showed that by utilizing these priors, which with the exception of γ, are still quite vague, the Bayesian E_{max} model could be fitted to virtually all of their cases. The prior for γ is of course still much less informative than the common practice of constraining it to be exactly one. The ability of a Bayesian E_{max} model with evidence based weakly informative priors to provide good fit to most clinical dose response data is in stark contrast to the difficulties typically encountered when using likelihood based methods. Of course, it is still important to check that these priors are credible for the particular study being run. If this is not deemed credible then the prior should be adjusted accordingly; our motivating example is one such case.

TABLE 7.1: Prior distributions for the E_{max} when used to model small molecule dose-response data in Phase IIb or III based on Thomas et al. (2014).

Parameter	Prior Distribution
E_0	When possible use informative prior for placebo response Otherwise, Normal (mean = 0, SD = very large relative to residual error)
E_{max}	Normal (mean = 0, SD = very large relative to residual error) Note that when the data does not cover both plateaus the E_{max} and ED_{50} parameters are highly correlated and hence, can be sensitive to each other's priors.
ED_{50}	$\log(ED_{50}) \sim$ t-distribution(mean = logP50, scale = 1.1, df = 4) logP50 = log of prior estimate of ED_{50} from previous clinical or preclinical studies or, if no reliable estimate, the geometric mean of lowest two active doses
γ	$\log(\gamma) \sim$ t-distribution(mean = 0, scale = 0.35, df = 4)

In some cases, we may have more informative priors either based on previous clinical studies of similar compounds, perhaps targeting the same mechanism of action, or based on earlier experiments using the same compound. The motivating example introduced earlier is of the latter type.

Bornkamp (2012) considers using *functional uniform priors* when it is not possible to use historical data or a properly elicited prior. He argues that in this situation using uniform priors in the parameter space is actually more informative than expected. This is due to the uniform prior being sensitive to the parameterization and the bounds used. He notes that the obvious alternative, the Jeffreys' prior has practical limitations in the setting of non-linear regression as the prior would need to be pre-specified. Therefore, he proposes the functional uniform distribution, which imposes a distribution on the parameters, so that it is uniform in the functional shapes underlying the nonlinear regression function. More detail on this approach can be found in Bornkamp (2012).

7.2.5 Dose-response in human trial based on pre-clinical data: Analysis of the data

In order to be confident that the next much larger study in patients could adequately test the scientific hypothesis underpinning the rationale for the treatment, it was considered important that blood concentrations at least as high as the ED_{50} could be obtained. Without undertaking any formal analysis, it is clear from Figure 7.1 that the concentration-response curve has not reached its upper plateau and the data alone would not be able to answer this question, since to estimate the ED_{50}, it is necessary to have reliable estimates of both the lower (E_0) and upper plateaus ($E_0 + E_{max}$). First, we will fit a simple E_{max} model using very flat priors for all except the γ parameter. The recommendations of Thomas et al. (see Table 7.1) are not appropriate here as this is not a traditional Phase IIb dose ranging study. In particular, the concentration range is at least an order of magnitude greater than that observed in the typical study included in their meta-analysis. Here we essentially use the default priors proposed by Woodward (2016): $E_0 \sim N(0, 100)$, $E_{max} \sim N(0, 100)$, $\log(ED_{50}) \sim N(\log(5.7), 4.4)$, $\log(\gamma) \sim N(0, 0.35)$ and $\sigma^2 \sim \text{Inv-Gamma}(0.001, 0.001)$.

The priors for E_0, E_{max} and σ are those conventionally used to represent vague prior knowledge. The prior for ED_{50} is weakly informative, having median in the center of the concentration range (more specifically the geometric mean of the lowest and highest concentrations observed) and a Log-Normal distribution implying 50% prior probability of lying inside the range of the concentrations being studied. The prior for γ is relatively strong, with median of 1 and prior probability of 95% of lying between 0.5 and 2.

`OpenBUGS` (Lunn et al., 2009) was used to fit the model using a burn-in of 25,000 followed by 4,000 samples with 25−th thinning. Although the history plots indicated convergence, there were occasional spikes in the plots for ED_{50} and E_{max} almost certainly due to the priors being too weak to overcome the paucity of information with which to estimate these parameters in the data. Posterior estimates are shown in Table 7.2 and the fitted model, obtained using the `Excel GUI BugsXLA` (Woodward, 2016), is displayed in Figure 7.3.

TABLE 7.2: Summarized posterior distributions using relatively weak priors.

Parameter	Mean	SD	2.5%ile	Median	97.5%ile
E_0	1.5	0.26	0.9	1.5	1.9
E_{max}	9.2	9.2	3.4	6.0	42
ED_{50}	350	1300	28	74	2700
γ	1.2	0.45	0.6	1.1	2.3
σ	0.74	0.099	0.57	0.73	0.95

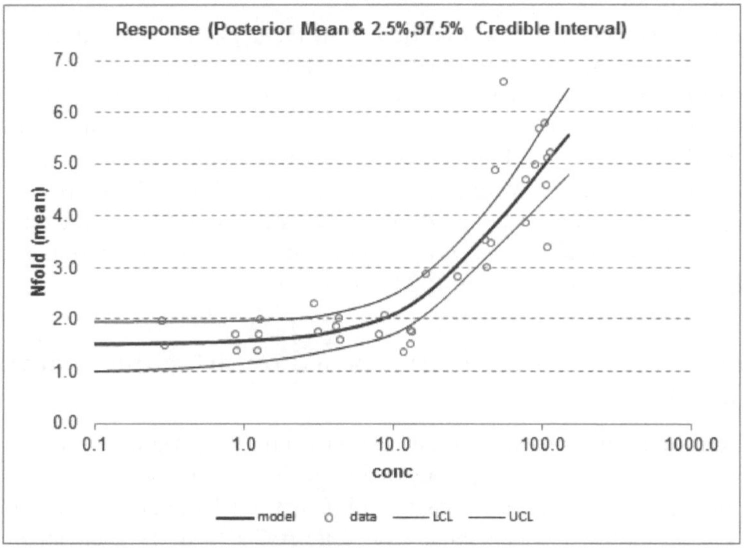

FIGURE 7.3: E_{max} model summarized in Table 7.2 (weak priors).

Inspection of both the E_{max} and the ED_{50} parameters shows that neither is estimated very precisely, both having credible values that are well outside the range of the data.

Results such as these should alert the user to the strong possibility that the priors are influential, which is of concern when they are not based on justifiable prior beliefs.

There was some reason to believe that the maximum possible effect should be the same in both the pre-clinical laboratory experiment and the clinical study. If so, the posterior for the E_{max} parameter obtained from the pre-clinical experiment could be justified as a prior for the clinical study. After some discussion, it was decided that the additional uncertainty in the translation of the pre-clinical experiment should be incorporated by inflating the variance of the posterior based on the pre-clinical data. The posterior for the E_{max} parameter in the pre-clinical study could be summarized by a mean of 3.38 and a standard deviation of 0.32, which was used to justify a Normal prior distribution for the E_{max} in the clinical study with a mean of 3.4 and a standard deviation of 1. This prior implies that, before running the clinical study, we believe the E_{max} lies between 1.4 and 5.4 with probability 95%. The posterior estimates and fitted model using this more informative prior are shown in Table 7.3 and Figure 7.4.

TABLE 7.3: Summarized posterior distributions using informative prior for E_{max}.

Parameter	Mean	SD	2.5%ile	Median	97.5%ile
E_0	1.6	0.20	1.2	1.6	2.0
E_{max}	4.1	0.59	3.1	4.0	5.4
ED_{50}	40	11	23	38	67
γ	1.7	0.44	1.0	1.6	2.8
σ	0.71	0.097	0.55	0.70	0.92

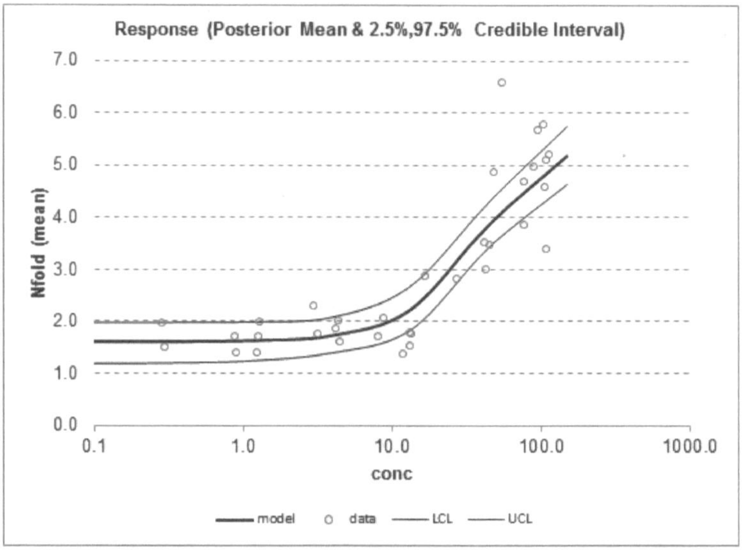

FIGURE 7.4: E_{max} model summarized in Table 7.3 (informative prior for E_{max}).

Not surprisingly, the posterior for the E_{max} parameter is much more precise than before, with a mean that has been shrunk towards the prior mean. Although none of the other prior distributions were changed from the defaults, the additional information regarding the value of the E_{max} parameter has also greatly increased the posterior precision for the

ED_{50} parameter. This should not be a surprise either, since this parameter defines the concentration that gives a response half-way between E_0 and $(E_0 + E_{max})$. This shows that an informative prior of E_{max} is essential, because in the majority of cases the data do not exist in the study with which to estimate E_{max} precisely.

It is informative to compare the estimated Bayesian models with that obtained using classical methods. Table 7.4 shows the parameter estimates obtained using the `nls` package in `R` to fit the same four parameter E_{max} model. The most obvious difference is the γ estimate, which is effectively equivalent to fitting a step function at the ED50 concentration. More concerning is the apparent precision with which the E_{max} has been estimated. Even a cursory inspection of the data indicates that these inferences do not appear to be justified.

TABLE 7.4: Non-linear least squares estimates using `nls` routine in `R`.

Parameter	Mean	SD
E_0	1.9	0.14
E_{max}	3.1	0.25
ED_{50}	43	1.4
γ	17	11
σ	0.63	(30 df)

One might argue that a fairer comparison would be one in which the γ parameter is constrained in a similar manner to how the strong prior affects the Bayesian posterior distributions. One method is to set lower and upper bounds to the estimates using the port algorithm in the `nls` package. If these bounds are set equal to the three standard deviation limits of the prior distributions, the constrained least squares estimates shown in Table 7.5 are obtained.

TABLE 7.5: Non-linear least squares estimates using `nls` routine in `R` with constraints on the estimates based on the initial Bayesian priors used.

Parameter	Mean	SD
E_0	1.7	0.19
E_{max}	3.4	0.48
ED_{50}	34	6.1
γ	2.8	1.3
σ	0.67	(30 d.f.)

Although there is now more uncertainty in the E_{max} estimate, it is still indicating that we can be reasonably confident that it lies between 2.4 and 4.4. Based on the data alone, this still appears to be an unreasonably precise estimate of the upper asymptote of the concentration response curve. We argue that the initial Bayesian analysis more appropriately accounts for the uncertainty in the fitted model based on the data in the study alone. Also, if the informative prior for the E_{max} parameter can be justified then the Bayesian approach can be used to demonstrate that it is possible to achieve concentrations of the compound in the blood that are almost certainly higher than the ED_{50}, this being the primary objective of the study. The Bayesian analysis makes it clear that we cannot draw this conclusion from the study data alone, but only if we accept the more informative prior for the E_{max} parameter appropriately represents our knowledge following the pre-clinical experiment.

7.2.6 MCP-Mod methodology

Recently, interest has been raised in the *MCP-Mod method* (Multiple Comparison Procedure - Modeling) first proposed by Bretz et al. (2005). This methodology has also been endorsed by the CHMP in their Qualification Opinion of MCP-Mod as an efficient statistical methodology for model-based design and analysis of Phase II dose finding studies under model uncertainty (EMA, 2014) and designated by the FDA as a fit for purpose method of dose finding (U.S. Food and Drug Administration, 2016). In this approach a candidate set of potentially relevant parametric dose-response models is proposed and a multiple comparison procedure is used to choose one of them. The aim of this model selection technique is to preserve the family-wise error rate without losing the benefits of making inferences via a good fitting smooth curve. The procedure begins by testing the null hypothesis of no dose-response for each candidate model individually using a test statistic derived from a model specific optimal linear combination of the dose group mean responses. Multiplicity adjustment is made that accounts for the multivariate joint distribution of all these test statistics. Of the models that have a significant contrast test statistic one is chosen to be the best fit to the data; typically, this is the one with the smallest P-value although other considerations may come into play, e.g. the numerical stability of the model fit. This best model is then used in the usual way to determine the doses to take into the next stage of development, e.g. the minimal effective dose might be chosen as the one that has expected effect greater than some pre-specified clinically relevant difference. The main motivation of the MCP-Mod procedure appears to be that it provides strong family-wise error control of the significance test for a dose-response. If Type I error rate control is of primary concern when designing the study, then it is true by definition that a frequentist approach should be preferred to the Bayesian. We argue that dose-response studies should be primarily considered part of the learning, rather than confirming, stage of drug development, which gives us the flexibility to use Bayesian methods with the advantages discussed in this chapter. Also, given that Thomas and Roy (2017) have shown that the E_{max} curve provides an adequate fit for the vast majority of Phase IIb dose-response studies, the MCP-Mod procedure appears to be overly cautious. However, if one was persuaded of the need to consider alternative models as part of a single analysis plan, Bayesian Model Averaging (see also Chapter 1), which would also accommodate the uncertainty in the final choice of model, is a natural approach to adopt, see Ohlssen and Racine (2015).

7.3 Dose escalation trials in oncology

The goal of *dose escalation trials* for oncology drugs is to identify the range of safe doses to be used for further development of the drug. The upper limit of the range is called the *maximum tolerated dose* (MTD). These trials are usually testing the drug for the first time in human and hence, usually no prior information on the toxicity of the compound is available. Such trials are typically small (in the range of 10-60 patients) and conducted in an heterogeneous population (e.g. with different tumor types at different stages of the disease). An introduction to such trials is discussed in Chapter 10 of Piantadosi (2005).

The design of dose escalation trials defines which doses are tested, in which sequence and in how many subjects. The designs are all sequential in nature. Namely, doses are tested in a group of patients (called a cohort, with typical sizes from 1 to 6). A decision based on the observed data is then made for the next cohort until a stopping rule is reached at which time the MTD is defined. In addition, the assumption is made that higher doses lead to higher toxicity. The designs are typically based on the observation of *dose limiting toxicities* (DLT), which is a set of predefined toxic effects attributable to the drug considered to be unacceptable and to limit the dose escalation (Le Tourneau et al., 2009).

The section is organized as follows. We first describe a motivating example. Then follows the introduction of the classical approach and the issues related to this approach. The *Bayesian Continual Reassessment Method* (CRM) is introduced next. An important aspect of the CRM is its flexibility, allowing for a variety of extensions, which we will also describe. We then illustrate the use of the CRM on our motivating example. We end with a conclusion.

7.3.1 MTD for a new immunotherapy: Background

The goal of this trial was to determine the Maximum Tolerated Dose of a new immunotherapy to treat patients with solid tumors. The compound under investigation was a genetically modified version of a natural signaling molecule of the immune system. This trial was the first-in-human experiment with this molecule. The starting dose of 0.1mg was defined as 3 to 4 times higher than the *minimum anticipated biological effect level* (MABEL) to avoid a too long dose escalation. The doses to be tested were initially 0.1, 0.5, 1.5 and 3mg. Subsequent doses were to be chosen by the dose escalation design from a grid starting at 10mg with increments of 5mg. Pharmaco-kinetic (PK) characteristics of the drug obtained from animal data suggested a high patient to patient PK variability. Patients treated with doses differing by less than 5mg would have similar PK parameters. The same animal data predicted an MTD in humans of 70mg.

7.3.2 "3+3" dose escalation designs

The most frequently used Phase I dose escalation design is the "3+3" design (Rogatko et al., 2007; Le Tourneau et al., 2012). It is a rule-based design by which a set of pre-specified rules define what dose to give to the next cohort. The model-based design, which will be treated in Section 7.3.3 relies on a model to calculate the best dose to administer to the next cohort.

The "3+3" design pre-specifies the starting dose and escalation steps. A first cohort is treated at the starting dose. If no DLT is observed, the next pre-defined dose is tested in a cohort of 3 patients. If one DLT is observed, the current cohort is expanded to 6 patients at the same dose to confirm the toxicity finding. If 2 or more DLTs out of 3 or 6 patients are experienced, the MTD is defined as the dose prior to the dose at which these 2 or more DLTs were observed. This ensures that the observed proportion of DLT is less than 33% at the MTD. We refer to Storer (1989) for the statistical properties of this design.

The main benefit of this design is that it is easy to implement in practice, does not require complex computation and so does not need the input of statisticians. For these reasons, the design is still popular among clinical researchers. However, the literature reports the following pitfalls for the 3+3 design (Le Tourneau et al., 2009; Lin and Shih, 2001; Reiner et al., 1999). Namely, too many subjects are treated at sub-therapeutic doses; there is slow escalation of the doses and small precision of the MTD estimate; there is use of the last cohort only (3 to 6 patients) to derive the risk of DLT and most importantly a poor MTD estimate is obtained due to early stopping. To address those pitfalls, many modifications to the original design and other ruled-based approaches were proposed and are cited in the thorough review from Sverdlov et al. (2014).

7.3.3 Bayesian model-based dose escalation designs

To overcome the limitations outlined in Section 7.3.2, model-based approaches have been introduced. These approaches use the entire set of observed data to derive the best dose to be administered in either the next cohort or as MTD. The CRM was introduced by O'Quigley et al. (1990) as the first Bayesian model-based approach for a dose escalation design.

O'Quigley et al. (1990) proposed to compute the next dose as the one for which the posterior expectation of the toxicity rate is the closest to a given threshold (denoted θ). The choice of θ is based on the type of drug (and mechanism of action) and the disease for which it is developed. It typically lies between 20 and 35% and is consistent with the "3+3" design, which derives the MTD based on a 33% DLT rate. Formally, let x_i be the dose given to the i−th patient ($i = 1, \ldots, m$) and $y_1, \ldots, y_m$ be the corresponding observed toxicities ($y_i = 1$ when i−th patient has experienced a DLT and 0 otherwise). Let also $\Psi(x; \alpha)$ be a model for the dose-toxicity curve with parameter α. O'Quigley et al. (1990) used in their examples a one parameter power "skeleton" model for $\Psi(x; \alpha)$, i.e. $\Psi(x; \alpha) = [(\tanh x + 1)/2]^{\alpha}$. Then for the $(m + 1)$−th patient, the dose x_{m+1} will be chosen such that

$$\theta_{m+1} = \int \Psi(x_{m+1}; \alpha) p(\alpha \mid D_m) d\alpha \tag{7.2}$$

is the closest to the given threshold θ.

In Equation (7.2), $p(\alpha \mid D_m)$ is the posterior density of α given the observed data D_m up to the m−th patient. Bayes Theorem tells us that

$$p(\alpha \mid D_m) = \frac{p(\alpha) \prod_1^m \Psi(x_i; \alpha)^{y_i} [1 - \Psi(x_i; \alpha)]^{1-y_i}}{\int p(\alpha) \prod_1^m \Psi(x_i; \alpha)^{y_i} [1 - \Psi(x_i; \alpha)]^{1-y_i} d\alpha}, \tag{7.3}$$

where $p(\alpha)$ is the prior density for α. For the one parameter power "skeleton" model $\Psi(x; \alpha) = ((\tanh x + 1)/2)^{\alpha}$, the prior $p(\alpha) = \exp(-\alpha)$ is suggested (O'Quigley et al., 1990). See Chapters 5 and 6 for a broader discussion of choosing priors. O'Quigley et al. (1990) looked at the operating characteristics of a design that decides about the dose after each patient (cohorts of 1 patient) and enrolls a fixed number of 25 patients.

In Goodman et al. (1995); Korn et al. (1994); Tighiouart and Rogatko (2012) three issues were reported with the original CRM. Firstly, a cohort size of 1 imposes that the recruitment is halted after each patient, this to allow the time (called DLT observation period) to observe the toxicity. This period often leads to significant delays in the conduct of the trial. Secondly, the proposed doses by the CRM may be too large and thus investigators may feel uncomfortable to follow the dose recommendations. Thirdly, the fixed predefined number of patients does not allow to stop the trial earlier even when sufficient evidence is available for a given dose. We will now describe a variety of extensions of the original CRM design that deal with the above objections against the original CRM design.

For the first issue, Goodman et al. (1995) suggested the enrollment of larger cohorts. This allows to gather more evidence on the toxicity between each interruption of the recruitment. Tighiouart and Rogatko (2012) studied the effect of cohort size on the performance. They reported a similar performance for a design with cohorts of 3 patients compared to 1 patient cohorts.

For the second issue, Korn et al. (1994) suggested to impose a limit on the dose escalation (e.g. $\mid \theta_{m+1} - \theta_m \mid / \theta_m < 1$).

Babb et al. (1998) suggested a modification of the dose calculation strategy. They proposed an escalation design that controls the overdose, called the *Escalation with Overdose Control* (EWOC) design. The EWOC design ensures a sufficiently high probability that the next dose is below the MTD. The following strategy is installed. Let the unknown MTD be x^* and $0 \leq \rho \leq 1$ be the unknown toxicity at the starting dose x_{min}. In Babb et al. (1998)

a two-parameter model for the dose-toxicity model is assumed and this model is reparameterized as a function of x^* and ρ leading to the model $\overline{\Psi}(x; x^*, \rho)$. Using this approach, the dose x_{m+1} is chosen such as

$$\Pr(x^* < x_{m+1} \mid D_m) < \epsilon \tag{7.4}$$

where

$$\Pr(x^* < x_{m+1} \mid D_m) = \int_{x_{min}}^{x_{m+1}} \int_0^1 p(x^*, \rho \mid D_m) d\rho dx^*. \tag{7.5}$$

Expression (7.5) makes use of the posterior

$$p(x^*, \rho \mid D_m) = \frac{p(x^*, \rho) \prod_1^m \overline{\Psi}(x; x^*, \rho)^{y_i} [1 - \overline{\Psi}(x; , x^*, \rho)]^{1-y_i}}{\int p(x^*, \rho) \prod_1^m \overline{\Psi}(x; x^*, \rho)^{y_i} [1 - \overline{\Psi}(x; , x^*, \rho)]^{1-y_i} d\rho dx^*},$$

with $p(x^*, \rho)$ the joint prior for x^* and ρ (see Babb et al. (1998) for suggestions).

Another dose calculation method with the same goals has been proposed by Neuenschwander et al. (2008). They proposed to use the following loss function for the determination of the next dose:

$$l(x; \alpha) = \begin{cases} l_1 = 1 & \text{if } \Psi(x; \alpha) \in (0, 0.2] \\ l_2 = 0 & \text{if } \Psi(x; \alpha) \in (0.2, 0.35] \\ l_3 = 1 & \text{if } \Psi(x; \alpha) \in (0.35, 0.6] \\ l_4 = 2 & \text{if } \Psi(x; \alpha) \in (0.6, 1] \end{cases}$$

From the loss function, a Bayes risk is computed that penalizes over- or undershooting of the function $\Psi(x; \alpha)$, i.e. when it is outside the interval (0.2, 0.35]. The Bayes risk is here defined as $B(x) = l_1 \Pr(\Psi(x, \alpha) \in (0, 0.2]) + l_1 \Pr(\Psi(x, \alpha) \in (0, 0.2]) + l_2 \Pr(\Psi(x, \alpha) \in (0.2, 0.35]) + l_3 \Pr([\Psi(x, \alpha) \in (0.35, 0.6]) + l_4 \Pr(\Psi(x, \alpha) \in (0.6, 1])$ is minimized to compute the dose for the next cohort.

The third issue involves the stopping rule. Many authors have proposed adaptation to allow for early stopping. We describe now some suggested changes. Korn et al. (1994) proposed to stop dose escalation when a minimum of 6 patients have been treated at the MTD. Goodman et al. (1995) suggested to use the width of the credibility interval for the toxicity at the MTD as an indication of the accuracy of the estimation. Heyd and Carlin (1999) proposed a stopping rule based on the credibility interval for α. Zohar and Chevret (2001) investigated seven stopping rules through simulations. They concluded that using a stopping rule allows effectively reducing the sample size required for the dose escalation trial but observed that there were no uniformly best stopping rule adapted to all situations. O'Quigley (2002) suggested to stop the dose escalation based on the probability that the recommended dose does not change, given the current data. They show that this stopping rule works well in reducing the sample size but no comparative study between a variety of stopping rules was reported. Finally, Neuenschwander et al. (2008) suggested stopping the dose escalation when the recommended dose has a sufficiently high probability to be in the target toxicity range, i.e. $\Pr(\Psi(x; \alpha) \in (0.2, 0.35])$ is above a pre-specified threshold.

In addition to the above three issues, the choice of the model $\Psi(x; \alpha)$ and the prior for α are discussed in the literature. For instance, Cheung and Chappell (2002) proposed conditions for consistency of the CRM and Paoletti et al. (2004) proposed a theoretical framework to compare approaches.

The original CRM introduces a "skeleton" probability power model. Neuenschwander et al. (2008) proposed a two-parameter logistic model and compared it to the "skeleton" power model. They argue that the operating characteristics for the two models are the same and that the two-parameter logistic is more realistic. Yin and Yuan (2009) proposed a model averaging strategy. Model averaging improves the operating characteristics of the design compared to the skeleton model with acceptable computation complexity. Curve-free approaches have been introduced (see (Sverdlov et al., 2014) for details). For the prior specification, O'Quigley and Conaway (2010) described three options: 1) postulate a suitable prior density $\pi(\alpha)$. In Neuenschwander et al. (2008) one way is reported to define this prior based on the elicitation of quantities that are easy to grasp for clinicians. 2) Introduce a set of pseudo-data (see (Murphy and Hall, 1997)) and 3) Introduce a 2-stage approach whereby the initial approach is used to calibrate the CRM run at the second stage (see (Sverdlov et al., 2014) for references on this topic).

7.3.4 Benefits of the CRM approaches

In this section, we highlight the benefits of using the Bayesian CRM design over the classical "3+3" approach. We discuss: i) the theoretical and large sample properties of the CRM and the MTD estimator; ii) the small sample properties of the CRM versus the "3+3" approach; and iii) the flexibility of the CRM framework.

Firstly, while Shen and O'Quigley (1996) showed that the classical "3+3" design is inconsistent, the consistency and asymptotic Normality of the MTD estimator was established by the authors under some regularity conditions. These conditions have been relaxed by Azriel (2012). Further, based on these results Cheung (2013) developed a method for sample size determination for CRM designs.

Secondly, small sample properties were examined in many simulation studies. Most publications report better operating characteristics for the CRM design. Ahn (1998) compared the original "3+3" approach together with various modifications against several CRM designs. They concluded that the CRM design recommends the correct MTD more frequently than the classical "3+3" approach. Iasonos et al. (2008) reported on an extensive simulation study comparing different CRM designs with the classical "3+3" design. They concluded that the different CRM designs are improved over the classical method in terms of accuracy and optimal dose allocation. One publication reports better operating characteristic for the "3+3" design: Korn et al. (1994) concluded that 1) the CRM design requires more time to define the MTD and 2) the CRM appears less conservative in the sense that it treats more patients at too high dose levels. However, this work did not account for the modifications suggested by Babb et al. (1998) and Neuenschwander et al. (2008). In addition, the conclusions of Korn et al. (1994) were questioned by O'Quigley (1999) who highlighted peculiar choices for design parameters for this simulation.

Thirdly, to illustrate the flexibility of the CRM framework, we show here various adaptations of the original design in specific settings. Thall et al. (2003) and Wages and Conaway (2013) proposed extensions of the CRM design to dose finding for a combination of drugs. Dejardin et al. (2014) proposed a randomized CRM design in dose finding for a combination of drugs where the dose of one drug is fixed. In Zhang et al. (2006); Bekele and Thall (2004); Yuan et al. (2007); Lee et al. (2011); Iasonos et al. (2011); Tighiouart et al. (2012); Van Meter et al. (2012) modifications to the CRM were proposed to account for the severity of observed toxicities. Ursino et al. (2017) reviewed designs that incorporate PK parameters and introduced a CRM design based on PK parameters. Braun et al. (2007) and Zhang and Braun (2013) optimized the dose and schedule simultaneously in CRM-like designs. Cheung and Chappell (2000) and Liu et al. (2013) proposed a CRM design that allows accounting for DLT's that may occur outside of the DLT observation period.

7.3.5 MTD for a new immunotherapy: Design and data

In the motivating example, doses were to be tested from a grid starting as low as 0.1mg and potentially up to 80 mg with 5mg increments. In this context, a "3+3" design would require 17 cohorts if the MTD predicted on the preclinical data is true. This calls for a design that allows a more efficient dose escalation.

As the compound was not tested in humans before, a careful initial run-in phase was set up and consisted in 4 cohorts of 1 patient investigating doses of 0.1, 0.5, 1.5 and 3mg. After the run-in phase, the CRM dose escalation was started to optimize the finding of the MTD. The trial used a simplified version of dose calculation described by Neuenschwander et al. (2008) in that it is based on limiting the probability of overdose $\Pr(\Psi(x,\alpha) \in (0.35,1])$ to 25% at most and maximizes the probability to be in the target toxicity range $\Pr(\Psi(x,\alpha) \in (0.20, 0.35])$. The model for toxicity was chosen as a bivariate logistic model (as used in Neuenschwander et al., 2008), i.e.

$$\Psi(x;\boldsymbol{\alpha}) = \frac{\exp[\alpha_0 + \alpha_1 \ln(x/\overline{x})]}{1+\exp[\alpha_0 + \alpha_1 \ln(x/\overline{x})]},$$

where $\boldsymbol{\alpha} = (\alpha_0, \alpha_1)^\top$ is a bivariate set of parameters and $\overline{x}$ is the reference dose set to 56mg. Following Neuenschwander et al. (2008), a bivariate Normal prior was chosen for

$$\begin{pmatrix} \alpha_0 \\ \ln(\alpha_1) \end{pmatrix} \sim \mathrm{N}\left(\begin{pmatrix} -0.85 \\ 1 \end{pmatrix}, \begin{pmatrix} 1 & -0.5 \\ -0.5 & 1 \end{pmatrix} \right).$$

These values were elicited from clinical experts according to the following considerations:

- Given the marginal distribution of α_0, the probability of toxicity (i.e. DLT) at the median dose $\overline{x}$ is approximately 0.3, with a corresponding 95% confidence range of 0.057 to 0.75 for the DLT rate.

- Given the joint distribution of α_0 and $\ln(\alpha_1)$, the prior distribution conservatively assumes that a dose of 70 mg (the anticipated MTD) leads to a DLT rate of approximately 0.50, with a corresponding 95% confidence range of 0.15 to 0.94 for the DLT rate. This should ensure a conservative prior for the dose escalation strategy.

- A fixed correlation of -0.5 is assumed between α_0 and $\ln(\alpha_1)$.

Cohorts were to include at least three patients. Note that due to the fact that some patients drop out at the screening because of non-compliance to inclusion/exclusion criteria, the number of patients screened for a specific cohort is usually higher than the number of patients treated in the cohort. It may happen that no patients drop out and due to the delay between screening and treatment in the cohort, this can lead to cohorts of more than 3 patients. The CRM can handle these practical constraints. The classical "3+3" design does not typically allow for variable cohort sizes. Further, the design allows for a doubling of the dose. Finally, the dose escalation was to stop when the probability to be in the target range $\Pr(\Psi(x;\alpha) \in (0.35, 1]) > 0.50$ and at least 2 cohorts are accrued at a dose within 20% of the MTD).

Table 7.6 presents the data collected during the study. Along with the cohort size, the dose tested and the number of patients with the DLT, the dose decisions are detailed.

Note that the clinical decision differs sometimes from the recommended dose from the CRM. This is due to 1) maximum increments for CRM that may have been too high 2) the fact that the study team accounted for data beyond the DLTs definition and data outside of the study (a parallel imaging substudy was conducted at the same time and informed the study team on potential risks). The run-in of 4 cohorts of 1 patient served as calibration of

TABLE 7.6: Trial observation and data collected: C = cohort number, Dose tested = dose administered in patients in the cohort, Size = size of the cohort, Number of DLTs = number of patients who experienced a DLT, Dose by CRM = Dose recommended by CRM based on data from the cohort, Decision by Study Team = Decision made by the study team for the next cohort. NA = not applicable (run-in phase of the study).

C	Dose (mg) tested	Size	Number of DLT's	Dose (mg) by CRM	Decision by study team
1	0.1	1	0	NA	Run-in
2	0.5	1	0	NA	Run-in
3	1.5	1	0	NA	Run-in
4	3	1	0	10	CRM run the run-in phase allow the starting dose of CRM dose escalation
5	10	4	0	20	Low grade toxicities (no DLT) lead to the opening of a cohort at the same dose to confirm safety
6	10	6	0	20	The dose tested is the recommended dose from CRM
7	20	5	0	40	The dose tested is the recommended dose from CRM
8	40	3	1	50	The dose tested is the recommended dose from CRM
9	30	3	1	45	In the presence of one DLT in C8, the dose recommended by CRM (reduction compared to previous recommended dose) was deemed too high and decision was to test 30mg
10	30	3	1	40	In the presence of one DLT in C9, the dose recommended by CRM (reduction compared to previous recommended dose) was deemed too high and decision was to test 30mg
11	30	5	0	45	In the presence of one DLT in C10, the dose recommended by CRM was deemed too high and decision was to test 20mg
12	20	3	3	30	The CRM recommends the MTD at 30 mg

the CRM. At the start of the 5th cohort, the CRM was run and the starting dose of the CRM dose escalation part of the trial was cleared by the data. At the end of cohort 12, 3 DLTs out of 3 patients were observed at the dose of 20mg. The study team assessed this occurrence as "extreme" given the observations made at higher doses and the follow up of previous cohorts. The stopping rules of the CRM (accounting for those 3 exceptional DLTs) were then met and the MTD was defined as 30mg.

In this example, we see that the CRM was not always followed completely. However, we note that the CRM adapted the dose properly in the sense that in a presence of DLT, the dose is reduced or the increment is small (defined as coherence, see Cheung, 2005). We note that, with the same increments, the "3+3" design would not have been safer. Further, the exceptional findings in cohort 12 would have led to a definition of the MTD of 10mg in a "3+3" design. Accounting for the data on all cohorts, the CRM leads to a more reasonable recommendation for the CRM.

7.4 Conclusions

Dose response trials and dose escalation trials are a critical part of the drug development cycle.

Traditionally, dose response trials would be analyzed using an assumption-weak approach; however, ICH E4 suggests that it is the elucidation of the whole of the dose response which is important and not just the dose which is significantly different to control. Bayesian methods can help with dose response models, particularly if the modeling is done using an assumption-rich approach. It has been shown that in the vast majority of Phase IIb studies the dose-response data obtained can be adequately characterized by a Bayesian E_{max} model with weakly informative priors based on historical data.

The literature on dose escalation designs for oncology studies is vast and an exhaustive review of the work is beyond the scope of this chapter. This introduction is focused on the CRM as this approach has attracted the most interest and developments. Other Bayesian approaches exist and an overview can be found in Sverdlov et al. (2014). They however lack the flexibility of the CRM to adapt to different settings. We have tried to provide an introduction to CRM designs and justify why the Bayesian CRM approaches make more sense than the classical "3+3" design. Namely, CRM designs have better theoretical properties, have better small sample properties and a variety of extensions to specific situations have been developed. Challenges in the implementation of such designs lie in the wide range of possibilities (with techniques even beyond the CRM). No design has been found to be best for the majority of situations and it takes time to determine which design is best in each case.

In both dose response trials and dose escalation trials, this chapter has tried to highlight the possibilities and advantages of the Bayesian approaches.

Bibliography

Ahn, C. (1998). An evaluation of Phase I cancer clinical trial designs. *Statistics in Medicine*, 17(14):1537–1549.

Azriel, D. (2012). A note on the robustness of the continual reassessment method. *Statistics & Probability Letters*, 82(5):902 – 906.

Babb, J., Rogatko, A., and Zacks, S. (1998). Cancer Phase I clinical trials: Efficient dose escalation with overdose control. *Statistics in Medicine*, 17(10):1103–1120.

Bekele, B. and Thall, P. (2004). Dose-finding based on multiple toxicities in a soft tissue sarcoma trial. *Journal of the American Statistical Association*, 99(465):26–35.

Bornkamp, B. (2012). Functional uniform priors for nonlinear modeling. *Biometrics*, 68(3):893–901.

Braun, T., Thall, P., Nguyen, H., and de Lima, M. (2007). Simultaneously optimizing dose and schedule of a new cytotoxic agent. *Clinical Trials*, 4(2):113–124.

Bretz, F., Pinheiro, J. C., and Branson, M. (2005). Combining multiple comparisons and modeling techniques in dose-response studies. *Biometrics*, 61(3):738–748.

Cheung, Y. (2005). Coherence principles in dose-finding studies. *Biometrika*, 92(4):863–873.

Cheung, Y. (2011). *Dose Finding by the Continual Reassessment Method.* Chapman & Hall/CRC, Boca Raton, FL.

Cheung, Y. (2013). Sample size formulae for the Bayesian continual reassessment method. *Clinical Trials*, 10(6):852–861.

Cheung, Y. and Chappell, R. (2000). Sequential designs for Phase I clinical trials with late-onset toxicities. *Biometrics*, 56(4):1177–1182.

Cheung, Y. and Chappell, R. (2002). A simple technique to evaluate model sensitivity in the continual reassessment method. *Biometrics*, 58(3):671–674.

Committee for Medicinal Products for Human Use (2014). *Qualification Opinion of MCP-Mod as an efficient statistical methodology for model-based design and analysis of Phase II dose finding studies under model uncertainty.* European Medicines Agency.

Dejardin, D., Lesaffre, E., Hamberg, P., and Verweij, J. (2014). A randomized Phase I Bayesian dose escalation design for the combination of anti-cancer drugs. *Pharmaceutical Statistics*, 13(3):196–207.

Gelman, A., Stern, H., Carlin, J., Dunson, D., Vehtari, A., and Rubin, D. (2013). *Bayesian Data Analysis.* Chapman and Hall/CRC.

Goodman, S., Zahurak, M., and Piantadosi, S. (1995). Some practical improvements in the continual reassessment method for Phase I studies. *Statistics in Medicine*, 14(11):1149–1161.

Heyd, J. and Carlin, B. (1999). Adaptive design improvements in the continual reassessment method for Phase I studies. *Statistics in Medicine*, 18(11):1307–1321.

Iasonos, A., Wilton, A., Riedel, E., Seshan, V., and Spriggs, D. (2008). A comprehensive comparison of the continual reassessment method to the standard 3 + 3 dose escalation scheme in Phase I dose-finding studies. *Clinical Trials*, 5(5):465–477.

Iasonos, A., Zohar, S., and O'Quigley, J. (2011). Incorporating lower grade toxicity information into dose finding designs. *Clinical Trials*, 8(4):370–379.

Korn, E., Midthune, D., Chen, T., Rubinstein, L., Christian, M., and Simon, R. (1994). A comparison of two Phase I trial designs. *Statistics in Medicine*, 13(18):1799–1806.

Le Tourneau, C., Gan, H., Razak, A., and Paoletti, X. (2012). Efficiency of new dose escalation designs in dose-finding Phase I trials of molecularly targeted agents. *PLOS One*, 7(12):e51039.

Le Tourneau, C., Lee, J., and Siu, L. (2009). Dose escalation methods in Phase I cancer clinical trials. *Journal of the National Cancer Institute*, 101(10):708–720.

Lee, S., Cheng, B., and Cheung, Y. (2011). Continual reassessment method with multiple toxicity constraints. *Biostatistics*, 12(2):386–398.

Lin, Y. and Shih, W. (2001). Statistical properties of the traditional algorithm-based designs for Phase I cancer clinical trials. *Biostatistics*, 2(2):203–215.

Liu, S., Yin, G., and Yuan, Y. (2013). Bayesian data augmentation dose finding with continual reassessment method and delayed toxicity. *The Annals of Applied Statistics*, 7(4):1837.

Lunn, D., Spiegelhalter, D., Thomas, A., and Best, N. (2009). The BUGS project: Evolution, critique and future directions. *Statistics in Medicine*, 28(25):3049–3067.

Murphy, J. and Hall, D. (1997). A logistic dose-ranging method for Phase I clinical investigations trials. *Journal of Biopharmaceutical Statistics*, 7(4):635–647.

Neuenschwander, B., Branson, M., and Gsponer, T. (2008). Critical aspects of the Bayesian approach to Phase I cancer trials. *Statistics in Medicine*, 27(13):2420–2439.

Ohlssen, D. and Racine, A. (2015). A flexible Bayesian approach for modeling monotonic dose–response relationships in drug development trials. *Journal of Biopharmaceutical Statistics*, 25(1):137–156.

O'Quigley, J. (1999). Another look at two Phase I clinical trial designs. *Statistics in Medicine*, 18(20):2683–2690.

O'Quigley, J. (2002). Continual reassessment designs with early termination. *Biostatistics*, 3(1):87–99.

O'Quigley, J. and Conaway, M. (2010). Continual reassessment and related dose-finding designs. *Statistical Science*, 25(2).

O'Quigley, J., Pepe, M., and Fisher, L. (1990). Continual reassessment method: A practical design for Phase I clinical trials in cancer. *Biometrics*, 46(1):33–48.

Paoletti, X., O'Quigley, J., and Maccario, J. (2004). Design efficiency in dose finding studies. *Computational Statistics and Data Analysis*, 45(2):197 – 214.

Piantadosi, S. (2005). *Clinical Trials: A Methodologic Perspective.* Wiley-Blackwell.

Reiner, E., Paoletti, X., and O'Quigley, J. (1999). Operating characteristics of the standard Phase I clinical trial design. *Computational Statistics and Data Analysis*, 30(3):303 – 315.

Rogatko, A., Schoeneck, D., Jonas, W., Tighiouart, M., Khuri, F., and Porter, A. (2007). Translation of innovative designs into Phase I trials. *Journal of Clinical Oncology*, 25(31):4982–4986.

Schmidli, H., Neuenschwander, B., and Friede, T. (2017). Meta-analytic-predictive use of historical variance data for the design and analysis of clinical trials. *Computational Statistics and Data Analysis*, 113:100–110.

Shen, L. and O'Quigley, J. (1996). Consistency of continual reassessment method under model misspecification. *Biometrika*, 83(2):395–405.

Storer, B. (1989). Design and analysis of Phase I clinical trials. *Biometrics*, 45(3):925–937.

Sverdlov, O., Wong, W., and Ryeznik, Y. (2014). Adaptive clinical trial designs for Phase I cancer studies. *Statistical Surveys*, 8:2–44.

Thall, P. F., Millikan, R. E., Mueller, P., and L., S.-J. (2003). Dose-finding with two agents in Phase I oncology trials. *Biometrics*, 59(3):487–496.

Thomas, N. and Roy, D. (2017). Analysis of clinical dose–response in small-molecule drug development: 2009–2014. *Statistics in Biopharmaceutical Research*, 9(2):137–146.

Thomas, N., Sweeney, K., and Somayaji, V. (2014). Meta-analysis of clinical dose–response in a large drug development portfolio. *Statistics in Biopharmaceutical Research*, 6(4):302–317.

Tighiouart, M., Cook-Wiens, G., and Rogatko, A. (2012). Escalation with overdose control using ordinal toxicity grades for cancer Phase I clinical trials. *Journal of Probability and Statistics.*

Tighiouart, M. and Rogatko, A. (2012). Number of patients per cohort and sample size considerations using dose escalation with overdose control. *Journal of Probability and Statistics*, pages 1–12.

Ursino, M., Zohar, S., Lentz, F., Alberti, C., Friede, T., Stallard, N., and Comets, E. (2017). Dose finding methods for Phase I clinical trials using Pharmacokinetics in small populations. *Biometrical Journal*, 59(4):804–825.

U.S. Food and Drug Administration (2016). *Drug Development Tools: Fit-for-Purpose Initiative, MCP-Mod for dose finding.*

Van Meter, E., Garrett-Mayer, E., and Bandyopadhyay, D. (2012). Dose-finding clinical trial design for ordinal toxicity grades using the continuation ratio model: an extension of the continual reassessment method. *Clinical Trials*, 9(3):303–313.

Wages, N. and Conaway, M. (2013). Specifications of a continual reassessment method design for Phase I trials of combined drugs. *Pharmaceutical Statistics*, 12(4):217–224.

Woodward, P. (2016). *Bayesian Analysis Made Simple: An Excel GUI for WinBUGS.* Chapman and Hall/CRC.

Wu, J., Banerjee, A., Jin, B., Menon, S., Martin, S., and Heatherington, A. (2018). Clinical dose-response for a broad set of biological products: A model-based meta-analysis. *Statistical Methods in Medical Research*, 27(9):2694–2721.

Yin, G. and Yuan, Y. (2009). Bayesian model averaging continual reassessment method in Phase I clinical trials. *Journal of the American Statistical Association*, 104(487):954–968.

Yuan, Z., Chappell, R., and Bailey, H. (2007). The continual reassessment method for multiple toxicity grades: A Bayesian quasi-likelihood approach. *Biometrics*, 63(1):173–179.

Zhang, J. and Braun, T. (2013). A Phase I Bayesian adaptive design to simultaneously optimize dose and schedule assignments both between and within patients. *Journal of the American Statistical Association*, 108(503):892–901.

Zhang, W., Sargent, D., and Mandrekar, S. (2006). An adaptive dose-finding design incorporating both toxicity and efficacy. *Statistics in Medicine*, 25(14):2365–2383.

Zohar, S. and Chevret, S. (2001). The continual reassessment method: comparison of Bayesian stopping rules for dose-ranging studies. *Statistics in Medicine*, 20(19):2827–2843.

8

Bayesian Adaptive Designs in Drug Development

Gary L. Rosner

Johns Hopkins University, US

This chapter contains a discussion of adaptive clinical trials that incorporate Bayesian statistical considerations. An adaptive design for a clinical study includes one or more possible modifications to the study's design or conduct where the possible modifications are planned prospectively and result from (planned) analyses of data accruing during the course of the study. The adaptations may change the size or duration of the study (e.g. early stopping for efficacy or futility); the types of patients eligible to enter (i.e. adaptive enrichment); or aspects of the design, such as the randomization probabilities for assigning treatments to incoming study participants. A key feature of adaptive designs is the prospective planning of any proposed modifications that may occur while the study is ongoing. The discussion includes a brief history of adaptive designs for clinical studies.

Whereas group sequential designs have been in use for decades, response adaptive randomization has received a lot of attention thanks, in part, to several high-profile clinical trials. We discuss ways to implement response adaptive randomization from a Bayesian perspective, as well as other forms of trial adaptation. We present some approaches for avoiding several potential pitfalls and include examples of several adaptive trials.

While the chapter provides some of the reasons one might consider applying an adaptive design, there are ethical, practical, and statistical considerations that may temper one's enthusiasm toward adaptive trials in all instances, especially trials that incorporate response adaptive randomization. Overall, adaptive study designs incorporate formal learning from the accruing data and offer many potential benefits.

8.1 Introduction

This chapter presents an overview of Bayesian adaptive designs in clinical studies. Clinical studies across the drug development spectrum have included various forms of pre-specified adaptation for a long time, sometimes in an *ad hoc* manner (e.g. the so-called 3+3 dose escalation design — see Chapter 7) and often based on frequentist considerations (e.g. the O'Brien-Fleming group sequential design, O'Brien and Fleming, 1979). Interest in applying Bayesian considerations when designing clinical studies began to grow during the last quarter of the twentieth century. Part of the reason interest has grown is the greater flexibility afforded by the Bayesian approach to statistical inference. The Bayesian paradigm is one of learning. The paradigm provides the inferential tools to use information, be it data-derived or opinion-based, to increase certainty about treatment effects, associations, or whatever the focus of the analysis is. Much of the recent interest stems from interest in adaptive randomization, in which data from earlier enrollees influence treatment assignment probabilities for later study participants.

The main considerations for a clinical study with a Bayesian adaptive design are the structure of interim decisions, the statistical models that will inform these decisions, the evaluation of design criteria, the actual conduct of the study, and the presentation of the study's results. In this chapter, we review these considerations, primarily focusing on the design side. A good source for more details about adaptive clinical trials is the book by Berry et al. (2010a).

8.2 Brief history of adaptive designs

Many people credit a paper by W. R. Thompson as offering the earliest proposal for adapting the proportion of patients receiving each treatment in a study according to the posterior probability that one treatment is superior to the other (Thompson, 1933). Thompson used Bayes rule with a Beta-Binomial model to find the probability that a patient is more likely to respond to one treatment over the other, i.e. that one treatment's response probability is greater than that of the other treatment. Several decades later, interest in adaptive designs increased as proposals appeared for formal sequential decision making in clinical trials. Sequential monitoring rules arose for monitoring quality in manufacturing (Dodge and Romig, 1929; Barnard, 1946; Wald, 1945). P. Armitage proposed applying the sequential approach to clinical trials and adapting some of the sequential methods for this purpose (Armitage, 1960). In his review of the Armitage book for the *Journal of the American Statistical Association*, F. J. Anscombe took issue with the frequentist approach underlying the designs in the book (Anscombe, 1963). Anscombe argued for use of the likelihood in the analysis of the clinical trial, not on basing inference on error probabilities that consider what might have been observed but was not.

It does not appear that many trials incorporated sequential designs until the second half of the 1970s, when a large number of papers appeared in the statistical literature. Group sequential clinical trials appeared as an alternative to fully sequential designs (Pocock, 1977; O'Brien and Fleming, 1979; Jones and Whitehead, 1979). An additional push came as researchers showed how to extend the theory underlying the distribution of test statistics in sequential clinical trials from Normally distributed outcome data to other types of endpoints, particularly time-to-event outcomes (Tsiatis, 1981, 1982). All of these group sequential designs were based on frequentist inference, meaning that the boundaries all had to preserve the overall Type I error probability at or below some pre-specified value. Because of the frequentist concern with outcomes that could have occurred but did not, data analysis became complicated, with no clear single way to order the sample space for frequentist inference (Rosner and Tsiatis, 1988). Bayesian statisticians following a purely Bayesian approach are less concerned about Type I error probabilities and are not forced to perform the acrobatics necessary to maintain a Type I error probability below some arbitrary value (Berry, 1985). Around the same time that group sequential design methodology was appearing in the literature, several proposals for Bayesian sequential clinical trials began to appear, including several influential papers from researchers at the Medical Research Council Biostatistics Unit (Freedman and Spiegelhalter, 1989; Spiegelhalter et al., 1994).

Other types of adaptive designs also appeared in the literature, and a few studies incorporated them. A particular adaptive design that caught the attention of several clinical trialists was a design that sought to alter treatment assignments over time to "play the winner" (Zelen, 1969). In its simplest form, a play-the-winner rule assigns each patient to whichever treatment is achieving greater success at the time the patient enters the study. If no treatment appears better (or best if there are three or more treatment arms), then the study randomizes patients equally across treatments.

An interesting study of historical merit that used an urn scheme-form of a play-the-winner rule for adaptive randomization was the study of extra-corporeal membrane oxygenation or ECMO (Bartlett et al., 1985). This study randomized newborn babies in respiratory distress to the conventional therapy at the time or to ECMO, which was a new but highly invasive therapy. The investigators started with an imaginary urn that contained two balls, one for ECMO and one for the standard treatment. A ball chosen at random from the urn determined which treatment the baby would receive. The ball would be returned to the urn. Additionally, if the baby survived, then another ball representing the baby's treatment would be added to the urn. If, however, the baby died, then a ball representing the alternative treatment would be added.

In the ECMO trial, the first baby's treatment assignment was ECMO. The baby survived, which meant that there were now two ECMO balls and one ball for conventional therapy in the urn. The next baby's assignment was conventional therapy. Unfortunately, this baby died, leading to three ECMO balls in the urn and one ball for the standard therapy. The next baby, assigned to ECMO, survived. All subsequent babies received ECMO treatment assignments and survived. The pre-specified stopping rule, based on frequentist considerations, occurred with eleven babies treated with ECMO and one baby receiving conventional therapy. All of the ECMO-treated babies survived, but the one baby who received conventional therapy died.

The study raised many questions, not the least of which referred to its use of a play-the-winner type of adaptive randomization. In fact, because just one baby had received conventional therapy—and died—many researchers questioned the validity of the study. The controversy led to a subsequent study at the Children's Hospital of Boston that used a modified adaptive randomization (O'Rourke et al., 1989).

Another issue that arose with the ECMO study concerned frequentist inference. As pointed out by Begg (1990) and the discussion following that paper, there are many ways to approach inference following a trial that incorporated adaptive randomization via urn sampling. Each approach could lead to a different p value and, thereby, a different inference. As pointed out by Royall in his discussion of Begg's paper (Royall, 1990), the problem rests on inference based on significance tests and other inferential approaches that consider probability over parts of the sample space that include values not observed. Inference should rest on the likelihood, according to the Likelihood Principle (Berger and Wolpert, 1988). Briefly, this means that experiments that give rise to the same likelihood function for a given parameter should lead to the same inference about that parameter. Frequentist approaches to inference in the context of the ECMO trial do not obey the Likelihood Principle. Bayesian inference, on the other hand, does obey the Likelihood Principle, highlighting an advantage of the Bayesian approach for adaptive trial design.

One important lesson to take from the ECMO experience is the importance of ensuring that the study does not start to change the randomization probabilities too soon. Even with Bayesian response adaptive trial designs, experience has taught us not to start adapting randomization until the study has accrued, treated, and followed sufficient patients to ensure that the community will accept the study results. There is no fixed rule to determine what a "sufficient" number of patients is. The answer to that question will depend on the context. For example, a randomized trial evaluating therapies for relatively rare diseases may start adapting randomization sooner than would a randomized trial that is enrolling patients with diseases having higher incidence rates.

8.3 What is an adaptive clinical trial?

What do we mean when we say that a clinical trial is "adaptive"? A useful definition is given by the Food and Drug Administration (FDA) of the United States in a 2010 draft guidance (U.S. Food and Drug Administration, 2010). "An adaptive design clinical study is defined as a study that includes a prospectively planned opportunity for modification of one or more specified aspects of the study design and hypotheses based on analysis of data (usually interim data) from subjects in the study."

Let us consider some of the more important points given in the definition. "...**prospectively planned opportunity**...": an adaptive study design allows one to make certain modifications to the conduct of the trial while it is running. The study investigators need to consider all modifications they may make to the study, when such modifications may occur, and what might trigger such modifications *before* the start of the study. This definition does not allow one to call a trial design "adaptive" if modifications to its design occur during the course of the trial based on information that became available after it began, unless the individuals designing the study considered that sort of information and worked out how it might lead to modifications prior to enrolling the first patient. The document that describes the plan of the study (i.e. the study protocol) will present the evaluations and decisions of how and when to make these modifications.

"...**modification of one or more specified aspects of the study design and hypotheses**...": the investigators must specify what part or parts of the study may change during the course of the study before the study begins. Changes to the study design would include, for example, the timing of analyses, the randomization probabilities, and which treatments to evaluate. The FDA definition allows for changes to the study hypotheses, as well as to the design. For example, one may plan a study to provide evidence that a new treatment is not worse than a current standard therapy—a so-called non-inferiority study. After the study has begun, the study's goal may change. The trial may now seek to show that the new treatment is actually better than the standard. Thus the hypothesis of non-inferiority has changed to a hypothesis of superiority. Another example of a change to a study hypothesis might occur if the accruing data suggest that a subset of the patient population does not benefit from the treatment. Although the study began with a formal hypothesis that the treatment is beneficial for all patients with the disease, that might not be the case. When designing the study, the investigators may consider the possibility that some patients do not benefit from the treatment. The protocol may include appropriate considerations to allow the study's hypothesis to change, including the possibility of restricting future enrollment to enrich for the patients who seem to be benefitting and limiting or excluding future enrollment of patients whose characteristics are associated with lack of efficacy. Additionally, one may not change study endpoints during the course of the study without having considered and evaluated the effects of such a change during the trial's planning stage.

...**analysis of data**...**from subjects in the study**...: This part of the definition clearly states that the preplanned modifications are based on data internal to the study and not from outside sources. The protocol will describe how and when these analyses will occur, as well as what study data will be included in the interim analyses.

One other point is worth noting when it comes to Bayesian clinical trials. While many study designs are fully Bayesian, others include Bayesian calculations but are not truly Bayesian. A fully Bayesian design would be one that bases decisions on maximizing the expected value of a study-specific utility function or on posterior probabilities of key variables. An example of a design that is not fully Bayesian, what one might call stylistically

Bayesian or calibrated Bayes (Little, 2006), is one that calibrates the parameters in a prior distribution to make the design achieve certain desired frequentist operating characteristics. We present both kinds in this chapter.

8.4 Types of adaptation

Clinical studies include various targets for adaptation, leading to various types of adaptive designs. The following are the most important categories of adaptive trial designs, although there are many ways in which a trial's design may allow modifications after the study has begun.

- Group sequential: allows for early stopping;
- Sample size re-estimation: increases the sample size to achieve statistical significance;
- Response adaptive: randomization probabilities change over time to favor better treatments;
- Adaptive enrichment: entry criteria for patients change over time to enrich the study entrants in favor of those who appear more likely to benefit from the study treatment.

8.4.1 Group sequential designs

Adaptive clinical trial designs allow the trial to change in response to accumulating data. The most common adaptive design is a sequential design that includes interim analyses of the accruing data. So-called group sequential studies allow for early termination of a randomized clinical trial once there is clear evidence of the superiority of one treatment over the other treatments in the study. A group sequential trial might also incorporate early stopping for futility. Futility in this context is usually defined as a low probability of ultimately finding a "significant" difference between the treatments if the study continues to its planned end.

Bayesian inference is particularly suited for interim analyses of data while a study is ongoing. Frequentist methods for group sequential designs require preservation of the overall Type I error probability at some pre-specified level in light of the multiple looks at the data. In essence, the group sequential designs force the analyst to pay a price (hence the so-called "spending functions") for looking at the accruing data. That price means that the nominal significance level required at an interim analysis is smaller than what would be required without interim looks if one wants the overall Type I error probability to remain no greater than some prespecified number α (e.g. the ubiquitous 0.05). The calculations that lead to these designs can be somewhat complex, since they may require numerical integration (Armitage et al., 1969). As we pointed out in the ECMO example, frequentist inference violates the Likelihood Principle in the case of sequential designs (Berger and Wolpert, 1988). For clinical trials, the Likelihood Principle means that one need not consider the interim analyses when inferring the treatment effect, unless the likelihood function includes components relating to the interim analyses that are functions of the treatment effect parameter. In general, the stopping boundaries in group sequential trials partition the sample space but do not contribute information about the treatment effect beyond the information in the data. Thus, the likelihood from a trial with a group sequential design for interim analyses is proportional to the likelihood from a trial with a single analysis at the end of the trial, with respect to the parameter of interest. Therefore, according to the Likelihood Principle, the inference about the treatment effect should not change whether one analyzed the data once, twice, or however many times prior to the end of the study. Bayesian inference does obey the Likelihood Principle, so the Bayesian analysis is unaffected by the number of interim analyses.

Bayesian approaches for monitoring interim data in a clinical study tend to be of three kinds. One approach bases decisions on posterior probabilities, such as stopping if the posterior probability that the new treatment is superior to the standard treatment (or placebo) is high (e.g. greater than 90%). A second approach uses predictive probability calculations in interim analyses to determine the probability that the study will ultimately find a strong treatment effect, given the data in hand, as well as any external information. The third approach uses decision theory and at each interim analysis chooses the action (e.g. stop or continue) that maximizes the expected utility. In all cases, the decisions might be to continue the study until the next planned analysis or to stop the study before the planned end of the study and declare one treatment superior to the other (assuming just two treatments in the trial) or declare little difference between the two treatments (futility).

Suppose we let θ represent the treatment effect (e.g. a difference in some continuous measure, a relative risk, a hazard ratio, etc.). We assume that there is a value that corresponds to equivalence (e.g. $\theta = 0$ for a log odds ratio or $\theta = 1$ for a hazard ratio) and that values larger than this value reflect superiority of the new treatment over its comparator. We might want to design the study to stop and declare the new treatment superior when we see that $\Pr(\theta > 0 \mid \text{Data}) > \gamma$, with $\gamma > 0.5$, assuming that treatment equivalence for the study's outcome corresponds to $\theta = 0$. The closer γ gets to 1, the more certainty we require that the new treatment is superior (i.e. that $\theta > 0$).

There are two elements of the design and model that are separate from the data and that will affect the ease with which the study stops early based on the results of an interim analysis. One element is the probability threshold (γ) that we set as a minimum degree of certainty we wish to have to declare that the new treatment is superior, stopping the study as a result. The second element is the prior distribution for θ. Suppose we consider a range of indifference for the treatment effect: $(\theta_0 - \varepsilon, \theta_0 + \varepsilon)$. For example, the treatment effect might be measured in terms of the difference between two treatments in a randomized clinical trial with respect to the change in blood pressure after four weeks of treatment. Then θ_0 might be zero, and we might set ε to 5 mm Hg. We would say that we would not consider the two treatments to be meaningfully different if the blood pressure change for the old treatment minus the change for the new treatment was within ± 5 mm Hg of zero. If we specify a somewhat skeptical prior for the treatment difference, we might assign much of the prior probability over the indifference region. With such a symmetric skeptical prior centered at θ_0, there will be relatively less prior probability assigned to regions in which one treatment is superior to the other. If a prior distribution puts less probability on a region of the treatment's effect that corresponds to superiority, then the stopping rule will require greater evidence in the data to recommend study termination based on a posterior probability of superiority that exceeds a pre-specified threshold value. On the other hand, if the prior distribution has relatively less mass over the indifference region and more over the regions that correspond to superiority, then the study may stop earlier and declare a treatment preference, since the data do not have to provide as much precision as in the former case.

The literature is full of Bayesian design proposals that set the threshold γ to a value very close to 1 (e.g. 0.98) or that incorporate a prior distribution that has relatively little probability in the region beyond the null value, such as the one-sided region $(\theta_0 + \varepsilon, \infty)$. These proposed designs set the prior distributions this way in an effort to control the frequentist operating characteristics, such as incorrectly declaring a treatment difference. Such modifications to the decision rules—especially to the prior distribution—to obtain desired frequentist properties (e.g. a Type I error probability of 0.05) are examples of calibrated Bayes (Little, 2006). Although the design uses Bayesian calculations, the prior distribution is calibrated to achieve acceptable frequentist characteristics. A major reason to calibrate the design is to meet regulatory conditions for the trial. With such modifications to the prior, however, the prior distribution no longer reflects prior beliefs or uncertainties about the treatments' effects.

Similarly, one may carry out predictive probability calculations at the interim analyses and base decisions on the predictive probability that continuing the study will lead to a decision that the new treatment is superior. The predictive probability may project to a decision based on the ultimate probability of superiority or it may project to the final analysis which may be a statistical hypothesis test (Lee and Liu, 2008). Again, one has to set a threshold corresponding to the level of certainty one will require at an interim analysis to stop the study early. One might use a predictive probability approach to set a futility boundary. That is, if the predictive probability that the ultimate hypothesis test is unlikely to declare a statistically significant difference between the treatments, then one would conclude that it would be futile to continue the study and decide to stop.

Decision-theoretic designs have appeared in the literature but do not seem to have gained as wide acceptance as the approaches based on posterior and predictive probabilities. Likely reasons include the computational burden associated with sequential decision making (see Section 8.6), the challenge of defining a utility function that represents the viewpoints of multiple stakeholders, and relative unfamiliarity with this approach to study design. The field would benefit from more research into Bayesian decision-theoretic designs and their application in adaptive clinical trials.

8.4.2 Sample size re-estimation

Sample size re-estimation occurs when the investigators increase the target accrual goal for the study after the study has begun accruing patients. Reasons that may lead to the decision to increase accrual generally relate to a realization based on an interim analysis that there will be fewer events than originally planned in the study protocol. For example, an interim analysis for a trial with a failure-time primary endpoint might reveal that the study's patients are experiencing a lower event rate than originally expected. One can determine the overall event rate from pooled data without carrying out a statistical test comparing the treatments. In this example, the original statistical hypotheses in the protocol do not change.

Another type of sample size re-estimation occurs when the study investigators learn at an interim or at the final analysis that the treatment appears to be more efficacious than the control therapy but its benefit over the control is not as large as originally assumed in the protocol's power calculation. The investigators may want to increase the study's sample size from that given in the protocol to provide adequate power to show that the interim estimate of the treatment effect is statistically significant. In this example, the statistical hypotheses change as a result of an analysis of the study's primary endpoint. Most methods in the literature for re-estimating a study's sample size in response to an analysis of the study's primary endpoint are frequentist. That is, they are concerned with using available data at the time of an interim or final analysis to decide how many more subjects to enroll in order to achieve a statistically significant finding. Because the final analysis will include data from the cohort of subjects whose data formed the basis of the re-estimation calculations, the frequentist has to pay a price in order to preserve the Type I error probability of the final analysis. The few publications that present a Bayesian approach to this problem propose using predictive probabilities to calculate the probability of ultimately rejecting the statistical null hypothesis, e.g. Wang (2007) and Zhong et al. (2013). The goal is to find a rule that keeps this predictive probability from exceeding the preset Type I error probability. Thus, sample size re-estimation is a wholly frequentist issue, and we will not discuss it further.

8.4.3 Adaptive randomization

A design approach that has received a lot of attention since the end of the twentieth century is a randomized clinical trial in which the randomization probabilities change dynamically during the course of the study. The theory for such approaches goes back to what were called "bandit problems" — see Berry and Fristedt (1985) and Gittins et al. (2011). Frequentist approaches for adaptive randomization have included urn sampling schemes and play-the-winner rules (Zelen, 1969, 1974), as in the ECMO study (Section 8.2).

Adaptive randomization can also include dose finding in Phase I studies. In a typical Phase I study, one can think of allocation of patients (or cohorts of patients) to various dose levels as randomization with assignment probabilities alternating between 0 and 1 as the study gathers toxicity information from patients already enrolled and treated at various dose levels.

8.4.4 Adaptive enrichment

Situations arise when one is not sure if only a subset of the patient population will benefit from the treatment. One would like to be able to investigate this question while also assessing the clinical benefit of the treatment. If the benefit is restricted to a subpopulation and one evaluates the treatment in the whole population, the estimate will be attenuated. The trial might lead the clinical community to overlook a treatment that provides benefit to the appropriate patient subgroup. Adaptive enrichment trials include decision rules regarding patient inclusion criteria that the investigators apply during the course of the trial. If the study's data indicate that the treatment's benefit is restricted to a subgroup of patients, then the trial may begin only enrolling patients who belong to this subgroup. Bayesian decision rules may require predictive probability calculations alone or within the context of a decision-theoretic design. We discuss adaptive enrichment designs further in Section 8.7

8.5 Reasons we might consider adaptive designs

There are many reasons to consider an adaptive design. Benefits apply over a broad range of clinical trials, including studies that occur early in the drug development process. These reasons include some ethical arguments, such as providing information about the superiority (or inferiority) of a new treatment option earlier than one might if one waited until the planned end of the study. Providing this information as soon as the evidence supports the conclusion allows patients and their caregivers to benefit from this knowledge. Patients participating in the study may benefit if the design includes pre-planned modifications to drop apparently less effective therapies during the study, while retaining the more effective or less toxic treatment arms for continued evaluation.

Phase I study designs, especially in oncology, have long been adaptive but not necessarily Bayesian. The once universal 3+3 design is a decision rule that treats incoming cohorts of patients with particular doses, depending on how previous patients tolerated the doses they received. Since the publication of the continual reassessment design (CRM) (O'Quigley et al., 1990), many new designs for dose finding have appeared in the literature. Most of these new designs incorporate a Bayesian model. Notable examples include dose escalation with overdose control (EWOC; Babb et al., 1998), application of Bayesian model averaging to dose finding (Yin and Yuan, 2009b), model-based approaches that consider risk intervals rather than a single risk target for the maximally-targeted dose (Neuenschwander et al., 2008), the use of copulæ for dose finding with combinations of drugs (Yin and Yuan, 2009a), and rule-based approaches that achieve nearly the simplicity of the 3+3 design (Ji et al., 2010; Liu and Yuan, 2015; Guo et al., 2017b). These papers and others have consistently demonstrated through simulation studies that these designs provide superior operating characteristics to the standard 3+3 and common frequentist designs. See also Chapter 7 for more details on such designs.

Another advantage of an adaptive design would be the efficiency with which the study might provide evidence from a randomized clinical trial that one subgroup of patients benefits more from a treatment than other patients. In the study's design, enrollment criteria may change to enrich the study population in favor of patients who appear to be deriving benefit and to stop enrolling patients who may not be benefiting or who may be suffering harm. Such an adaptive study could provide randomized evidence to support individualizing therapies.

An ethical argument for modifying randomization probabilities based on interim results revolves around a desire to increase the number of patients in the study who receive superior therapy and decrease the number receiving inferior treatment. The ethical arguments in favor of adaptive randomization are not universally accepted, however. Discussions relating to the ethics of adaptive randomization have appeared in several journals (e.g. see Bather, 1985, and Hey and Kimmelman, 2015, along with the discussion following these articles). The arguments the authors present in the discussions highlight several of the viewpoints that exist in the community of clinical trialists related to this question.

8.5.1 Randomization probabilities

A key element of response adaptive designs is the calculation of the randomization probabilities as functions of the patient outcomes. Several algorithms have appeared in the literature for dynamically determining randomization probabilities during the course of the randomized clinical trial. There is no consensus regarding which approach is better. It is useful to look at several of the proposals to see what they are and if there are any weaknesses or concerns. We do that in this section.

Let us first consider a trial with just two treatment arms, A and B. One relatively straightforward approach uses the posterior probability that outcome with one treatment is better than the other. That is, one may wish to set the probability a patient is randomized to treatment A to be $\Pr(A > B \mid \mathrm{D}_t)$ at time t, where D_t represents all data available at time t. A shortcoming of this approach is that the estimate of this probability that one uses to alter randomization can have quite a large variance and may lead to assigning more patients to the inferior treatment, especially early in the study. Equal randomization during the initial part of the study could reduce the risk of creating such an imbalance, since the posterior probability would be based on a more data.

Another approach for stabilizing the randomization probabilities is one that discounts them by smoothing them out to affect how quickly these probabilities change with accruing information. Specifically, the probability a patient entering at time t receives treatment A as the treatment assignment might be

$$R_A(t) = \frac{\Pr(A > B \mid \mathrm{D}_t)^\phi}{\Pr(A > B \mid \mathrm{D}_t)^\phi + \Pr(B > A \mid \mathrm{D}_t)^\phi}, \tag{8.1}$$

where $0 \leq \phi \leq 1$. If $\phi = 0$, then the study assigns treatments to patients with equal probability. If $\phi = 1$, then treatment assignment is based on the posterior probability the treatment is superior to the other treatment. Values of ϕ between 0 and 1 lead to randomization probabilities between the extremes of equal randomization and full use of the posterior probabilities of superiority. Of course, whenever $\Pr(A > B \mid \mathrm{D}_t) = 0.5$, treatment assignment will follow equal randomization. Discounting the posterior probabilities may be viewed as somewhat contrary to Bayesian inference, since the posterior distribution is supposed to characterize one's current state of knowledge about the response probability. The discount factor is added to provide better operating characteristics to address potential concerns among regulators and other stakeholders. This discounting of posterior probabilities leads to more of a stylistically (or calibrated) Bayesian design rather than a fully Bayesian one.

One can also let the exponent ϕ change over time. A particularly useful application of dynamically changing the exponent is to keep the randomization close to equal randomization early in the trial, with the randomization probabilities changing as the trial accrues more and more patients. Thall and Wathen (2007) proposed setting $\phi = \phi(t, n) = \frac{n}{2N}$, where n is the current number of patients who have enrolled into the trial by time t, and N is the target maximum accrual to the study. With this exponent in Equation (8.1), the fraction $\frac{n}{2N}$ will be very small at the start of the study, when there are few patients in the trial, and equal to 1/2 at the end of the study.

Naturally, one can incorporate outcome adaptive randomization in trials that evaluate more than two treatments. One way to accomplish this is to pick a fixed threshold, p^*, against which the trial evaluates the treatments. Suppose there are K treatments and that p_j denotes the probability of response associated with treatment $j = 1, \ldots, K$. One might use the following as the basis of the randomization probabilities

$$r_j = \frac{\Pr(p_j > p^* \mid \mathrm{D}_t)^\phi}{\sum_{k=1}^K \Pr(p_k > p^* \mid \mathrm{D}_t)^\phi}, \quad j = 1, \ldots, K \tag{8.2}$$

for $K \geq 2$ treatment arms.

With three or more treatment arms, one might choose one of the treatments as a reference treatment. For example, a trial that compares two or more experimental treatments to a standard-of-care control therapy might naturally use the control therapy as a fixed reference. For ease of presentation, suppose the trial's primary clinical endpoint is binary and is available relatively quickly as a measure of response to treatment. Furthermore, suppose the trial is evaluating two new treatments against a standard of care. Let p_1 be the probability a patient has a successful clinical outcome if the patient receives the standard of care. Let p_2 and p_3 be the probabilities of clinical benefit associated with the two experimental treatments. Extrapolating from Equation (8.2) to three treatments, we might want to allocate patients to treatment $j = 1, 2, 3$, say, with probability equal to

$$r_j = \frac{\Pr(p_j > p_1 \mid \mathrm{D}_t)^\phi}{\sum_{k=1}^3 \Pr(p_k > p_1 \mid \mathrm{D}_t)^\phi}.$$

The denominator in the formula includes $\Pr(p_1 > p_1 \mid \mathrm{D}_t)$, a logically difficult probability to consider. One may arbitrarily set this probability to 0.5, to allow the calculations to proceed. It turns out, however, that the probability of assigning a patient to arm 1 will never go below 20% in this situation, regardless of how much worse the response probability is for arm 1, the reference arm, relative to the other treatments.

This approach has another problem. A disadvantage of picking one of the treatment arms as a fixed reference arm is that the allocation ratio may depend on which treatment is considered the reference group. Suppose one uses treatment arm 1 as the reference group. Consider the scenarios, shown in Table 8.1 with 50 patients and independent uniform prior distributions for each of the 3 arms. In Scenario 1, the reference arm has the lowest underlying response probability (10%) and arms 2 and 3 each have a 50% probability of response. The randomization probabilities for arms 2 and 3 are the same, on average, and larger than the probability of assigning a patient to arm 1, as we would expect. In Scenarios 2 and 3, however, the randomization probability for arm 1 is always higher than the probability of assigning a patient to either arm 2 (Scenario 2) or to arm 3 (Scenario 3), even though the response probabilities are the same. We see, then, that the randomization probabilities are not indifferent to which treatment arm serves as the reference arm with this approach.

TABLE 8.1: Average randomization probabilities based on 1000 simulations with the exponent $\phi = 1$ and 50 patients per treatment arm.

Scenario	Underlying response probabilities (p_1, p_2, p_3)	Average randomization probabilities (Arm 1, Arm 2, Arm 3)
1	(0.10, 0.50, 0.50)	(0.20, 0.40, 0.40)
2	(0.50, 0.50, 0.10)	(0.55, 0.45, 0.00)
3	(0.50, 0.10, 0.50)	(0.55, 0.00, 0.44)
4	(0.10, 0.70, 0.85)	(0.20, 0.40, 0.40)

Yet another issue may arise if, say, p_1 is considerably smaller than the response probabilities for the other treatment arms (Scenario 4). In this case, the randomization probabilities for the other treatment arms become close to each other, making it difficult to distinguish between these better performing treatments.

One way to make the adaptive randomization probabilities indifferent to the label of the reference treatment arm is called moving-reference adaptive randomization (Yuan and Yin, 2011). The method works by finding randomization probabilities among progressively smaller groups of treatments. One starts with all treatments under consideration and computes the posterior mean response probability among the pooled treatments. The treatment with the smallest posterior probability of being larger than the pooled average receives a randomization probability based on this posterior probability relative to the similar posterior probabilities for the other treatments in the set. One then removes this treatment from consideration and finds the posterior average response probability of the remaining set of treatments. Again, one sets aside the treatment in this reduced set, assigning to it a randomization probability according to its posterior probability of being larger than the average response probability in the reduced set. The process continues, removing a treatment from consideration at each step after finding its posterior probability of exceeding the average, until one has randomization probabilities for each treatment.

An advantage of the moving-reference adaptive randomization approach is that the randomization probabilities are no longer sensitive to which treatment is considered the control or reference treatment. A disadvantage is the added computation. Additionally, the computation based on peeling away the apparently less effective treatments tends to make the randomization probabilities reflect underlying differences more quickly.

Another way to compute randomization probabilities aims to increase accrual to the treatment that has the highest posterior probability of being the best. That is, instead of comparing each treatment's response probability to a fixed reference or to a control treatment's response probability, one computes the posterior probability that each treatment is the best from among the treatments in the study. If we define $r_j = \Pr(p_j = \max_k(p_k) \mid \mathrm{D}_t)$, then we can use these probabilities to determine the treatment assignment for the next patient. That is, at time t, we set the probability π_j of assigning a patient to treatment j equal to $\frac{r_j}{\sum_{k=1}^{K} r_k}$ or $\frac{r_j^{\phi}}{\sum_{k=1}^{K} r_k^{\phi}}$ as discussed earlier in this chapter.

Thus far, we have looked at binary outcomes for which we based randomization probabilities on the posterior probabilities that each treatment is either better than a fixed value or a reference (control) treatment arm. One can apply similar considerations for continuous outcomes and time-to-event outcomes. For continuous outcome measures, one can randomize patients to each treatment with probabilities proportional to the posterior probability that the treatment is associated with the best outcome. For example, consider a randomized trial comparing various doses of a drug or different drugs to treat high blood pressure. The treatment that induces the largest decline in blood pressure from baseline would be the treatment to which the trial should assign more patients. Suppose Δ_j is the mean change in blood pressure from baseline for treatment $j, j = 1, \ldots, K$. Randomization probabilities based on the treatment-specific posterior means could serve the goal of adaptive randomization in this case. For example, let r_j be the current (at time t) posterior probability that treatment j is associated with the biggest decline in blood pressure among the K treatments, i.e. $r_j = \Pr(\Delta_j > \Delta_{max} \mid \mathrm{D}_t)$, where $\Delta_{max} = \max\{\Delta_1, \ldots, \Delta_K\}$. Then, the randomization probability to treatment j, π_j would be $\frac{r_j^{\phi}}{\sum_{k=1}^{K} r_k^{\phi}}$, as before, with $0 \leq \phi \leq 1$.

For time-to-event endpoints, things get a bit more complicated, primarily because posterior distributions may no longer be available in closed form. When one is collecting failure-time data, observations come in pairs for each person, (T_i, δ_i), where T_i is the observed time on study for the i-th patient, and δ_i is an indicator of whether or not the patient experienced the event. For example, if overall survival (time from randomization until death) is the primary endpoint for the study, then a patient may die before the data analysis, in which case $\delta_i = 1$, or the patient may still be alive at the time of analysis and $\delta_i = 0$. Suppose we assume that the patients' times until they experience the event of interest follow an Exponential distribution and the distribution's rate parameter depends on the treatment. The statistical model for the observations is $T_i \mid \lambda_j \sim \mathrm{Exp}(\lambda_j)$ when patient i receives treatment j. If one posits a Gamma distribution prior for λ_j, then the posterior distribution will also be a Gamma distribution. The form of the posterior for this model is as follows.

$$\begin{aligned} \lambda_j &\sim \mathrm{Gamma}(\alpha, \beta); \\ T_i \mid \lambda_j &\sim \mathrm{Exp}(\lambda_j); \\ \lambda_j \mid \mathrm{D}_t &\sim \mathrm{Gamma}(\alpha', \beta'). \end{aligned}$$

The parameters in the posterior Gamma distribution are $\alpha' = \alpha + \sum_{i=1}^{n} \delta_i$ and $\beta' = \beta + \sum_{i=1}^{n} T_i$. If there are two treatments, A and B, say, then the randomization probability for treatment A may simply be the posterior probability that treatment A is better than treatment B with respect to the primary endpoint. For example, one could consider the mean time to failure, μ_{A}, or the median failure time, $\log(2)/\lambda_{\mathrm{A}}$. For the mean, the probability a patient is assigned treatment A might be $\Pr(\mu_{\mathrm{A}} > \mu_{\mathrm{B}} \mid (T_1, \delta_1), \ldots, (T_n, \delta_n))$. One could use the same sort of computation to make the randomization probability a function of the posterior distributions of the treatment-specific medians. The posterior distributions of the treatment-specific means are available directly from the parameters in the posterior distributions of the treatment-specific hazard functions or of the Exponential distributions' rate parameters. That is, $\mathrm{E}[\lambda \mid \mathrm{Data}] = \alpha'/\beta'$, where (α', β') are the parameters of the posterior Gamma distribution as shown above. If one is using the median as the summary statistic, then one can use an Inverse-Gamma prior distribution for the median (instead of a Gamma distribution as the prior for the rate parameter) and the posterior will again be Inverse-Gamma. Conjugacy follows, since the median is inversely proportional to the rate parameter in the Exponential sampling distribution.

The Exponential distribution is particularly easy to work with when analyzing failure-time data. Exponentially distributed data are positive and the posterior distribution is available directly if one uses a Gamma prior distribution for the rate parameter, since this distribution is conjugate for an Exponential sampling distribution or likelihood. In most cases, however, the Exponential distribution may not characterize the patients' failure times well and one will use a different probability model for the observations, such as another parametric model (e.g. the Weibull distribution) or a semi-parametric proportional hazards regression model. Even if one uses a different model when one analyzes the study's data, the Gamma-Exponential model may be adequate for adapting the randomization probabilities. As part of developing the study design and writing the protocol, one should explore the robustness of the Gamma-Exponential model via simulation studies that may use alternative sampling distributions to characterize likely study data.

If the randomized trial includes more than two treatments, then one has similar choices to those discussed earlier for binary endpoints. For example, one of the treatments may be designed as the control treatment, in which case it would be reasonable to allocate patients to a treatment with probability proportional to the probability that the treatment is superior to the control. That is, if there are three treatment arms in the trial and treatment 1 is the control, then one might compute $r_j = \Pr(\mu_j > \mu_1 \mid \mathrm{D}_t), j = 1, 2, 3$, and use randomization probabilities $\pi_j \propto r_j^c$ as discussed previously. Of course, one could do the same thing with the median.

Often, we compare two failure-time distributions with the hazard ratio, which corresponds to the inverse of the ratio of medians when hazards are constant over time. Using the hazard ratios (or median ratios) again with treatment 1 as the control, we could use the following to determine the randomization probabilities. Let $\nu_j = \lambda_j/\lambda_1, j = 2, 3$ be the treatment effect of treatment j on the failure-time endpoint, relative to treatment 1. The Bayesian model could be as follows. Assume an Inverse-Gamma prior for the median time to failure with treatment 1 (m_1, say) and Gamma prior distributions for the ratios $\nu_j, j = 2, 3$. Define $\tau_j = m_1/\nu_j, j = 2, 3$, with $\tau_1 = m_1$. Assign a patient to treatment j at time t with probability proportional to $\Pr(\tau_j = \max(\tau_1, \tau_2, \tau_3) \mid \mathrm{D}_t)$.

The failure-time data models above assume Exponentially distributed outcomes. Assuming that the failure times follow an Exponential distribution may be useful in practice, such as when the time from randomization until the event is relatively quick. For other situations, however, a more general model may be more appropriate. One extension would model the hazard function as piecewise constant with fixed change points, leading to a piecewise Exponential sampling model. If one is willing to assume proportional hazards for the treatments, then one may still use adaptive randomization based on the posterior distribution of the hazard ratio. If one does not want to assume that the hazards are proportional to each other, then one might base randomization probabilities on the treatment-specific posterior probabilities that a patient survives past a fixed but relatively early time point, such as one year. The equations for setting the randomization probabilities would incorporate these (posterior) survival probabilities in much the same way we used the response probabilities to determine the allocation ratios in Equation (8.2). If there is an intermediate measure that is associated with the event of interest and that is available more quickly, then one might be able to incorporate this intermediate measure to improve the way the randomization probabilities change over time, making them more sensitive to treatment differences (Huang et al., 2009).

8.6 Example of an adaptive design

One particularly instructive study that included an adaptive design was the Acute Stroke Therapy by Inhibition of Neutrophils (ASTIN) Trial (Krams et al., 2003). ASTIN was a fairly complex study, and many of the decisions and solutions provide insight into what one might accomplish with an adaptive Bayesian design and the challenges one may face when designing such a trial. ASTIN was a double-blind randomized trial that sought to determine the best dose of the agent while simultaneously comparing the therapy to a placebo. The design provided for a seamless transition from a dose-finding phase to a randomized Phase II study. The agent under evaluation was a neutrophil inhibitory factor, and the trial design included adaptive allocation to one of 15 doses of the agent or placebo during dose finding. Over time, as data accrued, the randomization probabilities changed to favor the doses that appeared to be improving patient outcomes. The study's primary outcome measure was the change in the Scandinavian Stroke Scale (SSS) from baseline to day 90. As shown in the paper, the randomization probabilities changed over time and tended to assign patients to placebo or to one of the three highest doses. A key feature of the study design was that the placebo arm always remained, allowing for the possibility that no dose of the agent would show superiority to placebo. The study enrolled 966 patients, of whom 248 received an assignment to the placebo arm. The trial stopped early for futility, because there was little evidence that any dose of the agent provided superior benefit to patients, relative to the placebo.

Several of the features of the ASTIN Trial are informative and applicable to other Bayesian adaptive trials. The study consisted of two phases. In the first phase, the investigators sought to learn about the drug's dose-response relationship. This relationship was not known, and a determination of the drug's activity should evaluate the drug at its best dose. The investigators chose to consider a relatively large number of doses, namely, 15 doses plus placebo, during the first part of the study. According to the design, randomization to the various doses would change as the study progressed to increase allocation of patients to doses appearing to be superior and reduce allocation to inferior doses. Since the ultimate comparison would be to placebo, the randomization would always include some probability of assigning placebo to a patient.

The investigators used a flexible model to characterize the unknown dose-response relationship. Rather than assuming a parametric model, such as a linear or loglinear regression, the investigators used a flexible Normal dynamic linear model (NDLM) to characterize the dose-response curve (West and Harrison, 1997). This model considers the relationship to be locally linear but allows for random deviations from linearity across the range of doses. In fact, the NDLM would even allow one to infer the dose-response relationship, even if it would turn out to be non-monotone.

The goal of the initial dose-finding phase of the study was to determine the dose of the drug to use in the second phase of the study, viz., the randomized comparison of the drug to placebo. The target of dose finding was the ED_{95}, which is the dose that provides 95% of the maximum activity above what placebo achieved. Dose finding proceeded with adaptive randomization. The algorithm that drove the adaptive randomization chose doses to minimize the posterior variance of the mean or expected response at the estimate of the ED_{95}. The mean response, in turn, was an estimate that came from the NDLM that estimated the dose-response relationship. The posterior variance of the mean response at the ED_{95}, therefore, incorporated the posterior variance of the ED_{95} and the uncertainty of the dose-response relationship at this value.

During the dose-finding phase, the study randomized patients to all doses within 10% of the estimated ED_{95}, with a minimum of 15% probability of assignment to placebo. The thought was that as the estimate of the ED_{95} would become more precise, the set of doses to which the study would randomize patients would get smaller. Thus, randomization to the various doses would change over time to increase allocation to doses appearing to be superior and reduce allocation to inferior performing doses.

Periodically during the dose-finding phase, the trial investigators had to decide whether to continue that phase of the study, stop the trial and abandon the drug, or stop dose finding and move to the confirmatory Phase II part of the study. This decision required repeated calculation of the expected utility for each action. Optimizing repeated decision making during the study required the use of backward induction to determine the optimal sequential design. Backward induction is a computational procedure for determining optimal decisions in a sequential decision problem (Berger, 1985). A clinical trial that includes interim analyses leading to decisions, such as stopping the study, dropping a treatment, etc. is a sequential decision problem. As the name implies, backward induction works by determining the optimal decisions in reverse sequential order.

First, one determines the optimal decision for each possible outcome at the end of dose finding. The choices are to continue to the randomized second phase of the study or stop the study and declare that the treatment does not offer enough benefit to continue. The optimal decision to make for a given outcome at the end of dose finding is the action that maximizes the expected utility given this outcome. For example, if there appears to be little benefit over placebo at the estimated ED_{95}, it will likely be better to stop the study than to continue to a randomized comparative trial.

After determining the optimal decisions for the final set outcomes, the algorithm considers outcomes at the next-to-last interim analysis during dose finding. For each of these outcomes, one chooses among three actions: (i) continue enrolling patients; (ii) start the randomized trial; or (iii) stop the study and abandon the drug. Again, the algorithm finds the expected utility for each action at each outcome. If the choice is to continue enrolling patients in dose finding, then the algorithm will consider possible outcomes at the time of the next (i.e. the final) analysis. We already know the optimal action for each outcome at the final dose-finding analysis, and the algorithm uses this information to decide on the optimal action at the penultimate analysis for each possible outcome. The process continues backwards until it reaches the first analysis during the dose-finding phase. In the end, we learn the optimal action for each outcome at each of the planned interim analyses during dose finding.

Clearly, the computational burden increases quickly as there are more interim analyses, more decisions, and more possible outcomes at each analysis. In this study, the possible outcomes (i.e. benefit over placebo in terms of the 90-day SSS) at each analysis exist along a continuum, making the computation unwieldy. The ASTIN investigators addressed the computational burden by constraining the set of outcomes informing the decision process, thereby reducing the computational burden. They constrained the outcomes by working on a finite grid rather than a continuum. By considering outcomes over time constrained to fixed values and determining the optimal decisions backwards in time, the procedure approximated the optimal sequential decision rule in a computationally feasible manner. Other examples of the use of this dual strategy for optimal sequential study design are in (Carlin et al., 1998; Rossell et al., 2007; Ding et al., 2008). Once the accrued information indicated that a dose-response does exist for the drug, and the evidence in favor of this dose-response relationship reached some minimal level of precision, the study would move to the confirmatory phase. This phase would be a balanced randomized clinical trial that would compare the drug at its estimated ED_{95} dose to placebo.

The decision to embark on the second phase also relied on a decision-theoretic calculation. The utility function in this calculation balanced the potential gain of an improvement over placebo in the primary outcome against the cost of sampling and treating patients in the trial. The benefit in the utility function only applied if the predicted confirmatory phase would lead to a statistically significant test at the end of the study. The calculation of the expected utility of going ahead with the confirmatory study required the predictive distribution of the outcome of the future confirmatory phase if the study would switch. This calculation involved predicting outcomes for future enrollees and for patients already in the study who have not yet reached their 90-day evaluation. The ASTIN investigators used a longitudinal model for the change in the SSS over time to facilitate these calculations. The longitudinal model allowed computation via the predictive distribution for future observations which include incomplete information from patients who had not yet reached their 90-day assessments, as well as future enrolling patients. The predictive model was an autoregressive Normal model with prior distributions for the parameters based on a historical database. Therefore, the predictive distribution with the longitudinal model allowed the calculation of the expected utility, conditional on currently available data and possible future observations via a predictive model.

The ASTIN trial was very innovative and helped set the stage for later adaptive trials, such as the study of dulaglutide versus sitagliptin to treat type 2 diabetes (Skrivanek et al., 2012; Geiger et al., 2012). Further details of the two-stage design approach that includes adaptive dose finding can be found in Berry et al. (2010b).

8.7 Adaptive enrichment designs

Sometimes, one wants to see if a treatment's benefit is limited to patients with certain characteristics or whose disease exhibits certain features. For example, development of anticancer drugs since the end of the twentieth century has focused on targeting specific molecular characteristics of the cancers, either attempting to disrupt molecular pathways the cancer cells are using to survive and multiply. One might want to carry out such investigations retrospectively, using data from one or several completed clinical trials. Alternatively, one may want to proceed prospectively to determine whether all patients experience a treatment's beneficial effects or if clinical benefit is confined to a subset of patients who share one or more observable characteristics. Adaptive enrichment designs seek to simultaneously determine prospectively whether a treatment benefits all patients or only a subgroup of the patients with the disease and to modify the trial's eligibility criteria or randomization probabilities to favor assigning the drug to treat the patients who appear to be benefiting from it. The study subgroups may be defined prior to starting the study or dynamically through the course of the trial. Again, the investigators must determine and evaluate the rules for these possible modifications to the study before opening the study to accrual.

Frequentist proposals have appeared in the literature (Freidlin and Simon, 2005; Mandrekar and Sargent, 2009; Rosenblum and van der Laan, 2011; Rosenblum et al., 2016). These designs are concerned with determining which patients benefit from a treatment while maintaining a pre-specified Type I error probability below some nominal level. A truly Bayesian design, on the other hand, will base enrichment decisions on either a utility function or on some function of the posterior (or predictive) probability of benefit. Brannath et al. (2009) present a hybrid Bayesian-frequentist design for carrying out an adaptive Phase II/III trial. The hybrid aspect is that they propose embedding Bayesian decision tools within a frequentist designed randomized group sequential clinical trial. In this design, one chooses the subpopulations of interest at the start of the trial. The study includes a single interim analysis at which time one will decide whether to continue enrolling patients from the full population or restrict future enrollment to patients who belong to a pre-specified subpopulation. This analysis will occur before the group sequential interim efficacy or futility analyses. The design calls for using Bayesian calculations to inform this decision. The calculations include the predictive probabilities of ultimately rejecting the study's statistical null hypothesis if enrollment continues with the full population or if future enrollment is restricted to members of the pre-specified subpopulation. Simulations help determine thresholds against which one compares the predictive probabilities when making the decision whether to enrich future enrollment or not. Final determination of the thresholds for the study will be based on consideration by the study team of the right balance of risk of incorrect decisions against the likelihood of correct decisions under various likely or plausible scenarios. The BATTLE (Kim et al., 2011; Zhou et al., 2008) and I-SPY2 (Barker et al., 2009; Alexander et al., 2013) studies are examples of clinical trials that utilize Bayesian computations to adapt randomization probabilities to match patient subgroups with treatments that appear to provide better outcomes for this group of patients.

While sometimes one may have an idea ahead of time which characteristics may confer greater sensitivity to the drug, quite often one does not know before the study begins if a specific population might be more sensitive to the treatment. In such a situation, a researcher may be interested in finding the set of patient or disease characteristics that define subgroups of patients who benefit most from the treatment and, in the same study, determining the treatment effect. In this case, the potential subgroups for possible enrichment are not specified before the study starts, and one may be concerned that a decision to restrict further accruals to a subgroup may be based on a random extreme observation. Such studies have become more common, especially in cancer, as the use of technologies for high-throughput analysis of tens of thousands of genetic material or other biologic material has increased. Several Bayesian designs have already appeared in the literature (Xu et al., 2016; Guo et al., 2017a; Zhang et al., 2016; Schnell et al., 2017).

Let us look at the Subgroup-Based Adaptive or SUBA design (Xu et al., 2016). The name is derived from its goal of simultaneously learning which treatments work best for which subpopulations and adapting randomization during the trial to preferentially allocate patients who belong to a particular subpopulation to the treatment that appears to provide more benefit to that subgroup. We suppose that treatment evaluation is based on a binary clinical outcome that is available relatively quickly and with which one wishes to assess treatment effects. The authors of SUBA assume that the researchers propose a set of continuous biomarkers with which to form the subgroups of patients who benefit from among the treatments under study.

The underlying model is fully Bayesian. Imagine partitioning the range of each biomarker by dividing the range of values into two subregions. A subgroup of the patients consists of a combination of one subregion from each biomarker. SUBA assumes a prior distribution on the space of partitions formed from the biomarkers' possible values. The prior distribution over the partitions is formed based on all possible partitions that one can form by splitting the biomarkers at their medians. The split for a biomarker may be over its entire range or over the range within a part of the partition that already consists of a sub-interval of the biomarker's range. The space of possible partitions is reduced by restricting the number of splits that form the partition to a small number (three, for example). There is also a prior distribution for the probability of response for each treatment within each of the subgroups based on the partitions. The prior distributions for the subgroup-specific probabilities of clinical benefit are Beta distributions.

Initially, the SUBA trial will randomize patients to treatments with equal probability. After enrolling a pre-set number of patients, randomization will start to adapt according to outcomes within the subgroups. The randomization probabilities will relate to predictive probabilities as follows. Conditional on a given partition, we can compute the predictive probability that a new patient will respond to each treatment, given the patient's biomarker values. That is, the patient's biomarker values determine in which part of the partition the patient belongs, and given the observations from patients already in that subgroup, one can compute the predictive probability of response. Averaging the subgroup-specific predictive probabilities with respect to the posterior distribution of each partition in the space of partitions gives the predictive probability that the patient will respond to each treatment. The decision rule for assigning a given treatment to a new patient uses these treatment-specific predictive probabilities. One can assign the patient to the treatment with the largest predictive probability of response or use the predictive probabilities in an adaptive randomization approach along the lines discussed in Section 8.5.1.

8.8 Some criticisms of adaptive designs

Most of the criticisms and controversy surrounding adaptive designs relate to adaptive randomization. Some of the concerns are ethical and some are statistical. An early critique of adaptive randomization questioned the stated optimality of data-dependent randomization (Armitage, 1985). The critique was a reaction to a comparison of fixed allocation to data-dependent allocation in a clinical trial, where the comparison focused on precision of estimation and minimizing the number of patients receiving an inferior treatment (Bather, 1985). In the critique, Armitage (1985) noted that such data-dependent adaptive allocation rules had found little application in practice, although much theoretical work had appeared in the statistical literature. The problems with data-dependent allocation rules that he pointed out include the ethical concern related to loss of equipoise, the role that randomization plays in avoiding covariate imbalance between the treatment groups, and the inherent complexity of these designs. Debate regarding ethical issues relating to adaptive randomization continues, as in (Hey and Kimmelman, 2015) and the discussion papers that follow that article.

The main ethical concern relates to the concept of equipoise. Given the responsibility of a physician to recommend to the patient the therapy that the physician thinks is the best, the ethical justification for randomized clinical trials rests on the notion that the physician is unsure which of the treatments under study is best. The physician is in a state of equipoise regarding the therapeutic options for the patient. One can expand the notion of equipoise from that of the individual physician to the state of knowledge in the physician's larger medical community to justify randomized clinical trials. This broader definition of equipoise that considers the medical community's attitude rather than an individual physician's state of uncertainty is called clinical equipoise (Freedman, 1987). If, as the trial collects data, evidence accrues that indicates that one treatment is better than the other treatments in the study, then there may come a point when the state of equipoise no longer holds. The altered randomization probabilities will reflect the evidence supporting the superiority of one (or more) of the treatments under study, and this evidence may be enough to move a participating physician from a state of equipoise to a clear preference as to which treatment to recommend to the next patient seeking care for the disease targeted by the treatment. Should this physician no longer participate in the randomized trial? What level of evidence of superiority is sufficient to remove the medical community from its state of equipoise? Do changes in the randomization probabilities themselves provide enough evidential weight for some physicians to convince them that one treatment is better than another? How do ethical arguments relating to equipoise balance against the ethical arguments relating to the desire to maximize the number of benefiting patients and minimize the number of patients exposed to inferior therapies? These discussions will likely continue, especially as more trials incorporate adaptive randomization.

An inferential concern about adaptive randomization is the potential biased estimation of a treatment effect at the conclusion of the trial. Causes of the bias may be stochastic in nature or systematic. The former cause might occur if random extreme outcomes appear early in the trial among patients receiving one of the treatments. The final estimate of the treatment's benefit may reflect the better outcomes early in the trial, which were random highs, and any actual benefit that may be seen later in the trial. One way to minimize the risk of random extreme outcomes inflating (or deflating) the randomization probabilities and subsequent estimation is by postponing adaptation until the trial has enrolled and treated a fixed number of patients. Thinking back to the ECMO example in Section 8.2, we can imagine how the investigators who designed the first study might have avoided the ensuing controversy had they included more balls of each color in the urn at the start of the study. Had there been, say, three or more balls of each color in the urn when the first patient entered the study, it would have been far less likely that the trial would have assigned just one baby to one of the two treatments. The same reasoning applies to the recommendation to postpone adapting randomization probabilities.

A particularly problematic systemic cause of bias is called *drift* and occurs when the prognostic characteristics of patients who enter the study in the later stages of the trial, namely after randomization has changed from 1:1, differ from those already in the trial. Since the randomization now favors one treatment, the prognoses of these later enrolling patients may act to reinforce or weaken the appearance of superior outcomes with the treatment already receiving a larger fraction of treatment assignments. The drift may be random but may also be an operational problem. For example, if physicians begin to think that the treatment receiving more patient assignments is really better than the comparator, they may begin to enroll patients with worse prognoses to the study.

Simulation studies have illustrated potential problems that may occur with outcome adaptive randomization (Thall et al., 2015; Wathen and Thall, 2017). One problem that may arise is assigning more patients to the inferior treatment—the antithesis of the goal with adaptive randomization. One recommendation to avoid such an outcome is to wait until adapting randomization probabilities, as already stated, and restricting randomization probabilities to lie between a suitable range, such as $[0.1, 0.9]$. Additionally, deviations from equal randomization reduce efficiency, meaning that estimates at the end of the study may be less precise if the randomization probabilities to the treatments are far from equal.

Aside from risks of bias arising from drift in the types of patients entering the study over time and from overestimation, there are practical issues that one has to address when designing any Bayesian clinical trial, especially an adaptive clinical trial. First of all, these designs tend to be more complex than standard group sequential designs. Often, one has to carry out interim calculations that require Markov chain Monte Carlo or other methods to estimate posterior probabilities. One also has to determine appropriate stopping criteria to ensure that the trial behaves as desired under a variety of scenarios. Quite often, clinical trial simulation is required to determine appropriate values for these design parameters.

An adaptive clinical trial also requires computational and data management infrastructure to support its design and conduct. The process of simulating the study under multiple scenarios requires a large computational effort in all but the simplest of cases. While the study is ongoing, the study team has to be able to enter patient data quickly and without error to ensure that computations that may lead to adaptations reflect up-to-date trial data accurately. If the study's database primarily reflects data from patients who suffer ill effects of the treatments without also including good outcomes, interim decisions may be inappropriate and not the ones that would occur with complete data. Aside from having the infrastructure in place to support the adaptive design, the study team should test and evaluate the infrastructure prior to enrolling patients. This exercise, similar to the many *in silico* clinical trials that provide estimates of the design's operating characteristics, will reveal if there are any potential problems or weaknesses that could affect the integrity of the study.

The importance of clinical trial simulation to evaluate the properties of adaptive trials cannot be overstated. Many adaptive trials involve complicated decision rules based on approximating models with many calculations occurring throughout the course of the study. Non-statistical collaborators may not understand the complicated modeling or the implications of the mathematical models underlying the study's design. Simulations under numerous possible or plausible scenarios provide a way to communicate to the study investigators the properties and characteristics of the adaptive trial. It is not unusual for protocols to include many tables summarizing simulations assuming certain "truths" for the treatments and/or patients entering the study. For example, one can model a drift in patient characteristics to see how robust the design may be against the effects of changes in the patient population over the course of the trial or the extent of any ensuing bias. It is also worth emphasizing the need to include simulations of the clinical trial under the so-called null situation in which all treatments produce similar outcomes. The null case results provide a background with which one can calibrate the trial's properties under the various non-null scenarios.

8.9 Summary

Adaptive clinical trials offer many benefits. They often will have a smaller average sample size than would a corresponding non-adaptive trial, thereby providing the opportunity for a clinical trial to reach a conclusion before enrolling the full target sample size. For many people, the twin goals of increasing the fraction of patients receiving the better treatment and reducing the number of patients receiving inferior therapy provide strong incentive to include outcome adaptive randomization in a trial. Patients may find outcome adaptive randomization appealing, since the trial will tend to treat fewer patients with inferior therapies. Such attitudes can improve patient acceptance and lead to greater accrual to the trial.

The benefits of adaptive clinical trials do come at a cost, however. These trials are complex, require a lot of work during the planning stages of the trials, more oversight during the course of the trial, and specialized expertise throughout the course of the study. An important consideration is how the wider community of physicians and clinical trialists will receive the trial. With careful evaluation of a proposed design via extensive simulation studies, one can feel more confident that the trial will behave as it should under a wide variety of circumstances. Ongoing evaluation of how the trial is proceeding once patients start to enroll in the study, including checks of the randomization probabilities once adaptation begins, will help ensure the success of the randomized trial. In the end, the investigators need to weigh the ethical and practical arguments in favor of and against different ways of incorporating adaptation in a trial's design and decide what will be the best design for addressing the particular clinical question of interest.

Bibliography

Alexander, B., Wen, P., Trippa, L., Reardon, D., Yung, W., Parmigiani, G., and Berry, D. (2013). Biomarker-based adaptive trials for patients with glioblastoma-lessons from I-SPY 2. *Neuro-Oncology*, 15(8):972–978.

Anscombe, F. (1963). Sequential medical trials. *Journal of the American Statistical Association*, 58(302):365–383.

Armitage, P. (1960). *Sequential Medical Trials.* Thomas, Springfield, IL.

Armitage, P. (1985). The search for optimality in clinical trials. *International Statistical Review*, 53(1):15–24.

Armitage, P., McPherson, C., and Rowe, B. (1969). Repeated significance tests on accumulating data. *Journal of the Royal Statistical Society — Series A*, 132(2):235–244.

Babb, J., Rogatko, A., and Zacks, S. (1998). Cancer Phase I clinical trials: Efficient dose escalation with overdose control. *Statistics in Medicine*, 17(10):1103–1120.

Barker, A., Sigman, C., Kelloff, G., Hylton, N., Berry, D., and Esserman, L. (2009). I-SPY 2: An adaptive breast cancer trial design in the setting of neoadjuvant chemotherapy. *Clinical Pharmacology and Therapeutics*, 86(1):97–100.

Barnard, G. (1946). Sequential tests in industrial statistics (with discussion). *Journal of the Royal Statistical Society*, 8(suppl.):1–26.

Bartlett, R., Roloff, D., Cornell, R., Andrews, A., Dillon, P., and Zwischenberger, J. (1985). Extracorporeal circulation in neonatal respiratory failure: a prospective randomized study. *Pediatrics*, 76(4):479–487.

Bather, J. (1985). On the allocation of treatments in sequential medical trials. *International Statistical Review*, 53(1):1–13.

Begg, C. (1990). On inferences from Wei's biased coin design for clinical trials (with discussion). *Biometrika*, 77(3):467–484.

Berger, J. (1985). *Statistical Decision Theory and Bayesian Analysis.* Springer-Verlag, 2nd edition.

Berger, J. and Wolpert, R. L. (1988). *The Likelihood Principle.* Institute of Mathematical Statistics, Hayward, CA:, 2nd edition.

Berry, D. (1985). Interim analyses in clinical trials: Classical vs. Bayesian approaches. *Statistics in Medicine*, 4(4):521–526.

Berry, D. and Fristedt, B. (1985). *Bandit Problems: Sequential Allocation of Experiments.* Chapman and Hall, New York, NY.

Berry, S., Carlin, B., Lee, J., and Müller, P. (2010a). *Bayesian Adaptive Methods for Clinical Trials.* CRC Press, Boca Raton, FL.

Berry, S., Spinelli, W., Littman, G., Liang, J., Fardipour, P., Berry, D., Lewis, R., and Krams, M. (2010b). A Bayesian dose-finding trial with adaptive dose expansion to flexibly assess efficacy and safety of an investigational drug. *Clinical Trials*, 7(2):121–135.

Brannath, W., Zuber, E., Branson, M., Bretz, F., Gallo, P., Posch, M., and Racine-Poon, A. (2009). Confirmatory adaptive designs with Bayesian decision tools for a targeted therapy in oncology. *Statistics in Medicine*, 28(10):1445–1463.

Carlin, B., Kadane, J., and Gelfand, A. (1998). Approaches for optimal sequential decision analysis in clinical trials. *Biometrics*, 54(3):964–975.

Ding, M., Rosner, G., and Müller, P. (2008). Bayesian optimal design for phase II screening trials. *Biometrics*, 64(3):886–894.

Dodge, H. and Romig, H. (1929). A method of sampling inspection. *The Bell System Technical Journal*, 8(4):613–631.

Freedman, B. (1987). Equipoise and the ethics of clinical research. *New England Journal of Medicine*, 317(3):141–145.

Freedman, L. and Spiegelhalter, D. (1989). Comparison of Bayesian with group sequential methods for monitoring clinical trials. *Controlled Clinical Trials*, 10(4):357–367.

Freidlin, B. and Simon, R. (2005). Adaptive signature design: An adaptive clinical trial design for generating and prospectively testing a gene expression signature for sensitive patients. *Clinical Cancer Research*, 11(21):7872–7878.

Geiger, M., Skrivanek, Z., Gaydos, B., Chien, J., Berry, S., and Berry, D. (2012). An adaptive, dose-finding, seamless phase 2/3 study of a long-acting glucagon-like peptide-1 analog (dulaglutide): trial design and baseline characteristics. *Journal of Diabetes Science and Technology*, 6(6):1319–1327.

Gittins, J., Glazebrook, K., and Weber, R. (2011). *Multi-Armed Bandit Allocation Indices.* John Wiley & Sons, Ltd., Chicester, UK, 2nd ed. edition.

Guo, W., Ji, Y., and Catenacci, D. (2017a). A subgroup cluster-based Bayesian adaptive design for precision medicine. *Biometrics*, 73:367–377.

Guo, W., Wang, S.-J., Yang, S., Lynn, H., and Ji, Y. (2017b). A Bayesian interval dose-finding design addressing Ockham's razor: mTPI-2. *Contemporary Clinical Trials*, 58:23–33.

Hey, S. P. and Kimmelman, J. (2015). Are outcome-adaptive allocation trials ethical? *Clinical Trials*, 12(2):102–106.

Huang, X., Ning, J., Li, Y., Estey, E., Issa, J.-P., and Berry, D. A. (2009). Using short-term response information to facilitate adaptive randomization for survival clinical trials. *Statistics in Medicine*, 28(12):1680–1689.

Ji, Y., Liu, P., Li, Y., and Bekele, B. N. (2010). A modified toxicity probability interval method for dose-finding trials. *Clinical Trials*, 7(6):653–63.

Jones, D. and Whitehead, J. (1979). Sequential forms of the log rank and modified Wilcoxon tests for censored data. *Biometrika*, 66(1):105–113.

Kim, E. S., Herbst, R. S., Wistuba, I., Lee, J. J., Blumenschein, G. R., J., Tsao, A., Stewart, D. J., Hicks, M. E., Erasmus, J., J., Gupta, S., Alden, C. M., Liu, S., Tang, X., Khuri, F. R., Tran, H. T., Johnson, B. E., Heymach, J. V., Mao, L., Fossella, F., Kies, M. S., Papadimitrakopoulou, V., Davis, S. E., Lippman, S. M., and Hong, W. K. (2011). The BATTLE trial: personalizing therapy for lung cancer. *Cancer Discovery*, 1(1):44–53.

Krams, M., Lees, K. R., Hacke, W., Grieve, A. P., Orgogozo, J. M., and Ford, G. A. (2003). Acute stroke therapy by inhibition of neutrophils (ASTIN): an adaptive dose-response study of uk-279,276 in acute ischemic stroke. *Stroke*, 34(11):2543–2548.

Lee, J. J. and Liu, D. D. (2008). A predictive probability design for phase II cancer clinical trials. *Clinical Trials*, 5(2):93–106.

Little, R. J. (2006). Calibrated Bayes: A Bayes/frequentist roadmap. *The American Statistician*, 60(3):213–223.

Liu, S. and Yuan, Y. (2015). Bayesian optimal interval designs for phase I clinical trials. *Journal of the Royal Statistical Society — Series C*, 64(3):507–523.

Mandrekar, S. J. and Sargent, D. J. (2009). Clinical trial designs for predictive biomarker validation: one size does not fit all. *Journal of Biopharmaceutical Statistics*, 19(3):530–542.

Neuenschwander, B., Branson, M., and Gsponer, T. (2008). Critical aspects of the Bayesian approach to Phase I cancer trials. *Statistics in Medicine*, 27(13):2420–39.

O'Brien, P. C. and Fleming, T. R. (1979). A multiple testing procedure for clinical trials. *Biometrics*, 35(3):549–556.

O'Quigley, J., Pepe, M., and Fisher, L. (1990). Continual reassessment method: a practical design for phase 1 clinical trials in cancer. *Biometrics*, 46.

O'Rourke, P. P., Crone, R. K., Vacanti, J. P., Ware, J. H., Lillehei, C. W., Parad, R. B., and Epstein, M. F. (1989). Extracorporeal membrane oxygenation and conventional medical therapy in neonates with persistent pulmonary hypertension of the newborn: a prospective randomized study. *Pediatrics*, 84(6):957–963.

Pocock, S. J. (1977). Group sequential methods in design and analysis of clinical trials. *Biometrika*, 64(2):191–200.

Rosenblum, M., Luber, B., Thompson, R., and Hanley, D. (2016). Group sequential designs with prospectively planned rules for subpopulation enrichment. *Statistics in Medicine*, 35(21):3776–3791.

Rosenblum, M. and van der Laan, M. J. (2011). Optimizing randomized trial designs to distinguish which subpopulations benefit from treatment. *Biometrika*, 98(4):845–860.

Rosner, G. L. and Tsiatis, A. A. (1988). Exact confidence intervals following a group sequential trial - a comparison of methods. *Biometrika*, 75(4):723–729.

Rossell, D., Müller, P., and Rosner, G. L. (2007). Screening designs for drug development. *Biostatistics*, 8(3):595–608.

Royall, R. M. (1990). On inferences from Wei's biased coin design for clinical trials – discussion. *Biometrika*, 77(3):473–476.

Schnell, P., Tang, Q., Müller, P., and Carlin, B. (2017). Subgroup inference for multiple treatments and multiple endpoints in an Alzheimer's disease treatment trial. *The Annals of Applied Statistics*, 11(2):949–966.

Skrivanek, Z., Berry, S., Berry, D., Chien, J., Geiger, M. J., Anderson, J. H., and Gaydos, B. (2012). Application of adaptive design methodology in development of a long-acting glucagon-like peptide-1 analog (dulaglutide): statistical design and simulations. *Journal of Diabetes Science and Technology*, 6(6):1305–1318.

Spiegelhalter, D., Freedman, L., and Parmar, M. (1994). Bayesian approaches to randomized trials. *Journal of the Royal Statistical Society — Series A*, 157:357–387.

Thall, P., Fox, P., and Wathen, J. (2015). Statistical controversies in clinical research: scientific and ethical problems with adaptive randomization in comparative clinical trials. *Annals of Oncology*, 26(8):1621–1628.

Thompson, W. R. (1933). On the likelihood that one unknown probability exceeds another in view of the evidence of two samples. *Biometrika*, 25:285–294.

Tsiatis, A. A. (1981). The asymptotic joint distribution of the efficient scores test for the proportional hazards model calculated over time. *Biometrika*, 68(1):311–315.

Tsiatis, A. A. (1982). Repeated significance testing for a general-class of statistics used in censored survival analysis. *Journal of the American Statistical Association*, 77(380):855–861.

U.S. Food and Drug Administration (2010). Guidance for industry: Adaptive design clinical trials for drugs and biologics.

Wald, A. (1945). Sequential tests of statistical hypotheses. *The Annals of Mathematical Statistics*, 16:117–186.

Wang, M.-D. (2007). Sample size reestimation by Bayesian prediction. *Biometrical Journal*, 49(3):365–377.

Wathen, J. K. and Thall, P. F. (2017). A simulation study of outcome adaptive randomization in multi-arm clinical trials. *Clinical Trials*, 14(5):432–440.

West, M. and Harrison, J. (1997). *Bayesian Forecasting and Dynamic Models*. Springer, New York, NY, 2nd ed. edition.

Xu, Y., Trippa, L., Müller, P., and Ji, Y. (2016). Subgroup-based adaptive (SUBA) designs for multi-arm biomarker trials. *Statistics in Biosciences*, 8(1):159–180.

Yin, G. and Yuan, Y. (2009a). Bayesian dose finding in oncology for drug combinations by copula regression. *Journal of the Royal Statistical Society — Series C*, 58:211–224.

Yin, G. and Yuan, Y. (2009b). Bayesian model averaging continual reassessment method in phase I clinical trials. *Journal of the American Statistical Association*, 104(487):954–968.

Yuan, Y. and Yin, G. (2011). Bayesian phase I/II adaptively randomized oncology trials with combined drugs. *The Annals of Applied Statistics*, 5:924–942.

Zelen, M. (1969). Play the winner rule and the controlled clinical trial. *Journal of the American Statistical Association*, 64(325):131–146.

Zelen, M. (1974). The randomization and stratification of patients to clinical trials. *Journal of Chronic Diseases*, 27(7):365–375.

Zhang, Y., Trippa, L., and Parmigiani, G. (2016). Optimal Bayesian adaptive trials when treatment efficacy depends on biomarkers. *Biometrics*, 72(2):414–421.

Zhong, W., Koopmeiners, J. S., and Carlin, B. P. (2013). A two-stage Bayesian design with sample size reestimation and subgroup analysis for phase II binary response trials. *Contemporary Clinical Trials*, 36(2):587–596.

Zhou, X., Liu, S., Kim, E. S., Herbst, R. S., and Lee, J. J. (2008). Bayesian adaptive design for targeted therapy development in lung cancer–a step toward personalized medicine. *Clinical Trials*, 5(3):181–193.

9

Bayesian Methods for Longitudinal Data with Missingness

Michael J. Daniels
University of Florida, US

Dandan Xu
U.S. Food and Drug Administration, US

This chapter reviews Bayesian methods for longitudinal data with missingness. We start out by briefly describing frequentist approaches and then move on to Bayesian approaches. For the latter, we focus on specification of prior distributions, models for the covariance structure, and Bayesian nonparametric methods. Next, we provide an overview of how to address ignorable and nonignorable missingness (with sensitivity parameters), including a discussion of approaches for missing covariates. Computational approaches for posterior inference as well as approaches for model selection and assessment are then reviewed. Finally, a careful case study analysis is performed for a drug clinical trial.

9.1 Introduction

There is extensive literature on approaches for the analysis of longitudinal data. The two major features of longitudinal data that need to be addressed in modeling include the fact that repeated observations on the same unit over time are correlated and that it is typical that the complete vector of longitudinal responses is not collected on all subjects. The approaches for modeling longitudinal data can be dichotomized into *non-likelihood-based* and *likelihood-based.*

The non-likelihood-based approaches try to minimize parametric assumptions (e.g. Liang and Zeger, 1986) and are often based solely on moments, while the likelihood-based approaches model the full probability distribution of the longitudinal data (Laird and Ware, 1982; Heagerty, 1999). The latter allows inference about any function of the distribution of the longitudinal data (simultaneously). Likelihood-based approaches either use frequentist inference (Fitzmaurice et al., 2012; Diggle et al., 2002; Verbeke and Molenberghs, 2000) or Bayesian inference (Gelman et al., 2014; Weiss, 2005). There is also extensive literature on joint modeling of longitudinal data with a time to event outcome (e.g. survival or dropout); we will not discuss these approaches here but we refer the reader to (2012) for details.

The main focus of the chapter will be likelihood-based approaches that use Bayesian inference. There is much literature on Bayesian longitudinal data; nice reviews are presented in Weiss (2005) and Chapter 15 of Lesaffre and Lawson (2012), as well as priors for longitudinal covariance structures (Pourahmadi and Daniels, 2002; Daniels and Pourahmadi, 2002, 2009; Wang and Daniels, 2013; Gaskins et al., 2014; Wong et al., 2003).

Missing data are the norm in longitudinal studies. Bayesian approaches allow automatically for certain types of missingness which might realistically hold for longitudinal data. Frequentist approaches based on moment-type restrictions require modifications (e.g. introduction of weights) to be valid for any reasonable missingness assumption (for longitudinal data) and are designed for a specific summary of the full probability distribution (e.g. the mean). There has been considerable research on missingness in longitudinal data; a very nice overview of Bayesian parametric approaches can be found in Daniels and Hogan (2008) and non-Bayesian approaches in Molenberghs and Kenward (2007) and Ibrahim and Molenberghs (2009). Recently, there has been work on Bayesian nonparametric approaches using Dirichlet process mixture models for dropout in longitudinal studies (Linero and Daniels, 2015; Daniels and Linero, 2015; Quintana et al., 2016; Linero and Daniels, 2018).

9.1.1 Motivating examples

We will discuss several examples of longitudinal studies throughout the chapter, including a careful analysis of a longitudinal clinical trial in an elderly population in Section 9.8. But we provide a brief snapshot of two of the examples here that will be referred to at times in the chapter:

Natural history study of Duchenne muscular dystrophy

This is an ongoing study that aims to better understand and measure progression in boys with Duchenne muscular dystrophy (DMD; Willcocks et al., 2016). Boys generally visit the clinic annually and various functional tests are conducted as well as Magnetic Resonance (MR) imaging. It is of interest to understand how these MR imaging biomarkers change with age and how well they capture a boy's progression. For the individual MR parameters, we have been building longitudinal models which we briefly describe previously. An ultimate goal of this study is to formally use MR parameters as biomarkers and to potentially assess new interventions based on the impact on these longitudinal biomarkers.

Schizophrenia clinical trial

This was a randomized, double blind, multicenter clinical trial designed to assess three different interventions: test drug, active drug, and placebo on schizophrenia, as measured by the Positive and Negative Syndrome Scale (PANSS) scores. Subjects were assessed at baseline, day 4, and weeks 1-4. Major issues for this trial included standard parametric approaches not providing good fit and the thought that some types of dropout were related to the unobserved longitudinal responses. A thorough analysis of this trial is provided in Daniels and Linero (2015) using Bayesian nonparametric models and the missing data framework described in Section 9.4.

9.1.2 Notation

We now introduce some notation. Let $\{Y_i(t) : t \geq 0\}$ be the underlying longitudinal response process in continuous time for the ith subject. In practice, longitudinal data are only observed at a discrete set of time points $\mathscr{T} = \{t_1, \ldots, t_J\}$ with resulting column vector of responses $\boldsymbol{Y}_i = \{Y_i(t) : t \in \mathscr{T}\} = (Y_{i1}, \ldots, Y_{iJ})^\top$. Covariates $\boldsymbol{X}_i = (\boldsymbol{X}_{i1}^\top, \ldots, \boldsymbol{X}_{iJ}^\top)^\top$ are also observed at the same time points, where $\boldsymbol{X}_{ij} = (X_{ij1}, \ldots, X_{ijp})^\top$ are covariates observed at time $j \in \{1, \ldots, J\}$ for the ith subject.

9.1.3 Overview of chapter

Section 9.2 provides a quick review and some key references for non-likelihood based approaches. Section 9.3 discusses likelihood-based approaches, focusing on Bayesian inference. Bayesian approaches to address missing data are reviewed in Section 9.4 and posterior computations in Section 9.5. Sections 9.6 and 9.7 discuss model selection and assessing model fit, respectively. Section 9.8 includes a detailed pharmaceutical case study to illustrate key concepts. Open issues/problems are briefly discussed in Section 9.9.

9.2 Common frequentist approaches

Frequentist approaches can be divided into moment-based approaches and likelihood-based (full probability model based) approaches. We will briefly survey the former in this section. In the next section, we will discuss likelihood-based approaches in the context of Bayesian inference.

Moment-based approaches in the context of longitudinal data typically specify a parametric model for the mean and estimate parameters using an appropriate set of estimating equations; Liang and Zeger (1986) called these generalized estimating equations (GEEs). These approaches offer inference robust to mis-specification of the covariance structure in many cases and do not make assumptions about the entire distribution of the longitudinal responses. Related approaches using estimating equations have also been used for quantiles (Koenker, 2004).

The 'moment-based' estimators are typically valid only under missingness that is completely at random (MCAR), i.e. missingness is independent of the longitudinal response conditional on covariates; for details, see Section 9.4. When this does not hold (and it would be very unusual for it to hold in longitudinal data), the equations need to be adjusted (typically with weights). The weights are computed from a model for the probability of missingness given observed responses and covariates. The modified equations are typically called inverse probability weighted (Robins et al., 1994). These can be made more efficient (and robust) in a variety of ways (Scharfstein et al., 1999; Qu et al., 2000; Gruber and Van Der Laan, 2009).

Repeated measures ANOVA (RMANOVA) is related to multivariate Normal models with a structured covariance matrix (which are discussed in Section 9.3). The induced structured correlation matrix assumes all the longitudinal measurements on a subject are equally correlated. This is not a reasonable assumption for longitudinal data where (some) serial correlation is anticipated. In addition, implementation of RMANOVA in standard software does not allow missing data and throws away incomplete cases (so only valid under MCAR which very rarely holds; for details see Section 9.4). So arguably, given the issues with missing data and the restrictive correlation structure, RMANOVA should not be used in settings with missing data and/or with at least three longitudinal time points.

9.3 Bayesian approaches

In this section, we review common models for longitudinal data and discuss the choice of priors for Bayesian inference. Bayesian inference for longitudinal models offers numerous advantages. Using approaches that sample from the posterior distribution (details in Section 9.5), 'exact' inference about any functional of the distribution of full data response, $\widetilde{\boldsymbol{Y}}_J = (Y_1, \ldots, Y_J)^\top$ including 'exact' credible intervals can be obtained easily; thus, large sample results like the delta method are unnecessary. Efficiency gains over frequentist approaches can be realized by specifying full probability models and/or including informative priors when historical information or expert information (by elicitation) is available. Uncertainty from the covariance structure estimation is naturally propagated into uncertainty about mean parameters. Flexible modeling of the data by Bayesian nonparametrics is possible, often without loss of efficiency. We provide details on all these in what follows.

The most common likelihood based approaches for longitudinal data are conditional approaches, which specify a mean model for responses conditional on other random variables, such as previous response in transition models, or parameters, such as random effects for mixed models. We start by discussing different types of random effects models, which induce correlations in the vector of longitudinal responses of each unit through the random effects.

Linear mixed models (LMMs) (LMMs) specify a multivariate Normal model for continuous longitudinal responses conditional on random effects $\boldsymbol{b}_i$ with linear mean function $\mathrm{E}(Y_{ij} \mid \boldsymbol{x}_{ij}, \boldsymbol{w}_{ij}, \boldsymbol{\beta}, \boldsymbol{b}_i) = \boldsymbol{x}_{ij}^\top \boldsymbol{\beta} + \boldsymbol{w}_{ij}^\top \boldsymbol{b}_i$ and $\mathrm{Var}(\boldsymbol{Y}_i \mid \boldsymbol{b}_i, \boldsymbol{x}_i, \boldsymbol{w}_i) = \sigma^2 \boldsymbol{I}$ (independence is not necessary here), where $\boldsymbol{\beta}$ is the regression parameter and $\boldsymbol{w}_{ij}$ is a design vector for the subject-specific random effects $\boldsymbol{b}_i$. The random effects are specified as $\boldsymbol{b}_i \sim \mathrm{N}(0, \boldsymbol{\Omega})$ which introduces dependence among the components of $\boldsymbol{Y}_i$. $\boldsymbol{x}_{ij}$ can include temporal and/or subject specific covariates. For example, in the analysis of the schizophrenia clinical trial in Chapter 7 in Daniels and Hogan (2008), a separate quadratic temporal trend was assumed over weeks for each treatment with random components of a quadratic orthogonal polynomial in the number of weeks.

Nonlinear mixed models (NLMMs) specify a nonlinear mean function $\mathrm{E}(Y_{ij} \mid \boldsymbol{x}_{ij}, \boldsymbol{\theta}, \boldsymbol{b}_i) = h(\boldsymbol{x}_{ij}, \boldsymbol{\theta}, \boldsymbol{b}_i)$, where $\boldsymbol{\theta}$ are model parameters and $h(\cdot)$ is a nonlinear function. Typically parameters $\boldsymbol{\theta}$ are interpretable and appropriately capture the nonlinearity, along with $h(\cdot)$. Similarly to LMM, random effects $\boldsymbol{b}_i$ are typically assumed to follow a (multivariate) Normal model.

An example of this type of model is one recently used for a natural history study to assess MR imaging as a biomarker for progression in boys with Duchenne Muscular Dystrophy (Rooney et al., ??), as discussed in Section 9.1.1. We assume the response, Y_{ij} for $j = 1, \ldots, 7$ measured at time t_j (months) where $(t_1, \ldots, t_7) = (0, 3, 6, 12, 24, 36, 48)$, is Normally distributed conditional on random effects with conditional mean model

$$\mathrm{E}(Y_{ij} \mid \boldsymbol{\theta}, \boldsymbol{b}_i, \mathrm{age}_{ij}) \;=\; A\sqrt{\frac{\tau_i}{2\pi}} \int_{-\infty}^{\mathrm{age_{ij}}} \exp\left(-\frac{(x-\mu_i)^2 \tau_i}{2}\right) dx,$$

where age_{ij} is age at t_j for the ith boy, $\mu_i = \mu_0 + b_{i1}$ and $\tau_i = \tau_0 b_{i2}$, and $\boldsymbol{\theta} = (A, \mu_0, \tau_0)^\top$, $\boldsymbol{b}_i = (b_{i1}, b_{i2})^\top$. This mean model was chosen for its S-shape and interpretable parameters. A represents the amplitude (maximum outcome progression). The parameter μ_i represents the centroid position/inflection point (here, the age at maximum progression rate). Finally, the parameter τ_i is precision of the distribution and represents the progression 'slope' at the age of the maximum progression rate.

Generalized linear mixed models (GLMMs) are commonly used to model binary and count responses. The conditional mean model is specified as $g(\mathrm{E}[Y_{ij} \mid \boldsymbol{x}_{ij}, \boldsymbol{w}_{ij}, \boldsymbol{\beta}, \boldsymbol{b}_i]) = \boldsymbol{x}_{ij}^\top \boldsymbol{\beta} + \boldsymbol{w}_{ij}^\top \boldsymbol{b}_i$, where $g(\cdot)$ is the link function, such as logit function for binary responses and log function for count responses, and similar to above, $\boldsymbol{b}_i$ are random effects with

$\boldsymbol{b}_i \sim \mathrm{N}(\mathbf{0}, \boldsymbol{\Omega})$. The induced marginal mean, obtained by integrating out the random effects, is typically not equal to $g(\boldsymbol{x}_{ij}^\top \boldsymbol{\beta})$; thus the attractive interpretation of the covariate effects in the conditional mean model is lost after the integration in terms of the interpretation of the marginal mean.

Transition (Markov) models specify a generalized linear model (GLM) for a binary response Y_{ij} conditional on k previous responses. The dependence between responses on the same unit is clearly induced by this conditioning. A transition model was used in Chapter 7 in Daniels and Hogan (2008) for a clinical trial designed to study the effect of exercise on smoking cessation. Women were randomized to one of two treatment groups, $Z \in \{0, 1\}$, and quit status $\boldsymbol{Y} = (Y_1, \ldots, Y_{12})^\top$ was recorded weekly over 12 weeks and the target for quitting was week 5. The main inferential objective was to compare time averaged (over weeks 5-12) quit rate between treatments. Given the design with a target quit week, it was thought the Markov dependence might differ at the quit week versus subsequent weeks. This could easily be accomplished in these models by allowing the Markov dependence parameter to depend on the quit week. We specify the model below:

$$\mathrm{logit}\,(\mathrm{E}[Y_{ij} \mid Y_{i,j-1} = y_{i,j-1}, Z_i = z_i]) = \mathbb{I}(j < 5)\alpha + \mathbb{I}(j \geq 5)(\beta_0 + \beta_1 z_i) + \gamma_i y_{i,j-1}$$

with a location change at the target quit week. The following serial dependence model was specified for γ_i for weeks 5 to 12, $\gamma_i = \gamma_{i1}\mathbb{I}(j = 5) + \gamma_{i2}\mathbb{I}(j > 5)$ for $j = 5, \ldots, 12$, where $\gamma_{ik} = \phi_{0k} + \phi_{1k} z_i$, $k = 1, 2$ and which allows a different dependence parameter at the target quit week.

Marginal approaches. In the current development, we have described conditional models. Another class of models that are sometimes used are marginal models. Marginal approaches directly specify a joint probability model for the longitudinal responses $\boldsymbol{Y}_i = (Y_{i1}, \ldots, Y_{iJ})^\top$. We briefly review some marginal mean models below. Multivariate Normal models (MVNs) are often directly specified for continuous responses as opposed to indirectly via a LMM. In particular, $\boldsymbol{Y}_i \sim \mathrm{N}(\boldsymbol{\mu}_i, \boldsymbol{\Sigma}_i)$ with covariance matrix, $\boldsymbol{\Sigma}_i = \boldsymbol{\Sigma}_i(\boldsymbol{\phi})$ and mean, $\boldsymbol{\mu}_i = \boldsymbol{x}_i^\top \boldsymbol{\beta}$, where $\boldsymbol{\phi}$ and $\boldsymbol{\beta}$ are parameters. $\boldsymbol{x}_{ij}$ can include temporal structure, e.g. $\boldsymbol{x}_{ij} = (1, t_j)^\top$, and/or subject specific covariates as with LMMs. We discuss models for $\boldsymbol{\Sigma}_i$ in Section 9.3.1; specification of $\boldsymbol{\Sigma}_i$ is particularly important for incomplete longitudinal data which we discuss in Section 9.4. We illustrate these models in a drug trial in Section 9.8. We also note that LMMs induce a specific form for Σ_i as discussed earlier. Some recent developments of marginal models include longitudinal models for Skew-Normal data (Tang et al., 2015). The *multivariate probit model (MVP)* is a generalization of the MVN for binary data. The likelihood cannot be written in closed form; however by introduction of appropriate latent Normal random variables, posterior sampling can be done quite easily using data augmentation (see Section 9.5).

'Marginalized' models for longitudinal binary data have also been developed based on both transition and random effects models (Heagerty, 1999; Schildcrout and Heagerty, 2005). We refer the reader to these references for further details as well as Case study 2 in Chapter 10 of Daniels and Hogan (2008).

When interest is in the marginal mean, marginal models are often preferred to conditional models. The marginal means of responses for conditional models can be derived by integrating the conditionals over the distribution of the random effects or previous responses. However the marginal means (except for linear mixed models) often do not have closed forms and/or the parameters do not have the same interpretation (e.g. if the conditional mean model has additive covariate effects, the marginal mean model often will not).

All the models described in this section can include smooth functions (e.g. splines) in the covariate matrix, $\boldsymbol{x}_{ij}$ for nonlinear smooth time trends or nonlinear covariate effects (Crainiceanu et al., 2005).

9.3.1 Models for the covariance structure and priors

In Markov models, parsimonious structure and covariates can be added to the covariance structure through the appropriate regression coefficients as shown in Section 9.3. Here, we review a popular approach for a covariance matrix, often referred to as the GARP/IV parameterization, which has easy to interpret parameters and avoids positive definiteness concerns. For this parameterization, we first reparametrize the covariance matrix, $\boldsymbol{\Sigma}$ (of a multivariate Normal model). This can be best understood by factoring the multivariate Normal distribution sequentially as $p(y_1, \ldots, y_J) = p(y_1) \prod_{j=2}^{J} p(y_j \mid \widetilde{\boldsymbol{y}}_{j-1})$ where $\widetilde{\boldsymbol{y}}_{j-1} = (y_1, \ldots, y_{j-1})^\top$. The covariance matrix $\boldsymbol{\Sigma}$ can be reparameterized into generalized autoregressive parameters (GARP), ϕ_{jk} for $j = 2, \ldots, J$ and $k = 1, \ldots, j-1$, which are regression coefficients in the conditional means, i.e. $\mathrm{E}[Y_j \mid \widetilde{\boldsymbol{Y}}_{j-1} = \widetilde{\boldsymbol{y}}_{j-1}] = \mu_j + \sum_{k=1}^{j-1} \phi_{jk}(y_k - \mu_k)$ and innovation variances (IV), σ_j^2 for $j = 1, \ldots, J$, which are the conditional variances, i.e. $\mathrm{Var}[Y_j \mid \widetilde{\boldsymbol{Y}}_{j-1} = \widetilde{\boldsymbol{y}}_{j-1}] = \sigma_j^2$. To ensure positive definiteness of $\boldsymbol{\Sigma}$, ϕ_{jk} have no restrictions and σ_j^2 only needs to be positive. This reparameterization has been called the modified Cholesky decomposition (Pourahmadi, 1999). With this parameterization, it is easy to introduce structure and/or covariates in $\boldsymbol{\Sigma}$ by modeling GARP with $\phi_{jk} = \boldsymbol{A}_{jk}^\top \boldsymbol{\gamma}$ and modeling IV with $\log(\sigma_j^2) = \boldsymbol{L}_j^\top \boldsymbol{\lambda}$ where $\boldsymbol{A}_{jk}$ and $\boldsymbol{L}_j$ are design matrix and $\boldsymbol{\gamma}$ and $\boldsymbol{\lambda}$ are regression parameters. There are no constraints on $\boldsymbol{\gamma}$ and $\boldsymbol{\lambda}$ for positive definiteness of $\boldsymbol{\Sigma}$. We discuss priors on these parameters in Section 9.3.2 and show its implementation in practice in the case study in Section 9.8. In addition to the developments in multivariate Normal response models, these covariance models have been implemented for the random effects covariance matrix in linear mixed models (Daniels and Zhao, 2003), generalized linear mixed models (Lee et al., 2012) and marginalized models (Lee et al., 2013).

Other approaches to model the covariance structure include the partial correlations/marginal variances parameterization, which first decomposes the covariance matrix into the marginal variances and the correlation matrix. Similar modeling can be done with the marginal variances as is done with the IVs above and there are not positive definiteness concerns. Further details can be found in the following papers: Daniels and Pourahmadi (2009); Wang and Daniels (2013); Su and Daniels (2015). This approach can also be used for the correlation matrix in multivariate probit models and has been used in marginalized random effect models (MREMs) (Lee et al., 2013). Zhang et al. (2015) proposed an alternative parameterization that also ensures positive definiteness but the resulting parameters are not easy to interpret. Related models have also been developed using the moving average parameters, instead of the autoregressive parameters in the GARP/IV used above (Zhang and Leng, 2011) and by combining both sets of dependence parameters (Lee et al., 2017).

9.3.2 Priors

We briefly discuss priors for the parameters in the models we have discussed so far. In the marginal and conditional approaches, when there is little prior information, the linear coefficients $\boldsymbol{\beta}$ are typically assumed to have diffuse Normal priors, i.e. $\boldsymbol{\beta} \sim \mathrm{N}(\boldsymbol{\beta}_0, \boldsymbol{\Omega}_\beta)$ with $\boldsymbol{\beta}_0 = \boldsymbol{0}$ and $\boldsymbol{\Omega}_\beta$ being a diagonal matrix with large values. In the multivariate Normal model, the covariance matrix is typically assumed to have an inverse Wishart prior, i.e. $\boldsymbol{\Sigma}^{-1} \sim \mathrm{Wishart}(\rho, \boldsymbol{\Sigma}_0)$ where parameter ρ controls the uncertainty and is bounded from below at dimension of $\boldsymbol{\Sigma}$, with $\boldsymbol{\Sigma}_0$ proportional to a prior guess. However, due to the lack of flexibility, flexible GARP/IV priors can be used for the covariance matrix based on the GARP/IV parameterization introduced in Section 9.3.1 (Daniels and Pourahmadi, 2002); in particular, Normal priors on the GARP (or the corresponding regression coefficients) and Gamma priors on $1/\sigma_j^2$ or Half-Normal or Uniform priors on σ_j can be used. Normal priors on the former are conditionally conjugate and are also on the latter for Gamma priors in a Normal regression. Priors for the correlation matrix in the multivariate probit model are discussed in Daniels and Pourahmadi (2009) and Gaskins et al. (2014). The prior for the covariance matrix $\boldsymbol{\Omega}$ for the random effects can be specified as an Inverse-Wishart prior or GARP/IV priors (Daniels and Zhao, 2003). For marginalized random effects models, similar flexible priors for the covariance matrix of the random effects can be used.

An important advantage of Bayesian inference is the incorporation of external information via priors. Historical information can easily be introduced via, for example, power priors (Ibrahim and Chen, 2000; Hobbs et al., 2011) that increase precision in a data dependent way; simple elicitation of prior information based on scientific information is nicely described in Christensen et al. (2011). In addition, (informative) priors are necessary for *incomplete* longitudinal data under nonignorable missingness, which we discuss in Section 9.4; a nice example of elicitation in this context can be found in Daniels and Hogan (2008, Chapter 9).

9.3.3 Use of Bayesian nonparametric models

The models discussed here in Section 9.3 can be made more flexible by using Bayesian nonparametric (BNP) models for the full data response or the random effects (Chapter 7 in Hjort et al., 2010). Some examples include Dirichlet process mixtures (DPM) for continuous and binary responses (Linero and Daniels, 2015; Quintana et al., 2016; Linero and Daniels, 2018), Beta shrinkage priors for longitudinal binary responses (Wang et al., 2010), and DPM for random effects (Kleinman and Ibrahim, 1998a,b; Li et al., 2010) among many other examples. See also Chapter 1 for an introduction to these models.

9.4 Ignorable and nonignorable missingness

It is rare to not have any missing data in longitudinal studies. Bayesian inference offers many advantages for missingness. Missingness can be handled 'automatically' when appropriate (under ignorable missingness, which can be a reasonable misingness assumption in longitudinal data); under this assumption, explicit specification of the missing data mechanism is not necessary, unlike non-likelihood, frequentist approaches. All of the models discussed above provide valid inference under ignorable missingness. In addition, uncertainty about the distribution of the missing data can be incorporated via informative priors under nonignorable missingness. Details are provided in what follows.

9.4.1 Missing data mechanisms

We need to introduce some additional notation for missingness. We define observed data indicators for each longitudinal response, $\boldsymbol{R} = (R_1, \ldots, R_J)^\top$ where $R_j = \mathbb{I}\{Y_j \text{ is observed}\}$. The full data are $(\boldsymbol{Y}, \boldsymbol{R})$. Any model for the full-data can be factored as

$$p(\boldsymbol{y}, \boldsymbol{r} \mid \boldsymbol{x}, \boldsymbol{\omega}) = p\left(\boldsymbol{y} \mid \boldsymbol{x}, \boldsymbol{\theta}(\boldsymbol{\omega})\right)\ p\left(\boldsymbol{r} \mid \boldsymbol{y}, \boldsymbol{x}, \boldsymbol{\psi}(\boldsymbol{\omega})\right),$$

where $\boldsymbol{\omega}$ are the parameters of the full data model. The factor $p\left(\boldsymbol{r} \mid \boldsymbol{y}, \boldsymbol{x}, \boldsymbol{\psi}(\boldsymbol{\omega})\right)$, parameterized by $\boldsymbol{\psi}$, which is a function of $\boldsymbol{\omega}$, is the missing data mechanism with the other term the full data response model, parameterized by $\boldsymbol{\theta}$. It is useful to rewrite the missing data mechanism as $p(\boldsymbol{r} \mid \boldsymbol{y}, \boldsymbol{x}, \boldsymbol{\psi}) = p(\boldsymbol{r} \mid \boldsymbol{y}_{\text{obs}}, \boldsymbol{y}_{\text{mis}}, \boldsymbol{x}, \boldsymbol{\psi})$, where $\boldsymbol{Y}$ is partitioned into observed and missing responses, $\boldsymbol{Y}_{\text{obs}}$ and $\boldsymbol{Y}_{\text{mis}}$. Missing data mechanisms are typically classified into one of three types: (1) missing completely at random (MCAR) when dropout is unrelated to all elements of $\boldsymbol{Y}$, i.e. $p(\boldsymbol{r} \mid \boldsymbol{y}, \boldsymbol{x}, \boldsymbol{\psi}) = p(\boldsymbol{r} \mid \boldsymbol{x}, \boldsymbol{\psi})$; (2) missing at random (MAR) when dropout is unrelated to $\boldsymbol{Y}_{\text{mis}}$, conditionally on $\boldsymbol{Y}_{\text{obs}}$, i.e. $p(\boldsymbol{r} \mid \boldsymbol{y}, \boldsymbol{x}, \boldsymbol{\psi}) = p(\boldsymbol{r} \mid \boldsymbol{y}_{\text{obs}}, \boldsymbol{x}, \boldsymbol{\psi})$; (3) missing not at random (MNAR) when dropout may depend on $\boldsymbol{Y}_{\text{mis}}$ after conditioning on $\boldsymbol{Y}_{\text{obs}}$, i.e. $p(\boldsymbol{r} \mid \boldsymbol{y}_{\text{obs}}, \boldsymbol{Y}_{\text{mis}} = \boldsymbol{y}_{\text{mis}}, \boldsymbol{x}, \boldsymbol{\psi}) \neq p(\boldsymbol{r} \mid \boldsymbol{y}_{\text{obs}}, \boldsymbol{Y}_{\text{mis}} = \boldsymbol{y}'_{\text{mis}}, \boldsymbol{x}, \boldsymbol{\psi})$ for some $\boldsymbol{y}_{\text{mis}} \neq \boldsymbol{y}'_{\text{mis}}$. In the context of a fully Bayesian model-based approach, it is more practical to consider ignorable vs. nonignorable missingness.

9.4.2 Ignorable missingness

In what follows, we will suppress $\boldsymbol{x}$ from the conditioning for clarity. A missing data mechanism is ignorable if the following three conditions hold: (1) the missing data mechanism is MAR; (2) the full data parameter $\boldsymbol{\omega}$ can be decomposed as $\boldsymbol{\omega} = (\boldsymbol{\theta}, \boldsymbol{\psi})$, where $\boldsymbol{\theta}$ indexes the full-data response model $p(\boldsymbol{y} \mid \boldsymbol{\theta})$, and $\boldsymbol{\psi}$ indexes the missing data mechanism $p(\boldsymbol{r} \mid \boldsymbol{y}, \boldsymbol{\psi})$; (3) the parameters $\boldsymbol{\theta}$ and $\boldsymbol{\psi}$ are a-priori independent; i.e. $p(\boldsymbol{\theta}, \boldsymbol{\psi}) = p(\boldsymbol{\theta})p(\boldsymbol{\psi})$. The key implications of ignorability (as alluded to above) are that the missing data mechanism $p(\boldsymbol{r} \mid \boldsymbol{y}, \boldsymbol{\psi})$ does not have to be specified (detail can be found in Chapter 6 of Daniels and Hogan, 2008). Thus the models in Section 9.3 can be used directly with the likelihood being based on the observed responses. In addition, the correct specification of the covariance structure — e.g. using models in Section 9.3.1 — is essential to avoid bias in the mean parameters (Daniels and Hogan, 2008; Little and Rubin, 2014) and of course, have accurate measures of uncertainty.

9.4.3 Nonignorable missingness and full-data models

It is very difficult to be certain about the ignorability assumption (in particular, MAR). To address uncertainty about or deviations from MAR, we need to model the joint distribution of the full data, $(\boldsymbol{Y}, \boldsymbol{R})$ to make valid inference on functions of the full-data response distribution, $p(\boldsymbol{y} \mid \boldsymbol{\theta})$. Full data models are typically classified based on how $p(\boldsymbol{y}, \boldsymbol{r} \mid \boldsymbol{\omega})$ is factored: (1) selection models (SMs; Diggle and Kenward, 1994):

$$p(\boldsymbol{y}, \boldsymbol{r} \mid \boldsymbol{\omega}) = p\,(\boldsymbol{y} \mid \boldsymbol{\theta}(\boldsymbol{\omega}))\;\, p\,(\boldsymbol{r} \mid \boldsymbol{y}, \boldsymbol{\psi}(\boldsymbol{\omega}))\,;$$

(2) pattern mixture models (PMMs; Little, 1994):

$$p(\boldsymbol{y}, \boldsymbol{r} \mid \boldsymbol{\omega}) = p\,(\boldsymbol{y} \mid \boldsymbol{r}, \boldsymbol{\alpha}(\boldsymbol{\omega}))\;\, p\,(\boldsymbol{r} \mid \boldsymbol{\phi}(\boldsymbol{\omega}))\,;$$

and (3) shared parameter models (SPMs; Wu and Carroll, 1988):

$$p(\boldsymbol{y}, \boldsymbol{r} \mid \boldsymbol{\omega}) = \int p\,(\boldsymbol{y}, \boldsymbol{r} \mid \boldsymbol{b}, \nu(\boldsymbol{\omega}))\, dF(b).$$

We advocate PMMs here (details in what follows).

Note that every full-data model uses an extrapolation that can be seen by factoring it as

$$p(\boldsymbol{y}, \boldsymbol{r} \mid \boldsymbol{\omega}) = p(\boldsymbol{y}_{\text{obs}}, \boldsymbol{r} \mid \boldsymbol{\omega}_{\text{O}}) \times p(\boldsymbol{y}_{\text{mis}} \mid \boldsymbol{y}_{\text{obs}}, \boldsymbol{r}, \boldsymbol{\omega}_{\text{E}}),$$

where $\boldsymbol{\omega} = g(\boldsymbol{\omega}_{\text{E}}, \boldsymbol{\omega}_{\text{O}})$. The first term is the observed data distribution and the second term is the missing data extrapolation (Daniels and Hogan, 2008); there is no information about the second term in the data. As an example, consider a longitudinal clinical trial with two longitudinal outcomes, Y_1 and Y_2 and assume there is only missingness in Y_2. Then the extrapolation distribution would be $p(y_2 \mid y_1, R = 0)$ and the observed data distribution would be composed of the following factors: $p(y_2 \mid y_1, R = 1)$, $p(y_1 \mid R = 0)$, $p(y_1 \mid R = 1)$, and $p(R = 1)$. Under MAR, the extrapolation of missing data from observed data does not depend on missing data pattern, i.e, $p(\boldsymbol{y}_{\text{mis}} \mid \boldsymbol{y}_{\text{obs}}, \boldsymbol{r}) = p(\boldsymbol{y}_{\text{mis}} \mid \boldsymbol{y}_{\text{obs}})$; in the simple example, $p(y_2 \mid y_1, R = 0) = p(y_2 \mid y_1)$. In general, since there is no information available in the data about the extrapolation distribution, it is important to incorporate uncertainty about it. This is typically done by introducing sensitivity parameters (that are given informative priors). Sensitivity parameters are parameters that when varied do not impact the fit of the model to the observed data, and when fixed, identify the full data model. A formal definition can be found in Daniels and Hogan (2008, Chapter 9).

9.4.4 Identification of the extrapolation distribution under monotone missingness

In practice, the extrapolation distribution $p(\boldsymbol{y}_{\text{mis}} \mid \boldsymbol{y}_{\text{obs}}, \boldsymbol{r}, \boldsymbol{\omega}_{\text{E}})$ typically corresponds to several conditional distributions. We illustrate this here for monotone missingness for longitudinal data. Monotone missingness (in the context of longitudinal data, this is missingness only due to dropout) is such that if $R_j = 0$, then $R_{j+k} = 0$ for $k = 1, \ldots, J - j$. Let $S \in \{1, \ldots, J\}$ be the number of observed responses; S captures all the information contained in $\boldsymbol{R}$ when missingness is monotone. Let $p_k(\boldsymbol{y}) = p(\boldsymbol{y} \mid S = k)$ be pattern specific distribution, which can be sequentially factored, i.e. $p_k(\boldsymbol{y}) = p_k(y_1)\Pi_{j=2}^{J} p_k(y_j \mid \widetilde{\boldsymbol{y}}_{j-1})$, where $\widetilde{\boldsymbol{y}}_{j-1} = (y_1, \ldots, y_{j-1})$. Also let $p_{\geq k}(\boldsymbol{y}) = p(\boldsymbol{y} \mid S \geq k)$. Recall, the extrapolation distribution cannot be identified from the observed data.

Table 9.1 shows identifiable distributions of a pattern-mixture model when $J = 4$ with nonidentifiable distributions labeled using '?'. Here, the extrapolation distribution consists of six conditional distributions. As such, a sensible, somewhat automatic, way to identify these distributions (that will allow sensitivity parameters) is needed. We advocate using restrictions (that allow sensitivity parameters) to identify these (Little, 1994; Thijs et al., 2002; Linero and Daniels, 2018).

TABLE 9.1: Identifiable distributions and nonidentifiable distributions (labeled using '?') of a pattern-mixture model with $J = 4$ and dropout. S is the number of observed responses.

	$j = 2$	$j = 3$	$j = 4$
$S = 1$	?	?	?
$S = 2$	$p_2(y_2 \mid y_1)$	?	?
$S = 3$	$p_3(y_2 \mid y_1)$	$p_3(y_3 \mid y_1, y_2)$	?
$S = 4$	$p_4(y_2 \mid y_1)$	$p_4(y_3 \mid y_1, y_2)$	$p_4(y_4 \mid y_1, y_2, y_3)$

We briefly introduce two commonly used identifying restrictions for monotone missingness: available case missing value (ACMV) and non-future dependence restrictions (NFD).

ACMV (Little, 1994) sets $p_k(y_j \mid \widetilde{\boldsymbol{y}}_{j-1}, \boldsymbol{\omega}) = p_{\geq j}(y_j \mid \widetilde{\boldsymbol{y}}_{j-1}, \boldsymbol{\omega})$, for all $k < j$ and $2 \leq j \leq J$ and identifies the entire extrapolation distribution. This restriction states that the conditional distribution of Y_j given the past, $\widetilde{\boldsymbol{Y}}_{j-1}$ for those that dropout before or at time j is the same as the conditional distribution of Y_j, given the same past among those still in the study at time j. As an example, in Table 9.1, the unidentified distribution, $p_2(y_3 \mid y_1, y_2)$, represented by a '?' in the $j = 3$ column, is set equal to a weighted combination, $p_{\geq 3}(y_3 \mid y_1, y_2)$ of $p_3(y_3 \mid y_1, y_2)$ and $p_4(y_3 \mid y_1, y_2)$, the two identified distributions in the $j = 3$

column; $p_1(y_3 \mid y_1, y_2)$ is set to the same weighted distribution. ACMV is equivalent to the MAR restriction under monotone missingness (Molenberghs et al., 1998), $p(S = s \mid \boldsymbol{Y}, \boldsymbol{\omega}) = p(S = s \mid \widetilde{\boldsymbol{Y}}_s, \boldsymbol{\omega})$; so the ACMV restrictions implies that the missingness only depends on the observed history. A MAR restriction (here ACMV) is often a good starting point for introducing sensitivity parameters as all distributions of interest are identified under such a restriction and we can consider how to structure deviations from it. We describe a way to do this next.

NFD (Kenward et al., 2003) assumes that the probability of dropout at time $(s + 1)$ depends only $\widetilde{\boldsymbol{Y}}_{s+1}$, $p(S = s \mid \boldsymbol{Y}, \boldsymbol{\omega}) = p(S = s \mid \widetilde{\boldsymbol{Y}}_{s+1}, \boldsymbol{\omega})$. In particular, dropout at time $s + 1$ depends on the past, $\widetilde{\boldsymbol{Y}}_s$, the 'present' Y_{s+1} but not the future, $\{Y_{s+2}, \dots, Y_J\}$ (conditional on the past and the present). This form for the missing data mechanism holds if and only if $p_k(y_j \mid \widetilde{\boldsymbol{y}}_{j-1}, \boldsymbol{\omega}) = p_{\geq j-1}(y_j \mid \widetilde{\boldsymbol{y}}_{j-1}, \boldsymbol{\omega})$, for $k < j - 1$ and $2 < j \leq J$. Note this restriction does not identify all the distributions in Table 9.1 as one component distribution on the left hand side, $p_{j-1}(y_j \mid \widetilde{\boldsymbol{y}}_{j-1})$ is not identified from the observed data. This distribution is the distribution of Y_j conditional on the past, $\widetilde{\boldsymbol{Y}}_{j-1}$ for those that dropout at time j; in Table 9.1 it is the last '?' in each column. As an example, for the $j = 3$ column, the distribution $p_1(y_3 \mid y_1, y_2)$ is set to the weighted combination of $p_j(y_3 \mid y_1, y_2) : j = 2, 3, 4$, $p_{\geq 2}(y_3 \mid y_1, y_2)$; this weighted combination contains one unidentified distribution, $p_2(y_3 \mid y_1, y_2)$ (the last '?' in the $j = 3$ column). As stated above, NFD leaves one distribution unidentified per pattern; restrictions like this which do not completely identify the extrapolation distribution have been called *partial restrictions* (Linero and Daniels, 2018). MAR is a special case of NFD when $p_{j-1}(y_j \mid \widetilde{\boldsymbol{y}}_{j-1}, \boldsymbol{\omega}) = p_{\geq j}(y_j \mid \widetilde{\boldsymbol{y}}_{j-1}, \boldsymbol{\omega})$.

Sensitivity parameters based on the NFD restriction can be introduced in several ways. As discussed above, there is one unidentified conditional distribution in each pattern. A natural anchor for this distribution is the MAR special case. Sensitivity parameters can be introduced which represent deviations from this MAR restriction via either a location shift (Wang and Daniels, 2011; Linero and Daniels, 2015) or exponential tilting (Birmingham et al., 2003; Linero and Daniels, 2018). We provide details of the former in the example in Section 9.8.

The above restrictions allow for non-monotone (intermittent) missingness to be partially ignorable (Harel and Schafer, 2009). An alternative would be to use non-monotone restrictions; a nice review can be found in Linero and Daniels (2018).

A careful data analysis in the setting of nonignorable missingness can be found in Section 9.8 for a growth hormone drug longitudinal trial and for drug trials for breast cancer prevention in Wang et al. (2010), and schizophrenia with multiple reasons for dropout (introduced in Section 1.2) in Linero and Daniels (2015).

9.4.5 Missing covariates

Within a fully Bayesian model, a simple way to accomodate missing covariates is to specify a model for them. Here we quickly review approaches for dealing with missing baseline covariates in longitudinal data. Early work along these lines was done by Ibrahim et al. (1999) using parametric models and more flexible additive models using splines (Chen and Ibrahim, 2006). A disadvantage of these models is that they are parametric and require effort to 'build' a good fitting model. Recently, a more flexible, default approach using Bayesian additive regression trees (BART) was proposed in (Xu et al., 2016b) for a non-longitudinal setting. This approach is valid under ignorable missing covariates. Missing covariates are ignorable if $\boldsymbol{X}_{\text{mis}} \perp\!\!\!\perp \boldsymbol{R}_x \mid \boldsymbol{X}_{\text{obs}}, \boldsymbol{Y}$ where $\boldsymbol{R}_x$ is the observed covariate indicator and the parameters of the missing data mechanism are distinct (and a priori independent) from the parameters of the models for $\boldsymbol{Y} \mid \boldsymbol{X}$ and $\boldsymbol{X}$.

To flexibly model the covariate distribution, Xu et al. (2016b) recommend factoring the marginal distribution of the covariates into univariate (sequential) conditionals and specifying each univariate conditional to be a BART model; they call this *sequential BART*. We refer the reader to the original paper for further details. We also note that with exogeneous time-varying covariates, the covariates can be first ordered by time and for a given time j, the covariates can be ordered as in Xu et al. (2016b). Finally, we point out that building a separate imputation model for missing covariates often results in uncongeniality (Meng, 1994) and bias in parameter estimates of the full data response model (Bartlett et al., 2015; Daniels and Luo, 2019).

9.5 Posterior inference

Markov chain Monte Carlo (MCMC) algorithms can be used to obtain a sample from the posterior distribution of the parameters for all the models considered here. `BUGS` (`WinBUGS`, `OpenBUGS`) (Lunn et al., 2000), `JAGS` (Plummer et al., 2003) and Stan (Gelman et al., 2015) are commonly used software for Bayesian inference and can interface to `R` (with `R` packages such as `R2WinBUGS`, `R2OpenBUGS`, `R2jags`, `rjags` and `rstan`). `SAS` now has an `MCMC procedure` (`Proc MCMC`) (Gunes and Chen, 2014).

Gibbs sampling (used by `BUGS` and `JAGS`) can be used for most of the models considered here, such as the MVN model and conditional models in Section 9.3. When the posterior of the parameters of interest $p(\boldsymbol{\theta} \mid \boldsymbol{y})$ is difficult to directly sample, data augmentation is often used to simplify the computations by introducing latent variables $\boldsymbol{z}$ such that $p(\boldsymbol{\theta} \mid \boldsymbol{y}, \boldsymbol{z})$ and $p(\boldsymbol{z} \mid \boldsymbol{y}, \boldsymbol{\theta})$ are easy to sample. For example, computations are simplified by sampling the latent Normal variables at each iteration. See Chapter 1 for MVP models and the random effects for LMMs. Depending on the model parameterization for the missing data model, it can sometimes be helpful to sample the missing responses; thus, alternating between sampling from the posterior of the parameters of the full data (response) model given the full data and the missing responses given the model parameters and observed responses at each iteration, see also Chapter 1 for further details.

Since some models cannot be fit or be efficiently sampled using `BUGS/JAGS/STAN`, `R` packages or special software/sampling algorithms are sometimes needed. The function `rmvpGibbs` in the `R` package `Bayesm` can be used for MVP model. For some of the non-ignorable missingness models described above, a post-hoc sampling step is required. Details can be found in Linero and Daniels (2015). For the sequential BART approach to missing covariates, there is an `R` package at `https://github.com/mjdaniels/SequentialBART` with details in (Xu et al., 2016b).

For GARP/IV models in Section 9.3.2, the regression parameters $\boldsymbol{\gamma}$ have full conditional distributions that are Normal when Normal priors are specified. To specify these models in `JAGS` or `BUGS`, the sequential specification of the model is more convenient (see example in Section 9.8) but standard software does not use the most efficient algorithm (Daniels and Pourahmadi, 2002) that uses conditionally conjugate updates for both $\boldsymbol{\beta}$ *and* $\boldsymbol{\gamma}$.

9.6 Model selection

There are numerous approaches for model selection in the Bayesian framework. Here we review two commonly used approaches and discuss how they should be implemented for longitudinal data models: the deviance information criterion (DIC) and the log pseudo-marginal likelihood (see Chapter 1).

DIC is very popular due to its ease of computation. Its standard form has two components: a goodness of fit term and a complexity (penalty) term. One would select the model that minimizes the DIC. The DIC is easy to compute from posterior samples using the MCMC output from standard software like BUGS or JAGS. However there are some caveats with using the DIC as were discussed in Chapter 3 of Daniels and Hogan (2008) and also in Chapter 1. We recommend using the DIC for marginal models such as MVN, marginalized transition model (MTM), and MVP. For conditional models, including random effects models, the likelihood for the DIC should be marginalized; if this is too difficult computationally, the DIC should not be used. When there is missing data, we strongly recommend using the observed data likelihood (Wang and Daniels, 2011), not the formulations recommended in Celeux et al. (2006) for 'missing data' (which are really for latent data like random effects, mixture model component indicators, etc.). Finally, caution should be used when using the 'default' DIC in different packages to ensure the DIC output is the one of interest; as an example, for incomplete data models, the DIC using the observed data likelihood is typically *not* the default.

An alternative to the DIC is the log pseudo-marginal likelihood (LPML; Geisser and Eddy, 1979), see also Chapter 1. It has the following form: $\widehat{p}(\boldsymbol{y}) \equiv \prod_{i=1}^{n} p_i(\boldsymbol{y}_i \mid \boldsymbol{y}_{-i})$ where $\boldsymbol{y}_{-i}$ is the full set of responses with $\boldsymbol{y}_i$ excluded, and $p_i(\boldsymbol{y}_i \mid \boldsymbol{y}_{-i})$ is termed the ith conditional predictive ordinate (CPO). LPML is defined as the logarithm of PML, i.e. LPML $= \sum_{i=1}^{n} \log(\text{CPO}_i)$. One selects the model that maximizes LPML. LPML is invariant to the parameterization and choice of likelihood unlike the DIC. For missing data, $\boldsymbol{y}_i$ is the vector of observed responses.

There are two straightforward ways to compute LPML. If high performance computing is available, a brute force way can be used, by refitting the model n times, or an approximation can be used that requires only fitting the model once (Gelfand and Dey, 1994; Vehtari et al., 2017).

9.7 Model checking and assessment

In the previous section, we discussed criteria to select among models. However, we also need to determine how well the model fits the observed data in an absolute sense. To check whether the model is consistent with the observed data, posterior predictive checks (see also Chapter 1) are commonly used. The idea is if the model fits well, the replicated data ($\boldsymbol{y}^{\text{rep}}$) generated under the model, $p(\boldsymbol{y}^{\text{rep}} \mid \boldsymbol{y}) = \int p(\boldsymbol{y}^{\text{rep}} \mid \boldsymbol{\theta}, \boldsymbol{y}) p(\boldsymbol{\theta} \mid \boldsymbol{y}) d\boldsymbol{\theta}$ should look similar to the observed data. For a chosen discrepancy $T(\boldsymbol{y}, \boldsymbol{\theta})$, posterior predictive probabilities,

$$\begin{aligned} p_B &= \Pr(T(\boldsymbol{y}^{\text{rep}}, \boldsymbol{\theta}) \geq T(\boldsymbol{y}, \boldsymbol{\theta}) \mid \boldsymbol{y}) \\ &= \int\int I_{T(\boldsymbol{y}^{\text{rep}}, \boldsymbol{\theta}) \geq T(\boldsymbol{y}, \boldsymbol{\theta})} p(\boldsymbol{y}^{\text{rep}} \mid \boldsymbol{\theta}, \boldsymbol{y}) p(\boldsymbol{\theta} \mid \boldsymbol{y}) d\boldsymbol{y}^{\text{rep}} d\boldsymbol{\theta} \end{aligned} \tag{9.1}$$

can be computed to quantify lack of fit. A common default choice of $T(\boldsymbol{y}, \boldsymbol{\theta})$ to examine 'overall fit' is the χ^2 discrepancy, $T(\boldsymbol{y}, \boldsymbol{\theta}) = \sum_i \frac{(y_i - \text{E}[Y_i \mid \boldsymbol{\theta}])^2}{\text{Var}(Y_i \mid \boldsymbol{\theta})}$; modifications of this for longitudinal models can be done by standardizing using the covariance matrix (instead of the variance) or by conditioning the mean on the random effects, as appropriate. Posterior predictive probabilities based on the χ^2 discrepancy can be computed to assess whether variability in the observed data is consistent with variability in the replicated data. In the context of ignorable missingness, the approach can be used to replicate the 'observed' data (implicitly conditional on the vector of observed data indicators); however this has some drawbacks including not accounting for the uncertainty in the observed data indicators.

A more comprehensive approach in the setting of incomplete longitudinal data would be to also account for the uncertainty in the observed data indicators (which are also random variables). Under nonignorable models (Section 9.4), the full data distribution is modeled so this can be done by doing checks based on *replicated observed data* (Xu et al., 2016a). To create the replicated observed data, we first replicate the full data, $(\boldsymbol{y}^{\text{rep}}, \boldsymbol{r}^{\text{rep}})$. Then, we compute replicated observed data as $\boldsymbol{y}_{\text{obs}}^{\text{rep}} = \{y_i^{\text{rep}} : r_i^{\text{rep}} = 1\}$, i.e. the components of $\boldsymbol{y}^{\text{rep}}$ (the replicated complete response data sets) for which the corresponding replicated observed data indicators, $\boldsymbol{r}^{\text{rep}}$ are equal to one.

Checks based on replicated observed data are invariant to the extrapolation distribution (Daniels et al., 2012); thus, they provide the same conclusions as the extrapolation distribution is (sensitivity parameters are) varied. In addition, such checks can assess any features of the joint distribution of $(\boldsymbol{y}_{obs}, \boldsymbol{r})$.

9.8 Practical example: Growth hormone trial

We will illustrate some of the approaches introduced in Sections 9.3—9.7 on a pharmaceutical clinical trial. In particular, we analyze data from a randomized clinical trial to examine the effects of recombinant human growth hormone (GH) therapy for increasing muscle strength in the elderly. The trial enrolled 160 participants who were randomized to one of four treatments, $Z \in \{1, 2, 3, 4\}$, Growth hormone plus exercise (EG), Growth hormone (G), Placebo plus exercise (EP), Placebo (P). The outcome of interest is quadriceps strength (QS) measured in foot-pounds of torque exerted against a resistance device which were recorded at baseline, 6 months and 12 months, $(Y_1, Y_2, Y_3)^\top$ with $(t_1, t_2, t_3)^\top = (0, 6, 12)^\top$. The primary objective is to compare the treatments on mean QS at 12 months following randomization. The dropout rate was 25%. Let $\boldsymbol{R} = (R_1, R_2, R_3)^\top$ be the observed data indicators associated with $(Y_1, Y_2, Y_3)^\top$. Since the missingness is monotone in this trial, we can replace $\boldsymbol{R}$ with S, the number of observed responses. Further summaries of the data can be found in Daniels and Hogan (2008). This case study expands on the original results presented in Daniels and Hogan (2008) including consideration of NFD (partial) identifying restrictions as well as Bayesian nonparametric models for the observed data.

9.8.1 Ignorable dropout

We first assume ignorable dropout and compare the four treatments at 12 months. We use an MVN model for the responses for each treatment, i.e. $\boldsymbol{Y}_i \mid Z_i = k \sim \text{N}(\boldsymbol{\mu}_k, \boldsymbol{\Sigma}_k)$, where $\boldsymbol{\mu}_k = (\mu_{1k}, \mu_{2k}, \mu_{3k})^\top$ and we use GARP/IV to parameterize $\boldsymbol{\Sigma}_k$, specifically,

$$\begin{array}{lcl} Y_{i1} \mid Z_i = k & \sim & \text{N}(\mu_{1k}, \sigma_{1k}^2) \\ Y_{i2} \mid Y_{i1} = y_{i1}, Z_i = k & \sim & \text{N}(\beta_{0k} + \phi_{21,k} y_{i1}, \sigma_{2k}^2) \\ Y_{i3} \mid Y_{i2} = y_{i2}, Y_{i1} = y_{i1}, Z_i = k & \sim & \text{N}(\beta_{1k} + \phi_{31,k} y_{i1} + \phi_{32,k} y_{i2}, \sigma_{3k}^2), \end{array}$$

where $\boldsymbol{\phi}_k = (\phi_{21,k}, \phi_{31,k}, \phi_{32,k})^\top, k = 1, \ldots, 4$ is the set of generalized autoregressive parameters (GARP) for each treatment, $\boldsymbol{\sigma}_k^2 = (\sigma_{1k}^2, \sigma_{2k}^2, \sigma_{3k}^2)^\top, k = 1, \ldots, 4$ is the set of innovation variances (IV) for each treatment and $\mu_{jk} = \beta_{j-2,k} + \sum_{l=1}^{j-1} \phi_{jl,k}\mu_{lk}$ for $j = 2, 3$ and $k = 1, \ldots, 4$. We assume three models for the covariance structure: model 1 specifies distinct and unstructured covariance matrix $\boldsymbol{\Sigma}_k$ for each treatment, i.e. $(\boldsymbol{\phi}_k, \boldsymbol{\sigma}_k^2)$, $k = 1, \ldots, 4$; Model 2 assumes common $\boldsymbol{\Sigma}$ across treatments, i.e. $\{\boldsymbol{\phi}_k, \boldsymbol{\sigma}_k^2) = (\boldsymbol{\phi}, \boldsymbol{\sigma}^2)$: $k = 1, \ldots, 4\}$; and Model 3 specifies the structure based on the observed covariance matrix: $(\sigma_{1k}^2, \phi_{31,k}, \phi_{32,k}) = (\sigma_1^2, \phi_{31}, \phi_{32})$ for $k = 1, \ldots, 4$, $(\sigma_{2k}^2, \sigma_{3k}^2) = (\sigma_2^2, \sigma_3^2)$ for $k = 2, 3, 4$ and $\phi_{21,k} = \phi_{21}$ for $k = 1, 2, 3$. Model 3 is based on examining the maximum likelihood estimators of the group specific covariance matrices, which suggest that σ_{21}^2 and σ_{31}^2 for EG are different from the other treatments and $\phi_{21,4}$ for P is different from the other treatments. Diffuse priors are used for all the parameters.

We also consider BNP models, in particular, Dirichlet process mixture (DPM) of Normal models analogous to the above three parametric model specifications. Specifically BNP Model 1 assumes DPM of Normal models for each treatment by specifying a DP prior on the distribution of the parameters $(\boldsymbol{\mu}_k, \boldsymbol{\Sigma}_k)$, i.e. $\boldsymbol{Y}_i \mid Z_i = k \sim \mathrm{N}(\boldsymbol{\mu}_{ik}, \boldsymbol{\Sigma}_{ik})$, $(\boldsymbol{\mu}_{ik}, \boldsymbol{\Sigma}_{ik}) \sim G_k$, $G_k \sim DP(H_k, \alpha_k)$, where H_k is a Normal-GARP/IV distribution and α_k is a precision parameter (as $\alpha_k \to \infty$, the distribution goes to MVN). BNP Model 2 specifies a DP prior on the distribution of $(\boldsymbol{\mu}_1, \boldsymbol{\mu}_2, \boldsymbol{\mu}_3, \boldsymbol{\mu}_4, \boldsymbol{\Sigma})$ and BNP Model 3 specifies a DP prior on the distribution of $(\boldsymbol{\mu}_1, \boldsymbol{\mu}_2, \boldsymbol{\mu}_3, \boldsymbol{\mu}_4, \sigma_1^2, \phi_{31}, \phi_{32}, \sigma_2^2, \sigma_3^2, \sigma_{2,1}^2, \sigma_{3,1}^2, \phi_{21}, \phi_{21,4})$. Prior specification of hyperparameters is based on Taddy (2008) with details in a similar setting to here given in the supplementary materials of Daniels and Linero (2015). This model can be re-written (and approximated) as a finite mixture of Normals (Ishwaran and James, 2002), which can facilitate posterior computation and sampling using software such as `BUGS/JAGS`.

`WinBUGS` was used to generate samples from the posterior distribution of parameters in the model. Table 9.2 shows the posterior mean and 95% credible intervals (CIs) of the mean parameters for the EG treatment (which had the highest dropout rate, 16/38) under the MVN and the BNP model specifications; there are differences in the posterior means (due to the importance of the covariance structure with missing data) with more notable changes in the CIs. All six models suggest that EG has largest mean QS at 12 months. Posterior probabilities that each of the pairwise treatment differences at 12 months is greater than zero suggest that EG treatment has a larger effect than G and P (posterior probabilities of .01 and .00 respectively), and P has a larger effect than EP (.03).

DIC using the observed data likelihood is calculated for the three MVN models in Table 9.3 with the smallest for Model 3 suggesting the best fit; we did not compute the DIC for the BNP models as the standard version is not appropriate. To compare the parametric and nonparametric specifications, we use LMPL which is also calculated in Table 9.3. These results suggest that BNP models perform similarly to the corresponding MVN models and Model 3 is slightly better than other specifications. But we also point out that for this data, where the parametric models appear to provide adequate fit, the BNP specifications do not result in a loss of efficiency (as the credible intervals are of similar length to their parametric alternatives). For model checking, we computed the χ^2 discrepancy using the observed data standardized by the covariance matrix for Model 3. The posterior predictive probability was 0.55, indicating good model fit.

TABLE 9.2: Posterior mean and 95% CI of the mean response at month 12 for treatment EG under three MVN and three BNP model specifications

(1)	(2)	(3)	BNP (1)	BNP (2)	BNP (3)
79(65,92)	81(73,90)	81(71,92)	80(69,91)	80(69,89)	80(71,91)

TABLE 9.3: LMPL and DIC comparing three MVN and three BNP model specifications.

Model	(1)	(2)	(3)	BNP (1)	BNP (2)	BNP (3)
LPML	-1705	-1701	-1693	-1705	-1696	-1694
DIC	3402.6	3398.5	3382.3			

9.8.2 Nonignorable dropout

It is likely that dropout is nonignorable in this trial. We illustrate such an analysis only using treatments EG and EP. We specify a pattern mixture model for each treatment separately. For simplicity, we drop the treatment indicator (k) in the model specification below. The pattern indicator S has a Multinomial distribution, i.e. $S \sim \text{Mult}(\boldsymbol{\phi})$ where $\boldsymbol{\phi} = (\phi_1, \phi_2, \phi_3)$. The model for $Y_1 \mid S$ is specified as a Normal distribution, i.e. $Y_1 \mid S = s \sim \text{N}(\mu_s, \sigma_s^2)$ for $s = 1, 2, 3$. The model for $Y_2 \mid Y_1, S$ is specified as $Y_2 \mid Y_1, S = 1 \sim \text{N}(\alpha_{2\cdot 1}^{(0)} + \beta_{2\cdot 1}Y_1, \sigma_{2\cdot 1}^2)$ and $Y_2 \mid Y_1, S \geq 2 \sim \text{N}(\alpha_{2\cdot 1}^{(1)} + \beta_{2\cdot 1}Y_1, \sigma_{2\cdot 1}^2)$.

Finally we specify $Y_3 \mid Y_1, Y_2, S$ in two ways (corresponding to two MNAR scenarios): MNAR (1) specifies $Y_3 \mid Y_1, Y_2, S = 1, 2 \sim \text{N}(\alpha_{3\cdot 21}^{(0)} + \beta_{3\cdot 21}Y_1 + \gamma_{3\cdot 21}Y_2, \sigma_{3\cdot 21}^2)$ and $Y_3 \mid Y_1, Y_2, S = 3 \sim \text{N}(\alpha_{3\cdot 21}^{(1)} + \beta_{3\cdot 21}Y_1 + \gamma_{3\cdot 21}Y_2, \sigma_{3\cdot 21}^2)$. Here the intercepts, $\alpha_{3\cdot 21}^{(0)}$ and $\alpha_{3\cdot 21}^{(1)}$ differ in patterns $S = \{1, 2\}$ from pattern $S = 3$ (where the intercept is identified). MNAR (2) specifies $Y_3 \mid Y_1, Y_2, S$ under an NFD assumption but $Y_3 \mid Y_1, Y_2, S = 2$ is identified the same way as in MNAR (1). Under NFD, one of the three unidentified distributions in MNAR (1) is now identified, $Y_3 \mid Y_1, Y_2, S = 1$ by

$$
\begin{aligned}
P(Y_3 \mid Y_1, Y_2, S = 1) &= P(Y_3 \mid Y_1, Y_2, S \geq 2) \\
&= P(Y_3 \mid Y_1, Y_2, S = 2)\frac{P(S = 2 \mid Y_1, Y_2)}{P(S \geq 2 \mid Y_1, Y_2)} \\
&\quad + P(Y_3 \mid Y_1, Y_2, S = 3)\frac{P(S = 3 \mid Y_1, Y_2)}{P(S \geq 2 \mid Y_1, Y_2)}.
\end{aligned}
$$

Since the distributions $Y_2 \mid Y_1, S = 1$, $Y_3 \mid Y_1, Y_2, S = 1$ and $Y_3 \mid Y_1, Y_2, S = 2$ cannot be identified using observed data, $(\alpha_{2\cdot 1}^{(0)}, \alpha_{3\cdot 21}^{(0)})$ are sensitivity parameters for both MNAR specifications. Let $\alpha_{2\cdot 1}^{(0)} = \alpha_{2\cdot 1}^{(1)} + \Delta_1$ and $\alpha_{3\cdot 21}^{(1)} + \Delta_2$. MAR is induced by setting $\Delta_1 = \Delta_2 = 0$ (for an alternative sensitivity analysis, see Daniels and Hogan, 2008, Chapter 9).

We examine how the mean difference in Y_3 between the two treatments, $\theta = E_{EG}(Y_3) - E_{EP}(Y_3)$, changes with the two MNAR model specifications. We specify diffuse priors for identified model parameters. For the sensitivity parameters, we calibrate priors as follows, $\Delta_1 \sim U(-\sigma_1, 0)$ and $\Delta_2 \sim U(-\sigma_2, 0)$ where $\sigma_1 = SD(Y_2 \mid Y_1)$ and $\sigma_2 = SD(Y_3 \mid Y_2, Y_1)$ are estimated from the observed data. These priors correspond to the conditional mean for dropouts being uniformly lower than for non-dropouts (up to one standard deviation); in the GH data, $\sigma_1 \approx 15$ and $\sigma_2 \approx 20$. Table 9.4 shows the posterior mean and standard deviation (SD) of the mean response at 12 months for EP and EG and the mean difference at 12 months between the two treatments based on MAR and the above two MNAR assumptions. The mean responses at 12 months in the MNAR models are smaller than in the MAR model as expected, since we assume dropouts have lower means through the sensitivity parameters. The mean response at 12 months in the MNAR (1) model is slightly lower than the MNAR (2) model. The MNAR models have slightly higher posterior standard deviations at 12 months due to the use of non-degenerate priors on the sensitivity parameters. All the models suggest that EG has higher weight at 12 months than EP but with 95% CIs covering zero. The MAR model has a slightly higher mean difference than MNAR models.

TABLE 9.4: Posterior mean and SDs of the mean response at 12 months for treatment EP and EG and the change from baseline to 12 months in pattern mixture models

		Pattern Mixture Models		
Trt	Month	MAR	MNAR 1	MNAR 2 (NFD)
EP	12	73 (4.9)	70 (5.1)	71 (5.0)
EG	12	78 (7.2)	73 (7.9)	75 (7.6)
Diff. at 12 mos.		5.4 (8.8)	3.0 (9.4)	3.7 (9.1)

9.9 Wrap-up and open problems

We have reviewed Bayesian approaches for longitudinal data (with missingness) including classes of model, priors, computations and model selection and assessment of fit. We have also illustrated some of these approaches using a data example. The code for the example can be found at `https://github.com/mjdaniels/Book_Chapter`.

More work is needed on nonignorable dropout for non-mean regression, e.g. quantile regression, that allows sensitivity parameters building on previous approaches (Liu et al., 2015; Yuan and Yin, 2010) and nonignorable missingness in covariates building on the work in Xu et al. (2016b), Murray and Reiter (2016) and Roy et al. (2018). Also, further development of flexible covariance models for multivariate longitudinal data, including using BNP models, and intuitive approaches for sensitivity analysis in shared parameter models building on work in Su et al. (2019) are needed.

Bibliography

Bartlett, J. W., Seaman, S. R., White, I. R., and Carpenter, J. R. (2015). Multiple imputation of covariates by fully conditional specification: accommodating the substantive model. *Statistical Methods in Medical Research*, 24(4):462–487.

Birmingham, J., Rotnitzky, A., and Fitzmaurice, G. M. (2003). Pattern–mixture and selection models for analysing longitudinal data with monotone missing patterns. *Journal of the Royal Statistical Society — Series B*, 65(1):275–297.

Celeux, G., Forbes, F., Robert, C. P., and Titterington, D. M. (2006). Deviance information criteria for missing data models. *Bayesian Analysis*, 1(4):651–673.

Chen, Q. and Ibrahim, J. (2006). Semiparametric models for missing covariate and response data in regression models. *Biometrics*, 62(1):177–184.

Christensen, R., Johnson, W., Branscum, A., and Hanson, T. E. (2011). *Bayesian Ideas and Data Analysis: an Introduction for Scientists and Statisticians*. CRC Press.

Crainiceanu, C. M., Ruppert, D., and Wand, M. P. (2005). Bayesian analysis for penalized spline regression using WinBUGS. *Journal of Statistical Software*, 14:1–24.

Daniels, M., Chatterjee, A. S., and Wang, C. (2012). Bayesian model selection for incomplete data using the posterior predictive distribution. *Biometrics*, 68(4):1055–1063.

Daniels, M. and Hogan, J. (2008). *Missing Data in Longitudinal Studies: Strategies for Bayesian Modeling and Sensitivity Analysis*. CRC Press.

Daniels, M. and Linero, A. (2015). Bayesian Nonparametrics for Missing Data in Longitudinal Clinical Trials. In Mitra, R. and Müller, P., editors, *Nonparametric Bayesian Inference in Biostatistics*, pages 423–446. Springer International Publishing, Cham.

Daniels, M. J., and Luo, X. (2019). A note on compatibility for inference with missing data in the presence of auxiliary covariates. *Statistics in medicine*, 38(7):1190–1199.

Daniels, M. and Pourahmadi, M. (2002). Bayesian analysis of covariance matrices and dynamic models for longitudinal data. *Biometrika*, 89(3):553–566.

Daniels, M. and Pourahmadi, M. (2009). Modeling covariance matrices via partial autocorrelations. *Journal of Multivariate Analysis*, 100(10):2352–2363.

Daniels, M. and Zhao, Y. D. (2003). Modelling the random effects covariance matrix in longitudinal data. *Statistics in Medicine*, 22(10):1631–1647.

Diggle, P., Heagerty, P., Liang, K., and Zeger, S. (2002). *Analysis of Longitudinal Data*. Oxford University Press, Oxford, UK.

Diggle, P. and Kenward, M. G. (1994). Informative drop-out in longitudinal data analysis. *Journal of the Royal Statistical Society — Series C*, 43(1):49–93.

Fitzmaurice, G. M., Laird, N. M., and Ware, J. H. (2012). *Applied Longitudinal Analysis*. John Wiley & Sons.

Gaskins, J., Daniels, M., and Marcus, B. (2014). Sparsity inducing prior distributions for correlation matrices of longitudinal data. *Journal of Computational and Graphical Statistics*, 23(4):966–984.

Geisser, S. and Eddy, W. F. (1979). A predictive approach to model selection. *Journal of the American Statistical Association*, 74(365):153–160.

Gelfand, A. E. and Dey, D. K. (1994). Bayesian model choice: asymptotics and exact calculations. *Journal of the Royal Statistical Society — Series B*, 56(3):501–514.

Gelman, A., Carlin, J. B., Stern, H. S., Dunson, D. B., Vehtari, A., and Rubin, D. B. (2014). *Bayesian Data Analysis*, volume 2. CRC press, Boca Raton, FL.

Gelman, A., Lee, D., and Guo, J. (2015). Stan: A probabilistic programming language for Bayesian inference and optimization. *Journal of Educational and Behavioral Statistics*, 40(5):530–543.

Gruber, S. and Van Der Laan, M. J. (2009). Targeted maximum likelihood estimation: A gentle introduction. *U.C. Berkeley Division of Biostatistics Working Paper Series*, 252.

Gunes, F. and Chen, F. (2014). Getting started with the MCMC procedure. `https://support.sas.com/rnd/app/stat/papers/2014/gettingstartedMCMC2014.pdf`.

Harel, O. and Schafer, J. L. (2009). Partial and latent ignorability in missing-data problems. *Biometrika*, 96(1):37–50.

Heagerty, P. J. (1999). Marginally specified logistic-normal models for longitudinal binary data. *Biometrics*, 55(3):688–698.

Hjort, N., Holmes, C., Müller, P., and Walker, S. (2010). *Bayesian Nonparametrics.* Cambridge University Press.

Hobbs, B. P., Carlin, B. P., Mandrekar, S. J., and Sargent, D. J. (2011). Hierarchical commensurate and power prior models for adaptive incorporation of historical information in clinical trials. *Biometrics*, 67(3):1047–1056.

Ibrahim, J. and Chen, M. (2000). Power prior distributions for regression models. *Statistical Science*, 15(1):46–60.

Ibrahim, J., Lipsitz, S. R., and Chen, M.-H. (1999). Missing covariates in generalized linear models when the missing data mechanism is non-ignorable. *Journal of the Royal Statistical Society — Series B*, 61(1):173–190.

Ibrahim, J. and Molenberghs, G. (2009). Missing data methods in longitudinal studies: A review. *Test*, 18(1):1–43.

Ishwaran, H. and James, L. F. (2002). Approximate Dirichlet process computing in finite normal mixtures:Smoothing and prior information. *Journal of Computational and Graphical statistics*, 11(3):508–532.

Kenward, M. G., Molenberghs, G., and Thijs, H. (2003). Pattern-mixture models with proper time dependence. *Biometrika*, 90(1):53–71.

Kleinman, K. P. and Ibrahim, J. (1998a). A semiparametric Bayesian approach to generalized linear mixed models. *Statistics in Medicine*, 17(22):2579–2596.

Kleinman, K. P. and Ibrahim, J. (1998b). A semiparametric Bayesian approach to the random effects model. *Biometrics*, 54(3):921–938.

Koenker, R. (2004). Quantile regression for longitudinal data. *Journal of Multivariate Analysis*, 91(1):74–89.

Laird, N. M. and Ware, J. H. (1982). Random-effects models for longitudinal data. *Biometrics*, 38(4):963–974.

Lee, K., Baek, C., and Daniels, M. (2017). ARMA Cholesky factor models for the covariance matrix of linear models. *Computational Statistics and Data Analysis*, 115:267–280.

Lee, K., Daniels, M., and Joo, Y. (2013). Flexible marginalized models for bivariate longitudinal ordinal data. *Biostatistics*, 14(3):462–476.

Lee, K., Lee, J., Hagan, J., and Yoo, J. K. (2012). Modeling the random effects covariance matrix for generalized linear mixed models. *Computational Statistics and Data Analysis*, 56(6):1545–1551.

Lesaffre, E. and Lawson, A. (2012). *Bayesian Biostatistics.* CRC Press.

Li, Y., Lin, X., and Müller, P. (2010). Bayesian inference in semiparametric mixed models for longitudinal data. *Biometrics*, 66(1):70–78.

Liang, K.-Y. and Zeger, S. L. (1986). Longitudinal data analysis using generalized linear models. *Biometrika*, 73(1):13–22.

Linero, A. and Daniels, M. (2018). A general Bayesian nonparametric approach for missing outcome data. *Statistical Science*, 33:198–213.

Linero, A. R. and Daniels, M. (2015). A flexible Bayesian approach to monotone missing data in longitudinal studies with nonignorable missingness with application to an acute schizophrenia clinical trial. *Journal of the American Statistical Association*, 110(509):45–55.

Little, R. J. (1994). A class of pattern-mixture models for normal incomplete data. *Biometrika*, 81(3):471–483.

Little, R. J. and Rubin, D. B. (2014). *Statistical Analysis with Missing Data.* John Wiley & Sons.

Liu, M., Daniels, M., and Perri, M. G. (2015). Quantile regression in the presence of monotone missingness with sensitivity analysis. *Biostatistics*, 17(1):108–121.

Lunn, D., Thomas, A., Best, N., and Spiegelhalter, D. (2000). WinBUGS - a Bayesian modelling framework: Concepts, structure, and extensibility. *Statistics and Computing*, 10:325–337.

Meng, X.-L. (1994). Multiple-imputation inferences with uncongenial sources of input. *Statistical Science*, 9(4):538–558.

Molenberghs, G. and Kenward, M. (2007). *Missing Data in Clinical Studies*, volume 61. John Wiley & Sons.

Molenberghs, G., Michiels, B., Kenward, M. G., and Diggle, P. J. (1998). Monotone missing data and pattern-mixture models. *Statistica Neerlandica*, 52(2):153–161.

Murray, J. and Reiter, J. (2016). Multiple imputation of missing categorical and continuous values via Bayesian mixture models with local dependence. *Journal of the American Statistical Association*, 111(516):1466–1479.

Plummer, M. et al. (2003). JAGS: A program for analysis of Bayesian graphical models using Gibbs sampling. In *Proceedings of the 3rd International Workshop on Distributed Statistical Computing*, volume 124, page 125. Vienna, Austria.

Pourahmadi, M. (1999). Joint mean-covariance models with applications to longitudinal data: Unconstrained parameterisation. *Biometrika*, 86(3):677–690.

Pourahmadi, M. and Daniels, M. (2002). Dynamic conditionally linear mixed models for longitudinal data. *Biometrics*, 58(1):225–231.

Qu, A., Lindsay, B. G., and Li, B. (2000). Improving generalised estimating equations using quadratic inference functions. *Biometrika*, 87(4):823–836.

Quintana, F. A., Johnson, W. O., Waetjen, L. E., and B. Gold, E. (2016). Bayesian nonparametric longitudinal data analysis. *Journal of the American Statistical Association*, 111(515):1168–1181.

Rizopoulos, D. (2012). *Joint Models for Longitudinal and Time-to-Event Data: With Applications in R.* Chapman and Hall/CRC.

Robins, J. M., Rotnitzky, A., and Zhao, L. P. (1994). Estimation of regression coefficients when some regressors are not always observed. *Journal of the American Statistical Association*, 89(427):846–866.

Rooney, W. D., Berlow, Y. A., Triplett, W. T., Forbes, S. C., Willcocks, R. J., Wang, D.-J., Harneet Arora, I. A., Senesac, C. R., Lott, D. J., Tennekoon, G. I., Finkel, R. S., Russman, B. S., Finanger, E. L., Chakraborty, S., O'Brien, E., Moloney, B., Barnard, A., Lee Sweeney H., Daniels, M. J., Walter, G. A., and Vandenborne, K. Modeling disease trajectory in duchenne muscular dystrophy. *Neurology*. DOI: https://doi.org/10.1212/WNL.0000000000009244.

Roy, J., and Lum, K. J., Zeldow, B., Dworkin, J. D., Re III, V. L., and Daniels, M. J. (2018). Bayesian nonparametric generative models for causal inference with missing at random covariates. *Biometrics*, 74(4):1193–1202.

Scharfstein, D. O., Rotnitzky, A., and Robins, J. M. (1999). Adjusting for nonignorable drop-out using semiparametric nonresponse models. *Journal of the American Statistical Association*, 94(448):1096–1120.

Schildcrout, J. S. and Heagerty, P. J. (2005). Regression analysis of longitudinal binary data with time-dependent environmental covariates: Bias and efficiency. *Biostatistics*, 6(4):633–652.

Su, L. and Daniels, M. (2015). Bayesian modeling of the covariance structure for irregular longitudinal data using the partial autocorrelation function. *Statistics in Medicine*, 34(12):2004–2018.

Su, L., Li, Q., Barrett, J. K., and Daniels, M. J. (2019). A sensitivity analysis approach for informative dropout using shared parameter models. *Biometrics*, 75(3):917–926.

Taddy, M. (2008). *Bayesian Nonparametric Analysis of Conditional Distributions and Inference for Poisson Point Processes*. PhD dissertation at UCSC.

Tang, Y., Sinha, D., Pati, D., Lipsitz, S., and Lipshultz, S. (2015). Bayesian partial linear model for skewed longitudinal data. *Biostatistics*, 16(3):441–453.

Thijs, H., Molenberghs, G., Michiels, B., Verbeke, G., and Curran, D. (2002). Strategies to fit pattern-mixture models. *Biostatistics*, 3(2):245–265.

Vehtari, A., Gelman, A., and Gabry, J. (2017). Practical Bayesian model evaluation using leave-one-out cross-validation and WAIC. *Statistics and Computing*, 27(5):1413–1432,

Verbeke, G. and Molenberghs, G. (2000). *Linear Mixed Models for Longitudinal Data*. Springer, New York, NY.

Wang, C. and Daniels, M. (2011). A note on MAR, identifying restrictions, model comparison, and sensitivity analysis in pattern mixture models with and without covariates for incomplete data. *Biometrics*, 67(3):810–818.

Wang, C., Daniels, M. J., Scharfstein, D. O., and Land, S. (2010). A Bayesian shrinkage model for incomplete longitudinal binary data with application to the breast cancer prevention trial. *Journal of the American Statistical Association*, 105(492):1333–1346.

Wang, Y. and Daniels, M. (2013). Bayesian modeling of the dependence in longitudinal data via partial autocorrelations and marginal variances. *Journal of Multivariate Analysis*, 116:130–140.

Weiss, R. E. (2005). *Modeling Longitudinal Data*. Springer Science & Business Media.

Willcocks, R., Rooney, W., Triplett, W., Forbes, S., Lott, D., Senesac, C., Daniels, M., Wang, D., Harrington, A., Tennekoon, G., Russman, B., Finanger, E., Byrne, B., Finkel, R., Walter, G., Sweeney, H., and K., V. (2016). Multicenter prospective longitudinal study of magnetic resonance biomarkers in a large duchenne muscular dystrophy cohort. *Annals of Neurology*, 79(4):553–547.

Wong, F., Carter, C. K., and Kohn, R. (2003). Efficient estimation of covariance selection models. *Biometrika*, 90(4):809–830.

Wu, M. C. and Carroll, R. J. (1988). Estimation and comparison of changes in the presence of informative right censoring by modeling the censoring process. *Biometrics*, 44(1):175–188.

Xu, D., Chatterjee, A., and Daniels, M. (2016a). A note on posterior predictive checks to assess model fit for incomplete data. *Statistics in Medicine*, 35(27):5029–5039.

Xu, D., Daniels, M., and Winterstein, A. G. (2016b). Sequential BART for imputation of missing covariates. *Biostatistics*, 17(3):589–602.

Yuan, Y. and Yin, G. (2010). Bayesian quantile regression for longitudinal studies with nonignorable missing data. *Biometrics*, 66(1):105–114.

Zhang, W. and Leng, C. (2011). A moving average Cholesky factor model in covariance modelling for longitudinal data. *Biometrika*, 99(1):141–150.

Zhang, W., Leng, C., and Tang, C. Y. (2015). A joint modelling approach for longitudinal studies. *Journal of the Royal Statistical Society — Series B*, 77(1):219–238.

10

Survival Analysis and Censored Data

Linda D. Sharples

London School of Hygiene and Tropical Medicine, UK

Nikolaos Demiris

Cambridge Clinical Trials Centre, University of Cambridge, UK

This chapter focuses on time-to-event data used as outcome measures, particularly in Phase III randomized trials. Analysis of time-to-event outcomes is typically based on the hazard function and an assumption that the hazards for different treatment groups are proportional through time. The baseline hazards for the control group (when all covariates take the value zero) may have a parametric or non-parametric form. The Bayesian approach to survival analysis is well developed and very flexible, with model fitting based on Markov Chain Monte Carlo methods available in both specialist Bayesian and general statistical packages. Using worked examples, this chapter shows that Bayesian models can accommodate a range of survival functions, as well as clustering between experimental units and, provided that missing at random is a plausible assumption, multiple imputation is straightforward. Simulation-based methods allow estimation of useful data summaries and functions of potentially correlated parameters; for example, the probability that the treatment effect is large enough to outweigh safety concerns, and restricted mean survival time for when the PH assumption is in doubt. We highlight analysis beyond the main trial results, including estimating joint posterior distributions for efficacy and safety outcomes in order to assess risk-benefit assessment and joint models of time to event outcomes and longitudinal measures of time-varying biomarkers. Challenges include the need to provide prior densities, while the requirement for simulation-based estimation means that analysis can be relatively slow. However, for trials involving medical devices, rare diseases, rare outcomes and small populations, a Bayesian approach has great potential to increase statistical efficiency, through synthesis of prior, likelihood and external data.

10.1 Introduction

Time-to-event data represent a common type of outcome and are concerned with the duration until a particular type of event occurs. The measurement of such data requires the definition of (i) a time-origin, such as the entry of an individual into a study or randomization in a clinical trial, (ii) an event, for example death, metastasis or stroke and (iii) the scale of measurement, usually time in days, months or years in medical research. The analysis of time-to-event outcomes is characterized by the distinct features of the data, notably the fact that they are non-negative, often revealing a highly variable right-skewed distribution and the presence of censoring. In most applications of survival methods, it is assumed that

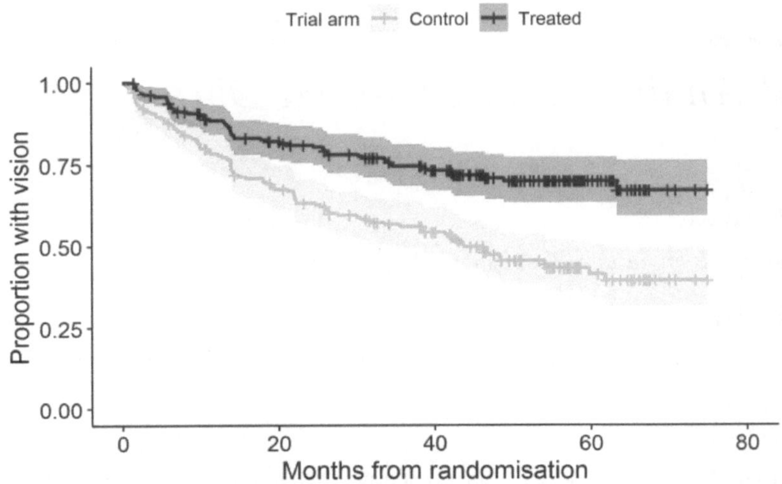

FIGURE 10.1: Diabetic retinopathy trial: Kaplan-Meier estimates of the survival curve.

censored individuals are representative of those who remain in the risk set, possibly conditional on covariates, in terms of their chance of survival. A further characteristic relates to the scale of modeling. Instead of specifying the model directly on the probability/density scale for both exploratory analyses and regression-type models, the statistical model for time-to-event data is typically defined via the hazard or survival functions.

10.2 Review of survival analysis

Descriptive analysis centers on plotting the non-parametric Kaplan-Meier estimator of the survival function, with consideration of the censored subjects through appropriate adjustment of the risk set at each event time. Figure 10.1 provides an example from a trial of laser treatment for diabetic retinopathy.

The effect of covariates is specified through the hazard function, with a Cox-type regression model (Cox, 1972) chosen for its flexibility in the majority of medical applications. We recall the standard notation for a continuous random variable T, representing time to the event of interest, with probability density function $f(t)$, such that $f(t) = h(t)S(t)$, where $S(t)$ denotes the survival function, which is related to the cumulative distribution function by $S(t) = 1-F(t)$, $h(t)$ the hazard rate at time t and $S(t) = \exp(-\int_0^t h(u)du)$, so that every distribution is uniquely characterized by any one of the $f(t), h(t)$ or $S(t)$ functions. That is, for a single event of interest there is a one-to-one relationship between these quantities.

10.2.1 Regression models

The two broad options for modeling the effect of covariates on survival data are (i) assuming a parametric distribution for the density of the data and (ii) adopting a semi-parametric approach like the *Cox model*, where the hazard function is of the form $h(t;\, \boldsymbol{z}) = h_0(t)\exp\left(\boldsymbol{\beta}^\top \boldsymbol{z}\right)$, with the baseline hazard $h_0(t)$ left unspecified and $\boldsymbol{z}$ representing the vector of covariates, including the treatment under investigation (see for example Kalbfleisch and Prentice, 2011, for details).

In the parametric approach to survival analysis the likelihood function is straightforward to define, provided that censoring is independent of the event of interest; that is, the hazard function for the censored individual is assumed to be the same as that for individuals who are observed beyond the censoring time. In this case, the contribution of a right-censored observation is given by the survival function evaluated at that particular time point. Specifically, given a random sample of time-to-event data $\{(t_i, \delta_i) : (i = 1, \ldots, n)\}$, where t_i denotes the observed duration and δ_i the event indicator, with $\delta_i = 1$ and $\delta_i = 0$ corresponding to an event and a censored individual respectively, the likelihood is given by:

$$\prod_{i=1}^{n} S(t_i)^{(1-\delta_i)} f(t_i)^{\delta_i} = \prod_{i=1}^{n} S(t_i) h(t_i)^{\delta_i}.$$

In the semiparametric case, parameter estimation is implemented using *Cox's partial likelihood* (Cox, 1975) since a formal justification for its use was given in Andersen and Gill (1982), using the *counting process* formulation. The latter provides a rigorous unified framework for extending the standard model in several directions, including time-dependent covariates and serves as the basis for the Bayesian analysis of semi-parametric survival models. As the *proportional hazards (PH) model* is the most commonly used regression model for estimating the effect of covariates on the hazard of the event, including the effects of interventions, it is adopted for the analyses in this chapter. While the PH assumption is often reasonable, it should not be accepted without testing. Plots of scaled Schoenfeld residuals over time (Grambsch and Therneau, 1994) may highlight time-varying patterns and plots of scaled score residuals can identify influential subjects. Such departures from standard model assumptions may manifest as non-proportional hazards and are sometimes addressed by allowing time-varying covariates, $h(t;\, \boldsymbol{z}) = h_0(t)\exp\left(\boldsymbol{\beta}^\top \boldsymbol{z}(t)\right)$. Other options for time-to-event data include the additive risk (relative survival) model, the accelerated failure time model, the proportional odds model and combinations thereof, see Kalbfleisch and Prentice (2011) or Hosmer et al. (2011) and references therein for an extensive treatment of such models.

10.2.2 The Bayesian approach to survival regression

Adopting the Bayesian paradigm necessitates the specification of prior distributions for all the model parameters. In PH models, the coefficients for treatment effects and other covariates, $\boldsymbol{\beta}$, representing log hazard ratios, are often assigned weakly-informative priors, for example Gaussian densities with large variance. If early phase trials are available then more informative priors for $\boldsymbol{\beta}$ may be derived, or the prior density may be elicited from experts (see Chapter 5 on expert prior elicitation and O'Hagan et al., 2006, for practical guidance and software).

The type of prior used for the baseline hazard has varied substantially. In the parametric setting, where a particular form for the hazard is assumed, weakly informative priors are often assigned, for example, large variance Gaussian distributions on the log-scale for the Weibull shape and scale/rate parameters. However, in the semi-parametric case, where the baseline hazard is a function, a suitable prior is not immediately apparent. The most common option is based on variations of the neutral-to-the-right (Doksum, 1974) class of continuous-time stochastic models, with the Gamma process being the default option in applications. The latter has been used in Kalbfleisch (1978) as a Bayesian justification for Cox's partial likelihood by allowing the prior precision to approach zero, see also Sinha et al. (2003) for an extension to time-dependent covariates. The *Gamma Process* is used as a prior on the cumulative baseline hazard $H_0(t) = \int_0^t h_0(u)du$, by first defining a partition of the time axis and then assuming that a-priori $H_0(t) \sim GP(c\gamma(t), c)$, with $\gamma(t)$ the mean and c the precision parameter. This prior then postulates that the increments of $H_0(t)$ over disjoint intervals are independent, with $H_0(t) - H_0(s) \sim \text{Gamma}(c\,(\gamma(t) - \gamma(s))\,, c)$ where Gamma(a, b) denotes the Gamma distribution with shape $a > 0$ and scale $b > 0$. This model is an alternative to the Dirichlet Process prior (and its variations) seen in Chapter 1.

The Bayesian approach to semi-parametric survival regression proceeds by employing the counting process framework where the likelihood stems from using the Cox model when defining the intensity function. Inference proceeds via the Poisson approximation to the number of events in a small time-interval, see for example Clayton (1991).

Right censoring is a characterizing feature of survival analysis and arises from the need to analyse results before all individuals have experienced the event. Left censoring and interval censoring, in which individuals go through a period of not being at risk of the event, are also encountered in some applications, particularly when modeling stages of progressive diseases such as cancer and HIV, see e.g. Bogaerts et al. (2017).

10.2.3 Use of Bayesian methods for trials with time to event outcomes

Although some Phase II trials have included time-to-event outcomes, see for example (Cotterill and Whitehead, 2015), they usually focus on short-term surrogates, such as tumor shrinkage or biomarkers. Time to clinical events are more common in 'definitive' Phase III randomized trials and a range of Bayesian methods for the design of such trials are available, see for example Spiegelhalter et al. (2004). Brard et al. (2017), conducted a systematic review of the use of Bayesian methods in trials with time-to-event outcomes in 2016. Only 28 Phase II and III trials were identified, most (25/28) in oncology patients and most (24/28) evaluated new pharmacological agents. No trials reported using informative priors for the treatment effect, although four did include historical data to inform priors of other parameters. Although regulatory bodies have traditionally been reluctant to accept Bayesian analyses for new pharmacological interventions, the U.S. Food and Drug Administration has published guidance, including Bayesian methods, for evaluation of drugs in rare diseases (U.S. Food and Drug Administration, 2015), for adaptive trials (U.S. Food and Drug Administration, 2010a) and for medical devices (U.S. Food and Drug Administration, 2010b). Moreover, the European Medicines Agency has mentioned using Bayesian sensitivity analysis for trials in small populations (European Medicines Agency, 2006) and the International Rare Cancers Initiative also recognized the value of Bayesian clinical trials for rare cancers (Bogaerts et al., 2015).

The consensus appears to be that Bayesian methods are most attractive when large Phase III trials are difficult due to small populations, rare diseases or rare outcomes (Billingham et al., 2016; Brard et al., 2017; Cannon et al., 2009, 2010). In these cases, inclusion of prior knowledge and a focus on reducing uncertainty in treatment effect estimate is of greater importance than hypothesis testing. The natural updating of posterior densities as new data emerge makes Bayesian methods attractive for sequential monitoring in clinical trials, and several authors have suggested that they may be more efficient than their classical analogues (Buzdar et al., 2005).

The Bayesian approach also facilitates the fitting of complex models, such as frailty models where clustering or other forms of heterogeneity are appropriately modeled. Survival models in which a subset of the population is not expected to have the event of interest (often named cure models) and other problems with discrete frailty distributions are often subject to identifiability issues, which can be addressed by introducing a realistic prior for the mixing proportion, see for example (Chen et al., 1999). Joint models of posterior distributions of survival times and longitudinal biomarkers, via correlated random effects, have also been developed (Rizopoulos, 2012). Notably, Rizopoulos provides an `R` package, `JMBayes`, that fits joint models in a Bayesian framework, and provides an application to a trial comparing Didanosine and Zalcitabine in HIV patients (Rizopoulos, 2018). Bogaerts et al. (2017) also shows how Bayesian methods can be used to model complicated (interval) censoring patterns, while avoiding strong assumptions about the nature of the survival models. In addition, the Bayesian paradigm offers a suitable framework for the synthesis of diverse sources of evidence: see Jackson et al. (2017) and references therein for a review of different methods for integrating distinct types of data, with the aim of extrapolating survival curves beyond the observed time-horizon of the clinical data, as is often necessitated in health economic evaluations.

10.3 Software

Practical implementation is commonly performed using Markov chain Monte Carlo (MCMC) methods. The `WinBUGS` software has hitherto been the standard tool for doing so. When fitting parametric models, censoring is accommodated through sampling of the missing event times from their appropriate distribution. Additional software, with similar syntax, has emerged, such as `JAGS` which is also based upon the Metropolis-Hastings class of MCMC samplers and is also available beyond the windows environment, including Mac and Linux. A more recent addition to the Bayesian toolkit is the `STAN` software, which uses a version of Hamiltonian Monte Carlo and also offers alternative approximate inference based on variational approximation or penalized maximum likelihood. `STAN` is also available across platforms and can be called from standard software like `R` and `Stata`, as can `BUGS` and `JAGS`. Additionally, generic Bayesian analysis tools have become available in mainstream statistical software; for example the procedure `PROC MCMC` in `SAS` uses a Metropolis algorithm to sample from posterior distributions (SAS Institute, 2014). `SAS` procedures `PROC LIFEREG` and `PHREG` also allow specific Bayesian parametric and semi-parametric survival models, estimated using Gibbs sampling. A similar generic MCMC package is available in `R` but this is most suited to simple continuous distributions (Geyer and Johnson, 2017). Specialist packages for more complex situations, such as joint survival and longitudinal biomarker models are also available in the CRAN library (Rizopoulos, 2018).

Model determination in this context is typically assessed in two related directions. Model comparison is performed using appropriate criteria such as the Deviance Information Criterion (Spiegelhalter et al., 2002). Model adequacy is inspected through graphical tools. These include the superposition of fitted functions over the observed equivalents, with the survival curve against the Kaplan-Meier estimator being a standard choice. This approach is often complemented by the investigation of suitably defined residuals.

10.4 Applications

The Bayesian approach to the analysis of time to event data is illustrated using two of the freely available data sets found in the R package `survival`.

10.4.1 Colon cancer trial

Data

The first example concerns a large trial of adjuvant chemotherapy for colon cancer patients who have had surgical removal of the tumor. When the trial first reported in Moertel et al. (1990), three groups were compared: (i) No chemotherapy, (ii) Levamisole and (iii) Levamisole+Fluorouracil. However, we restrict analysis to the 614 patients randomized to one of the two active chemotherapy arms. The trial outcome of interest was recurrence-free survival, defined as the time to the first of tumor recurrence or death. There were additional covariates included in the analysis but we focus on the effect of treatment, adjusting for other covariates.

Model and priors

The data were analysed using both a Weibull-based parametric model and a Cox-type semi-parametric approach. For the Weibull likelihood with shape r and rate λ, the baseline hazard was parameterized as $h_0(t) = \lambda r t^{(r-1)}$, and we assumed proportional hazards for the covariates for comparability with the Cox PH model. The shape parameter was assigned a Gamma(1,100) prior and covariate coefficients (on a log scale) modeled via the rate parameter were assigned weakly informative Gaussian priors with zero mean and variance set to 10^4. Note here that very large prior variances were chosen because no prior information was available; moreover, in this case the observed likelihood was rich enough to ensure convergence of the posterior. In practice, much smaller variances, say $5 - 10$ on the log scale are sufficiently uncertain, will result in robust posterior estimates in most cases and may improve the stability of the estimation procedure. The baseline hazard for the Cox PH model was flexible and a Gamma Process prior was adopted (see Section 10.2.3). We assumed a priori independent increments for the cumulative baseline hazard and used a small value for the precision parameter c. The reported results are based on $c = 0.1$, which reflects weak prior information for the baseline hazards, and allows the data primarily to influence the posterior through the likelihood. In addition to treatment, we included the following covariates in the models: days since surgery (> 20 compared to ≤ 20), obstruction of the colon, number of lymph nodes involved (> 4 compared to 0-4), extent of tumor invasion (3 levels) and histologic differentiation (3 levels). All covariates were centered around their mean value to promote convergence of the baseline hazards. Again, we placed weakly informative Gaussian priors on the covariate coefficients (on the log scale) with zero mean and variance 10^4.

Multiple imputation

A convenient feature of simulation-based Bayesian inference is the ability to accommodate missing measurements by simultaneously estimating the posterior distributions of the model parameters and the missing measurements, via a kind of multiple imputation. In the colon cancer data set, the three-level categorical covariate histologic differentiation was missing for 16 patients. Excluding patients from analysis of randomized trials may result in loss of statistical efficiency, as well as biased estimates if the missing data patterns vary by group. This can be a major issue in smaller trials or when several covariates are missing. When the mechanism leading to the missing values can be assumed missing at random (Little and Rubin, 2002), multiple imputation techniques enable inclusion of all the available evidence and retain all the subjects in the analysis. In the context of survival analysis, and more generally in non-linear models, multiple imputation is not straightforward but such methods are naturally catered for within the simulation-based approach we adopted. Specifically, using the `BUGS` software, the missing observations are denoted by `NA` and a sampling model for these is defined, from which the missing measurements are sampled. In the present analysis we assumed that histologic differentiation was a categorical covariate and the three different categories were given a vague Dirichlet(1,1,1) prior density. Note that `JAGS` deals with missing data in a similar way, while other packages such as `STAN` require estimation of the missing data likelihood for each pattern of missing covariates, which can be difficult to specify and estimate. `SAS` packages sample missing data directly from the sampling distribution at each simulation.

TABLE 10.1: Colon cancer trial: Posterior summary measures for regression coefficients from Bayesian models compared with the classical Cox model.

Covariate	Weibull Model	Cox Model	Classical Cox Model**
Levamisole+Fluorouracil	-0.49 (-0.71, -0.27)	-0.44 (-0.67, -0.22)	-0.44 (-0.67, -0.22)
> 4 Lymph Nodes Involved	0.91 (0.67, 1.14)	0.86 (0.61, 1.11)	0.88 (0.64, 1.12)
Obstruction of the Colon	0.33 (0.05, 0.59)	0.34 (0.08, 0.59)	0.38 (0.10, 0.65)
20 Days Since Surgery	0.36 (0.11, 0.60)	0.36 (0.12, 0.61)	0.35 (0.10, 0.60)
Tumor Differentiation			
Baseline well			
Moderate	0.22 (-0.15, 0.62)	0.19 (-0.14, 0.55)	0.20 (-0.18, 0.59)
Poor	0.47 (0.03, 0.92)	0.46 (0.05, 0.87)	0.49 (0.03, 0.94)
Extent of invasion			
Baseline Submucosa	-	-	-
Muscle	-	-	-
Serosa	0.41 (0.04, 0.81)	0.38 (0.01, 0.77)	0.38 (-0.01, 0.77)
Contiguous Structures	0.87 (0.24, 1.47)	0.84 (0.22, 1.42)	0.84 (0.21, 1.46)
Shape parameter	0.73 (0.66, 0.80)	-	-
Mean Deviance	6723 (6715, 6734)	5799 (5752, 5854)	-

** Note that 16 observations were deleted due to missing tumor differentiation

Results

The results are summarized in Table 10.1, alongside the classical Cox model estimates. The data set has some missing covariate values that are categorical, so that the DIC cannot be used to assess model fit; the DIC is based on the fit of the statistical model to the data, some of which are not observed but are estimated as part of the MCMC simulation. As a result it is not clear whether the missing observations should be included in the likelihood or prior component of the DIC; neither is it clear how to condition on missing categorical variables, since there is no obvious plug in value (note that the DIC for missing normally distributed data can be estimated by plugging in the posterior mean; Mason et al., 2012). The posterior mean deviance within the MCMC sampling process in `WinBUGS` is estimated from the observed data only and is provided for this example. The greater flexibility of the Bayesian Cox model resulted in a substantially lower mean deviance in this example, suggesting that it provides a better fit to the data than the Bayesian Weibull distribution. This is also evident from Figure 10.2, in which the fitted survival curves for each treatment

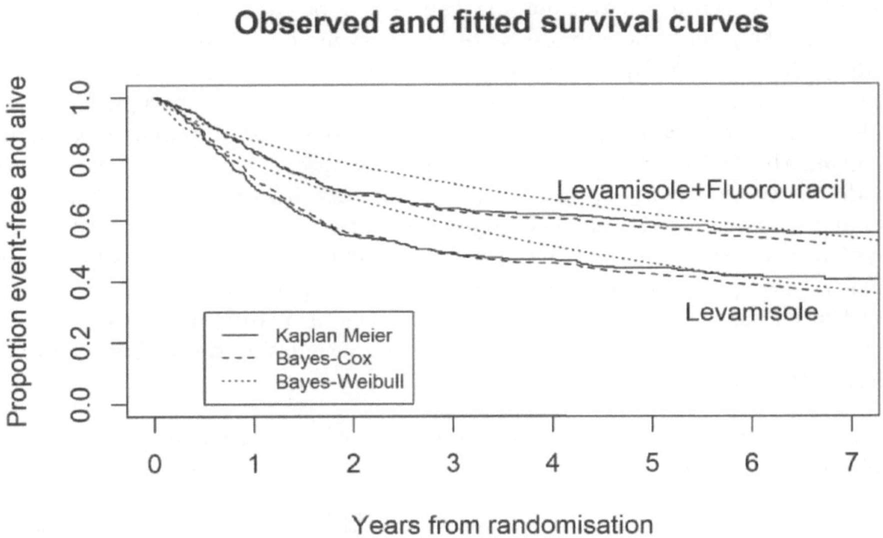

FIGURE 10.2: Colon cancer trial: Comparison of Kaplan-Meier and Bayesian models for recurrence-free survival.

group are estimated at the average values for the other covariates. The Weibull model, which has only two parameters, displays a substantial lack of fit in the middle part of the follow up period, before converging to the Kaplan-Meier curve, while the Bayesian Cox model is closer to the empirical survival function throughout. Despite the lack of fit, there were only small differences between the Weibull and the Cox models in the estimates of treatment effects, both showing that Levamisole combined with Fluorouracil significantly reduces the hazard compared to Levamisole alone. The posterior hazard ratio (95% credible interval) for the parametric and non-parametric models were 0.61 (0.49, 0.76) and 0.64 (0.51, 0.80) respectively; both were consistent with the large treatment effect found in the original trial analysis and a classical Cox regression (Table 10.1). For all models, the hazard was greater if there were more than 4 lymph nodes with detectable cancer, obstruction of the colon by tumor, prolonged time from surgery to randomization (> 20 days), poor tumor differentiation and greater local spread.

Although the Hazard Ratio (HR) is often the parameter of primary interest in pharmaceutical trials, the samples from the joint posterior distribution allow investigation of a range of other important quantities, such as functions of the basic model parameters. For example, the safety profile of the drug may be such that it would only be acceptable if the HR reached some threshold, say 0.75. Calculation of the relevant probabilities is straightforward from the MCMC output. The comparison of the two arms in the colon cancer trial estimated the HR as 0.64, with a 95% CI (0.51, 0.80), corresponding to a $\Pr(\text{HR} < 0.75 \mid \text{data})$ of 0.909, while $\Pr(\text{HR} < 0.5 \mid \text{data}) = 0.015$. *Restricted mean survival*, defined as the area under the survival curve, up to a specific time point, may be of interest if the PH assumption is in doubt; point and interval estimates for the Levamisole and combined treatment groups can be calculated from the survival functions. For the colon cancer example the difference in restricted mean survival over time is plotted using the Bayesian-Cox survival functions in Figure 10.3.

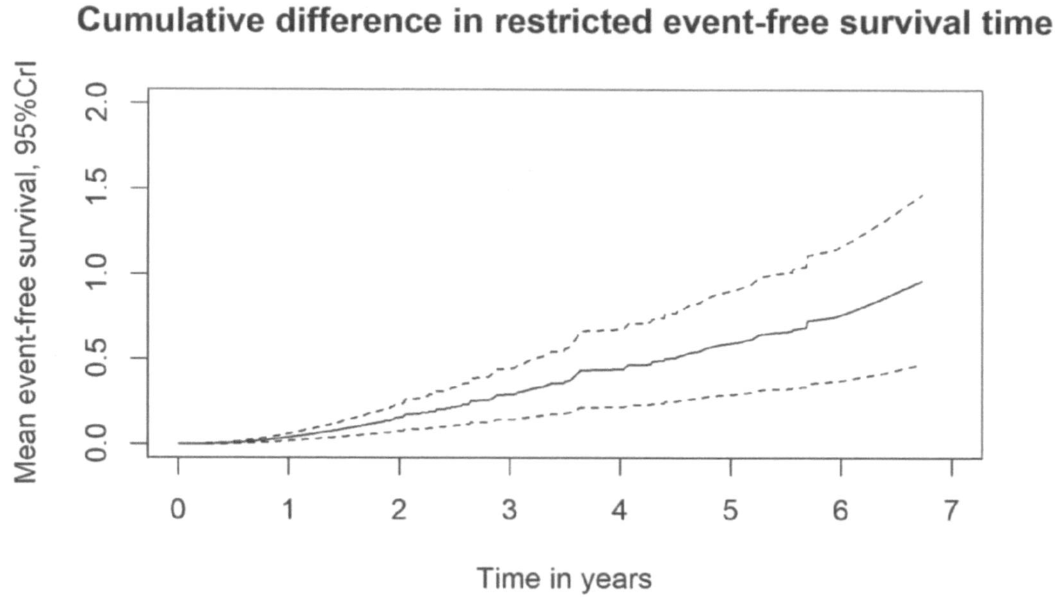

FIGURE 10.3: Colon cancer trial: Difference in restricted mean survival over time.

This shows that the difference is statistically significant and increases steadily over time with the Levamisole+Fluorouracil group having higher mean survival compared to Levamisole alone, gaining a little over one month over each year after the first. Although a point estimate of the restricted mean survival is available using a classical approach, confidence intervals are difficult to estimate; in contrast, they are available with little additional effort from the MCMC samples using the Bayesian approach.

10.4.2 Extensions using random effects

Clustering in trials is increasingly common. We illustrate a Bayesian model for clustered time to event data using a trial of laser coagulation as a treatment to delay diabetic retinopathy. The data set contains two observations for each of the 197 patients in the trial, with one eye randomized to laser treatment and the other eye receiving no treatment. The event of interest was the time (in months) from initiation of treatment until loss of vision, defined as visual acuity below 5/200 for two consecutive visits. The survival times in this data set are the actual time to vision loss, minus the minimum possible time to event (6.5 months). Censoring was potentially due to death, dropout, or the end of the study. The data were first reported in Blair et al. (1976) and re-analysed in Huster et al. (1989).

In addition to treatment arm, we used the covariates which were included in the design: age at diagnosis of diabetes, the type of laser used (argon or xenon), the eye treated (left or right), the type of diabetes (juvenile or adult) and a risk score ranging from 6 to 12.

In common with the colon cancer example, we fitted a Weibull parametric model and a Cox model to these data with and without random (individual) effects. The random effects represent patient-specific log hazard ratios which, in this example, are assumed to arise from a Gaussian distribution centered at zero, with variance σ^2. We assigned a Gamma(1,100) prior for the random effects variance; otherwise all model specifications are the same as in the colon cancer example.

TABLE 10.2: Diabetic retinopathy trial: Posterior summary measures for the model parameters compared with the classical Cox model. DIC = Deviance Information Criterion

Covariate	Weibull Model	Weibull Model with Random Effects	Cox Model	Cox Model with Random Effects	Classical Cox Model with Gamma Frailty
Treated	-0.80 (-1.14, -0.45)	-0.99 (-1.36, -0.62)	-0.76 (-1.10, -0.41)	-0.88 (-1.23, -0.52)	-0.91 (-1.26, -0.66)
Age per 10 years	0.10 (-0.10, 0.28)	0.15 (-0.12, 0.43)	0.10 (-0.10, 0.31)	0.13 (-0.11, 0.36)	0.15 (-0.12, 0.42)
Risk per unit increase	0.15 (0.02, 0.25)	0.17 (0.03, 0.31)	0.11 (0.00, 0.23)	0.14 (0.03, 0.24)	0.16 (0.02, 0.30)
Xenon Laser	-0.17 (-0.50, 0.18)	-0.27 (-.77, 0.21)	-0.23 (-0.54, 0.10)	-0.30 (-0.77, 0.08)	-0.25 (-0.69, 0.19)
Adult Diabetes	-0.12 (-0.69, 0.43)	-0.23 (-1.05, 0.54)	-0.18 (-0.79, 0.40)	-0.21 (-0.86, 0.47)	-0.26 (-1.06, 0.54)
Right Eye	-0.21 (-0.55, 0.11)	-0.27 (-0.78, 0.20)	-0.27 (-0.62, 0.08)	-0.31 (-0.71, 0.12)	-0.30 (-0.74, 0.06)
Sigma*		1.06 (0.65, 1.46)		0.84 (0.45, 1.20)	0.89
DIC	1677	1618	1587	1566	
Mean deviance	1662	1460	1498	1349	

* Random Effects Standard Deviation (log hazard ratio scale)

Results

The DIC and the parameter estimates for the treatment effect, with their equal tail 95% credible intervals for each model are summarized in Table 10.2, alongside the corresponding classical Cox model with log-normal random effects. The best fit according to the DIC was provided by the Bayesian Cox model with random effects (DIC = 1566), followed by the standard Bayesian Cox model (DIC = 1587), while the Weibull model with random effects had a worse fit with DIC = 1618 and the standard Weibull model had DIC=1677. The estimated numbers of parameters were 112, 46, 80 and 7.8 respectively, reflecting that the additional complexity of including the random effects and the baseline hazard provides a substantially better fit to the data. There is some debate over the use of the DIC for comparing models with and without random effects, see also Chapter 1. Using the asymptotic equivalence of cross-validation and AIC/DIC, the term of the DIC that penalizes for complexity depends on whether the model fit is intended to be used for prediction of results for a new measurement from a particular eye or person in the sample or for a new eye or person from the population outside of the sample. The DIC is appropriate for prediction of new results from a person within the current sample; the deviance, AIC or BIC would be more appropriate for prediction of results for a new person from the same population, since the distribution is marginalized (the random effects are integrated out) for these assessments of fit. For the diabetic retinopathy example, the corresponding measures of posterior mean deviance which exclude the penalty term are given in Table 10.2, confirming that the random effects models have improved fit.

Figure 10.4 shows the fitted and empirical survival curves for the two models, with both parametric and non-parametric models close to the empirical data.

Although the more flexible baseline hazard for the Cox models resulted in slightly bigger treatment effects than the Weibull models, with estimated hazard ratios (95% CI) of 0.42 (0.29, 0.59) compared with 0.45 (0.32, 0.64), the remaining regression coefficients were similar across different models, suggesting that the resulting estimates are reasonably robust. The random effects standard deviation is somewhat smaller for the Bayesian Cox model than for the Weibull model. This might be expected, since part of the between-patient hazards will be explained by the more flexible baseline of the semiparametric approach. Finally, there are only minor differences in the parameter point estimates between the Bayesian and classical Cox random effects models, but the Bayesian estimates are slightly more precise and have the added benefit that functions of parameters, and their posterior distributions, are available from the MCMC samples.

10.5 Reporting

The review of Bayesian survival analysis methods in clinical trials highlighted the lack of detailed reporting in these publications (Brard et al., 2017). The limited space allocated to each contribution to a clinical journal means that adequate reporting of the full model and sensitivity analyses in the main trial report is difficult. Moreover, clinicians find detailed statistical models difficult to understand and of low priority. On the other hand, adequate reporting of the statistical model and assumptions is crucial for robust analysis and can provide excellent examples of Bayesian clinical trial analysis for others to follow. Simple checklists such as the 7-item ROBUST criteria (Sung et al., 2005) provide a minimum set of information to be reported, while more detailed checklists such as BAYESWATCH (Spiegelhalter et al., 2000) and BaSiS (BaSis, 2001) can be followed and reported in supplementary

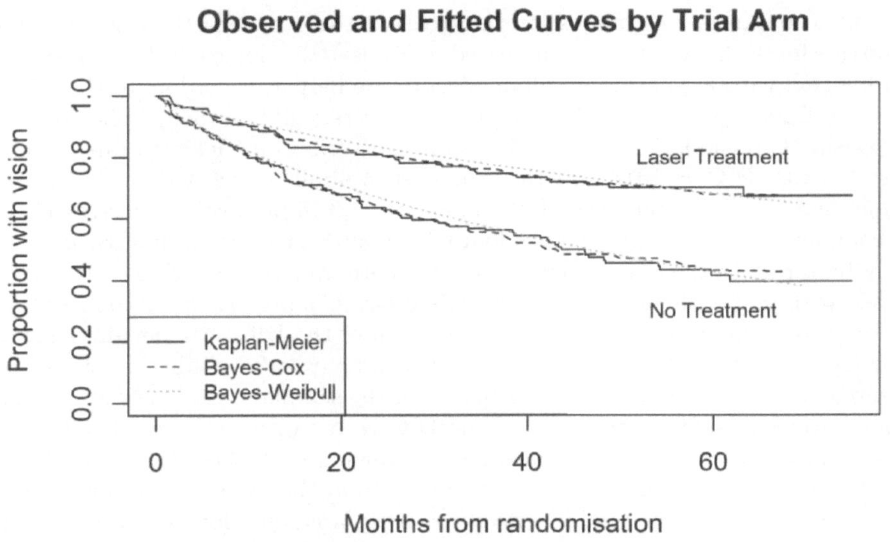

FIGURE 10.4: Diabetic retinopathy trial: Comparison of Kaplan-Meier and Bayesian models for time to loss of vision.

information online, or as part of protocol publications. A more sophisticated approach to prior specification, using expert elicitation, is enabled by packages such as SHELF (O'Hagan, 2008, see also Chapter 5) and these can be published in their own right (see for example Hampson et al., 2015).

10.6 Other comments

The Bayesian approach to survival analysis is very flexible and can accommodate a range of survival functions, clustering and, provided that missing at random is plausible, multiple imputation can be performed in a relatively straightforward manner. Simulation-based methods allow straightforward estimation of useful data summaries and functions of potentially correlated parameters; for example the probability that a particular hazard ratio exceeds the minimum treatment effect that will outweigh safety concerns and restricted mean survival when the PH assumption is in doubt. Rigorous estimation of this kind is not straightforward from a classical viewpoint and computer-intensive methods such as the bootstrap are typically employed.

Bayesian methods are particularly suited to more complex data structures. It is relatively straightforward to estimate joint posterior distributions for both efficacy and safety outcomes, perhaps assuming correlated random effects; estimates and plots of the joint posterior distribution may facilitate risk-benefit evaluations. As described above, time to event outcomes and longitudinal measures of time-varying biomarkers can be modeled jointly within a Bayesian framework; for example, Rizopoulos (2012) analyses serial measurements of C4 counts and survival, and provides associated `R` code. The need to provide prior densities for the range of parameters specified in survival models is problematic, especially for registration trials, and the frequent requirement for simulation-based estimation means that analysis will be relatively slow, even for experienced users. However, regulators and researchers have recognized a place for a Bayesian approach in trials involving medical devices, rare diseases, rare outcomes and small populations, as well as their value for early phase and adaptive trials, trial monitoring and sensitivity analysis. Where prior or external evidence is available, particularly for the baseline hazards, a Bayesian approach has the potential to increase statistical efficiency. The greater availability of tools to aid prior elicitation and MCMC functionality in standard software continues to open up these methods for use in more applied research settings, including clinical trials.

Bibliography

Andersen, P. K. and Gill, R. D. (1982). Cox's regression model for counting processes: A large sample study. *The Annals of Statistics*, 10(4):1100–1120.

BaSis (2001). The BaSis workshop: Bayesian Standards in Science. "`http://www.stat.cmu.edu/bayesworkshop/2001/BaSisGuideline.htm`".

Billingham, L., Malottki, K., and Steven, N. (2016). Research methods to change clinical practice for patients with rare cancers. *The Lancet Oncology*, 17(2):e70–e80.

Blair, A. L., Hadden, D. R., Weaver, J. A., Archer, D. B., Johnston, P. B., and Maguire, C. J. (1976). The 5-year prognosis for vision in diabetes. *Americal Journal of Ophthalmology*, 81:14.

Bogaerts, J., Sydes, M., Keat, N., McConnell, A., Benson, A., Ho, A., Roth, A., Fortpied, C., Eng, C., Peckitt, C., Coens, C., Pettaway, C., Arnold, D., Hall, E., Marshall, E., Sclafani, F., Hatcher, H., Earl, H., Ray-Coquard, I., Paul, J., Blay, J.-Y., Whelan, J., Panageas, K., Wheatley, K., Harrington, K., Licitra, L., Billingham, L., Hensley, M., McCabe, M., Patel, P., Carvajal, R., Wilson, R., Glynne-Jones, R., McWilliams, R., Leyvraz, S., Rao, S., Nicholson, S., Filiaci, V., Negrouk, A., Lacombe, D., Dupont, E., Pauporté, I., Welch, J., Law, K., Trimble, T., and Seymour, M. (2015). Clinical trial designs for rare diseases: studies developed and discussed by the International Rare Cancers Initiative. *European Journal of Cancer*, 51(3):271–281.

Bogaerts, K., Komárek, A., and Lesaffre, E. (2017). *Survival Analysis with Interval-Censored Data: A Practical Approach with Examples in R, SAS, and BUGS*. Chapman & Hall/CRC Interdisciplinary Statistics. CRC Press.

Brard, C., Le Teuff, G., Le Deley, M., and Hampson, L. (2017). Bayesian survival analysis in clinical trials: What methods are used in practice? *Clinical Trials*, 14(1):78–87.

Buzdar, A., Ibrahim, N., Francis, D., Booser, D., Thomas, E., Theriault, R., Pusztai, L., Green, M., Arun, B., Giordano, S., Cristofanilli, M., Frye, D., Smith, T., Hunt, K., Singletary, S., Sahin, A., Ewer, M., Buchholz, T., Berry, D., and Hortobagyi, G. (2005). Significantly higher pathologic complete remission rate after neoadjuvant therapy with trastuzumab, paclitaxel, and epirubicin chemotherapy: results of a randomized trial in human epidermal growth factor receptor 2-positive operable breast cancer. *Journal of Clinical Oncology*, 23(16):3676–3685.

Cannon, C., Dansky, H., Davidson, M., Gotto, A., Brinton, E., Gould, A., Stepanavage, M., Liu, S., Shah, S., Rubino, J., Gibbons, P., Hermanowski-Vosatka, A., Binkowitz, B., Mitchel, Y., Barter, P., and DEFINE investigators (2009). Design of the DEFINE trial: determining the EFficacy and tolerability of CETP INhibition with AnacEtrapib. *American Heart Journal*, 158(4):513–519.e3.

Cannon, C., Shah, S., Dansky, H., Davidson, M., Brinton, E., Gotto, A., Stepanavage, M., Liu, S., Gibbons, P., Ashraf, T., Zafarino, J., Mitchel, Y., and Barter, P. (2010). Safety of anacetrapib in patients with or at high risk for coronary heart disease. *New England Journal of Medicine*, 363(25):2406–2415.

Chen, M., Ibrahim, J., and Sinha, D. (1999). A new Bayesian model for survival data with a surviving fraction. *Journal of the American Statistical Association*, 94(447):909–919.

Clayton, D. (1991). A Monte Carlo method for Bayesian inference in frailty models. *Biometrics*, 47(2):467–485.

Cotterill, A. and Whitehead, J. (2015). Bayesian methods for setting sample sizes and choosing allocation ratios in Phase II clinical trials with time-to-event endpoints. *Statistics in Medicine*, 34(11):1889–1903.

Cox, D. R. (1972). Regression models and life-tables. *Journal of the Royal Statistical Society — Series B*, 34(2):187–220.

Cox, D. R. (1975). Partial likelihood. *Biometrika*, 62(2):269–276.

Doksum, K. (1974). Tailfree and neutral random probabilities and their posterior distributions. *The Annals of Probability*, 2(2):183–201.

European Medicines Agency (2006). Guideline on Clinical Trials in Small Populations. "http://www.ema.europa.eu/docs/en_GB/document_library/Scientific_guideline/2009/09/WC500003615.pdf".

Geyer, C. and Johnson, L. (2017). "https://cran.r-project.org/web/packages/mcmc/mcmc.pdf".

Grambsch, P. and Therneau, T. (1994). Proportional hazards tests and diagnostics based on weighted residuals. *Biometrika*, 81(3):515–526.

Hampson, L., Whitehead, J., Eleftheriou, D., Tudur-Smith, C., Jones, R., Jayne, D., Hickey, H., Beresford, M., Bracaglia, C., Caldas, A., Cimaz, R., Dehoorne, J., Dolezalova, P., Friswell, M., Jelusic, M.and Marks, S., Martin, N., McMahon, A.-M., Peitz, J., Royen-Kerkhof, A. v., Soylemezoglu, O., and Brogan, P. (2015). Elicitation of expert prior opinion: Application to the MYPAN trial in childhood polyarteritis nodosa. *PLOS One*, 10(3):e0120981.

Hosmer, D., Lemeshow, S., and May, S. (2011). *Applied Survival Analysis: Regression Modeling of Time-to-Event Data.* Wiley Series in Probability and Statistics. Wiley.

Huster, W., Brookmeyer, R., and Self, S. (1989). Modelling paired survival data with covariates. *Biometrics*, 45(1):145–156.

Jackson, C., Stevens, J., Ren, S., Latimer, N., Bojke, L., Manca, A., and Sharples, L. (2017). Extrapolating survival from randomized trials using external data: A review of methods. *Medical Decision Making*, 37(4):377–390.

Kalbfleisch, J. (1978). Non-parametric Bayesian analysis of survival time data. *Journal of the Royal Statistical Society — Series B*, 40(2):214–221.

Kalbfleisch, J. and Prentice, R. (2011). *The Statistical Analysis of Failure Time Data*. Wiley Series in Probability and Statistics. Wiley.

Little, R. and Rubin, D. (2002). *Statistical Analysis With Missing Data*. Wiley Series in Probability and Statistics - Applied Probability and Statistics Section Series. Wiley.

Mason, A., Richardson, S., and Best, N. (2012). Two-pronged strategy for using DIC to compare selection models with non-ignorable missing responses. *Bayesian Analysis*, 7(1):109–146.

Moertel, C., Fleming, T., Macdonald, J., Haller, D., Laurie, J., Goodman, P., Ungerleider, J., Emerson, W., Tormey, D., Glick, J., Veeder, M., and Mailliard, J. (1990). Levamisole and fluorouracil for adjuvant therapy of resected colon carcinoma. *New England Journal of Medicine*, 322(6):352–358.

O'Hagan, A. (2008). SHELF: the Sheffield Elicitation Framework. [Elicitation of expert judgements] . `http://www.tonyohagan.co.uk/shelf/`.

O'Hagan, A., Buck, C., Daneshkhah, A., Eiser, J., Garthwaite, P., Jenkinson, D., Oakley, J., and Rakow, T. (2006). *Uncertain Judgements: Eliciting Experts' Probabilities*. Statistics in Practice. Wiley.

Rizopoulos, D. (2012). *Joint Models for Longitudinal and Time-to-Event Data: With Applications in R*. Chapman & Hall/CRC Biostatistics Series. Taylor & Francis.

Rizopoulos, D. (2018). Joint Modeling of Longitudinal and Time-to-Event Data under a Bayesian Approach. `https://cran.r-project.org/web/packages/JMbayes/JMbayes.pdf`.

SAS Institute (2014). SAS/STAT_14.3_User's_Guide. `"http://documentation.sas.com/?docsetId=statug&docsetTarget=statug_mcmc_details01.htm&docsetVersion=14.3&locale=en"`.

Sinha, D., Ibrahim, J., and Chen, M. (2003). A Bayesian justification of Cox's partial likelihood. *Biometrika*, 90(3):629–641.

Spiegelhalter, D., Abrams, K., and Myles, J. (2004). *Bayesian Approaches to Clinical Trials and Health-Care Evaluation*. Wiley, New York, NY.

Spiegelhalter, D., Best, N., Carlin, B., and van der Linde, A. (2002). Bayesian measures of model complexity and fit (with discussion). *Journal of the Royal Statistical Society — Series B*, 64:1–34.

Spiegelhalter, D., Myles, J., Jones, D., and Abrams, K. (2000). Bayesian methods in health technology assessment: a review. *Health Technology Assessment*, 4(38):1–130.

Sung, L., Hayden, J., Greenberg, M., Koren, G., Feldman, B., and Tomlinson, G. (2005). Seven items were identified for inclusion when reporting a Bayesian analysis of a clinical study. *Journal of Clinical Epidemiology*, 58(3):261–268.

U.S. Food and Drug Administration (2010a). Guidance for Industry Adaptive Design Clinical Trials for Drugs and Biologics. "https://www.fda.gov/downloads/drugs/guidances/ucm201790.pdf".

U.S. Food and Drug Administration (2010b). The Use of Bayesian Statistics in Medical Device Clinical Trials: Guidance for Industry and Food and Drug Administration Staff. "https://www.fda.gov/downloads/MedicalDevices/DeviceRegulationandGuidance/GuidanceDocuments/ucm071121.pdf".

U.S. Food and Drug Administration (2015). Guidance on Rare Diseases: Common Issues in Drug Development Guidance for Industry. "https://www.fda.gov/downloads/Drugs/GuidanceComplianceRegulatoryInformation/Guidances/UCM458485.pdf".

11

Benefit of Bayesian Clustering of Longitudinal Data: Study of Cognitive Decline for Precision Medicine

Anaïs Rouanet
MRC Biostatistics Unit, UK

Sylvia Richardson
MRC Biostatistics Unit, UK

Brian Tom
MRC Biostatistics Unit, UK

Precision medicine is an emerging field that aims to improve disease prevention and treatment by accounting for individual variations in genes, lifestyle and environment. Extensive datasets are used to uncover subpopulations with different biological characteristics and susceptibility to the disease or response to treatment. This finer characterisation is ultimately directed towards the identification of clinical biomarkers, the prediction of the risk of disease and its progression, or the estimation of treatment effects at the individual level, based on the subject's shared characteristics with one of the identified subpopulations. This chapter focuses on the study of cognitive decline and brain imaging for precision medicine, and is based on data from the North American ADNI cohort. We aim to identify clusters of subjects with different susceptibility to cognitive decline, based on repeated cognitive scores and baseline MRI volumetric data. However, the clustering analysis of such an observational dataset raises a number of challenges. We describe in this chapter how Bayesian modelling can be used to overcome them successfully.

11.1 Introduction

Precision medicine is an emerging field that aims to improve disease prevention and treatment by accounting for individual variations in genes, lifestyle and environment. Extensive datasets are used to uncover subpopulations with different biological characteristics and susceptibility to the disease or response to treatment (National Research Council, 2011). This finer characterisation is ultimately directed towards the identification of clinical biomarkers, the prediction of the risk of disease and its progression, or the estimation of treatment effects at the individual level, based on the subject's shared characteristics with one of the identified subpopulations.

Statistical tools commonly used for precision medicine purposes include clustering methods, regression modelling, variable selection and dimension reduction techniques. They aim to integrate various data types. In particular, longitudinal data are a key resource for precision medicine when applied to chronic diseases; giving insight into the complex patterns of disease progression, quantifying time-varying exposure to treatments, or facilitating the development of individual-level dynamic disease prediction tools, updated as new biomarker information is collected. Individuals found to be at high risk may benefit from tailored healthcare management, or may be eligible for recruitment into clinical trials.

In the area of longitudinal data, mixture models have played a fundamental role in modelling. In particular, (continuously distributed) random effects in mixed models have been used to account for within patient correlation in repeated measurements and hierarchical (multi-level) structure. These models have been extended to cluster longitudinal data through the use of both discrete and continuously distributed random effects. For example, latent class mixed models (Verbeke and Lesaffre, 1996), which assume a finite mixture of normal distributions for the random effects, have been used extensively to identify a small number of subgroups where the outcome trajectories define these groups. These latent class mixed models have paved the way to several further developments, such as handling non-Gaussian outcomes (Proust-Lima and Jacqmin-Gadda, 2005; Spiessens et al., 2002), modeling multiple outcomes (Muthén and Shedden, 1999; Proust-Lima et al., 2009; Rouanet et al., 2016) and performing inference in a Bayesian setting (Komárek, 2009; Elliott et al., 2005).

This chapter focuses on the study of cognitive decline and brain imaging for precision medicine, and is based on data from the North American ADNI cohort (Mueller et al., 2005). We aim to identify clusters of subjects with different susceptibility to cognitive decline, based on repeated cognitive scores and baseline Magnetic Resonance Imaging (MRI) volumetric data. However, the clustering analysis of such an observational dataset raises a number of challenges. Firstly, there is no clinical evidence regarding the number of longitudinal profiles expected and no actual consensus as to the best statistical criterion for finite mixture model selection. Yet, "optimizing" the number of clusters is a critical part of the analysis to ensure clinical interpretability of results, as there is no single clustering solution. Secondly, quadratic trends are often specified for cognitive patterns but in the possible case these are too restrictive, they could compromise the final partition. Adoption of a flexible modeling approach would ensure the robustness of the model to the misspecification of the longitudinal trend. Finally, the interpretation of results should also account for the uncertainty of the clustering solution, as the clustering structure is latent and recovered from the data. The nonparametric Bayesian framework used in this chapter provides certain advantageous features for tackling these issues. Dirichlet Process Mixture models described by Lo (1984) deal with an unconstrained number of clusters using a nonparametric Dirichlet Process prior (Antoniak, 1974), thus allowing the propagation and quantification of the uncertainty of the clustering allocations. Molitor et al. (2010) extended this method to link nonparametrically an outcome to a set of correlated covariates in their 'profile regression' approach. Finally, Johnson et al. (2020), taking advantage of the flexibility afforded by the use of Gaussian Processes (Rasmussen and Williams, 2006), adapted the profile regression framework to the longitudinal outcome setting.

In the next section, we describe the ADNI dataset that will be used throughout this chapter to illustrate the use of the proposed mixture model. A mathematical representation of the Bayesian features of this model is presented in Section 11.3, followed by a standard frequentist analysis using latent class mixed models and the proposed nonparametric Bayesian profile regression alternative (Molitor et al., 2010) in Sections 11.4 and 11.5 respectively. Section 11.6 concludes the chapter.

11.2 Motivating example

Our work is motivated by the study of Alzheimer's Disease (AD) and cognitive decline. The repeated failure of promising AD drugs to obtain regulatory approval has shifted research towards secondary prevention and clinical trials in individuals at either the pre-clinical or asymptomatic stage of disease where individuals are biomarker positive for AD. There is currently a dearth of disease progression models capable of accurately identifying individuals at 'high risk' of progression to dementia or of rapid cognitive decline. Such models have the potential to reduce screen failures and increase the chance of demonstrating effectiveness in secondary prevention trials. Moreover, their use to identify potential biomarkers that can be surrogates of clinical outcomes in trials would be appealing, as changes in these biomarkers are expected to be seen earlier than the clinical endpoints (especially in pre-clinical and asymptomatic populations). This would enable shorter duration AD trials to be conducted.

The objective of our analysis was to identify meaningful subgroups of subjects with specific trends of cognitive decline and profiles of brain imaging, socio-demographics and genetic characteristics. The data to be used here were obtained from the Alzheimer's Disease Neuroimaging Initiative (ADNI) study (adni.loni.usc.edu). ADNI was launched in 2003 as a public-private partnership with the primary goal of testing whether imaging, biological markers, clinical and neuropsychological assessments can be combined to measure the progression of mild cognitive impairment (MCI) and early AD — for up-to-date information, see `www.adni-info.org`.

For our analysis, we randomly selected 199 subjects who are representative of the overall sample with respect to gender and baseline disease state (cognitively normal, early mild cognitive impairment, late mild cognitive impairment, AD). The selected subjects were aged 55 years and over and 41% were women. Thirty three percent of these subjects had fewer than 16 years of education, while 45% were APOE4 carriers, a genetic trait known to be a major risk factor of AD. Mean age at entry into the ADNI study was 76 years with standard deviation (SD) of 6.3 years. Subjects were followed up over a maximum duration of 8 years, with an average of 5.6 visits per subject (SD = 2 visits). A random subset of individuals was chosen for illustrative purposes and to reduce the computational burden of fitting a Bayesian clustering approach to the data from the full ADNI cohort.

11.2.1 Longitudinal cognitive marker

We considered cognitive functioning as our longitudinal response and focused on the Mini-Mental State Examination (MMSE) cognitive test (Folstein et al., 1975), a 30-point questionnaire assessing different cognitive functioning domains, such as registration, attention, calculation, recall and language. Higher scores indicate higher cognitive levels. The MMSE has ceiling and floor effects (Proust-Lima et al., 2007), thus presenting difficulty in discriminating among subjects with low scores or those with high scores. Moreover, this varying sensitivity to change indicates that a one-point difference in low scores does not have the same clinical meaning as a one-point change in high scores, which violates the linearity assumption of standard linear mixed models. To overcome this problem, we used the monotonic transformation in Figure 11.1, proposed by Philipps et al. (2014), to define a normalized MMSE between 0 and 100 points. Figure 11.2 presents the individual cognitive trajectories of the 199 subjects, on both the original and normalized MMSE scales. We observe that the latter better discriminates subjects for both high and low scores.

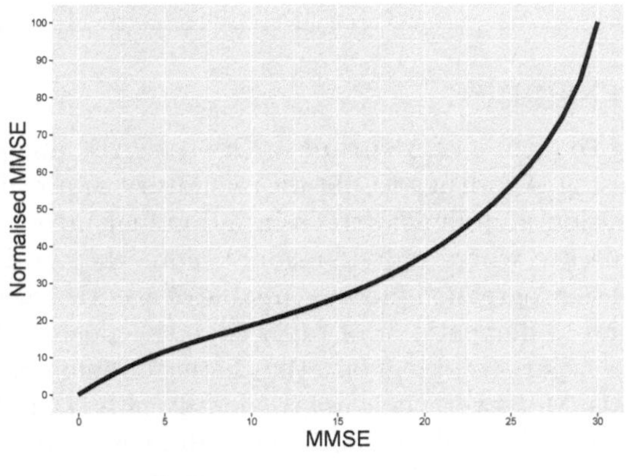

FIGURE 11.1: Normalising transformation for MMSE

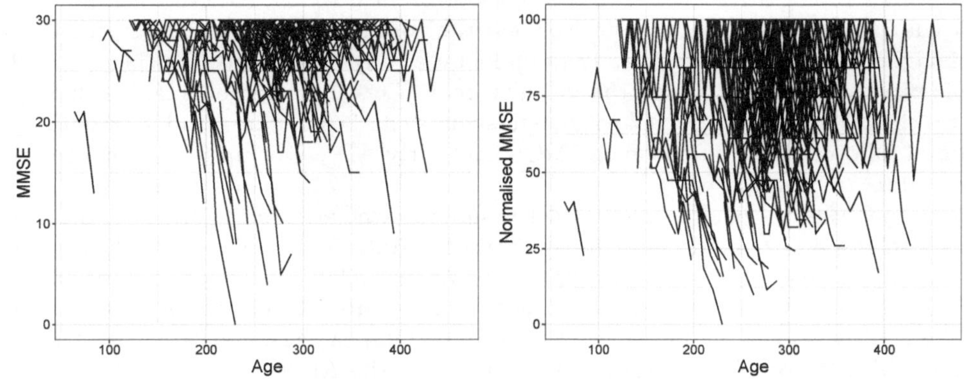

FIGURE 11.2: ADNI cohort: Observed cognitive trajectories of the 199 selected subjects on both the original and normalized MMSE scales.

11.2.2 Baseline imaging markers

ADNI also collected imaging data, including MRI volumetric biomarkers. We consider the volumes of 6 cerebral regions (in cm^3). The ventricles, which include four communicating cavities producing the cerebrospinal fluid; the hippocampus, which is a ridge of grey matter tissue involved in neurogenesis in adults; the entorhinal cortex, an outer layer of grey matter; the fusiform and the middle temporal gyri, which are folds in the cortex; and the whole brain. All these brain regions are known to play key roles in memory (Kempermann et al., 2015; Breteler et al., 1994). We standardized these 6 volumetric imaging biomarkers by the intracranial volume to make them comparable across individuals.

11.2.3 Methodological issues for precision medicine

Even though the concept of precision medicine was first proposed for cancer research, worldwide initiatives have targeted other common disease areas with large societal impact, such as dementia, auto-immune and infectious diseases. Pharmaceutical companies have also recognized the need to go beyond the "one-size-fits-all" paradigm for drug development and so have started to use biomarkers for guiding patient selection and patient population specification, and when designing clinical trials with targeted treatments. One of the main challenges of precision medicine is thus to identify subpopulations that differ in their disease susceptibility or treatment response. Integrating diverse types of data may help better capture the complexity of the disease and refine the granularity of the patient classification.

When using clustering approaches for dementia, the number of clusters has to be driven by the data as there is no prior knowledge or clinical evidence about the number of profiles expected. Several statistical criteria have been proposed for finite mixture model selection such as the Akaike Information Criterion (Akaike, 1998), Bayesian Information Criterion (BIC) (Schwarz, 1978), Deviance Information Criterion (Spiegelhalter et al., 2002), relative entropy (Muthén and Muthén, 2002) or the Minimum Information Ratio (Windham and Cutler, 1992) based on the Fisher information matrix. However, there is no actual consensus as to the best criterion even though the BIC is commonly recommended (Hawkins et al., 2001; Zhang and Cheng, 2004) because of its computational simplicity, effective performance across many modeling areas, connection to Bayes factors for model selection and its tendency to prefer more parsimonious models (Neath and Cavanaugh, 2012). Moreover other aspects, such as the size of the classes and the discriminative ability of the model, may also be considered when deciding on the number of clusters. Needless to say, model selection is a critical part of the analysis process as the estimation of the other parameters is done conditionally on the number of clusters, without necessarily accounting for the uncertainty of the clustering solution.

Furthermore, the estimation procedure should account for the correlation among the cognitive scores at the cluster level. Standard frequentist approaches define, given the cluster allocations, latent processes with cluster-specific polynomial time trends, linked to the individual mean trajectories via continuous link functions. If the polynomial trend is misspecified, the cluster-specific correlation will also be so; thus compromising the clustering solution. Nonparametric Bayesian priors on the cluster-specific underlying processes can offer more flexibility in order to lessen the impact of such misspecification.

In the following section, we mention Bayesian nonparametric features of the proposed model which allow for the uncertainty of the partition, and offer flexibility in modeling longitudinal data.

11.3 Nonparametric Bayesian models

In this section, we introduce the Bayesian Dirichlet Process and Gaussian Process (GP) priors and highlight their advantages for optimizing the number of clusters, quantifying the uncertainty of the clustering solution and modeling longitudinal data.

11.3.1 Dirichlet Process prior for unconstrained number of clusters

Let $\boldsymbol{W}_i$ be the vector of the nine baseline profile variables including the six standardized MRI brain imaging, Gender, Education and APOE4 carrier status, and $\boldsymbol{Y}_i$ be the vector of the longitudinal normalized MMSE for subject i, $i = 1, \dots, N$. A Dirichlet Process Mixture Model (DPMM) is a mixture model with a Dirichlet Process (distribution over probability measures) as prior for the cluster weights. It can be considered as the limit of the following parametric mixture model when the number of components G tends to infinity:

$$\begin{aligned} \boldsymbol{Y}_i, \boldsymbol{W}_i \mid c_i &\sim f(\boldsymbol{Y}_i, \boldsymbol{W}_i \mid \Theta_{c_i}) \\ \Theta_{c_i} &\sim F_0 \\ c_i \mid \boldsymbol{\pi} &\sim \text{Categorical}(\pi_1, \dots, \pi_G) \\ \boldsymbol{\pi} \mid \alpha &\sim \text{Dir}(\alpha/G, \dots, \alpha/G) \end{aligned} \tag{11.1}$$

The joint conditional density function $f(\cdot \mid \Theta_{c_i})$ is parameterized by the latent random parameter Θ_{c_i} with a prior distribution F_0; c_i denotes the latent cluster membership variable with a discrete distribution such that $\Pr(c_i = g \mid \boldsymbol{\pi}) = \pi_g$.

Although this formulation assumes an infinite number of clusters, the number of non-empty ones is actually finite. The positive concentration hyperparameter α, typically assumed fixed or drawn from a Gamma distribution as suggested by Escobar and West (1995), influences the distribution of the cluster weights and the probability to observe new non-empty clusters. Different ways to represent and build a Dirichlet Process (with parameters F_0 and α) have been proposed, the most commonly used being the Chinese restaurant process (Aldous, 1985) and the stick-breaking one (Sethuraman, 1994). DPMM have been used in various applications, handling different types of data and demonstrating good performance in recovering the clustering structure (Hejblum et al., 2019).

11.3.2 Gaussian Process prior for flexible longitudinal modelling

Let Y_{ij} denote the normalized MMSE score for individual i, $i = 1, \dots, N$ at occasion j, $j = 1, \dots, n_i$ and time t_{ij}. This observed score can be considered as a noisy measurement of the underlying cognitive process $\eta_g(\cdot)$, given the cluster g:

$$Y_{ij} = \eta_g(t_{ij}) + \epsilon_{ij}, \tag{11.2}$$

with Gaussian measurement errors $(\epsilon_{i1}, \dots, \epsilon_{in_i}) \sim \text{N}(0, \nu_{g,1}\, \boldsymbol{I}_{n_i \times n_i})$, where $\boldsymbol{I}$ denotes the identity matrix and $\nu_{g,1}$ the measurement error variance. A Gaussian Process prior (Rasmussen and Williams, 2006) can be adopted for the cluster-specific cognitive process to add flexibility. A GP is a distribution over functions, more specifically an infinite set of random variables of which every finite collection has a joint multivariate Gaussian distribution. It can be used within a Bayesian regression framework to flexibly model longitudinal outcomes. This distribution over functions is parameterized by mean and covariance functions. Thus, given cluster g,

$$\eta_g(\cdot) \sim \text{GP}\left(m_g(\cdot), \mathcal{K}_g(\cdot, \cdot)\right), \tag{11.3}$$

with the mean function for the GP prior, $m_g(\cdot)$, set to the null function (i.e. 0) and a class-specific squared exponential covariance function defined as $\mathcal{K}_g(t, t') = Cov\left(\eta_g(t), \eta_g(t')\right) = \nu_{g,2} \exp\big(-(t - t')^2/(2\nu_{g,3})\big)$ for any two timepoints t and t'. Figure 11.3 provides an illustration of samples from a Gaussian Process with non-null mean and squared exponential covariance functions. The hyperparameter $\nu_{g,2} > 0$ is the signal variance while the length scale $\nu_{g,3}$ controls the correlation decay rate between neighboring timepoints. Log-Normal priors can be adopted for $\nu_{g,1}$, $\nu_{g,2}$ and $\nu_{g,3}$ to ensure positivity. The correlation among the cognitive scores is captured at the individual and cluster levels via the $\mathcal{K}_g(\cdot, \cdot)$ function.

Finally, the mean and variance of the posterior Gaussian Process can be calculated analytically, providing a complete description of the distribution of the outcome predictions (including uncertainty measures). Gaussian processes are particularly popular in longitudinal modeling for their flexibility using only a few parameters, their simplicity and efficiency.

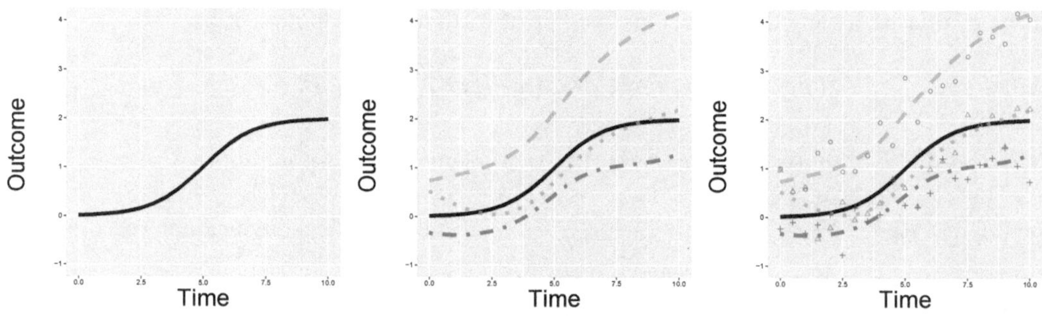

FIGURE 11.3: Illustration of samples from a Gaussian Process prior. Left: Cluster mean function (corresponding to m_g) in solid black line. Center: Three individual mean trajectories (corresponding to $\eta_g(t_i)$) in broken solid lines. Right: Individual measurements with error for the same 3 individuals (corresponding to $\eta_g(t_i) + \epsilon_i$) denoted as points.

11.3.3 Uncertainty propagation and quantification

In finite frequentist mixture models, we obtain a likelihood-based point estimate of the partition and, given this partition, subjects are assigned to the class with the highest membership probability (given their individual observations). In contrast, DP mixture models provide the full posterior distribution of the partition, propagating the uncertainty of the clustering solution to the estimation of the other parameters.

More specifically, the selection procedure for the final representative clustering structure is based on the $N \times N$ posterior similarity matrix S, which contains the estimated posterior co-clustering probabilities for all pairs of subjects. Each element (i, j) of this matrix is the proportion of iterations subjects i and j are allocated to the same cluster across all MCMC iterations. In order to find the optimal partition that best represents S, we apply the Partitioning Around Medoids (PAM) algorithm (Kaufman and Rousseeuw, 2005) to the posterior dissimilarity matrix $1 - S$, which robustly assigns individuals to clusters in a way consistent with S. That is, for a fixed number of clusters, PAM is applied to the dissimilarity matrix with the goal of minimising the overall dissimilarity between each cluster's center and its members. PAM is implemented for each possible number of clusters up to a prespecified maximum and for each number, a 'best' PAM partition is selected. The final representative/optimal partition is determined by maximizing the average silhouette width (Rousseeuw, 1987) across all the 'best' PAM partitions.

Once the optimal representative partition is selected, the parameters of each cluster are evaluated by averaging across all subjects allocated to that cluster over all the MCMC iterations. For example, the measurement error variance $\nu_{g,1}$ in cluster g is estimated by

$$\widehat{\nu}_{g,1} = \frac{1}{N_g^{opt}} \sum_{k=1}^{K} \sum_{i=1}^{N_g^{opt}} \nu_{c_i^{(k)},1}^{(k)} \tag{11.4}$$

where K is the total number of MCMC iterations, N_g^{opt} is the size of cluster g in the optimal representative partition and $\nu_{c_i^{(k)},1}^{(k)}$ is the sampled measurement error variance for the cluster $c_i^{(k)}$ that subject i (belonging to cluster g in the best partition) is allocated to in the $k-$th MCMC iteration. Summary estimates of cluster parameters for the profile variables can be obtained similarly. In addition, the representative longitudinal trajectories of these clusters can be evaluated at any T-dimensional vector of (ordered) timepoints $\boldsymbol{\tau}$ by

$$\widehat{\boldsymbol{Y}}_g(\boldsymbol{\tau}) = \boldsymbol{\mathcal{K}}_g\left(\boldsymbol{\tau}, \boldsymbol{\tau}^{(g)}\right) \left[\boldsymbol{\mathcal{K}}_g\left(\boldsymbol{\tau}^{(g)}, \boldsymbol{\tau}^{(g)}\right) + \widehat{\nu}_{g,1}\, \boldsymbol{I}\right]^{-1} \boldsymbol{Y}^{(g)}, \tag{11.5}$$

where the $T \times T^{(g)}$ matrix, $\boldsymbol{\mathcal{K}}_g\left(\boldsymbol{\tau}, \boldsymbol{\tau}^{(g)}\right)$, has (i,j) element corresponding to $\mathcal{K}_g\left(\tau_i, \tau_j^{(g)}\right) = Cov\left(\eta_g(\tau_i), \eta_g(\tau_j^{(g)})\right) = \widehat{\nu}_{g,2} \exp\Big(-\dfrac{(\tau_i - \tau_j^{(g)})^2}{2\widehat{\nu}_{g,3}}\Big)$; and the $T^{(g)}$-dimensional vectors $\boldsymbol{\tau}^{(g)}$ and $\boldsymbol{Y}^{(g)}$ correspond to the vectorization of the sets $\{t_i : i \in \text{cluster } g \text{ of the optimal partition}\}$ and $\{\boldsymbol{Y}_i : i \in \text{cluster } g \text{ of the optimal partition}\}$ respectively.

11.3.4 Profile regression for longitudinal data

Profile regression is a Bayesian infinite mixture model that nonparametrically links a response to a set of correlated covariates through cluster membership (Molitor et al., 2010). By capturing the heterogeneity among the covariates, the idea is to identify covariate profiles (combination of covariate values), representative of the clusters, and to associate them with the outcome via a regression model, hence the name 'profile regression'. Note that the joint modeling of the correlated covariates and the outcome enables the outcome to inform the clustering as well. Molitor et al. (2010) use a Dirichlet Process prior for the parameters of the mixture model, allowing the number of clusters to vary across the iterations of the MCMC sampler. This advantage is twofold as it enables the propagation of the uncertainty of the cluster allocations using the Markov Chain Monte Carlo sampler and assessment of the uncertainty of the final clustering solution via postprocessing methods. The `PReMiuM` package (Liverani et al., 2015) implements profile regression for Gaussian, binary, ordinal, categorical, Poisson or survival outcomes and Gaussian or discrete profile variables. Johnson et al. (2020) extended `PReMiuM` to accommodate a longitudinal Gaussian outcome, collected at subject-specific timepoints, using Gaussian Process priors. Figure 11.4 is a directed graph summarising the relationships between the components of the profile regression model for longitudinal data with irregular observation timepoints. Note that in this extension, the longitudinal outcome and the covariate profiles are no longer linked via a regression model, but through the cluster membership only.

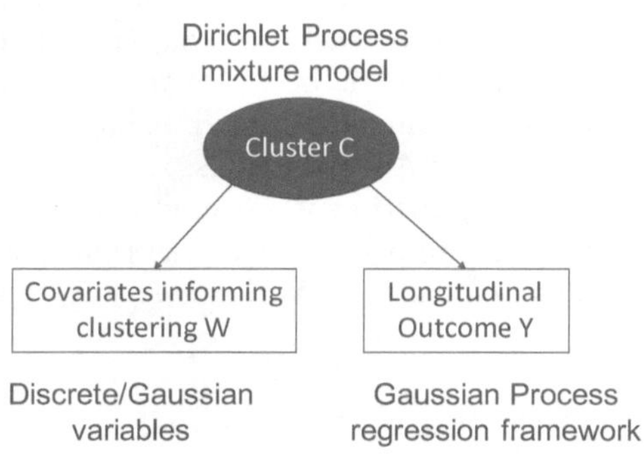

FIGURE 11.4: Graphical representation of profile regression. Ovals and squares represent unobserved and observed variables respectively.

The `PReMiuM` package handles Gaussian and/or discrete profile variables. In our application, the individual profile covariate vector $\boldsymbol{W}_i = (W_{i1}^\top, W_{i2}^\top)^\top$ is composed of W_{i1} the individual vector of the three binary covariates (Gender, Education and APOE4) and W_{i2}

the individual vector of the six continuous MRI variables. Assuming that W_{i1} and each of the profile variables are conditionally independent given the cluster g, we can write:

$$\begin{aligned} W_{i1q} &\sim \text{Bern}(\phi_{gq}), \ q = 1, 2, 3; \\ W_{i2} &\sim \mathcal{N}_6(\mu_g, \Sigma_g). \end{aligned} \tag{11.6}$$

The joint posterior distribution of the parameters and hyperparameters is thus written as follows:

$$\begin{aligned} p(\boldsymbol{c}, \boldsymbol{\Theta}, \boldsymbol{\pi}, \alpha \mid \boldsymbol{Y}, W) \propto \prod_{i=1}^{N} \{ & f_Y(\boldsymbol{Y}_i \mid \theta^Y_{c_i}) \times f_{\boldsymbol{W}_1}(W_{i1} \mid \theta^{W_1}_{c_i}) \times \\ & f_{\boldsymbol{W}_2}(W_{i2} \mid \theta^{W_2}_{c_i}) \times p(c_i \mid \boldsymbol{\pi}) \} \times \\ & \prod_{g=1}^{\infty} \{ p(\pi_g \mid \alpha) p(\Theta_g) \} p(\alpha), \end{aligned} \tag{11.7}$$

with $\boldsymbol{\Theta}$ the vector of all the parameters to be estimated by the model (but α) and $\mathbf{c}$ the vector of cluster allocations of the N subjects. Then, $f_Y(\cdot \mid \theta^Y_{c_i})$, $f_{\boldsymbol{W}_1}(\cdot \mid \theta^{W_2}_{c_i})$ and $f_{\boldsymbol{W}_2}(\cdot \mid \theta^{W_1}_{c_i})$ correspond to the distributions of $\boldsymbol{Y}_i$, W_{i1} and W_{i2} given c_i respectively, associated with the parameters $\theta^Y_{c_i}$, $\theta^{W_1}_{c_i}$ and $\theta^{W_2}_{c_i}$. Here θ^Y_g denotes the set $\{\eta_g(\cdot), \nu_{g,1}\}$ and $\theta^{W_1}_g$ and $\theta^{W_2}_g$ represent the sets $\{\mu_g, \Sigma_g\}$ and $\{\phi^q_g : q = 1, \ldots, 3\}$, respectively.

The profile regression model is fitted via Markov Chain Monte Carlo (MCMC) using a blocked Gibbs sampler. Details of the full conditionals are found in Johnson et al. (2020). A slice sampler (Kalli et al., 2011) is used to update the cluster allocations, and the hyperparameters of measurement errors and the GPs, $\nu_{g,1}$, $\nu_{g,2}$ and $\nu_{g,3}$, are sampled using Metropolis-within-Gibbs steps. We use the label switching move proposed by Hastie et al. (2015) to ensure good mixing behaviour in the MCMC sampler using the stick-breaking construction.

11.4 Standard frequentist analysis: Latent class mixed models

We begin by first considering the classical framework for mixture models. Here we fitted a latent class mixed model (Proust-Lima et al., 2017) to the 199 randomly sampled individuals from the ADNI cohort in order to identify meaningful clusters with different cognitive patterns, quantified by repeated normalized MMSE scores. Based on the assumption that the population can be divided into G unknown subgroups, called latent classes, this model combines a multinomial logistic regression model for the class membership probabilities and a mixed model for the longitudinal outcome. No covariates were included in the class membership probability model. A quadratic time trend was specified for the normalized MMSE cognitive marker, given each latent class $g = 1, \ldots, G$:

$$\begin{aligned} \text{normMMSE}_{ij} =& \beta_{0g} + \beta_{1g} \text{ age}_{ij} + \beta_{2g} \text{ age}^2_{ij} + u_{i0g} + u_{i1g} \text{ age}_{ij} + u_{i2g} \text{ age}^2_{ij} \\ & + \beta_3 \text{ Gender}_i + \beta_4 \text{ APOE4}_i + \beta_{5g} \text{ Learn}_{ij} + \beta_{6g} \text{ Educ}_i + \epsilon_{ij} \end{aligned}$$

with three random effects for the quadratic time trend $(u_{i0g}, u_{i1g}, u_{i2g})^T \sim \mathcal{N}_3(\mathbf{0}, \sigma^2_g B)$ and measurement errors $\epsilon_{ij} \sim \mathcal{N}(0, \sigma^2_\epsilon)$. Time t_{ij} for individual $i = 1, \ldots, N$, at occasion $j = 1, \ldots, n_i$ was defined as the age (in decades) centered around 55 years, men were the reference class for Gender and Educ and APOE4 were dichotomized (0 if fewer than 16 years of education and 1 otherwise; 0 if no APOE4 alleles, 1 otherwise). We accounted for a class-specific learning effect after the first interview, observed in previous studies on cognitive tests (Jacqmin-Gadda et al., 1997), using the covariate $\text{Learn}_{ij} = \mathbb{1}_{(t_{ij}>0)}$; and also included a class-specific education effect.

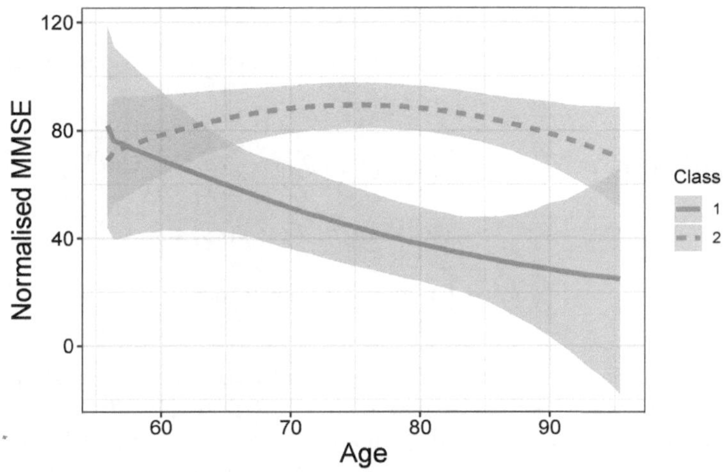

FIGURE 11.5: Class-specific mean trajectories estimated by the two-latent class mixed model, on the normalized MMSE scale, as a function of age for a man with no APOE4 alleles and fewer than 16 years of education. The shaded regions represent 95% confidence bands.

The number of latent classes was chosen based on the BIC criterion. We fitted latent class mixed models with 1 to 4 classes that gave BIC values of 9197, 9172, 9185 and 9210 respectively. We selected the model with the smallest BIC value. This separated the sample into two latent classes with different cognitive trends. The first class (48.2% of the sample) had a steep cognitive decline, as shown in Figure 11.5, and is referred to as a 'cognitive decliners' class. The second class (51.8% of the sample) experienced a steady cognitive evolution with age and was labelled as 'cognitively stable'. The discrimination of this model was found to be satisfactory as the mean posterior probability of belonging to Class 1 among subjects allocated to Class 1 was 91.1% and the corresponding mean posterior probability of belonging to Class 2 among those allocated to Class 2 was 85.2%. Estimates of the regression coefficients associated with the covariates are displayed in Table 11.1. APOE4 carriers, as expected, have, on average, lower normalized MMSE values than non-carriers, and women tend to have, on average, a higher cognitive level than men, controlling for the other covariates. Higher education is associated with higher cognitive level, especially in the 'cognitive decliners' class (Class 1).

On comparing the six standardized MRI volumetric imaging biomarkers between the two classes (Table 11.2), we observe that Class 1 of 'cognitive decliners' comprises individuals who, on average, have statistically significantly higher standardized volumetric measurements of ventricles and lower volumes of hippocampus, entorhinal cortex, fusiform and midtemporal gyri and whole brain, when compared to the Class 2 'cognitively stable' individuals.

These findings and the use of these models enable adoption of a precision medicine approach to identifying high risk individuals (e.g. those in Class 1) for recruitment into Alzheimer's Disease secondary prevention clinical trials and for predicting subjects'

TABLE 11.1: Regression parameter estimates, standard errors and P-values from the two-latent-class mixed model.

	$\widehat{\beta}$	SE($\widehat{\beta}$)	P-value
APOE4	-0.56	0.178	0.002
Gender	0.31	0.171	0.072
Educ Class1	1.73	0.673	0.010
Educ Class2	0.18	0.409	0.662

TABLE 11.2: Description of the standardized imaging markers using their means (standard deviations) by the two latent classes, with associated Student's 2-sample t-test P-values for comparing between classes.

Variable	Class 1	Class 2	P-value
s.Ventricles	0.20 (1.11)	-0.19 (0.84)	0.006
s.Hippocampus	-0.47 (0.94)	0.44 (0.85)	$< 10^{-3}$
s.Entorhinal	-0.47 (0.98)	0.44 (0.81)	$< 10^{-3}$
s.Fusiform	-0.33 (1.01)	0.31 (0.89)	$< 10^{-3}$
s.MidTemp	-0.33 (1.07)	0.31 (0.83)	$< 10^{-3}$
s.WholeBrain	-0.26 (1.03)	0.24 (0.91)	$< 10^{-3}$

subsequent trajectories based on MMSE, APOE4, gender and educational attainment. Our findings also suggest that baseline imaging biomarkers could help identify individuals belonging to the 'cognitive decliners' class.

11.5 Profile regression analysis

We applied the alternative nonparametric Bayesian profile regression to the same ADNI subsample. We considered two approaches to using profile regression with the ADNI data, to highlight the benefit of the Dirichlet Process prior and the Gaussian Process regression framework. We first considered a two-stage approach, whereby a summary of the normalized MMSE is used as the outcome, and then considered modeling the normalized MMSE with a GP. In both approaches, the correlation among cognitive scores was accounted for at both the cluster and the individual levels and the clustering structure was also profiled across the six standardized MRI volumetric imaging variables, APOE4 carrier status, gender and educational attainment status.

11.5.1 Integrative analysis of summarized cognitive and imaging data

In the two-step profile regression approach, we first fitted a linear mixed effects model to the normalized MMSE scores:

$$\text{normMMSE}_{ij} = \beta_0 + u_{i0} + \beta_1 \text{ age}_{ij} + u_{i1} \text{ age}_{ij} + \epsilon_{ij},$$

with $u_i \sim \mathcal{N}_2(0, B)$, $\epsilon_{ij} \sim \mathcal{N}_2(0, \sigma_e^2)$ and extracted the two-dimensional summary

$$\boldsymbol{Y}_i = (\widehat{u}_{i0}, \widehat{u}_{i1})^\top = \text{E}((u_{i0}, u_{i1})^\top \mid \boldsymbol{Y}_i; \widehat{\beta}_0, \widehat{\beta}_1, \widehat{B}, \widehat{\sigma}_e),$$

the empirical Bayes random effects estimates for the random intercept, u_{i0}, and random slope, u_{i1}.

In the second step, we used this bivariate summary $\boldsymbol{Y}$ as the outcome (instead of norm-MMSE) in profile regression, modelled by a multivariate normal distribution given the cluster g: $\boldsymbol{Y}_i \sim \mathcal{N}_2(\mu_g^u, \Sigma_g^u)$. The nine profile variables were modelled as in Equation (11.6).

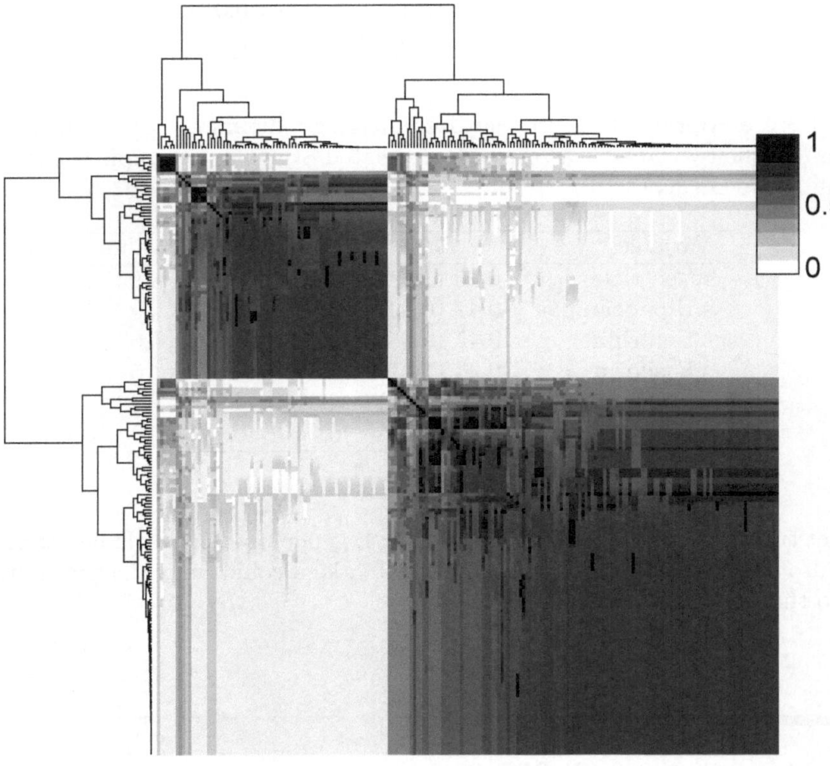

FIGURE 11.6: Posterior similarity matrix obtained by profile regression on random intercepts and slopes and profile variables. This identified 2 clusters comprising 70 (35.2%) and 129 subjects (64.8%) respectively.

Figure 11.6 displays the posterior similarity matrix across the 50,000 MCMC iterations. This suggests that there are 2 clusters of 70 and 129 subjects respectively. As shown in Figure 11.7, the first cluster is associated with lower random slopes compared to the second cluster, and relatively higher random intercepts. Thus, subjects in the first cluster experience a steeper decline, according to this linear approximation of the cognitive trajectories. Note that the fixed effect estimates of the intercept and slope from the fitted linear mixed effects model described in step 1 were 96.8 and -11.4 points per decade respectively. These estimates correspond to the zero values of the y-axes in the box-plots for the random intercept and random slope of Figure 11.7, respectively. Thus Cluster 1 can be characterized as a higher baseline cognitively functioning group with more rapid (relative to Cluster 2) cognitive decline. Cluster 2 can be described as a high baseline cognitive functioning group with a slower cognitive decline.

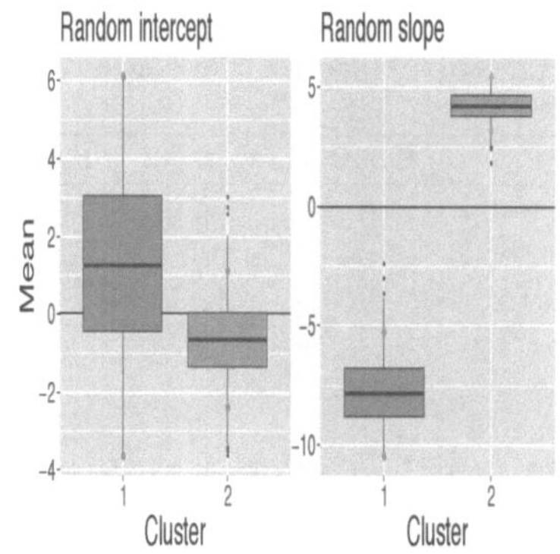

FIGURE 11.7: Posterior cluster-specific distributions of the mean of the multivariate outcome corresponding to random intercepts and random slopes, obtained by profile regression.

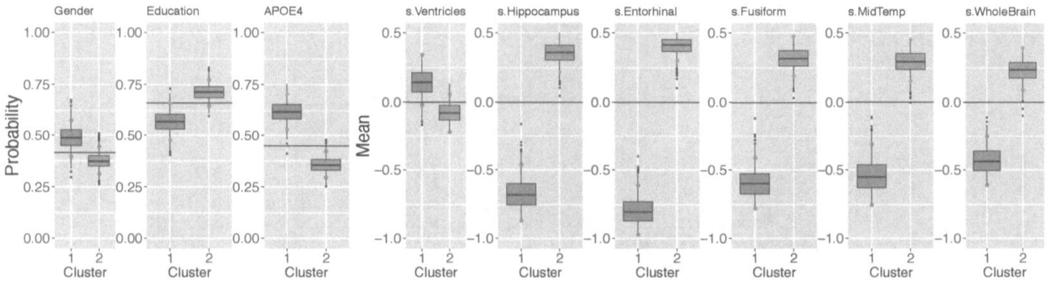

FIGURE 11.8: Posterior distributions of the mean parameters for brain volumetric variables for the representative clustering, for profile regression on random intercepts and slopes.

Figure 11.8 presents for the representative partition ($g = 1, 2$), the posterior distributions of the parameters for the continuous and binary profile variables. The first three graphs correspond to the probability of observing category 1 (female, 16 years or more of education, and at least one APOE4 allele), $\phi_g^q(1)$, for each binary variable $q = 1, 2, 3$ (gender, education and APOE4). The remaining six graphs show the mean parameter μ_g for each continuous brain volumetric imaging variable. We thus define the profile of each cluster by the combination of their mean profile variable values. Subjects in the first cluster have a higher standardized ventricle volume and lower standardized hippocampus, entorhinal cortex, fusiform and middle temporal gyri and whole brain volumes. These results are consistent with previous findings, showing that dementia is associated with a higher ventricle volume (Breteler et al., 1994) and an atrophy of the hippocampus (den Heijer et al., 2010), entorhinal cortex (Du et al., 2004; Velayudhan et al., 2013), fusiform gyrus (Galton et al., 2001), middle temporal gyrus (Convit et al., 2000) and the whole brain (Chan et al., 2003; Ridha et al., 2006). Moreover, we observe a higher proportion of women in the first cluster, as well as a higher prevalence of APOE4 carriers and a lower proportion with 16 years or more education. Table 11.3 compares this clustering structure to the latent class structure presented in Section 11.4 using the two-latent-class mixed model. The two derived partitions match on 79% of the sample.

TABLE 11.3: Cross-tabulation of the clustering structures obtained by latent class linear mixed model (Classes 1 and 2) and bivariate profile regression (Clusters 1 and 2).

	Class 1	Class 2	Total
Cluster 1	62	8	70
Cluster 2	34	95	129
Total	96	103	

11.5.2 Integrative analysis of longitudinal cognitive and imaging data

In our final analysis, we modelled the entire normalized MMSE trajectory using cluster-specific functions with Gaussian Process priors, as defined in (11.2) and (11.3), thus accounting for the correlation among the cognitive scores at both the individual and cluster levels. The 9 profile variables were modelled as in (11.6), as in the previous Profile Regression analysis.

Figure 11.9 shows the posterior similarity matrix. The identified optimal representative partition by the GP model consisted of four clusters comprising 57, 55, 44, and 43 subjects respectively.

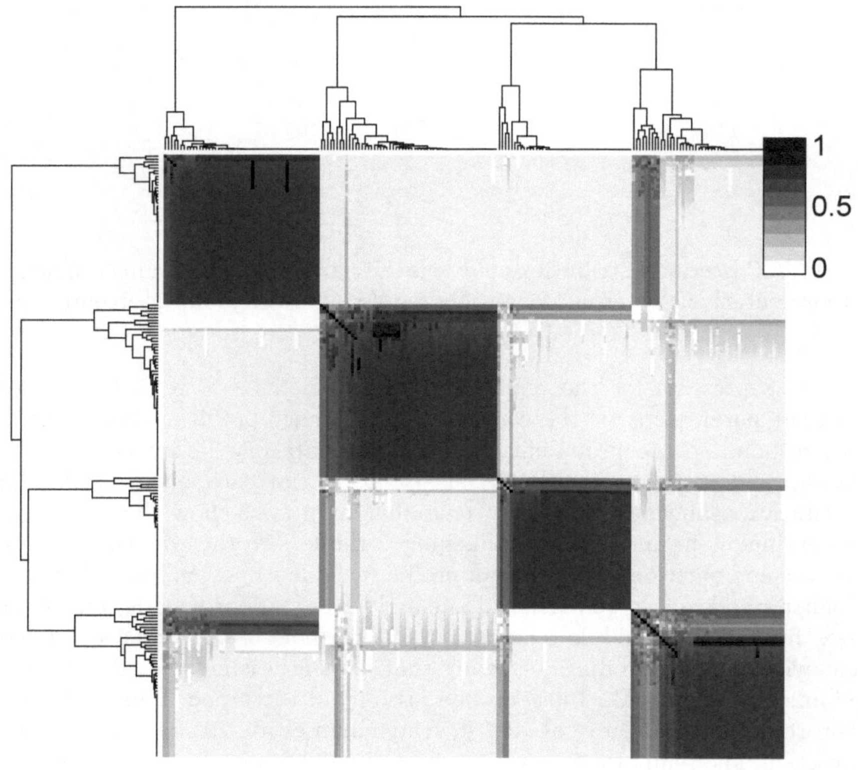

FIGURE 11.9: Posterior similarity matrix obtained by profile regression on repeated normalized MMSE scores and volumetric imaging biomarkers, identifying 4 clusters of 57 (28.6%), 55 (27.6%), 44 (22.1%) and 43 (21.6%) subjects, respectively.

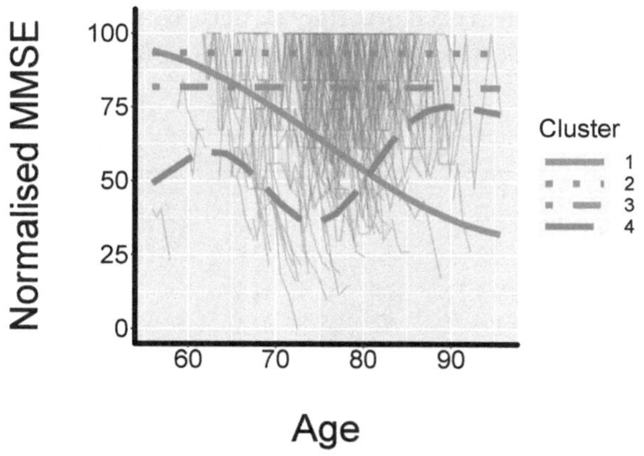

FIGURE 11.10: Class-specific trajectories obtained by the profile regression model (thick lines) and observed trajectories (thin lines) in the sub-sample, in the normalized MMSE scale.

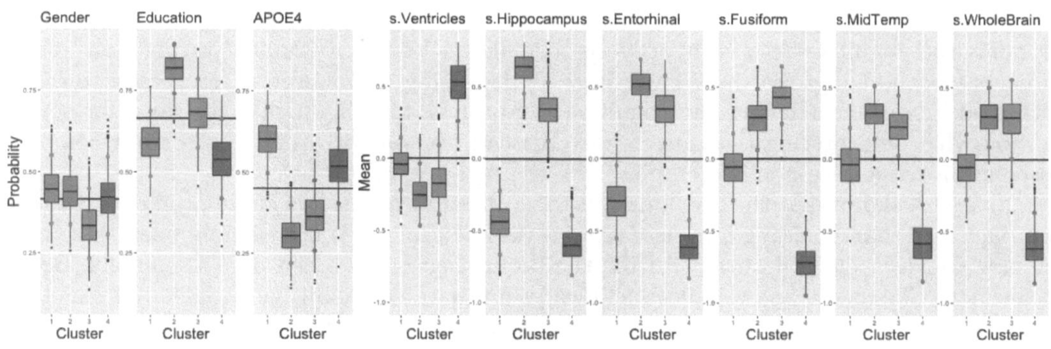

FIGURE 11.11: Posterior distributions of the mean parameters for imaging profile variables for the representative clustering, for profile regression on repeated normalized MMSE scores.

As shown in Figures 11.10 and 11.11, subjects in the first cluster on average have a steep cognitive decline and are characterized by 'average' levels of standardized volumes of ventricles, fusiform, middle temporal gyri and whole brain and low levels of standardized volumes of hippocampus and entorhinal cortex. Additionally, in this cluster, there is a high prevalence of APOE4 carriers and a relatively low proportion of individuals with 16 years or more of education. Gender does not seem to discriminate between the clusters.

The second and third clusters represent 'cognitively unimpaired' subjects, with stable cognitive evolutions but differing baseline cognitive levels that are within the cognitively normal ceiling range (75 to 100 points on the normalized MMSE scale; 28 to 30 points on MMSE scale). The imaging profiles of these two clusters are similar, with low standardized ventricle volume and high volumes for the 5 other brain regions. The second cluster has a higher proportion of highly educated subjects, which may explain the higher cognitive score, and a slightly lower proportion of APOE4 carriers.

TABLE 11.4: Cross-tabulation of the clustering structures obtained by profile regression based on a GP model (rows: Clusters 1 to 4) and the two-stage profile regression approach (columns: Clusters 1 and 2).

	Cluster 1	Cluster 2	Total
Cluster 1	33	24	57
Cluster 2	2	53	55
Cluster 3	6	38	44
Cluster 4	29	14	43
Total	70	129	

Finally, the fourth cluster has a peculiar pattern of cognitive evolution. Further investigations revealed that it contains two subgroups observed during two non-overlapping age ranges. A group with a steep cognitive decline, followed-up between 65 and 80 years old and a second one with a steady evolution, observed from 80 years onwards. However, these two subgroups were allocated to a common cluster as they both had particularly high standardized volumes of ventricles and as well as similarly low standardized volumes of hippocampus, entorhinal cortex, fusiform middle temporal gyri and whole brain. This supports the cognitive reserve hypothesis formulated by Stern (2009), stating that some subjects (second subgroup) may have more ability, using compensatory processes, to cope with brain damage, delaying the cognitive symptoms. This highlights the need for some caution when interpreting the clusters, as GPs can over-smooth the trajectories when the observation ranges are non overlapping.

Table 11.4 shows that the previous Cluster 1 obtained in our two-stage profile regression approach and characterising a rapid cognitive decline group has now mainly been split into the new Clusters 1 and 4 obtained from the profile regression based on a GP model. Both of the new Clusters 1 and 4 reflect 'clinically undesirable' cognitive profiles. Of the 129 subjects allocated to Cluster 2 based on the two-stage profile regression approach, 70.2% were allocated to new Clusters 2 and 3, which reflect stable cognitive evolution.

These results illustrate the potential gain of using directly the observed longitudinal cognitive measurements as the response over using a simple bivariate summary, such as the estimated random intercept and random slope, in profile regression. The information provided by the longitudinal outcome and the profile variables enabled a more refined stratification of the population. The profiles of the clusters give insight into the heterogeneity in the cognitive evolution and highlight significant differences between the declining and stable clusters in education, APOE4 carrier status and standardized volumes of the 6 cerebral regions. These results could be extended to account for genetic information to associate genetic profiles with these clusters and identify the genes that drive the mixture components, thus providing a further example of the benefit of using profile regression for precision medicine.

11.6 Conclusion

In conclusion, mixture models have considerable potential for precision medicine. They enable identification of homogeneous subgroups of the population from patterns of (repeated) data; provide individual-level probabilities for cluster membership, given a defined clustering structure; and allow the description and individual-level prediction of the longitudinal response over time. These clustering and prediction tools can be directed towards the recruitment into trials, used to target treatment or patient management strategies to the appropriate individuals, or to identify relevant biomarkers for disease evolution.

Both latent class mixed models and profile regression can handle longitudinal outcomes measured at subject-specific timepoints. However the Bayesian framework presents numerous advantages for recovering the clustering structure from longitudinal data. Firstly, non-parametric Bayesian Gaussian Process priors offer substantial flexiblity in the modeling of longitudinal data, with only a few parameters, and are easy to use as their predictions take the form of full posterior distributions, providing both mean and variability measures. Second, profile regression allows both the number and constitution of the clusters to vary across MCMC iterations. Thus uncertainty regarding the clustering can be quantified and propagated in the estimation of the other parameters. This helps characterise the discrimination of the model and confirm the interpretability of the results. Note that for predictive purposes, the interpretability of the results is less critical; however, the quantification of the predictions is of great interest.

Acknowledgements

We thank both Paul Kirk and Robert Goudie for their careful reading of the manuscript and helpful comments. Sylvia Richardson was funded by the UK Medical Research Council programme MRC_MC_UU_00002/10. Brian Tom was funded by the UK Medical Research Council programme MRC_MC_UU_00002/2. Anaïs Rouanet, Sylvia Richardson and Brian Tom were supported by the MRC-funded Dementias Platform UK (RG74590). Data collection and sharing for this project was funded by the Alzheimer's Disease Neuroimaging Initiative (ADNI) (National Institutes of Health Grant U01 AG024904) and DOD ADNI (Department of Defense award number W81XWH-12-2-0012).

ADNI is funded by the National Institute on Aging, the National Institute of Biomedical Imaging and Bioengineering, and through generous contributions from the following: AbbVie, Alzheimer's Association; Alzheimer's Drug Discovery Foundation; Araclon Biotech; BioClinica, Inc.; Biogen; Bristol-Myers Squibb Company; CereSpir, Inc.; Cogstate; Eisai Inc.; Elan Pharmaceuticals, Inc.; Eli Lilly and Company; EuroImmun; F. Hoffmann - La Roche Ltd and its affiliated company Genentech, Inc.; Fujirebio; GE Healthcare; IXICO Ltd.; Janssen Alzheimer Immunotherapy Research & Development, LLC.; Johnson & Johnson Pharmaceutical Research & Development LLC.; Lumosity; Lundbeck; Merck & Co., Inc.; Meso Scale Diagnostics, LLC.; NeuroRx Research; Neurotrack Technologies; Novartis Pharmaceuticals Corporation; Pfizer Inc.; Piramal Imaging; Servier; Takeda Pharmaceutical Company; and Transition Therapeutics.

Bibliography

Akaike, H. (1998). Information theory and an extension of the maximum likelihood principle. In *Selected Papers of Hirotugu Akaike*, pages 199–213. Springer.

Aldous, D. J. (1985). Exchangeability and related topics. In *École d'Été de Probabilités de Saint-Flour XIII-1983*, pages 1–198. Springer.

Antoniak, C. E. (1974). Mixtures of Dirichlet processes with applications to Bayesian nonparametric problems. *The Annals of Statistics*, 2(6):1152–1174.

Breteler, M., van Amerongen, N., van Swieten, J., Claus, J., Grobbee, D., van Gijn, J., Hofman, A., and van Harskamp, F. (1994). Cognitive correlates of ventricular enlargement and cerebral white matter lesions on magnetic resonance imaging. The Rotterdam study. *Stroke*, 25(6):1109–1115.

Chan, D., Janssen, J. C., Whitwell, J. L., Watt, H. C., Jenkins, R., Frost, C., Rossor, M. N., and Fox, N. C. (2003). Change in rates of cerebral atrophy over time in early-onset Alzheimer's disease: longitudinal MRI study. *The Lancet*, 362(9390):1121–1122.

Convit, A., de Asis, J., de Leon, M., Tarshish, C., De Santi, S., and Rusinek, H. (2000). Atrophy of the medial occipitotemporal, inferior, and middle temporal gyri in non-demented elderly predict decline to Alzheimer's disease. *Neurobiology of Aging*, 21(1):19–26.

den Heijer, T., van der Lijn, F., Koudstaal, P., Hofman, A., van der Lugt, A., Krestin, G., Niessen, W., and Breteler, M. (2010). A 10-year follow-up of hippocampal volume on magnetic resonance imaging in early dementia and cognitive decline. *Brain*, 133(4):1163–1172.

Du, A., Schuff, N., Kramer, J., Ganzer, S., Zhu, X., Jagust, W., Miller, B., Reed, B., Mungas, D., Yaffe, K., Chui, H., and Weiner, M. (2004). Higher atrophy rate of entorhinal cortex than hippocampus in AD. *Neurology*, 62(3):422–427.

Elliott, M. R., Gallo, J. J., Ten Have, T. R., Bogner, H. R., and Katz, I. R. (2005). Using a Bayesian latent growth curve model to identify trajectories of positive affect and negative events following myocardial infarction. *Biostatistics*, 6(1):119–143.

Escobar, M. D. and West, M. (1995). Bayesian density estimation and inference using mixtures. *Journal of the American Statistical Association*, 90(430):577–588.

Folstein, M. F., Folstein, S. E., and McHugh, P. R. (1975). Mini-mental state: A practical method for grading the cognitive state of patients for the clinician. *Journal of Psychiatric Research*, 12(3):189–198.

Galton, C., Patterson, K., Graham, K., Lambon-Ralph, M., Williams, G., Antoun, N., Sahakian, B., and Hodges, J. (2001). Differing patterns of temporal atrophy in Alzheimer's disease and semantic dementia. *Neurology*, 57(2):216–225.

Hastie, D., Liverani, S., and Richardson, S. (2015). Sampling from Dirichlet process mixture models with unknown concentration parameter: Mixing issues in large data implementations. *Statistics & Computing*, 25(5):1023–1037.

Hawkins, D. S., Allen, D. M., and Stromberg, A. J. (2001). Determining the number of components in mixtures of linear models. *Computational Statistics and Data Analysis*, 38(1):15–48.

Hejblum, B. P., Alkhassim, C., Gottardo, R., Caron, F., and Thiébaut, R. (2019). Sequential Dirichlet process mixture of skew t-distributions for model-based clustering of flow cytometry data. *The Annals of Applied Statistics*, 13(1):638–660.

Jacqmin-Gadda, H., Fabrigoule, C., Commenges, D., and Dartigues, J. (1997). A five-year longitudinal study of mini-mental state examination in normal aging. *American Journal of Epidemiology*, 145(6):498–506.

Johnson, R., Rouanet, A., Strauss, M., Richardson, S., Tom, B., White, S. and Kirk, P. (2020). Bayesian profile regression with a longitudinal response. Available at: `https://github.com/premium-profile-regression`.

Kalli, M., Griffin, J. E., and Walker, S. G. (2011). Slice sampling mixture models. *Statistics and Computing*, 21(1):93–105.

Kaufman, L. and Rousseeuw, P. (2005). *Finding Groups in Data: An Introduction to Cluster Analysis.* John Wiley, Hoboken.

Kempermann, G., Song, H., and Gage, F. H. (2015). Neurogenesis in the adult hippocampus. *Cold Spring Harbor Perspectives in Biology*, 7(9):a018812.

Komárek, A. (2009). A new R package for Bayesian estimation of multivariate normal mixtures allowing for selection of the number of components and interval-censored data. *Computational Statistics and Data Analysis*, 53:3932–3947.

Liverani, S., Hastie, D. I., Azizi, L., Papathomas, M., and Richardson, S. (2015). Premium: An R package for profile regression mixture models using Dirichlet processes. *Journal of Statistical Software*, 64(7):1–30.

Lo, A. (1984). On a class of Bayesian nonparametric estimates: I. Density estimates. *The Annals of Statistics*, 12(1):351–357.

Molitor, J., Papathomas, M., Jerrett, M., and Richardson, S. (2010). Bayesian profile regression with an application to the National Survey of Children's Health. *Biostatistics*, 11(3):484–498.

Mueller, S. G., Weiner, M. W., Thal, L. J., Petersen, R. C., Jack, C. R., Jagust, W., Trojanowski, J. Q., Toga, A. W., and Beckett, L. (2005). Ways toward an early diagnosis in Alzheimer's disease: the Alzheimer's Disease Neuroimaging Initiative (ADNI). *Alzheimer's & Dementia*, 1(1):55–66.

Muthén, B. and Shedden, K. (1999). Finite mixture modeling with mixture outcomes using the EM algorithm. *Biometrics*, 55(2):463–469.

Muthén, L. K. and Muthén, B. O. (2002). How to use a Monte Carlo study to decide on sample size and determine power. *Structural Equation Modeling*, 9(4):599–620.

National Research Council (2011). *Toward Precision Medicine: Building a Knowledge Network for Biomedical Research and a New Taxonomy of Disease.* National Academies Press.

Neath, A. A. and Cavanaugh, J. E. (2012). The Bayesian information criterion: background, derivation, and applications. *Wiley Interdisciplinary Reviews: Computational Statistics*, 4(2):199–203.

Philipps, V., Amieva, H., Andrieu, S., Dufouil, C., Berr, C., Dartigues, J.-F., Jacqmin-Gadda, H., and Proust-Lima, C. (2014). Normalized mini-mental state examination for assessing cognitive change in population-based brain aging studies. *Neuroepidemiology*, 43(1):15–25.

Proust-Lima, C., Amieva, H., Dartigues, J.-F., and Jacqmin-Gadda, H. (2007). Sensitivity of four psychometric tests to measure cognitive changes in brain aging-population-based studies. *American Journal of Epidemiology*, 165(3):344–350.

Proust-Lima, C. and Jacqmin-Gadda, H. (2005). Estimation of linear mixed models with a mixture of distribution for the random effects. *Computer Methods and Programs in Biomedicine*, 78(2):165–173.

Proust-Lima, C., Joly, P., Dartigues, J.-F., and Jacqmin-Gadda, H. (2009). Joint modelling of multivariate longitudinal outcomes and a time-to-event: A nonlinear latent class approach. *Computational Statistics and Data Analysis*, 53(4):1142–1154.

Proust-Lima, C., Philipps, V., and Liquet, B. (2017). Estimation of extended mixed models using latent classes and latent processes: The R package lcmm. *Journal of Statistical Software*, 78(2).

Rasmussen, C. and Williams, C. (2006). *Gaussian Processes for Machine Learning.* MIT Press, Cambridge, MA.

Ridha, B., Barnes, J., Bartlett, J., Godbolt, A., Pepple, T., Rossor, M., and Fox, N. (2006). Tracking atrophy progression in familial Alzheimer's disease: A serial MRI study. *The Lancet Neurology*, 5(10):828–834.

Rouanet, A., Joly, P., Dartigues, J.-F., Proust-Lima, C., and Jacqmin-Gadda, H. (2016). Joint latent class model for longitudinal data and interval-censored semi-competing events: Application to dementia. *Biometrics*, 72(4):1123–1135.

Rousseeuw, P. J. (1987). Silhouettes: A graphical aid to the interpretation and validation of cluster analysis. *Journal of Computational and Applied Mathematics*, 20:53–65.

Schwarz, G. (1978). Estimating the dimension of a model. *The Annals of Statistics*, 6(2):461–464.

Sethuraman, J. (1994). A constructive definition of Dirichlet priors. *Statistica Sinica*, 4(2):639–650.

Spiegelhalter, D. J., Best, N. G., Carlin, B. P., and Van Der Linde, A. (2002). Bayesian measures of model complexity and fit (with discussion). *Journal of the Royal Statistical Society — Series B*, 64(4):583–639.

Spiessens, B., Lesaffre, E., Verbeke, G., and Kim, K. (2002). Group sequential methods for an ordinal logistic random-effects model under misspecification. *Biometrics*, 58(3):569–575.

Stern, Y. (2009). Cognitive reserve. *Neuropsychologia*, 47(10):2015–2028.

Velayudhan, L., Proitsi, P., Westman, E., Muehlboeck, J., Mecocci, P., Vellas, B., Tsolaki, M., Kłoszewska, I., Soininen, H., Spenger, C., Hodges, A., Powell, J., Lovestone, S., Simmons, A., and dNeuroMed Consortium (2013). Entorhinal cortex thickness predicts cognitive decline in Alzheimer's disease. *Journal of Alzheimer's Disease*, 33(3):755–766.

Verbeke, G. and Lesaffre, E. (1996). A linear mixed-effects model with heterogeneity in the random-effects population. *Journal of the American Statistical Association*, 91(443):217–221.

Windham, M. P. and Cutler, A. (1992). Information ratios for validating mixture analyses. *Journal of the American Statistical Association*, 87(420):1188–1192.

Zhang, M.-H. and Cheng, Q.-S. (2004). Determine the number of components in a mixture model by the extended KS test. *Pattern Recognition Letters*, 25(2):211–216.

12

Bayesian Frameworks for Rare Disease Clinical Development Programs

Freda Cooner

Amgen Inc., US

Forrest Williamson

Eli Lilly and Company, US

Bradley P. Carlin

Counterpoint Statistical Consulting, US

Clinical development of orphan products in rare diseases poses unique clinical and statistical challenges, mainly surrounding the small population issue. Bayesian statistics naturally are adopted as a tool for both more efficient trial designs and more reliable treatment effect estimates. We start this chapter with an extensive summary of the global regulatory background that fosters clinical research in rare diseases, and which in turn has stimulated statistical innovations including the use of Bayesian methodologies in clinical trials. The use of natural history studies, long-term safety evaluation following marketing approval, and real-world data utilization are then discussed, with specific considerations in orphan products' clinical settings. The main focus of this chapter is the potential implementation of Bayesian approaches in confirmatory trials for orphan drug regulatory approvals. We briefly review trial designs that could incorporate Bayesian statistics and existing Bayesian approaches (e.g. two-step and power priors), and also introduce robust mixture priors. A case study in rare disease development is then investigated to illustrate the robust mixture approach with historical data. Advantages and caveats when using Bayesian statistics are discussed considerably throughout this chapter, focusing on the rare disease clinical development environment. Finally, we conclude this chapter with more encouraging recent regulatory updates and our current thinking on rare disease clinical development, with emphasis on the Bayesian framework.

12.1 Introduction

Rare diseases, intuitively, have very low prevalence as opposed to common diseases. The term's specific definition is bound by different regions through their respective regulatory health agencies. In the United States, a rare disease is defined as a condition affecting less than 200,000 of the individuals in the United States. As adopted by 28 member countries in the European Union, a disease is defined as rare when it affects fewer than 1 in 2,000 people. Japan requires a rare disease to affect fewer than 50,000 Japanese patients, which corresponds to a maximal incidence of 4 per 10,000. Singapore's Minister of Health describes a rare disease as a life threatening and severely debilitating illness affecting fewer than 20,000 people. Hence, a disease considered rare in one region is not necessarily rare in another.

These definitions arise from regional legislative acts. The earliest such regulation was established in United States, the 1983 Orphan Drug Act. The orphan drugs referred to in the act are for rare diseases or conditions, including biological products and antibiotics "orphaned" (abandoned) by drug companies due to their low sales potential, an obvious consequence of disease rarity. Following the establishment of this groundbreaking legislation, rare diseases are now often called "orphan diseases," and orphan drugs are inclusive of biologic products (though not medical devices). More than a decade later, the second major related legislative action was the 1999 Orphan Regulation adopted by the European Parliament. Both regulations include monetary incentives, marketing exclusivities, and clinical research assistance for rare disease medicinal product development. Other than drug product development, there are other regulations or government entities (e.g. the US Rare Diseases Act in 1992 and the Spanish Rare Diseases Research Institute) that aid patient support groups and fund research projects in rare diseases. Several papers, including Gupta (2012) and Gammie et al. (2015), synthesize details and comparisons across different legislations across nations. In fact, most developed countries and regions now have well-established rare disease or orphan product programs. The US remains one of the leaders and a key player in orphan product development and rare disease research.

Orphanet, a consortium of 40 countries originally established in France, estimates that roughly 6,000 to 7,000 rare diseases have been identified worldwide, while the World Health Organization (WHO) estimated there were about 5,000 to 8,000 rare diseases in 2013 (de Vrueh et al., 2013). Although the prevalence of each rare disease is of course low, together rare diseases affect a large number of populations. It is estimated that they affect 25 to 30 million people in the US alone and more than 300 to 400 million worldwide (de Vrueh et al., 2013). The majority (~80%) of rare diseases are believed to be genetic and chronic (Sanfilippo and Lin, 2014). Many rare diseases manifest early in life, and roughly 70% of the rare disease population are pediatric patients. Some rare conditions are defined within pediatric populations, as the same condition may be more common in adult populations, such as pediatric cancer.

According to the FDA Office of Orphan Products Development, there have been 600 orphan drugs and biologic products marketed since the 1983 Orphan Drug Act, as compared to fewer than ten from 1973–1983. This number continues to increase. In 2018, the FDA Center for Drug Evaluation and Research (CDER) approved 59 novel drugs with 34 (58%) of them developed to treat rare diseases. The European Commission Public Health Register for orphan medicinal products (EURODIS) counted 164 products gaining marketing authorization in EU during 2000-2017. It is great news to the patients and caregivers that there are more treatments available on the market. However, as a result it is now more competitive for a new drug to get approved or even recognized as an orphan product. Most of these marketed products were approved based on at least one parallel-group placebo-controlled study, similar to common disease treatments. An increasing number of available treatment options and genetic identifications sub-partition many diseases. Consequently, it becomes even more challenging to conduct a gold-standard adequate and well-controlled study in the targeted patient population. This is a critical time to keep investors motivated in orphan product development through novel yet more efficient clinical trial designs and analytic approaches. To this end, it seems prudent to make systematic use of our experience from past rare disease research. The Bayesian framework (Carlin and Louis, 2000) facilitates this, allowing us to build in simulation infrastructure that optimizes trial operations and incorporates post-marketing safety information. This can potentially alleviate the issues we face in orphan product development, such as small sample sizes, large variability, and the ever-changing clinical landscape in standard of care.

The next two sections in this chapter will evaluate some unique considerations in rare disease clinical trials and long-term safety commitment often tied with orphan products' approval. Then we will discuss and summarize a few orphan product trials with novel designs. We will also delve into Bayesian framework and its usage in rare disease researches with case examples. Finally we will provide a few concluding remarks and lay out future directions.

12.2 Natural history studies

Natural history in medicine means the usual course of development of a disease or condition without treatment. It is very difficult to understand the natural history of rare diseases, especially when a new rare disease is identified through a specific genetic sequence. The FDA emphasizes the importance of designing and conducting natural history studies at the earliest stages of drug development in its guidance document on rare diseases. Based on the guidance, the objectives of a natural history study should be to: 1) define the disease population; 2) understand and implement critical elements in clinical trial design; 3) select clinical endpoints and develop sensitive and specific outcome measures; and 4) identify new or validate existing biomarkers. Carrying out these fundamental aspects of planning a drug development program will deplete the already small number of subjects for some rare conditions just to run a proper natural history study. Confirmatory evidence will have to rely on a single-arm trial, which raises a different set of questions. A different section in the guidance discusses using historical or external controls when feasible. Intuitively, a historical or external control is not a concurrent comparator group, which puzzles many trialists who are accustomed to randomized concurrently controlled trials. Based on the natural history of a disease, we could derive an objective criterion for future single-arm trials to achieve. Alternatively, when subject-level natural history data can be accessed, we could attempt to mimic a randomized trial by extracting a "matching" cohort for future single-arm trials. Neither is an ideal solution.

Recently, Bayesian methods have been harnessed to either synthesize historical information or augment a small concurrent control group (Neuenschwander et al., 2010; Hobbs et al., 2011, 2012; Viele et al., 2013) — see also Chapter 6. Patient support groups and the research institutes (e.g. Spanish Rare Diseases Research Institute mentioned in Section 13.1) are the usual sources for natural history databases. Some data registries, many listed by the US National Organization for Rare Disorders, are other viable data sources; however, their data quality varies greatly, to say nothing about missing data issues. These data sources are often vulnerable under regulatory scrutiny and consequently considered unreliable.

As an example, Myozyme/Lumizyme (alglucosidase alfa) is an enzyme replacement therapy approved for Pompe disease. The original approval of Myozyme in 2006 was based on a historically controlled trial. The primary endpoint is time-to-death that starts from age 0 for both current trial subjects and the matching historical control cohort. Serving as the FDA statistical reviewer, Kammerman (2006) pointed out the decision was misleading, as the current trial subjects had to survive long enough to be enrolled into the trial, whereas all historical control subjects without any intervention were traced back to age 0. This is just one example where it is unachievable to mimic a randomized trial with a poorly matched historical control group. However, Bayesian statisticians could potentially build a simulator to generate a control group from the posterior distribution based on the whole historical group (inclusive of the matching cohort) and a noninformative prior. A second example is offered by Brineura (cerliponase alfa), the first treatment approved for a form of Batten disease. The approval in 2017 was also based on a single-arm historically-controlled study. The cohort was matched based on a physician rating, and the statistical reviewers (Min et al., 2017) spent much effort finding a suitable matching criteria to identify a "matching" historical control cohort. Through proper predictive modeling, Bayesian statistics may be introduced to provide a better estimate or distribution of the treatment effect through simulation. Unlike the Myozyme case, obtaining a consensus from clinical colleagues on the analysis model or acceptable treatment effect measurements may be challenging. Often, the so-called historical control is a simple literature review summary (e.g. Cholbam — cholic acid approval; U.S. Food and Drug Administration, 2015), and there is little statisticians can do to facilitate evaluation except design and produce simulations based on these summary data.

Patients and caregivers have raised awareness toward contributing to a good-quality data registry, and we expect more and better natural history data will become available for many rare diseases. With such data, statisticians and clinicians could better understand rare diseases, which in turn will better inform clinical development programs through identifying patient populations, endpoints and proper analysis models.

12.3 Long-term safety evaluation and usage of Real-World Data in rare diseases

Recognizing the limitations of pre-market clinical trials, such as refined clinical settings and relatively short observational periods, many if not all approved medicinal products undergo post-market surveillance. The purpose of post-market surveillance is usually to further confirm efficacy and its durability (including studies in minority populations), detect safety signals, and observe real-life patient usage of the products. Regulatory agencies have provided several guidance documents and general guidelines on post-approval studies and surveillance. Examples include the US FDA guidance for *Industry Post-Marketing Studies and Clinical Trials* in 2011 and for *Format and Content of a REMS Document* in 2017, as well as the EMEA *Good pharmacovigilance practices guidelines.*

Rare diseases are often serious and feature unmet medical needs. Hence, expedited programs are often adopted, and in fact recommended by regulatory agencies. Examples include the US FDA *Guidance for Industry: Expedited Programs for Serious Conditions – Drugs an Biologics* in 2014 and the EMEA *Guideline on the scientific application and the practical arrangements necessary to implement the procedure for accelerated assessment* in 2015 (European Medicine Agency, 2015). The most common approach is to gain conditional marketing approval/authorization through a surrogate endpoint and then commit to a confirmatory clinical outcome study. However, most of those post approval trials are projected to be conducted over a long period of time, and pharmaceutical companies are sometimes criticized for lacking the motivation to conduct these trials well and in a timely fashion (Fleming, 2005). In some cases, such as Mylotarg (reported by the US FDA News Release in 2017), the confirmatory trials fail to validate clinical benefit and subsequently the product is withdrawn from the market to better define the dose, formulation and/or regimen, and sometimes refine the target patient population.

The 21st Century Cures Act enacted in late 2016 by the US Congress has brought real-world data (RWD) and real-world evidence (RWE) onto the main stage of drug approval. These terms refer to observational data and evidence collected outside of controlled clinical trials, where data are often obtained from registries or electronic health records. Quality issues with these data have been discussed in earlier sections. Patient advocacy groups have contributed to these data registries in recent years and thus significantly increased the quantity of the database in terms of both the number of data registries and data entries in each database. However, this has not alleviated the data quality issue. Regulatory agencies have expressed some reservations in relying on RWD/RWE to support a drug approval, even though their utilization in post-approval safety evaluations has been practiced for decades.

In orphan drug post-approval validation trials, however, RWD/RWE could also be a viable option to salvage the long-running, never-ending clinical outcome trials mentioned above. The most common usage is very similar to the incorporation of natural history data discussed in Section 12.2, except that, should a company have real-time patient usage data from a similar version of the drug, those data will be viewed as RWD and not natural history. Outside of the RWD and natural history realm, researchers are seeking ways to incorporate data from previous clinical trials in the same class of drugs and similar indications with the emergence of the second generation of orphan products. Given the small patient populations, pre-approval data should not be discarded during post-approval evaluation. With all the data from these multiple sources, the Bayesian methods are ideally suited to synthesize all available data with built-in simulation tools.

12.4 Bayesian approaches in rare diseases

12.4.1 Clinical trial designs

Bayesian statistics could be introduced at different stages of a clinical development program — as early as pre-clinical studies or as late as post-market studies. It could also be incorporated into different aspects of a clinical trial. Many clinical programs have used posterior probabilities to inform dose selection, go/no-go decisions, subgroup identification and adaptation strategies. Moreover, as this platform trial engages multiple investigational treatments with a shared placebo control group, the Bayesian framework is implemented to properly evaluate the effect of each treatment.

Besides platform trial and adaptive designs, other clinical trial options that could be considered in orphan product development include cross-over (Zhang et al., 2017) and single-arm (Kammerman, 2006; Min et al., 2017; U.S. Food and Drug Administration, 2015) designs. Bayesian frameworks can be readily adapted to these settings. Some general aspects have already been discussed. In this section, more specific Bayesian models and case examples are illustrated.

12.4.2 Bayesian approaches

Historical data, if available, are almost always utilized when designing a clinical trial – for anything from identifying the right target population, to estimating accrual and dropout rates, to estimating effect size and variance to be used in sample size and power calculations. We wish to push beyond these applications and use this information as part of the analysis. To do this, the knowledge gained prior to starting a new trial must be quantified. Under the Bayesian approach, this information is summarized by the prior distribution, and we look at several forms it may take.

Use of historical data becomes even more critical in rare disease settings, by virtue of the small sample sizes that naturally accompany the disease's rarity. Chapter 6 is focused on the broader concept of using historical data in clinical trial design, and its connections to traditional meta-analytic methods. Without repeating the subject, it is prudent for us to point out a few aspects that are unique to the rare disease setting that we are discussing in this chapter. In particular, we note that most of the traditional criteria for effective use of such data recommended by Pocock (1976) are attempting to mimic a randomized controlled trial. Rare diseases usually cannot accommodate such restrictive matching criteria, and thus render some of these recommendations impractical or impossible. For instance, Pocock Criterion 4 states that, "the distributions of important patient characteristics in the group should be comparable with those in the new trial." Although there have been several attempts to meet this criterion in rare disease trials, the number of characteristics had to be very limited to ensure sufficient historical data to draw any inferential conclusions (Kammerman, 2006; Min et al., 2017). We may consider including covariate terms for any patient characteristics that may affect treatment effects, or using a propensity score as a covariate. Furthermore, Pocock Criterion 5 insists that, "the previous study must have been performed in the same organization with largely the same clinical investigators." Historical data for rare diseases, if they exist, are often not collected through pragmatic trials with organizations or clinical investigators involved, but rather from health records or a data registry. This fact will also almost surely lead to violating Pocock Criterion 2 ("the group must have been part of a recent clinical study which contained the same requirements for patient eligibility"). Acknowledging that these restrictions on historical data usage reduce the risk of bias in the results, we note that flexibility is typically required in rare disease settings. In what follows, we outline methods that may sacrifice some bias in exchange for a significant reduction in variability, which in turn will allow us to draw more definitive conclusions.

The most basic approach, then, would be to use all historical data directly by pooling them with the new trial data in a "two-step" fashion. To do this, we first use Bayes rule to generate a posterior on a parameter of interest θ using only the historical data D_0,

$$p(\theta \mid D_0) \propto L(\theta \mid D_0) p_0(\theta),$$

where $p_0(\theta)$ is the initial prior distribution of the response and is often chosen to be vague, and $L(\theta \mid D_0)$ is the likelihood of the historical data. In the second step, Bayes rule is applied again once data from the new trial, D, are obtained. The posterior distribution is then

$$p(\theta \mid D) \propto L(\theta \mid D) p(\theta \mid D_0)\ , \tag{12.1}$$

where $L(\theta \mid D)$ is the likelihood of the new data. Simple two-step pooling of historical data can be a valid approach, given that for many rare diseases there may be very little information available. However, it is likely that the historical data may be older or larger in size than the new data. In such cases, pooling the new data with the historical may put too much weight on the latter, discomfiting regulators and others.

As such, it may be desirable to downweight, or discount, the historical data. There are many ways to discount a prior distribution. A simple method of discounting is simply to increase the variance of the prior $p(\theta \mid D_0)$, and thus allow for more uncertainty in knowledge about θ *a priori*. Caution must be used when inflating the variance because too large an inflation will turn the historical prior into a vague (relatively noninformative) prior, whence little benefit will come from the previous information.

12.4.2.1 Power priors

A convenient and somewhat less arbitrary way to downweight the historical data is through the use of a power prior, which modifies Equation (12.1) by first raising the historical likelihood to a power $\alpha_0 \in (0, 1)$. Specifically, the power prior is derived as

$$p_P(\theta \mid D_0) \propto L\left(\theta \mid D_0\right)^{\alpha_0} p_0(\theta),$$

where for the moment we assume the power parameter α_0 is fixed in advance. Note that when $\alpha_0 = 0$, no historical data is used in the analysis, and only the initial (vague) prior remains. At the other extreme, when $\alpha_0 = 1$ the historical prior takes the same form as the pooling approach and no downweighting occurs. An α_0 strictly between 0 and 1 represents various degrees of discounting the historical data, where the closer α_0 is to 0 the more down-weighted the historical data is in the analysis. In the case of a Gaussian (Normal) historical likelihood with n_0 observations, it is easy to show that the effective historical sample size is $\alpha_0 n_0$ (Ibrahim and Chen, 2000).

Consider a situation where historical trial data is available on 50 patients, of which 20 are responders. The historical response rate is therefore 40%. For binary endpoints, the Beta distribution is particularly intuitive because for n subjects and r responses, the historical data likelihood is proportional to a Beta$(r, n-r)$. In this example, a Beta$(20, 30)$ can be used as the likelihood of response rate (θ) derived from historical data D_0. The initial prior, $p_0(\theta)$, is chosen to be uniform over the range $[0, 1]$. Figure 12.1 displays the densities of the power prior $p_P(\theta \mid D_0)$ using various values of the power coefficient α_0. Notice that when $\alpha_0 = 1$ this is the Beta$(20, 30)$ distribution representing the historical prior. As α_0 moves from 1 to 0, more discounting of the historical data occurs, until finally when $\alpha_0 = 0$ the prior is the initial prior with no utilization of historical information.

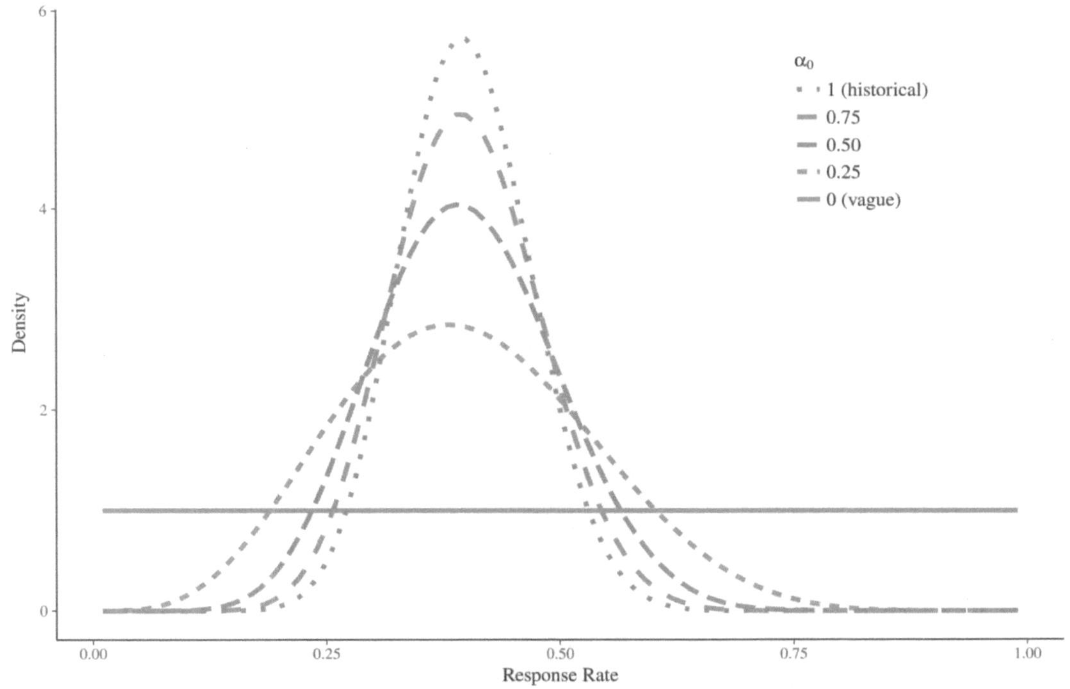

FIGURE 12.1: Impact of power prior coefficient on prior density.

To take this one step further, rather than selecting a fixed value for α_0, a hierarchical power prior structure may be used to introduce a distribution on the power parameter, $p(\alpha_0)$. The joint power prior for θ and α_0 based on the historical data might be expressed as

$$p_{\mathrm{JPP}}(\theta, \alpha_0 \mid D_0) \propto L(\theta \mid D_0)^{\alpha_0} p_0(\theta) p(\alpha_0), \tag{12.2}$$

where $p(\alpha_0)$ is often represented by a Beta distribution since α_0 must lie in (0,1). Adding a hyperprior on the power parameter will allow for greater uncertainty in the analysis compared to a fixed power prior. However, several authors (Duan et al., 2006; Neuenschwander et al., 2009; Hobbs et al., 2011) caution against the use of this joint power prior as it violates the Likelihood Principle (Birnbaum, 1962). This is because Equation (12.2) ignores a normalizing constant that cannot simply be discarded when computing the posterior, since it is a function of the unknown α_0. Instead, it is best to modify the joint power prior to the product of the *normalized* conditional power prior and an independent proper prior for α_0, producing the *modified power prior*

$$p_{\mathrm{MPP}}(\theta, \alpha_0 \mid D_0) \propto \frac{L(\theta \mid D_0)^{\alpha_0} p_0(\theta)}{\int L(\theta \mid D_0)^{\alpha_0} p_0(\theta) d\theta} p(\alpha_0). \tag{12.3}$$

Modified power priors obey the Likelihood Principle and produce marginal posteriors for α_0 that are proportional to products of familiar probability distributions. However, evaluating the integral in the normalizing constant of (12.3) can be difficult for nonconjugate model classes. Since we typically do not wish to use Markov chain Monte Carlo methods merely to specify a prior, in such cases we may turn to *commensurate prior* methods (Hobbs et al., 2011, 2012, 2013; Chen et al., 2018). Since these methods are presented and exemplified in Chapter 13 on methods for borrowing strength from adult data in pediatric clinical trials, we do not discuss them further here.

12.4.2.2 Robust mixture priors

The commensurate prior approach attempts to downweight the historical data when its message about θ is in conflict with that of the new data, i.e. when $p(\theta \mid D)$ turns out to be quite different from $p(\theta \mid D_0)$. Such historical-new data conflict may imply that the historical data should not be used. But how can one know in advance whether or not there will be such conflict? An approach called *robust mixture priors* adds a weakly informative component to a historical data prior, which allows for borrowing of information only when such borrowing is appropriate. That is, less historical-new data conflict means more borrowing from historical data, whereas more conflict results in heavier reliance on the weakly informative component (hence less historical data borrowing). Robust mixture priors can be particularly useful in a clinical trial setting where parties may be concerned about the impact excessive borrowing will have on trial operating characteristics.

A robust mixture prior is the addition of a weakly informative (robust) component to the historical data prior via a mixing weight to form a mixture distribution. In the case where a single historical study is being considered, the robust mixture prior has the form

$$p_{\mathrm{RMP}}(\theta, w \mid D_0) \propto (1-w)\, p(\theta \mid D_0) + w\, p_r(\theta),$$

where $p_r(\theta)$ is the robust component of the prior and $w \in (0,1)$ is a weight that can be thought of as the prior probability that the new trial differs systematically from the historical trial (Schmidli et al., 2014). If $w = 1$ then $p_{\mathrm{RMP}}(\theta, w \mid D_0)$ reduces to using only the robust prior; if $w = 0$ then only historical data are being used, equivalent to the simple pooling method first introduced in this section. For $w \in (0,1)$ the robust mixture prior allows for downweighting of the historical data in the Bayesian updating when historical-new data conflict is present. It does this via standard Bayesian calculations (Röver et al., 2019; Carlin and Louis, 2000); namely, by updating the prior weight w to a posterior weight,

$$\Pr(M_r \mid D) = \frac{p(D \mid M_r) w}{p(D \mid M_r) w + p(D \mid M_h)(1-w)},$$

where M_r denotes the robust prior model, M_h the historical prior model, and $p(D \mid M_i)$ is the marginal likelihood of the current data under model $i = r, h$, integrating out the model parameters (always possible in conjugate prior settings). Note that this expression makes clear that the amount of posterior belief in the robust component will monotonically increase as the marginal likelihood of the historical data decreases (i.e. as we see increasing "drift" between the historical and current data sources).

12.5 Case study

Progressive Supranuclear Palsy (PSP) is a rare neurodegenerative disorder characterized by the accumulation of aggregates of tau protein in the brain (Rossi, 2018). Several disease-modifying agents have been studied for the treatment of PSP. We consider two randomized, placebo controlled trials of putative disease-modifying agents in PSP. The first trial is a Phase II/III double-blind, parallel group trial of davunetide (30mg) versus placebo (Boxer and et al., 2014). The second trial is a Phase II, double-blind, parallel group trial of two doses of tideglusib (600 and 800mg) versus placebo (Tolosa and et al., 2014). Neither study met its 52-week primary outcome, but these trials have generated valuable data for our understanding of placebo response in PSP.

As PSP is a rare disease (prevalence of 1/16,600 according to *Orphanet*), we would like to use the placebo data from these two studies to augment the placebo arm in a new study, which could allow us to allocate fewer patients to placebo but achieve operating characteristics resembling a balanced design. We will build a historical prior based on the two trials mentioned above, and then robustify the prior by adding a vague prior to mix with the historical prior.

The primary endpoint is the PSP-Rating Scale (PSPRS). PSPRS is a quantitative measure of disability. It ranges from 0 to 100 comprising 28 items in six categories: daily activities, behavior, bulbar, ocular motor, limb motor, and gait/midline (Golbe and Ohman-Strickland, 2007). To determine if there is disease modification, patients are followed for 52 weeks and PSP severity is tracked throughout the course of treatment. For simplicity, we pool the placebo arms from the two trials and treat them as a single placebo cohort, and use change from baseline PSPRS at 52 weeks as the primary outcome measure. Note that when multiple sources of historical data are available, the meta-analytic predictive (MAP) prior can be constructed, and then used as the informative component in a robust mixture prior. For more details on robust MAP Priors, see Chapter 6. For our simpler pooled historical placebo approach, the change from baseline at 52-weeks of PSPRS for the combined placebo groups has mean 11.24 and standard deviation 9.95, from a sample size of 144 PSP patients (Stamelou et al., 2005).

We use a Normal distribution to approximate the historical control prior,

$$\theta \mid D_0 \sim \mathrm{N}(\mu = 11.24, \sigma = 9.95/\sqrt{144}),$$

and for the robust prior we use the same mean as the historical prior for consistency, but a much larger standard deviation,

$$\theta_{robust} \sim \mathrm{N}(\mu = 11.24, \sigma = 40),$$

with mixing weight of 0.5. Therefore, the robust mixture prior is

$$0.5 \times \mathrm{N}(11.24, 9.95/\sqrt{144}) + 0.5 \times \mathrm{N}(11.24, 40).$$

The choice of weight $w = 0.5$ is purely for illustrative purposes. In practice, the choice of w should be thoughtful and sensitivity analyses should be used to justify this choice.

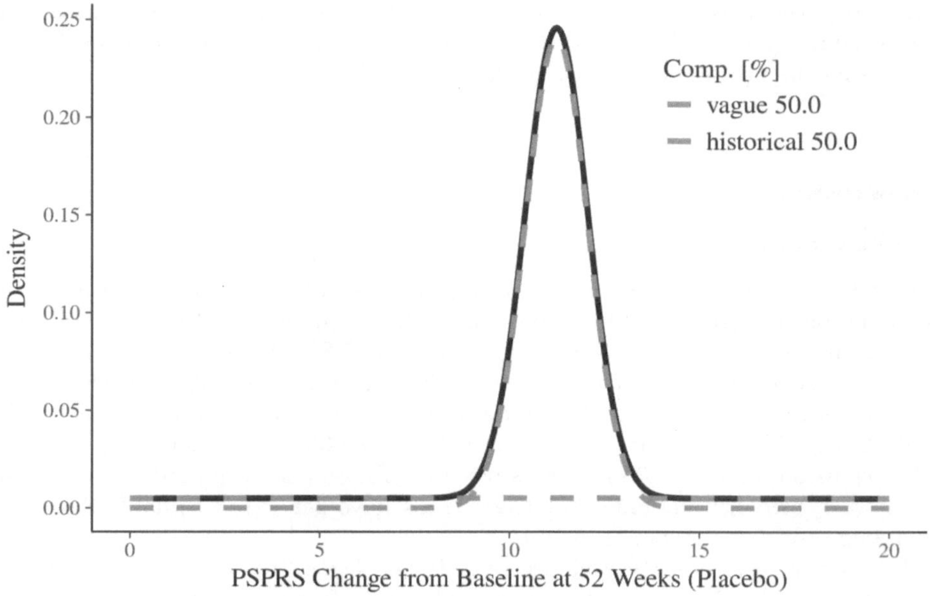

FIGURE 12.2: Robust mixture prior, with mixture components.

The robust mixture prior, and the relative contributions of the two components which make up the mixture, are plotted in Figure 12.2. Note that the two components, vague and historical, are not proper densities and integrate to their respective weights in the mixing equation (0.5 for each, in this case). The mixture distribution is a heavy-tailed version of the historical distribution, where in the tails the mixture matches the robust component, and around the mean historical response the mixture resembles the informative component. This structure allows for cautious and data-driven borrowing. That is, if the placebo response in a new trial is close to what was observed previously then historical information will be borrowed, but if the response in the new trial is in the tails of the historical response (i.e. prior-data conflict), little or no borrowing will occur. As noted by Schmidli et al. (2014), this borrowing is both convenient and effective, since it preserves conjugate structure and uses fixed mixing weights while still not requiring advanced knowledge of the degree of agreement of the historical and concurrent control data.

We now consider a new PSP trial with $n = 40$ placebo patients. We are interested in what effect this robust mixture prior will have on the posterior under two scenarios: prior-data conflict, and no prior data-conflict. Figure 12.3 shows two example likelihoods from a trial of size $n = 40$ overlaid on the robust mixture prior. The likelihood which illustrates prior-data conflict is centered at a mean PSPRS change from baseline at 52 weeks of 0, and the likelihood illustrating no prior-data conflict is centered at the historical mean of 11.24. We acknowledge it is unlikely that a new trial will exactly replicate results of a previous trial, but we use this in our example to demonstrate how the robust mixture behaves under the "perfect" scenario.

First consider the case where there is no prior-data conflict, where we use the "agreement" likelihood from Figure 12.3 and there is no "drift" between the new and historical controls. We have made the claim that when the new data looks similar to the historical data the informative component of the robust mixture prior will be more influential in the

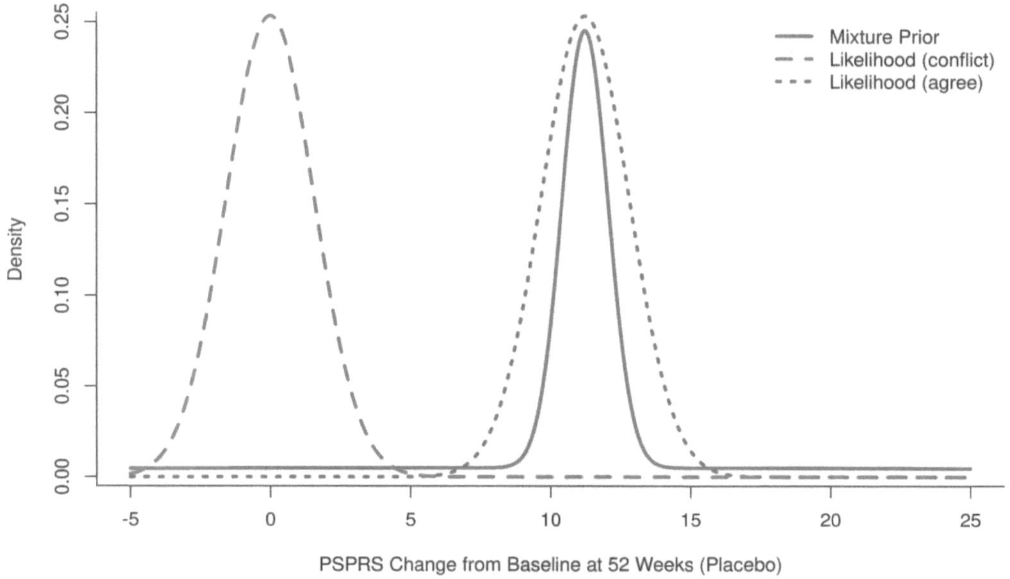

FIGURE 12.3: Two possible outcomes for a new trial.

posterior distribution. Figure 12.4 shows the resulting posterior distribution, as well as what the posterior distribution would have been using either the informative or robust components as a fixed prior. We can clearly see that the posteriors from the robust mixture and historical priors are nearly identical. This means that, when there is no prior-data conflict, the final analysis of the new trial data using the robust mixture is nearly equivalent to the posterior derived if using the historical prior alone, thus getting the maximal benefit from the historical information. If the historical data were not used and a vague prior was placed on PSPRS, Figure 12.4 shows that the resulting posterior distribution has much greater uncertainty due to the small sample size and relatively non-informative nature of the robust prior.

Figure 12.5 shows the posterior distribution that results from the robust mixture prior if prior-data conflict (from Figure 12.3) is observed in the new trial. It also shows what the posterior distribution would have been using either the informative or robust components as a fixed prior. The posteriors from the robust mixture and robust priors are indistinguishable — they are both plotted, but they are directly on top of one another. This shows that when there is prior-data conflict (in this case, relatively extreme conflict where most of the likelihood is in the tail of the mixture prior) the final analysis of the new trial data using the robust mixture is equivalent to the posterior derived if using the robust prior alone. This addresses one of the concerns that arose earlier: how do we develop a prior that is not overly influential if the new data shocks us and is not at all like data we have seen before? Figure 12.5 also shows what would have happened if the historical prior was used. In this case, the posterior is a pooled analysis of the historical data and new data, and therefore

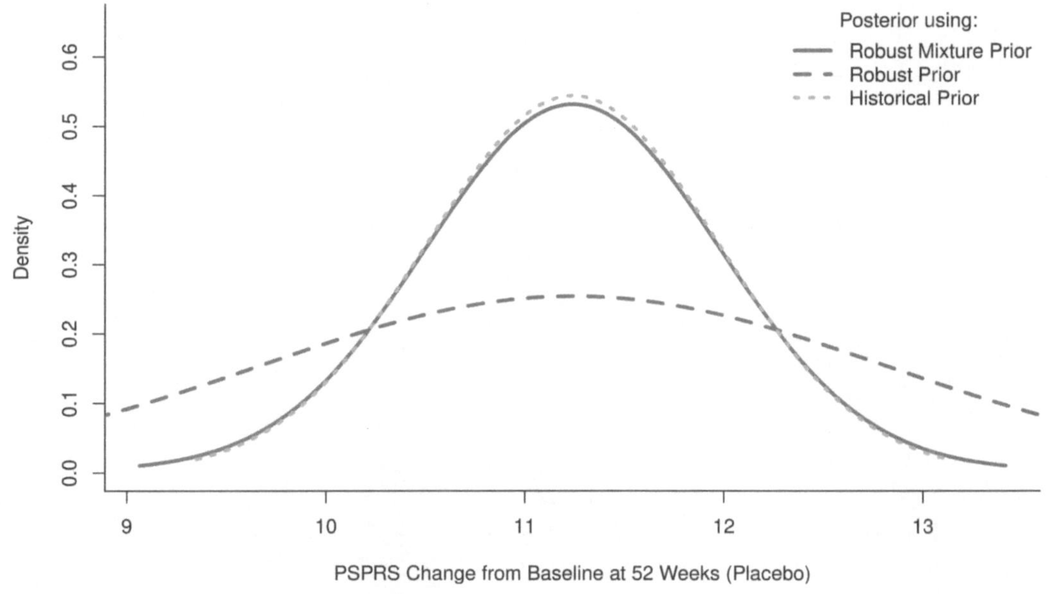

FIGURE 12.4: Example with prior-data agreement.

the density lies between the two. Because the historical data has more information ($n = 144$ compared to $n = 40$ in the new trial), the resulting posterior distribution is actually closer to the historical data. This is an outcome we'd like to protect against, and is one of the dangers of using a fixed prior structure.

These examples illustrate two extremes. More than likely, the new data could be overlapping partially with the historical data but still have some drift. Also, the choice of weight w has been described as a probability of applicability, and will also impact the amount of drift required before the robust component kicks in and takes over for the historical component. The robust mixture approach offers flexibility to inform the posterior based on the relevance of the historical data to the new data, without having to define in advance (other than through the choice of w) how different the data must be to be considered "close enough." Cautious borrowing methods such as the robust mixture prior may be preferred to two-step or fixed-downweighting power prior methods, because many fixed approaches determine the amount of discounting of prior information before seeing any data, therefore potentially losing precision when the data are similar but also potentially inflating bias when the data are dissimilar.

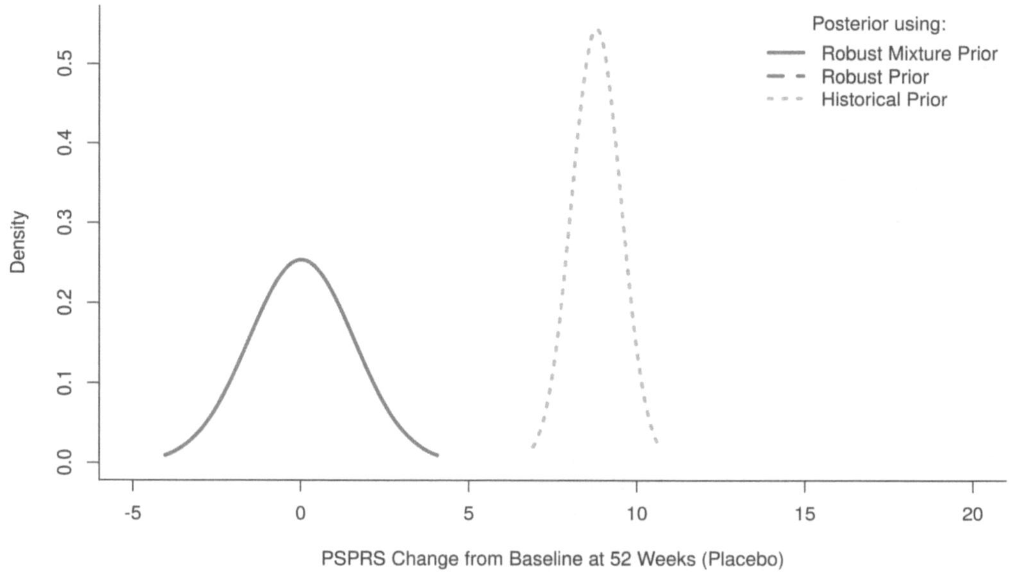

FIGURE 12.5: Example with prior-data conflict, with overlapping posteriors under the robust and robust mixture priors.

12.6 Conclusions and future directions

Rare disease research has come a long way since the first orphan product regulation (U.S. Food and Drug Administration, 1983), yet there is great room for further methodological improvement. Many current rare disease clinical programs either rely on traditional trial designs with few variations, or are purely based on clinical judgment. The deficiencies of these two options are obvious and become more prominent with new identifications of certain genetic mutations that define extremely small patient populations. The Scottish Medicines Consortium (SMC) has introduced an ultra-orphan definition associated with a new approach to decision-making on such medicines in 2018. The US FDA does not seem to be ready for such a regulatory definition, although it has requested additional budget for potential ultra-orphan incentives. Furthermore, the FDA initiated the Complex Innovative Trial Designs Pilot Program under the Prescription Drug User Fee Act (PDUFA) VI to support and facilitate novel trial designs including Bayesian trials. The first design was accepted for that program in early 2019 with placebo group augmentation components leveraging historical control data.

It is crucial to rethink the rare disease clinical development landscape, and Bayesian statistical approaches seem ideally suited to help reconstruct orphan products' evaluation frames. Through more frequent usage of Bayesian statistics, people not only become more comfortable with their properties, but also start to recognize their efficiency. With more practical and thoughtful Bayesian analysis models available, along with user-friendly software, we can readily envision the emergence of more trials with Bayesian components. Last but not least, understanding the importance of data in the advancement of public health, stakeholders invest more in data sharing. Such data afford more sensible prior distributions and more disease-specific analysis models. That said, there is much work to be done to implement the Bayesian methods in rare diseases clinical research. The growing awareness and understanding of this methodology can only increase the speed of its refinement and extension.

Bibliography

Birnbaum, A. (1962). On the foundations of statistical inference (with discussion). *Journal of the American Statistical Association*, 57:269–326.

Boxer, A., Lang, A.E., Grossman, M., Knopman, D.S., Miller, B., Schneider, L.S., Doody, R.S., Lees, A., Golbe, L.I., Williams, D.R., Corvol, J.-C., Ludolph, A., Burn, D., Lorenzl, S., Litvan, I., Roberson, E.D., Hoglinger, G.U., Koestler, M., Jack, C.R. Jr., Van Deerlin, V., Randolph, C., Lobach, I.V., Heuer, H.W., Gozes, I., Parker, L., Whitaker, S., Hirman, J., Stewart, A.J., Gold, M., and Morimoto, B.H. (2014). Davudentide for progressive supranuclear palsy: a multicenter, randomized, double-blind, placebo controlled trial. *The Lancet Neurology*, 13(7):676–685.

Carlin, B. and Louis, T. (2000). *Bayes and Empirical Bayes Methods for Data Analysis*. Chapman and Hall, Boca Raton, FL, 2nd edition.

Chen, N., Carlin, B., and Hobbs, B. (2018). Web-based statistical tools for the analysis and design of clinical trials that incorporate historical control. *Computational Statistics and Data Analysis*, 127:50–68.

de Vrueh, R., Baekelandt, E., and de Haan, J. (2013). Background Paper 6.19 Rare Diseases.

Duan, Y., Ye, K., and Smith, E. (2006). Evaluating water quality using power priors to incorporate historical information. *Environmetrics*, 17:95–106.

European Medicine Agency (2015). Guideline on the scientific application and the practical arrangements necessary to implement the procedure for accelerated assessment pursuant to Article 14(9) of Regulation (EC) No 726/2004. `https://tinyurl.com/yylqm3jt`.

Fleming, T. (2005). Surrogate endpoints and FDA's accelerated approval process. *Health Affairs*, 24(1).

Gammie, T., Lu, C., and Babar, Z.-D. (2015). Access to orphan drugs: A comprehensive review of legislations, regulations and policies in 35 countries. *PLOS One*, 10(10).

Golbe, L. and Ohman-Strickland, P. (2007). A clinical rating scale for progressive supranuclear palsy. *Brain*, 130:1552–1565.

Gupta, S. (2012). Rare diseases: Canada's "research orphans". *Open Medicine*, 1(6):e23–7.

Hobbs, B., Carlin, B., and Sargent, D. (2013). Adaptive adjustment of the randomization ratio using historical control data. *Clinical Trials*, 10:430–440.

Hobbs, B., Sargent, D., and Carlin, B. (2012). Commensurate priors for incorporating historical information in clinical trials using general and generalized linear models. *Bayesian Analysis*, 7(3):639–674.

Hobbs, B. P., Carlin, B. P., Mandrekar, S. J., and Sargent, D. J. (2011). Hierarchical commensurate and power prior models for adaptive incorporation of historical information in clinical trials. *Biometrics*, 67(3):1047–1056.

Ibrahim, J. and Chen, M. (2000). Power prior distributions for regression models. *Statistical Science*, 15(1):46–60.

Kammerman, L. (2006). `https://www.accessdata.fda.gov/drugsatfda_docs/nda/2006/125141s0000_Myozyme_StatR.pdf`. Accessed January 17, 2020.

Min, M., Chen, Y., Garrard, L., and Komo, S. (2017). `https://www.accessdata.fda.gov/drugsatfda_docs/nda/2017/761052Orig1s000StatR.pdf`. Accessed January 17, 2020.

Neuenschwander, B., Branson, M., and Spiegelhalter, D. (2009). A note of the power prior. *Statistics in Medicine*, 28:3562–3566.

Neuenschwander, B., Capkun-Niggli, G., Branson, M., and Spiegelhalter, D. (2010). Summarizing historical information on controls in clinical trials. *Clinical Trials*, 7(1):5–18.

Pocock, S. (1976). The combination of randomized and historical controls in clinical trials. *Journal of Chronic Diseases*, 29:175–188.

Rossi, K. (2018). Progressive supranuclear palsy treatment, ASN120290, gets orphan drug designation `https://tinyurl.com/y5thuzwm`. *Rare Disease Report.*

Röver, C., Wandel, S., and Friede, T. (2019). Model averaging for robust extrapolation in evidence synthesis. *Statistics in Medicine*, 38:674–694.

Sanfilippo, A. and Lin, J. (2014). *Rare Diseases, Diagnosis, Therapies, and Hope.* Blurb, Incorporated.

Schmidli, H., Gsteiger, S., Roychoudhury, S., O'Hagan, A., Spiegelhalter, D., and Neuenschwander, B. (2014). Robust meta-analytic-predictive priors in clinical trials with historical control information. *Biometrics*, 70:1023–1032.

Stamelou, M., Schöpe, J., Wagenpfeil, S., Ser, T. D., Bang, J., Lobach, I., Luong, P., Respondek, G., Oertel, W., Boxer, A., and Höglinger, G. (2005). Power calculations and placebo effect for future clinical trials in progressive supranuclear palsy. *Movement Disorders*, 31(5):742–747.

Tolosa, E. and et al. (2014). A phase 2 trial of the GSK-3 inhibitor tideglusib in progressive supranuclear palsy. *Movement Disorders*, 29(4):470–478.

U.S. Food and Drug Administration (1983). Code of Federal Regulation Title 21 Chapter 1 Subchapter D Part 316 Orphan Drugs.

U.S. Food and Drug Administration (2015). `https://www.accessdata.fda.gov/drugsatfda_docs/nda/2015/205750Orig1s000StatR.pdf`.

Viele, K., Berry, S., Neuenschwander, B., and et al. (2013). Use of historical control data for assessing treatment effects in clinical trials. *Pharmaceutical Statistics*, 13(1):41–54.

Zhang, Q., Toubouti, Y., and Carlin, B. (2017). Design and analysis of Bayesian adaptive crossover trials for evaluating contact lens safety and efficacy. *Statistical Methods in Medical Research*, 26:1216–1236.

13

Bayesian Hierarchical Models for Data Extrapolation and Analysis in Pediatric Disease Clinical Trials

Cynthia Basu
Pfizer, US

Bradley P. Carlin
Counterpoint Statistical Consulting, US

A pediatric population is one where the subjects are aged 18 years or less. The paucity of potential clinical trial enrollees and sensitivity of these patients, combined with a lack of sufficient natural history and experience, presents several economical, logistical and ethical challenges when designing trials for these populations. An increasingly well-accepted approach to address these challenges has been data extrapolation; that is, the leveraging of available data from adults or older age groups to help draw conclusions for the pediatric population. Bayesian hierarchical modeling facilitates the combining (or "borrowing") of information across disparate sources, such as adult and pediatric data. In this chapter, after a review of existing classical approaches to data extrapolation, we develop Bayesian hierarchical approaches to the problem. These include two-step, power prior, and commensurate prior methods. We then illustrate these approaches in the setting of a trial recording longitudinal observations that indicate the effectiveness of an experimental drug designed to treat secondary hyperparathyroidism in patients on dialysis for treatment of chronic kidney disease. We close with a brief discussion of the likely future usefulness of these methods in regulatory approvals in the US, Europe, and elsewhere.

13.1 Introduction

Pediatric diseases present a variety of challenges and limitations. The paucity of potential trial enrollees not only reduces the possible candidates and cases available for study and research, but also limits patient natural history and experience available. Rare diseases (a topic of an earlier chapter in this book) present similar challenges. Studies involving drugs targeted at pediatric or rare diseases thus require special attention, as they also present several economical, logistical and ethical problems (Roth-Cline et al., 2011; Knutsen et al., 2008).

The US federal government has taken action to promote research in these fields, including the Best Pharmaceuticals for Children Act (U.S. Food and Drug Administration, 2002), the Pediatric Research Equity Act (U.S. Food and Drug Administration, 2003), and the Orphan Drug Act (U.S. Food and Drug Administration, 2013). As the populations involved are often more sensitive as well as fewer in number, we wish to minimize the risk involved while maximizing the little information we have. We seek to borrow information from all available data sources, both to help substantiate the results of the current study as well as attempt to reduce the current pediatric study sample size. In the case of rare diseases, borrowing relevant information from historical data on the same disease has been proposed, and in fact reasonably well explored in the case of medical devices, with guidance documents available from FDA (U.S. Food and Drug Administration, 2010, 2015) and other regulatory agencies. However, borrowing information in the case of drugs is not as straightforward. This is especially true in pediatrics, since the pharmacokinetics (PK) and the pharmacodynamics (PD) of a drug may be very different in adults and children, and hence the children's responses may be quite different as well (Selevan et al., 2000).

Drugs are often approved for an adult population and subsequently prescribed off-label to children with only minimal understanding of the nuances of pediatric dosing and efficacy. Later, the sponsors may wish to conduct new studies to test the drug specifically in the pediatric population. In such studies, it is unethical to subject more children to experimentation than absolutely necessary, motivating incorporation of data from previous clinical trials on adults to strengthen our analysis and reduce the pediatric sample size. Many extrapolation techniques (Dunne et al., 2011) have been suggested and used to streamline rare or pediatric drug development and thus speed approvals of drugs for labeling.

Bayesian statistical methods facilitate adaptive dose-finding and other early-phase studies, permit formal borrowing of strength from other information sources, including expert opinion and previous data, and yield full probabilistic inference regarding model quantities of interest. Gamalo-Siebers et al. (2017) offer a recent review of Bayesian extrapolation methods useful in pediatric drug development, along with a corresponding regulatory perspective. In this chapter, we will look at Bayesian methods for data extrapolation techniques to facilitate more efficient and ethical pediatric clinical trial design and analysis. Our discussion will be conducted in the language of borrowing strength from adult data for pediatric approvals, but our methods apply equally well to the case of borrowing from historical control data in rare drug approval.

13.2 Classical statistical approaches to data extrapolation

The traditional approach to analyzing a trial for pediatric diseases, where the drug has already been approved for adults, is to carry out a study on children and analyze it without any information borrowed from adult data. Depending on the type of data set at hand, as well as the background clinical information, a wide variety of models can be fit to explain the dose-response relationship. These could be simple linear models, random or mixed effects survival models, piecewise linear regression models, or logit models for binary response data sets. Classical approaches include fitting simple frequentist random or mixed effects models to just the pediatric trial data, which is now routinely done using software packages such as `R` and `SAS`. An example for such a model is given in (13.1), where we regress the mean response μ_{ij} from the ith child's jth observation on the time from baseline, denoted here by $Time_{ij}$, the dose of the drug, denoted by $Dose_{ij}$, and introduce a subject-specific random intercept γ_i:

$$\mu_{ij} = \gamma_i + \boldsymbol{\beta}_1 Time_{ij} + \boldsymbol{\beta}_2 Dose_{ij} \ . \tag{13.1}$$

For a continuous observation Y_{ij}, a sensible sampling distribution (likelihood) is

$$Y_{ij} \stackrel{ind}{\sim} \mathrm{N}(\mu_{ij}, \sigma_Y^2),\ i = 1, \ldots, n_c,\ j = 1, \ldots, m_i, \tag{13.2}$$

for some $\sigma_Y^2 > 0$ where n_c is the number of children. However, this approach ignores the information in the adult data set.

An alternate but still naive approach would be to pool all adult and child observations into one big data set and then fit a model. This uncritical pooling of the pediatric and adult data sets may be inappropriate in many settings. A slight improvement to this procedure is to fit the regression once to the adult data and again to the pediatric data, and then take an appropriate weighted average of the pediatric and adult results. These weights could be based on the sample sizes of the two data sets, or perhaps expert opinion about the drug and the disease. However, the weight selection is crucial but difficult to justify in a traditional statistical framework.

A key aspect of such problems is the basis upon which extrapolation is deemed appropriate. Several pieces in the literature have discussed this issue (Dunne et al., 2011), where a systematic review of approaches for matching adult systemic exposures is often used as the basis for dose selection in pediatric trials submitted to the FDA. The literature refers to two categories of extrapolation, *full* and *partial* extrapolation. Full extrapolation is when adult data are used directly to establish pediatric safety or efficacy. These extrapolations rely on data supporting the assumptions that there are similar disease progressions, responses to intervention, and exposure-response relationships in the adult and pediatric populations. Pediatric development supported by pediatric pharmacokinetic and safety data or pediatric safety data alone can be considered adequate. By contrast, partial extrapolation is when adult data are statistically combined with pediatric data to make such determinations. By contrast, partial extrapolation of efficacy is used when there is uncertainty about at least one of the assumptions underlying complete extrapolation, as mentioned above. In such cases, pediatric development could be based on a PK-PD study to confirm response in the pediatric population, followed by a single, adequate, well-controlled pediatric trial to confirm the efficacy seen in adults.

13.3 Current Bayesian approaches

The approaches mentioned so far work well when we have a fairly rich pediatric data set and also understand the disease and drug mechanisms reasonably well. However when we are working with pediatric or rare diseases, we wish to use every bit of information available to us. In such cases, Bayesian methods can help strengthen our analysis through their ability to combine multiple information sources. Current Bayesian approaches include fitting hierarchical models (Berry et al., 2010; Carlin and Louis, 2008; Lindley and Smith, 1972) to both the adult and pediatric data together, where the parameters connecting the two data sets are related at some deeper level of the hierarchy. As an illustration, let us assume we have three data sets: two adult data sets D_1 and D_2, and a pediatric data set D_0. Let the numbers of patients in each of these data sets be n_1, n_2, and n_0, respectively, and let $i = 1, \ldots, n_1, \ldots (n_1 + n_2), \ldots, n$ denote the patient index, where $n = n_1 + n_2 + n_0$ denotes the total number of patients. Then assuming a simple linear fixed effects model like the one in (13.1) having sampling distribution (13.2), we can construct the following hierarchical model:

$$
\begin{aligned}
\mu_{ij} &= \gamma_{a,i} + \beta_{a,1} Time_{ij} + \beta_{a,2} Dose_{ij} \text{ for } i = 1, \ldots, (n_1 + n_2) \\
\mu_{ij} &= \gamma_{c,i} + \beta_{c,1} Time_{ij} + \beta_{c,2} Dose_{ij} \text{ for } i = (n_1 + n_2) + 1, \ldots, n, \\
\gamma_{a,i} &\sim \mathrm{N}(\gamma_{0a}, \sigma_a^2),\ \gamma_{c,i} \sim \mathrm{N}(\gamma_{0c}, \sigma_c^2),\ \gamma_{0a}, \gamma_{0c} \overset{ind}{\sim} \mathrm{N}(\gamma_0, \sigma_\gamma^2) \\
&\text{and } \beta_{a,k}, \beta_{c,k} \overset{ind}{\sim} \mathrm{N}(\boldsymbol{\beta}_k, \boldsymbol{\sigma}^2_{\boldsymbol{\beta}_k}) \text{ for } k = 1, 2.
\end{aligned} \tag{13.3}
$$

We may proceed to assign hyperpriors to $\boldsymbol{\gamma}_0, \boldsymbol{\beta}_1, \boldsymbol{\beta}_2$, and the variance parameters based on prior information from other data, such as crude auxiliary estimates of these numbers if possible, or using vague priors that let the data direct the values of these parameters. Such hierarchical models are widely used and often yield sensible results. These models can however be constructed to incorporate much more prior information than shown above, leading the hierarchy to become more complicated and possibly rely too much on the adult data. Viele (2016) and Hobbs et al. (2011) also stress that such "static borrowing" (where the amount of adult data incorporated is fixed ahead of time) can lead to biased estimates when the two data sources do not agree. Also, when we rely on vague hyperpriors, the model may be computationally improper and our MCMC algorithm may fail to converge, thus rendering the Bayesian approach futile. Care should thus be taken to incorporate all prior information and expert opinion regarding the problem at hand, as well as to be reasonably parsimonious with parameters. Note also that all borrowing is implicit through the exchangeability of the $\beta_{a,k}$ and $\beta_{c,k}$. Thus this method is simple, but doesn't allow us to explicitly control the amount of borrowing between the data sets.

13.3.1 Two-step approach

An alternative to fitting an exchangeable model for the data sets together is to take a two-step approach, where we first fit a hierarchical model to the adult data set, and then use its posterior estimates as the priors in a second statistical model for the pediatric data set. This method is illustrated in a real-life setting in Section 13.4.1. We might also downweight the adult information used by introducing various scaling parameters in the priors for the pediatric model.

In the longitudinal continuous data setting, suppose we first fit the adult model to our adult data and obtain posterior means and variances for γ_{0a}, $\beta_{a,1}$ and $\beta_{a,2}$, which we denote informally by $\widehat{\gamma}_{0a}$, $\widehat{\sigma}^2(\widehat{\gamma}_{0a})$, $\widehat{\beta}_{a,1}$, $\widehat{\sigma}^2(\widehat{\beta}_{a,1})$, $\widehat{\beta}_{a,2}$, and $\widehat{\sigma}^2(\widehat{\beta}_{a,2})$. Then in Step 2, we assume $\gamma_{0c} \sim \mathrm{N}\left(\widehat{\gamma}_{0a}, \alpha_0 \widehat{\sigma}^2(\widehat{\gamma}_{0a})\right)$, $\beta_{c,1} \sim \mathrm{N}\left(\widehat{\beta}_{a,1}, \alpha_1 \widehat{\sigma}^2(\widehat{\beta}_{a,1})\right)$, and similarly for $\beta_{c,2}$ using α_2 to scale the prior variance. The three hyperprior variance scaling parameters (α_0, α_1 and α_2) help us control the amount of borrowing from the adult data. In other words, we center our priors for these parameters at the posterior estimates we have obtained for the adults, but downweight this information by choosing α's bigger than 1. When these values equal 1, we assume full borrowing from the adult information.

13.3.2 Combined approach

A slightly more sophisticated and flexible method to facilitate data extrapolation while retaining control on the amount of borrowing is through the use of the *power prior* (Ibrahim and Chen, 2000). This approach downweights the supplemental (adult) likelihood by raising its likelihood in the posterior calculation to a power that is between 0 and 1. Assuming we wish to regress our response variable on some independent variables and the parameter of interest is θ, the power prior based on two adult data sets is

$$\pi(\theta, \boldsymbol{\lambda} \mid D_1, D_2) \propto \left[\prod_{k=1}^{2} L(\theta \mid D_k)^{\lambda_k}\right] \pi(\theta) , \tag{13.4}$$

where $\boldsymbol{\lambda} = (\lambda_1, \lambda_2)$ and the initial prior $\pi(\theta)$ is often vague. Note that λ_k controls how much information will be borrowed from auxiliary (adult) data set k to supplement the (fully-utilized) child data; e.g. $\lambda_k = 1$ means full borrowing from source k, while $\lambda_k = 0$ implies no borrowing from this source. Such control is important in cases where there is heterogeneity between the supplemental and primary data, or when equal weighting of primary and all supplemental data sources is inappropriate. In fact, for fixed power priors, there is a one-to-one relationship between the power parameter and the effective sample size in the prior. The relationship is particularly straightforward in the Normal likelihood setting; see for example Morita et al. (2008, 2012) and Pennello and Thompson (2016).

Finally, the *commensurate* prior approach (Hobbs et al., 2013, 2012, 2011) is an even more fully adaptive method to account for the *commensurability* between the adult and pediatric data sets. It essentially specifies a hierarchical model with posterior

$$p(\theta_c, \theta_a, \eta \mid D_0, D_1, D_2) \propto L(\theta_c \mid D_0) L(\theta_a \mid D_1, D_2) \pi(\theta_c \mid \theta_a, \eta) \pi(\theta_a) \pi(\eta) . \tag{13.5}$$

Hence the so-called *commensurate prior* for the child parameter vector θ_c, $\pi(\theta_c \mid \theta_a, \eta)$, is usually centered around the corresponding parameter for the adult data, e.g. $\mathrm{N}(\theta_c \mid \theta_a, \eta^{-1})$. The amount of borrowing can be modified by tuning the precision η of the prior around θ_a. A larger variance would imply we have less faith in the similarity of the pediatric and adult data, and therefore allow the pediatric estimate to be farther from that of the adult. Hobbs et al. (2011) recommend a “spike and slab” hyperprior for η, which helps crystallize the choice between borrowing and not borrowing. Both this method and the power prior method are also demonstrated in our subsection 13.4.2 case study.

All Bayesian models described above can be fit using standard Bayesian software such as `OpenBUGS` (Lunn et al., 2012), `Stan` (`mc-stan.org`), `Proc MCMC` in `SAS`, or in `R` using packages available in `CRAN` (`cran.r-project.org`) or those that call `BUGS` or its variants from `R`, such as `rjags`.

13.4 Practical example

Throughout this section our interest is driven by a data set on a drug we will call Drug A, which is being evaluated for the treatment of secondary hyperparathyroidism (HPT) in patients on dialysis for treatment of chronic kidney disease (CKD). In adult populations, Drug A has been shown to lower the parathyroid hormone (PTH) released by the parathyroid glands, which in turn reduces the level of calçium and phosphorous released from the bones. The iPTH (intact PTH) test level is of key interest, and is routinely monitored for people with chronic kidney disease; lowering it by some clinically significant percentage is a goal of many efficacy trials in this area.

Mimicking a real but confidential data set from a pharmaceutical partner, we simulate data sets from both adult and pediatric clinical studies of Drug A in the context of a linear mixed effects Bayesian hierarchical model to study the drug's effect on iPTH. The number of patients in the pediatric data set is just $n_c = 40$, whereas there are $n_a = 800$ patients in the adult study, a level of imbalance not uncommon in practice. Let X_{ij} be the percent change in the iPTH level of patient i $(i = 1, \ldots, n_c, \ldots, (n_c + n_a))$ in the week of the patient's jth observation, $j = 1, ..., m_i$ (where m_i varies from 3 to 25). That is:

$$X_{ij} = \frac{\text{iPTH}_{ij} - \text{baseline iPTH}_i}{\text{baseline iPTH}_i} \times 100 \, .$$

This percentage change will be our outcome variable in the linear model. Let t_{ij} denote the week after baseline for the jth observation on the ith patient. Since here we assume we don't have precise dosing information for every patient, our model (13.1) for the children becomes

$$\begin{aligned} X_{ij}^c &\sim \text{N}(\mu_{ij}^c, 1/\tau_e^c), \; i = 1, ..., n_c \\ \text{where } \mu_{ij}^c &= \mu_{1i}^c t_{ij}^c + \mathbb{I}(drug_i^c = 1)(\mu_d^c t_{ij}^c). \end{aligned} \tag{13.6}$$

Here μ_{1i}^c are the subject-level random effects, assumed to independently follow a $\text{N}(\eta_0^c, \tau_\eta^c)$ specification, and μ_d^c is the fixed effect of the drug on the child slope. Note we do not include intercepts in model (13.7) since X_{ij} is defined to be 0 at baseline $(t_{ij} = 0)$. Similarly for the adults, we assume

$$\begin{aligned} X_{ij}^a &\sim \text{N}(\mu_{ij}^a, 1/\tau_e^a), \; i = n_c + 1, ..., n_c + n_a \\ \text{where } \mu_{ij}^a &= \mu_{1i}^a t_{ij}^a + \mathbb{I}(drug_i^a = 1)(\mu_d^a t_{ij}^a). \end{aligned} \tag{13.7}$$

Now the μ_{1i}^a are subject-level random effects, assumed to independently follow a $\text{N}(\eta_0^a, \tau_\eta^a)$ specification, whereas μ_d^a is the fixed effect of the drug on the slope of the fitted iPTH percent change variable. Regarding hyperpriors, both η_0^c and η_0^a are assigned flat hyperpriors, μ_d^c and μ_d^a are assigned vague Normal priors, and we place vague Gamma(0.1, 0.1) hyperpriors on τ_e^c and τ_e^a.

13.4.1 Two-step approach

We first fit a two-step model along the lines of those described in Section 13.3. Specifically, in Step 1 we fit the adult model to our adult data and obtain posterior means and variances for η_0^a, and μ_d^a, which we denote by $\widehat{\eta}_0^a$, $\widehat{\sigma}^2(\widehat{\eta}_0^a)$, $\widehat{\mu}_d^a$, and $\widehat{\sigma}^2(\widehat{\mu}_d^a)$. Then in Step 2, we use these posterior estimates to guide our pediatric analysis. Specifically, we assume $\eta_0^c \sim \text{N}\left(\widehat{\eta}_0^a, \alpha_0 \widehat{\sigma}^2(\widehat{\eta}_0^a)\right)$ and similarly $\mu_d^c \sim \text{N}\left(\widehat{\mu}_d^a, \alpha_d \widehat{\sigma}^2(\widehat{\mu}_d^a)\right)$. The next question is therefore what the values of α_0 and α_d should be. They can be assigned based on expert knowledge, such as how similar clinicians think the two populations are likely to be and thus how much borrowing can be justified. As mentioned above, such static borrowing is straightforward but clearly somewhat subjective. Alternatively, we can assign hyperpriors to the α's, such as a vague Gamma or "spike and slab" distribution. However in some cases this may not be a good idea as it is often difficult to specify this hyperprior, and no information in our data exists to inform this decision.

A formula sometimes used to guide this decision is the *effective historical sample size* (EHSS; Hobbs et al., 2013). Various definitions exist, but a straightforward one (Pennello and Thompson, 2015) for a parameter of interest ξ is

$$\text{EHSS}(\xi) = n_c \left[\frac{\text{Var}(\xi \mid X^c)}{\text{Var}(\xi \mid X^c, X^a)} - 1 \right]. \tag{13.8}$$

In our case, we take the overall fitted slope in the drug group, $\eta_0^c + \mu_d^c$, as the parameter of interest ξ. Ideally the effective historical sample size should be no greater in magnitude than the pediatric sample size, since even though we are trying to borrow strength from the adult data, our analysis should be primarily driven by the pediatric data. However for our simulated data we often see EHSS values approaching or even exceeding the actual adult sample size of 800, since definition (13.8) is simple but may perform erratically in more complex hierarchical models, especially when implemented via MCMC. This is because (13.8) is simply the percent increase in precision provided by the addition of the adult data, and does not include any bounds to help control its magnitude in non-Gaussian models.

Tables 13.1—13.3 contain the results of the methods applied to our simulated data. We look at the estimated posterior mean and standard deviation (SD), the 95% equal tail Bayesian credible interval (CI), and the calculated EHSS corresponding to the placebo effect, η_0^c, and the overall slope in the treatment group, $\eta_0^c + \mu_d^c$. The latter is our primary parameter of interest, as it indicates whether or not the patients in the treatment group showed improvement over time.

In Table 13.1 we fit our two-step model using three different values of $\alpha = \alpha_0 = \alpha_d$ to show the effect of borrowing. The posterior estimates from Step 1 were $\widehat{\eta_0^a} = 0.5659$ and $\widehat{\mu_d^a} = -3.805$. Note that as α increases, the estimates for the children become more dissimilar to those of the adults. Note also that for the vaguest prior (α=100), we obtain the child data-only results (EHSS = 0), which also have the largest estimated SD's. It appears for around $\alpha = 15$, EHSS($\eta_0^c + \mu_d^c$) is fairly close to the actual size of the pediatric data set ($n_c = 40$). It should also be noted that based on the upper limit of the CI for $\eta_0^c + \mu_d^c$, for example, the significance of our findings change with α. In our case the change happens around $\alpha = 7$; smaller values lead to statistically significant findings, whereas larger values do not.

TABLE 13.1: Posterior estimates for the model coefficients using a two-step approach for various values of α.

	η_0^c				$\eta_0^c+\mu_d^c$			
α	mean	SD	95% CI	EHSS	mean	SD	95% CI	EHSS
1	0.67	0.35	(-0.04, 1.35)	1139.02	-3.12	0.53	(-4.15, -2.08)	703.1
7	1.13	0.86	(-0.59, 2.78)	102.17	-2.60	1.24	(-5.05, -0.19)	96.94
15	1.54	1.14	(-0.76, 3.74)	73.02	-2.24	1.59	(-5.39, 0.86)	42.86
100	3.05	1.92	(-0.76, 6.72)	0	-1.76	2.29	(-6.31, 2.69)	0

13.4.2 Combined approach

In this subsection we begin by fitting a commensurate prior model. We assume our model for the adults is as defined previously. We also model the pediatric data similar to before, but modify its prior to adaptively learn from the adult data based on their estimated similarity. Following (13.5), we assign the prior for η_0^c as $N(\eta_0^a, 1/\tau_c)$, and the prior for μ_d^c as $N(\mu_d^a, 1/\tau_{dc})$ to introduce the commensurability. We then proceed to assign spike and slab hyperpriors on τ_c and τ_{dc} as follows:

$$\tau_c \sim \begin{cases} N(200, 0.01) & \text{with probability } p; \\ \text{Uniform}(0.1, 5) & \text{with probability } 1-p, \end{cases}$$

$$\text{and } \tau_{dc} \sim \begin{cases} N(200, 0.01) & \text{with probability } p; \\ \text{Uniform}(0.1, 5) & \text{with probability } 1-p, \end{cases}$$

where we assume a common spike probability p for both τ_c and τ_{dc}. We can now vary the amount of borrowing by varying the value of p. An increase in p would mean a higher chance of the precision taking a value close to 200, our "spike", and hence more borrowing from the adult data. By contrast, small values of p encourage small τ values in the "slab", which discourages adult borrowing. Relatively little information on τ_c and τ_{dc} exist in the data, so the spike and slab parameters must be tuned carefully.

TABLE 13.2: Posterior estimates for the model coefficients using the commensurate prior for various values of p.

	η_0^c				$\eta_0^c+\mu_d^c$			
p	mean	SD	95% CI	EHSS	mean	SD	95% CI	EHSS
1	0.58	0.15	(0.29, 0.87)	7827.4	-3.23	0.15	(-3.53, -2.94)	9464.6
0.9	0.75	0.77	(0.29, 3.57)	244.54	-3.02	0.93	(-3.61, 0.15)	211.08
0.65	1.33	1.50	(0.19, 5.45)	35.36	-2.47	1.66	(-5.13, 1.66)	38.43
0.5	1.77	1.78	(0.14, 6.11)	13.73	-2.18	1.91	(-5.73, 1.98)	19.35
0	3.28	2.06	(-0.72, 7.38)	0	-1.72	2.32	(-6.36, 2.83)	0

Table 13.2 contains the results of this model for varying values of p. As can be seen, the results show the expected trends regarding borrowing between the data sets. For $p = 0$, we again get values consistent with no borrowing (EHSS = 0). The EHSS($\eta_0^c + \mu_d^c$) indicates a p of 0.65 delivers an EHSS approximately the size of the pediatric data set. However the EHSS does increase greatly for $p > 0.9$, becoming more than the available number of adult patients ($n_a = 800$). As noted in the case of the two-step approach, the significance of our findings changes with an increase in p, reemphasizing the caution with which the value of these parameters should be chosen. For $\eta_0^c + \mu_d^c$, the change seems to occur around p approximately 0.9; the CI contains zero for smaller p, and does not contain zero for very large p.

TABLE 13.3: Posterior estimates for the model coefficients using the power prior for various values of λ.

	η_0				$\eta_0+\mu_d$			
λ	mean	SD	95% CI	EHSS	mean	SD	95% CI	EHSS
0.1	0.78	0.16	(0.46, 1.09)	8504.4	-3.01	0.16	(-3.32, -2.71)	10706.6
0.001	2.24	1.11	(0.07, 4.40)	137.31	-2.57	1.12	(-4.72, -0.33)	169.99
0.00015	3.23	1.68	(-0.09, 6.52)	37.22	-2.11	1.76	(-5.52, 1.48)	44.43
0	4.11	2.34	(-0.39, 8.84)	0	-1.46	2.56	(-6.46, 3.47)	0

Finally we fit a power prior model. Here we may begin by assuming that $\eta_0^a = \eta_0^c = \eta_0$ and $\mu_d^a = \mu_d^c = \mu_d$. We then obtain the posterior $p(\mu_d \mid D_a, D_c)$ as proportional to $L(\mu_d \mid D_c)L(\mu_d \mid D_a)^\lambda \pi(\mu_d)$. For this method the EHSS was especially sensitive to the choice of λ. It appears that a very small λ of 0.00015 is needed to yield an EHSS close to the size of the pediatric data set. The CI for $\eta_0 + \mu_d$ again shows that the significance of our findings changes with a change of λ. The upper boundary of the CI for $\lambda = 0.001$ is close to zero, with this value roughly forming the break between Bayesian significance and insignificance.

If we fit a model as in the first step of the two-step approach to the pediatric data alone, the posterior estimate of η_0^c is 4.518 and $\eta_0^c + \mu_d^c$ is –2.02. As can be seen, for all three methods in Tables 13.1–13.3 as we move down the columns, the amount of borrowing from the adult data decreases and the obtained posterior estimates are now closer to those obtained by a hierarchical model on the pediatric data alone. In particular, the results in the no-borrowing (EHSS=0) cases are broadly similar across the models in all three tables; e.g. the posterior means for η_0^c are 3.05, 3.28 and 4.11, respectively (where the last value really pertains to η_0, since the adults and children are not parametrized separately by the power prior model). Other cross-table comparisons are harder to make, since EHSS values are not comparable and, again, the models parametrize things differently. Still, since p in the case of commensurate priors and λ in the case of power priors vary from 0 to 1, it is easier to intuitively set their values in accordance with our prior knowledge. EHSS performance is somewhat unstable in Table 13.3, suggesting the commensurate approach may be preferable. If we wish to limit the EHSS to roughly the pediatric sample size ($n_c = 40$), we must conclude the drug does not lead to a significant improvement in iPTH percent change under any of our three methods. However if we can tolerate a higher EHSS (say, greater than $5n_c$), for example due to added clinical justification or relaxed restrictions on borrowing, we can arrive at significant results and conclude that the drug shows improvement in pediatric populations as well.

13.5 Outlook

As demonstrated by our example in Section 13.4, several Bayesian modeling techniques exist to facilitate borrowing information between data sets for which we can control the degree of borrowing. Caution should be exercised when using these methods, especially when the data sets are very dissimilar and the adult or other historical data set has the potential to sway the answers overmuch. That being said, given sufficient familiarity with these methods and corresponding software, they can be used in a wide variety of problems to strengthen analysis, especially in studies of pediatric and rare disease where we have to work with smaller sample sizes for ethical and logistical reasons. As noted above, with an increase in α, decrease in p or decrease in λ, the statistical significance as seen in the CI changes, reemphasizing that the question of how to pick the degree of borrowing often remains hard to answer. The amount of borrowing can be based on several factors, such as expert opinion, or similarity between the adult and pediatric data sets. Our methods provide a way to quantify the trade-off between obtaining significant findings and fully justified adult data borrowing. However, more experience is needed with the spike and slab and other hyperpriors that control the degree of borrowing.

We also investigated individual mean levels for two individuals in our simulated data set, numbers 35 and 9. The 35th individual had relatively larger iPTH observations than the other pediatric patients, whereas the 9th patient was more or less randomly chosen and is not outlying. In both cases, EHSS could not be reliably estimated due to Monte Carlo error and the inherent smallness of these values. Thus EHSS does not seem to be a helpful tool in the case of individual random effects.

The outlook for Bayesian methods that borrow adaptively from adult data in pediatric approvals appears to be bright. In the US, the 21st Century Cures Act, passed by a bipartisan majority in late 2016 and signed into law by President Obama, encourages novel statistical approaches that may now be used to speed drug approvals. This in turn provided FDA with the "cover" to implement regulations that permit such approaches. More recently, in August 2017 President Trump signed into law the Food and Drug Administration Reauthorization Act (FDARA), a law that included the reauthorization of the Prescription Drug User Fee Act (PDUFA). The most recent version of this act (PDUFA VI) encourages the use of what the agency calls model-informed drug development (MIDD) and the use of complex adaptive, Bayesian, and other innovative clinical trial designs. FDA also plans to conduct several workshops on these topics, and indeed they have already begun in the past year with a series of meetings jointly sponsored by FDA and the Duke-Margolis Center for Health Policy. FDA statistical leadership is keenly aware of the problems presented by drug development and approval for pediatric and other rare diseases, and has encouraged novel applications in this area, as well as hired staff trained in Bayesian methods to read and react to these applications. Our experience with pediatric regulatory science in other countries is more limited, but it does appear that the European Medicines Agency (EMA) shares FDA's enthusiasm for novel approaches to pediatric approvals.

Of course, this modernization of a regulatory apparatus that has mostly served us well for 75 years is not without challenges. The most obvious is that the more complex Bayesian adaptive methods we advocate require us to simulate procedure operating characteristics (especially Type I error rate and power) for each possible collection of "true" parameter values. Note that, depending on the model, this in turn requires specific assumptions regarding both the effectiveness of the treatment in children and the commensurability of the pediatric and adult data. Determining a precise sample size ahead of time may not be possible, since at study outset we do not know if agreement between adult and pediatric data will be sufficient to justify borrowing strength from the former. In addition, simulation-based trial design is a time-consuming process that tends to create a mountain of tables, which is a lot of work to both create and to review. A second challenge is the natural resistance of sponsors to gamble on the use of novel approaches when they lack experience with them and often worry that regulators may scrutinize their results more carefully and, perhaps, more harshly. It will take some time for case studies and other experience with these approaches to percolate down to sponsors, providing them with the guidance and encouragement they need to implement them in their own studies.

Regarding future methodological work, a novel approach suggested by Basu et al. (2017) is to use another auxiliary data set, such as that from an earlier PK-PD analysis, to inform the degree of borrowing from the adult data. Since the PK-PD process captures the drug's mechanism of action in terms of its clearance as well as the dose-response relationship (Macdougall, 2006), it seems like a sensible metric for estimating the similarity in the way the drug should affect adults and children. The next development therefore may be a method to quantitatively assess auxiliary data similarity or dissimilarity, in order to come up with a more concrete justification for the degree of borrowing in such problems.

Bibliography

Basu, C., Ma, X., Mo, M., Xia, H., Brundage, R., Al-Kofahi, M., and Carlin, B. (2017). PK/PD data extrapolation models for improved pediatric efficacy and toxicity estimation, with application to secondary hyperparathyroidism. *Research Report, Division of Biostatistics.*

Berry, S., Carlin, B., Lee, J., and Müller, P. (2010). *Bayesian Adaptive Methods for Clinical Trials.* CRC Press, Boca Raton, FL.

Carlin, B. and Louis, T. (2008). *Bayesian Methods for Data Analysis.* CRC Press, Boca Raton, FL, 3rd edition.

Dunne, J., Rodriguez, W., Murphy, M., Beasley, B., Burckart, G., Filie, J., Lewis, L., Sachs, H., Sheridan, P., and Starke, P. (2011). Extrapolation of adult data and other data in pediatric drug-development programs. *Pediatrics*, 128(5):e1242–e1249.

Gamalo-Siebers, M., Savic, J., Basu, C., Zhao, X., Gopalakrishnan, M., Gao, A., Song, G., Baygani, S., Thompson, L., Xia, H., Price, K., Tiwari, R., and Carlin, B. (2017).

Statistical modeling for Bayesian extrapolation of adult clinical trial information in pediatric drug evaluation. *Pharmaceutical Statistics*, 16:232–249.

Hobbs, B., Carlin, B., Mandrekar, S., and Sargent, D. (2011). Hierarchical commensurate and power prior models for adaptive incorporation of historical information in clinical trials. *Biometrics*, 67(3):1047–1056.

Hobbs, B., Carlin, B., and Sargent, D. (2013). Adaptive adjustment of the randomization ratio using historical control data. *Clinical Trials*, 10(3):430–440.

Hobbs, B., Sargent, D., and Carlin, B. (2012). Commensurate priors for incorporating historical information in clinical trials using general and generalized linear models. *Bayesian Analysis*, 7(3):639–674.

Ibrahim, J. and Chen, M. (2000). Power prior distributions for regression models. *Statistical Science*, 15(1):46–60.

Knutsen, A., Butler, A., and Vanchieri, C. (2008). *Addressing the Barriers to Pediatric Drug Development: Workshop Summary*. National Academies Press.

Lindley, D. and Smith, A. (1972). Bayes estimates for the linear model (with discussion). *Journal of the Royal Statistical Society — Series B*, 34:14–46.

Lunn, D., Jackson, C., Best, N., Thomas, A., and Spiegelhalter, D. (2012). *The BUGS Book: A Practical Introduction to Bayesian Analysis*. CRC Press.

Macdougall, J. (2006). Analysis of dose–response studies — Emax model. In *Dose Finding in Drug Development*, N. Ting, ed., Statistics for Biology and Health series. New York: Springer.

Morita, S., Thall, P., and Müller, P. (2008). Determining the effective sample size of a parametric prior. *Biometrics*, 64(2):595–602.

Morita, S., Thall, P., and Müller, P. (2012). Prior effective sample size in conditionally independent hierarchical models. *Bayesian Analysis*, 7(3).

Pennello, G. and Thompson, L. (2015). Borrowing from adult data to make inferences about the effectiveness of medical devices in a pediatric population. *Technical report, Food and Drug Administration, Center for Devices and Radiological Health, Washington DC.*

Pennello, G. and Thompson, L. (2016). Design considerations for Bayesian clinical studies: Prior effective sample size and type 1 error level. *Proceedings of the ASA Biopharmaceutical Section FDA-Industry Statistics Workshop, Washington DC.*

Roth-Cline, M., Gerson, J., Bright, P., Lee, C., and Nelson, R. (2011). *Ethical Considerations in Conducting Pediatric Research*. Springer.

Selevan, S., Kimmel, C., and Mendola, P. (2000). Identifying critical windows of exposure for children's health. *Environmental Health Perspectives*, 108(Suppl 3):451.

U.S. Food and Drug Administration (2002). Best pharmaceuticals for children act. *Public Law*, pages 107–109. "https://www.fda.gov/regulatoryinformation/lawsenforcedbyfda/significantamendmentstothefdcact/ucm148011.htm". Accessed June 28 2017.

U.S. Food and Drug Administration (2003). Pediatric research equity act. *Public Law*, pages 108–155. "https://www.accessdata.fda.gov/scripts/cderworld/index.cfm?action=newdrugs:main&unit=4&lesson=1&topic=6". Accessed June 28 2017.

U.S. Food and Drug Administration (2010). Guidance for the Use of Bayesian Statistics in Medical Device Clinical Trials. "www.fda.gov/medicaldevices/deviceregulationandguidance/guidancedocuments/ucm071072.htm". Accessed Sept 18 2017.

U.S. Food and Drug Administration (2013). Orphan drug act. *Public Law*, pages 97–414. "https://www.fda.gov/regulatoryinformation/lawsenforcedbyfda/significantamendmentstothefdcact/orphandrugact/default.htm". Accessed June 28 2017.

U.S. Food and Drug Administration (2015). Leveraging existing clinical data for extrapolation to pediatric uses of medical devices: Draft guidance for industry and food and drug administration staff. "www.fda.gov/downloads/MedicalDevices/DeviceRegulationandGuidance/GuidanceDocuments/UCM444591.pdf". Accessed June 28 2017.

Viele, K. (2016). Issues in the incorporation of historical data in clinical trials. *Proceedings of the ASA Biopharmaceutical Conference, Washington DC.*

Part III

Post-marketing

14

Bayesian Methods for Meta-Analysis

Nicky J Welton

University of Bristol, UK

Hayley E Jones

University of Bristol, UK

Sofia Dias

University of York, and University of Bristol, UK

When considering clinical and cost-effectiveness of different treatment options, it is essential to consider all the relevant and available evidence. Combining evidence from different sources typically improves the precision of the estimates; in addition, by pooling evidence using a suitable model, it is possible to make the estimates more generalizable to account for potential differences in the underlying populations or design of the studies. Evidence synthesis is a general term to describe the pooling of results from multiple sources. Bayesian methods are convenient for evidence synthesis and generalized meta-analysis because of the hierarchical nature of the evidence and the ability to model complex relationships between the observed quantities (i.e. the data) and the underlying model parameters. In this chapter we describe Bayesian models for pairwise meta-analysis and network meta-analysis, highlighting some of the advantages of a Bayesian approach.

14.1 Introduction

When drawing conclusions about relative effectiveness and cost-effectiveness of different treatment options, it is important to consider all evidence relevant to the question (Claxton, 1999). There are several reasons why this might be desirable. Firstly, by combining evidence from multiple sources we can obtain greater precision in our estimates. Secondly, different studies may have been performed on slightly different populations and in different settings. By pooling evidence, the overall results may be more generalizable than if we just focused on one or a subset of studies. It is important for our conclusions to be fair, transparent, and reproducible, which is typically achieved through a process of systematic review where a clear rationale for inclusion/exclusion of studies according to the Population, Interventions and Comparators, and Outcomes (PICO) of interest is given (Egger et al., 2001). There are clearly also some disadvantages from pooling evidence across multiple studies. There may be a high degree of variability (heterogeneity) between the different study estimates, which can be due to a variety of factors: differences in patient populations, settings, and trial conduct, analysis, and reporting. If the populations and settings are so different that relative treatment effects differ between them, then we may be combining "apples with oranges", with the result that the pooled estimates are no longer interpretable and represent neither "apples" nor "oranges". It is therefore important to define study inclusion/exclusion criteria carefully to avoid excessive clinical or methodological heterogeneity. In addition, statistical checks can help to assess whether any statistical heterogeneity is present.

Evidence synthesis is a general term to describe the pooling of results from multiple sources. The most common example is pairwise meta-analysis (Egger et al., 2001) where all studies that compare two treatments A and B are combined to get a pooled estimate of the effect of A versus B (AvB). Network Meta-Analysis (NMA, Dias et al., 2018) extends this to the situation where there are multiple treatments A, B, C, ... and there is a network of evidence formed of randomized controlled trials (RCTs) (which may have more than 2 treatment arms) making various comparisons e.g. A versus B, A versus C, B versus C versus D, etc. This means that the estimate for each treatment comparison is informed by both direct head-to-head evidence as well as evidence from the rest of the network under the assumption of consistency, i.e. that the direct and indirect sources of evidence estimate the same "true" effect. However, the data may exhibit conflict between the direct and indirect evidence for a particular estimate, which is termed inconsistency (Lu and Ades, 2006). In NMA both heterogeneity and inconsistency may be present, and therefore need to be assessed.

Although RCTs are considered to be the gold standard study design to obtain causal estimates of relative treatment effects, the resulting estimates may be biased due to a lack of methodological rigour (internal validity) or a lack of generalisability to the population of interest (external validity). Methods to explore and adjust for biases are desirable, to produce robust and reliable treatment effect estimates.

Bayesian methods are convenient for meta-analysis for several reasons. The hierarchical nature of the evidence brings the need to estimate between-study variance and to also reflect the uncertainty in the estimate, which can be done naturally in a Bayesian context by specifying a prior distribution. Often there are only a few studies available, giving limited ability to estimate heterogeneity and the impact of bias. The ability to incorporate external evidence is therefore helpful. In cases where there are complex relationships between the observed quantities (i.e. the data) and the underlying model parameters that we wish to make inference on, the MCMC simulation environment often used to estimate Bayesian models provides the flexibility to fit complex models that are not otherwise possible. For example, it is only recently that frequentist methods have become available for NMA (White, 2009, 2011, 2015), and these are still only available for some outcome types and where all studies report the same quantity. Furthermore, the results from meta-analyses are often used in models to assess cost-effectiveness, where uncertainty is propagated from the meta-analysis into the decision model via simulation (probabilistic sensitivity analysis – see Section 15.4.2 and Claxton et al., 2005; Briggs et al., 2006). Estimating the meta-analysis model using an MCMC simulation framework automatically provides simulations from the required posterior distribution, for use in a cost-effectiveness model that captures all the correlations and uncertainties in the estimation process.

In this chapter we describe Bayesian models for pairwise meta-analysis and NMA highlighting some of the advantages of a Bayesian approach. We finish with a discussion of some further topics where a Bayesian approach is useful for evidence synthesis, indicating relevant literature.

14.2 Pairwise meta-analysis

In a pairwise meta-analysis each study compares the same two interventions, for a given population and outcome. For example, Hua et al. (2016) conducted a systematic review to identify RCTs assessing the ability of oral hygiene care to prevent ventilator-associated pneumonia (VAP) in critically ill patients receiving mechanical ventilation in intensive care. They identified 18 RCTs comparing chlorhezidine mouth rinse or gel versus placebo or usual care, where the outcome is the number of cases of VAP $y_{i,k}$ out of the total randomized individuals, $n_{i,k}$, in arm k of study i.

The Bayesian model for meta-analysis proposed by Smith et al. (1995) is described in the next section.

14.2.1 Likelihood, model and priors

As for any Bayesian analysis, we specify a sampling distribution $p(y \mid \boldsymbol{\theta})$. This represents how likely the observed data are for given parameter values but also shows the plausibility of the parameter values in the light of the observed data and we use the phrasing likelihood function to indicate this in the rest of this chapter. In addition, we consider a model linking the parameters we wish to estimate to the parameters that directly inform the likelihood. We give priors for those parameters that are not otherwise specified. There are two models that are usually used in meta-analysis (Egger et al., 2001), the common effect model (often termed a "fixed effect model") and the random effects model.

We assume that each arm of each study provides data that contribute to the likelihood according to a sampling distribution that reflects the data generating process:

$$Y_{i,k} \mid \theta_{i,k} \sim f(\theta_{i,k}).$$

For example, in the chlorhezidine example we have the number of patients who develop VAP out of the total number randomized as the outcome, so a Binomial distribution provides a good description of the data generating process:

$$Y_{i,k} \mid \theta_{i,k} \sim \text{Bin}(\theta_{i,k}, n_{i,k}), \tag{14.1}$$

where $\theta_{i,k}$ is the probability of relapse for study i in arm k.

A generalized linear model (McCullagh and Nelder, 1989; Dias et al., 2013a) is used for the parameter $\theta_{i,k}$, so that the model is linear on an appropriate scale:

$$g(\theta_{i,k}) = \mu_i + \delta_i \mathbb{I}_{k \neq 1}, \tag{14.2}$$

where $g(\cdot)$ is a link-function that transforms the parameter of interest to an appropriate scale, μ_i are effects on the reference treatment (arm 1) of study i (nuisance parameters, not of primary interest). δ_i is the study specific treatment effect, and $\mathbb{I}_{k \neq 1}$ is an indicator variable that indicates whether the data relate to the treatment arm 2 ($k = 2$), so that the treatment effect is not added on for the control arm ($k = 1$). For the chlorhezidine example the logit-link function is used, as this transforms probabilities onto the real number line. For models on rates, the log-link is commonly used, and for models on parameters that may take both positive and negative values, the identity link is often used.

The common effect model assumes that each study estimates the same underlying common effect:

$$\delta_i = d \tag{14.3}$$

and any differences in results observed between studies are simply the result of sampling error.

The random effects model relaxes this by assuming that each study estimates a different treatment effect, but that the treatment effects are exchangeable across studies, typically assumed to come from a common Normal distribution of study-specific treatment effects, with between-study standard deviation in study effects, τ:

$$\delta_i \sim \mathrm{N}(d, \tau^2). \tag{14.4}$$

Independent prior distributions are given to the study-specific reference treatment (arm 1) effects, μ_i, and the pooled treatment effect, d. Typically, these are given independent vague Normal priors:

$$\mu_i, d \overset{iid}{\sim} \mathrm{N}(0, 1000).$$

For the random effects model a prior distribution is also specified for the between-studies standard deviation τ, often a uniform prior with range appropriate to the scale of the relative treatment effect. For example, for the chlorhezidine example a range of (0,5) represents a very wide range for between-study standard deviation of log-odds ratios: $\tau \sim \mathrm{Uniform}(0, 5)$.

14.2.2 Model summaries and predictions

For the common effect model, the primary focus is on the pooled treatment effect, d, which can be summarized with the posterior mean, posterior median and credible interval (e.g. 95% CI).

For the random effects model, we estimate the distribution of study treatment effects, which can be summarized in a variety of ways, each with a different interpretation. The study-specific "shrunken effects" δ_i represent the modeled estimates for each study. These will differ from the raw effects observed in each study, because the exchangeability model shrinks study effects towards the overall random effect mean, d (this is a result of "borrowing strength" from the other study results).

The random effects distribution can be summarized by the mean, d, but note that we should interpret this as the treatment effect we would expect to see in a study that is similar to the "average" study, that is, a study in the middle of the distribution of effects (14.4). An alternative summary is to predict what we would expect to see in a new study population that is exchangeable with the studies included in our meta-analysis, by forming the predictive distribution:

$$\delta_{new} \sim \mathrm{N}(d, \tau^2). \tag{14.5}$$

The predictive distribution will still be centred in the same place as the posterior distribution for d, but the credible limits will be wider, reflecting our uncertainty as to where a new study population might lie in the random effects distribution, as well as reflecting parameter uncertainty in the values of d and τ (Ades et al., 2005).

Finally, we may consider one particular study population, (study i^*, say) to be most representative of the population that we wish to make inference for, in which case the shrunken estimate, δ_{i^*}, is the most appropriate summary to use from the random effects model (Welton and Ades, 2012; Welton et al., 2015).

Figure 14.1 shows the forest plot with the raw observed estimates for each study, the shrunken estimates for each study based on the random effects model, the common effect pooled estimate, the random effects mean estimate, and the predictive distribution from the random effects model. It can be seen that the shrunken estimates are closer to the random effects mean, and more precisely estimated than the raw study estimates, due to having borrowed strength across studies. For this example, the estimated random effects mean is practically identical to the common effect model estimate, but with a wider 95% CI due to accounting for potential statistical heterogeneity. Although the interval around the random effects mean indicates strong evidence of an intervention effect in an 'average' RCT, we see that the 95% predictive interval is much wider and crosses the null value of 1. This reflects a high level of uncertainty as to where in the random effects distribution the treatment effect in a new study population would fall.

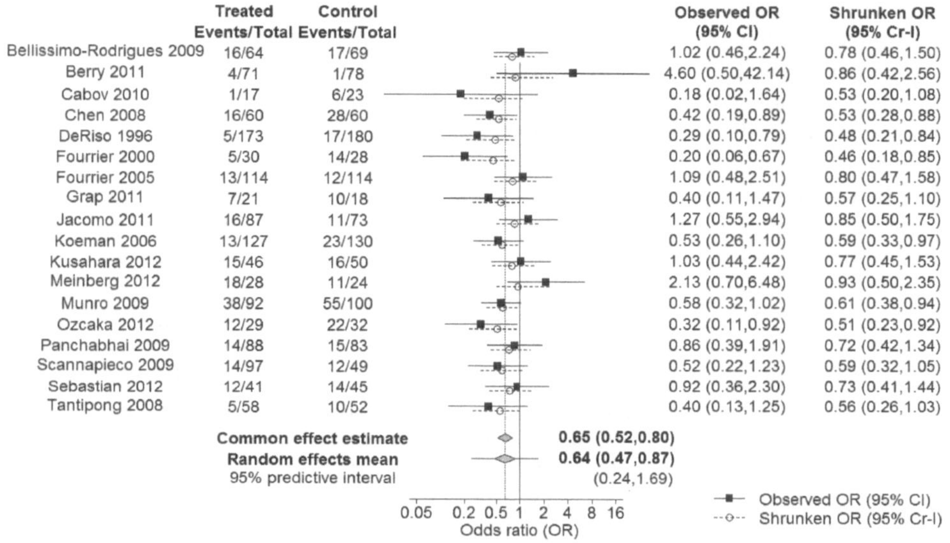

FIGURE 14.1: Chlorhezidine data set: Forest plot displaying results from Bayesian common effect and random effects meta-analyses.

14.2.3 Evidence based priors for variance parameters

Meta-analyses are often conducted with relatively small numbers of studies, which makes it challenging to estimate the between-studies standard deviation parameter τ. The Bayesian approach gives the opportunity to use external information to help estimate τ. In particular, Turner et al. (2012, 2015) estimated τ for 14,886 meta-analyses in the Cochrane library with binary outcomes, and fitted a random effects Log-Normal distribution to obtain a prediction for τ that might be expected to be seen in a new study exchangeable with those Cochrane meta-analyses. Turner et al. (2012, 2015) give predictions for τ in 80 different settings, according to the type of interventions compared, outcomes measured, and disease area. The appropriate prediction can be selected and used as an informative Log-Normal prior for τ.

For example, for the chlorhezidine example, with a vague Uniform(0,5) prior distribution τ was estimated to be 0.36, with 95% CI (0.03 to 0.85) (Table 14.1). For a meta-analysis of a pharmaceutical intervention versus placebo or control, with an outcome type of 'infection/onset of new disease' Turner et al. (2015) propose a $N(-2.49, 1.52^2)$ prior for τ. Applying this more informative prior to the chlorhezidine data, τ is estimated to be lower (0.11) and with a slightly narrower credible interval (0.00 to 0.57) (Table 14.1). The point estimate of the random effects mean is robust to this change in prior distribution, but its CI and the 95% predictive interval (PI) each become narrower due to the smaller estimate of τ (see Table 14.1 and Figure 14.1).

14.2.4 Exploring heterogeneity, meta-regression and subgroup analysis

It is important to assess whether there is evidence of statistical heterogeneity (in which case the random effects model is more appropriate than the common effect model), and if so to attempt to explain this heterogeneity, so that we can obtain more precise and interpretable results. In a Bayesian analysis, various statistics can be used to compare models. Here we present the posterior mean residual deviance as a measure of fit, the between studies standard deviation as a measure of heterogeneity, and the Deviance Information Criterion (DIC) which has been proposed as a measure of parsimony, balancing model fit with model complexity (Spiegelhalter et al., 2002, 2014). Models with smaller values for these statistics are preferred (Spiegelhalter et al., 2002, 2014). The deviance is defined as $-2\times$log-likelihood for a given fitted model. The residual deviance is defined as the deviance for the model minus the deviance for a saturated model (where each data-point is estimated exactly), to give a reference point. When comparing two models, we prefer the model with the lowest posterior mean deviance (or equivalently the model with the lowest posterior mean residual deviance). When considering the fit of a single model, we can compare the posterior mean of the residual deviance to the number of unconstrained data-points to get a measure of overall fit (models with values much larger than this indicate lack of fit). The DIC is the sum of the posterior mean deviance, $\bar{D}$, and the effective number of parameters, p_D, a measure of model complexity (Spiegelhalter et al., 2002) — see Chapter 1. For the common effect model, p_D can be counted directly as the number of studies N plus 1 (a μ_i for each study plus one d), e.g. 19 for the chlorhezidine data. For the random effects model, p_D will depend on the degree of heterogeneity, τ, with p_D similar to that from the common effect model when τ is close to 0, and p_D increasing to a maximum of $2N$ (a separate μ_i and δ_i for each study) as τ increases (Dias et al., 2018; Welton et al., 2012).

Table 14.1 compares these model summaries for the common and random effects models for the chlorhezidine example. We see that the posterior mean residual deviance is lower for the random effects model, indicating evidence of statistical heterogeneity. The posterior mean residual deviance for the random effects model is closer to 36 (the number of unconstrained data points, 18 studies $\times$ 2 arms) suggesting the random effects model provides a better fit. Note that this is nearly always the case, as random effects models can fit well simply by estimating a large value for τ. The DIC is also lower for the random effects model but only by one point. This suggests that the gain in model fit from the random effects model may not out weigh the increased complexity it introduces (increased effective number of parameters).

If possible, we wish to explain any heterogeneity that is apparent. Two main approaches are usually taken: sub-group analysis and meta-regression (Dias et al., 2013b; Sutton et al., 2000). In a sub-group analysis we simply perform the meta-analysis separately for different groups of studies, defined according to some criteria. For example, we might have concerns about bias according to a lack of methodological rigour in some of the included studies. To demonstrate the approach, we stratify the chlorhezidine studies into two groups: those assessed to be at high or unclear risk of bias due to lack of concealment of allocation to treatment arm in the randomisation (8 studies) versus those at low risk of bias (10 studies). Table 14.2 shows the results. We find that treatment effects favour chlorhezidine more strongly in the studies at high risk of bias.

Meta-regression estimates a regression coefficient that describes an interaction between treatment effect and some numerical characteristic of the included studies, x_i, with the model:

$$g(\theta_{i,k}) = \mu_i + (\delta_i + \beta x_i)\mathbb{I}_{k\neq 1}. \tag{14.6}$$

TABLE 14.1: Deviance Information Criterion (DIC) for the common effect and random effects model applied to the chlorhezidine data. $\bar{D}$ = posterior mean deviance, p_D = effective number of parameters. CI = credible interval; PI = predictive interval.

	$\bar{D}$	p_D	DIC	Posterior mean (95%CI) for τ	OR (95% CI) (95% PI)
Common effect model	48.4	19.1	67.5	—	0.65 (0.52, 0.80)
Random effects model with $N(-2.49, 1.52^2)$ prior for $\log(\tau)$, based on Turner et al. (18)	45.1	22.1	67.2	0.11 (0.00, 0.57)	0.64 (0.51, 0.83) PI: (0.37, 1.12)
Random effects model (with U(0,5) prior for τ)	40.3	26.1	66.4	0.36 (0.03, 0.85)	0.64 (0.47, 0.87) PI: (0.24, 1.69)

TABLE 14.2: Results from subgroup analyses of the chlorhezidine data according to risk of bias for allocation concealment.

		RCTs at low risk of bias for allocation concealment (n=10)	RCTs at high / unclear risk of bias for allocation concealment (n = 8)
Common effect meta-analysis	OR (95% CI)	0.78 (0.59, 1.03)	0.51 (0.37, 0.71)
Random effects meta-analysis*	RE mean OR (95% CI)	0.79 (0.56, 1.11)	0.51 (0.36, 0.70)
	95% predictive interval for the OR in a new trial	0.40 to 1.63	0.31 to 0.80
	τ (95% CI)	0.12 (0.00, 0.74)	0.06 (0.00, 0.49)

*Random effects results shown are from analyses with a $N(-2.49, 1.52^2)$ prior for $\log(\tau)$ (see Turner et al., 2015, as well as Section 14.2.3)

In the above equation, β is interpreted as the change in treatment effect for a unit change in study characteristic x, and δ_i is the study-specific treatment effect when $x_i = 0$, which can be modeled either as a common effect (14.3), or as a random effects model (14.4), representing residual heterogeneity after accounting for x. Note that if x is a binary indicator, then the meta-regression model (14.6) is almost equivalent to performing a random effects subgroup analysis, with the exception that between-study heterogeneity τ can be shared across the subgroups. For the chlorhezidine example, if x_i is 1 for studies at high/unclear risk of bias due to inadequate allocation concealment, and 0 otherwise, then β is the difference in log-odds ratios for studies at high/unclear risk of bias compared with studies at low risk of bias. Table 14.3 gives the results from this analysis, which are seen to be very similar to the results obtained from sub-group analysis.

Models can be compared on the basis of posterior mean (residual) deviance and DIC to assess whether there is any evidence of effect modification by inclusion of covariates x_i. In the ideal case, all heterogeneity would be explained by observed covariates, so that the remaining model reduces to a common effect model (Welton et al., 2015), although this is likely to be unusual in practice. For the chlorhezidine example, model fit statistics indicate only a slight improvement in model fit, and between-study standard deviation is only very slightly reduced by incorporating the risk of bias indicator (Table 14.3). This indicates that there is only weak evidence of the bias indicator being an important predictor of estimated treatment effect, which is consistent with the 95% CI for the ratio of ORs (Table 14.3) crossing the null value of 1. Adjusting for risk of bias moves the estimated OR closer to 1, and the 95% credible interval overlaps 1.

TABLE 14.3: Results from a meta-regression of the chlorhezidine data, with high/unclear risk of bias for allocation concealment (versus low risk) as a covariate compared with a meta-analysis that does not account for risk of bias. A $N(-2.49, 1.52^2)$ prior was used for $\log(\tau)$ in both cases (Turner et al., 2015, see also Section 14.2.3). $\bar{D}$ = posterior mean deviance, p_D = effective number of parameters. CI=credible interval; PI=predictive interval

Model	$\bar{D}$	p_D	DIC	τ (95%CI)	OR (95% CI) (95%PI)	Ratio of ORs for high/unclear vs. low risk of bias (95%CI)
Random effects, no adjustment for risk of bias	45.1	22.1	67.2	0.11 (0.00, 0.57)	0.64 (0.51, 0.83) (0.37, 1.12)	—
Meta-regression adjusting for risk of bias	43.2	22.4	65.6	0.09 (0.00, 0.55)	0.77 (0.57, 1.09) (0.46, 1.37)	0.65 (0.39, 1.03)

14.2.5 Sparse data

When events are either very rare or very common, standard frequentist approaches to meta-analysis run into difficulties, because they first form the empirical log-odds ratio before combining in meta-analysis (using a Normal likelihood, Sweeting et al., 2004). Approaches, such as Bayesian MCMC, that allow specification of an exact Binomial likelihood for each arm are preferred in this case (as described above for the chlorhezidine example). This means that studies which have a zero count on one arm (or equivalently all participants experience the event), can be included in the meta-analysis without needing to make a crude adjustment (such as the custom of adding 0.5 to each arm in a standard frequentist analysis, Sweeting et al., 2004). Note that if there are zero counts on both arms in a study, then we know that the event is relatively rare and that study is not sufficiently powered to detect differences in treatment effects for the event under question. Such a study provides information on the overall probability of the event, but the observed results are just as consistent with odds ratios that are much less than 1 as they are with odds ratios that are much more than 1 or equal to 1. Such studies therefore provide no information on the *relative* treatment effects and may be excluded from the meta-analysis (regardless of whether a Bayesian or frequentist analysis is conducted).

14.2.6 Shared parameter models

Studies often measure and report study outcomes in different ways, reflecting different (but related) quantities. Frequentist approaches to meta-analysis tend to either exclude studies for which a common summary measure (e.g. log-odds ratio) cannot be obtained, or use approximations to obtain common summary measures (e.g. converting from standardized mean differences to log-odds ratios, Chinn, 2000). A Bayesian approach allows us to combine information on an underlying parameter that fully reflects the data-generating process, even if outcomes have been reported differently in different studies (Dias et al., 2018; Welton et al., 2008, 2010). For example, suppose that we are looking at treatments to prevent relapse in patients with schizophrenia. We recognise that the relapse rate will depend on follow-up time, so the underlying parameters of interest are relapse rates, with treatment effects modeled as log-rate ratios. Some studies may provide direct information on rates, by reporting the total number of events, $y_{i,k}$, over an observed person-years at risk exposure, $E_{i,k}$. This data generating process is well described by a Poisson likelihood and model on the log-rate scale:

$$\begin{aligned} Y_{i,k} &\sim \text{Pois}(\theta_{i,k} E_{i,k}) \\ \log(\theta_{i,k}) &= \mu_i + \delta_i \mathbb{I}_{k \neq 1}. \end{aligned}$$

Other studies may report number of events $y_{i,k}$ out $n_{i,k}$ randomized over a follow-up period of s_i. The generating process that describes this data is Binomial, but the probability of an event is derived as the complementary log-log link function:

$$\begin{aligned} Y_{i,k} &\sim \text{Bin}(\theta_{i,k}, n_{i,k}) \\ \text{cloglog}(\theta_{i,k}) &= \mu_i + \delta_i \mathbb{I}_{k \neq 1}. \end{aligned}$$

The effects on the reference treatment (arm 1), μ_i, have a different interpretation for the two sets of studies, but the relative treatment effects δ_i are log-rate ratios in both cases, and can be combined through either a common effect (14.3) or random effects model (14.4) as described above. In this case the parameters are shared across both model statements.

Shared parameter models can also be used to include a combination of studies that report separately for each arm (with Binomial likelihood) and studies that report summary measures across arms (e.g. log odds ratios and their standard errors, with a Normal likelihood; Dias et al., 2018, 2013a; Franchini et al., 2012; Keeney et al., 2018). Shared parameters can also be used to combine evidence from studies where some report aggregate data summaries and some studies report individual patient level data (Donegan et al., 2013; Riley et al., 2008).

14.3 Network meta-analysis

Network Meta-Analysis (Higgins and Whitehead, 1996; Caldwell et al., 2005; Lu and Ades, 2004) is an extension of pairwise meta-analysis to combine information from RCTs on multiple treatments, where each RCT compares 2 or more interventions. For example, Figure 14.2 shows a network of treatment comparisons made in RCTs of pharmacological treatments for acute depression in bipolar disorder (National Collaborating Centre for Mental Health, National Institute for Health and Care Excellence, 2014), where each connected edge represents two treatments that have been compared head-to-head in at least one RCT. NMA allows evidence on multiple treatments to be pooled using methodology that respects the randomisation in the RCTs, delivering a set of estimates comparing any pair of treatments in the network, even for treatments that have not been compared head-to-head in an RCT. NMA does however require a connected network of treatment comparisons. In other words, we require that there is a path (i.e. at least one RCT) between any two treatments in the network plot. No estimates can be derived between treatments that are not connected in the network plot. We can verify that the network in Figure 14.2 is connected as there is a path from each treatment to every other.

NMA makes the assumption that the evidence is "consistent", meaning that the effects that were seen in an AC trial would have also been seen in an AB trial if it had included a C arm. This can be thought of as an assumption that there are no important differences in treatment effect modifiers between the populations in the different studies. Note that this is essentially the same exchangeability assumption that is also made in the pairwise random effects meta-analysis model (Section 14.4), extended to include more than two treatments (Lu and Ades, 2006).

NMA is commonly used in Health Technology Assessment (HTA; see Chapter 15) to support policy makers and healthcare providers making decisions between multiple treatment options. NMA delivers a set of coherent treatment effect estimates, and correlations between them, that can then be accounted for in subsequent decision models to determine which treatments are most likely to be effective and cost-effective. Even if we are only interested in a comparison between 2 treatments, NMA may be necessary if the treatments of interest have not been compared directly, but indirect evidence exists from a network of comparisons. Historically, frequentist methods for NMA were not available, and so Bayesian methods have been routinely employed for NMA, especially within a HTA context, where results are to be used in an economic model (Dias et al., 2018).

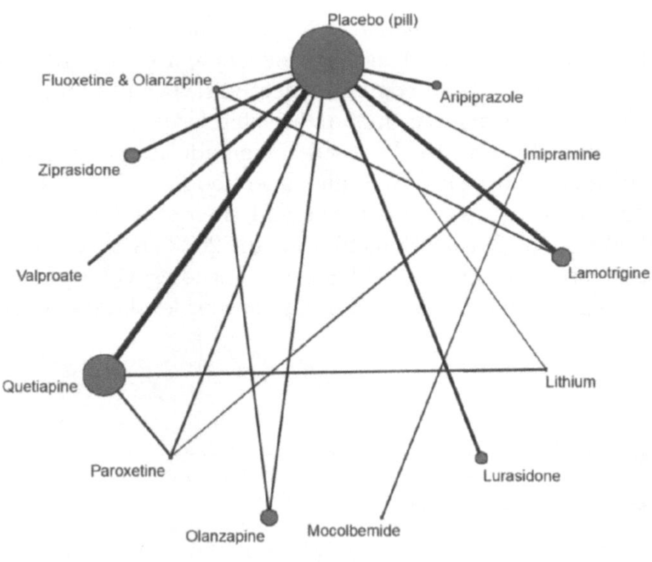

FIGURE 14.2: Network of treatment comparison for the discontinuation outcome in the Bipolar disorder example.

14.3.1 Likelihood, model and priors

The definition of the likelihood is exactly as for pairwise meta-analysis. We describe the model in a generalized linear modelling framework, as set out by Dias et al. (2018, 2013a), who also provide `WinBUGS` code for a wide range of outcomes and link functions (Dias et al., 2011). In the acute depression in bipolar disorder example analyses were presented for two different outcomes (i) discontinuation for any reason, and (ii) response given continued with treatment (National Collaborating Centre for Mental Health, National Institute for Health and Care Excellence, 2014). Here we present the results for the discontinuation outcome. This is a binary outcome, and the data are therefore well described by a Binomial likelihood, as given by Equation (14.1). As for pairwise meta-analysis, the model is put on an appropriate scale using a link function $g(\cdot)$ with the following generalized linear model, which is identical to Equation (14.2), except that the relative treatment effect, $\delta_{i,k}$, depends on study and arm to allow for the fact that some studies may have more than 2 arms:

$$g(\theta_{i,k}) = \mu_i + \delta_{i,k}\mathbb{I}_{k\neq 1}. \tag{14.7}$$

The relative treatment effects may be given a common effect or a random effects model. The common effect model has:

$$\delta_{i,k} = d_{1,t_{i,k}} - d_{1,t_{i,1}}, \tag{14.8}$$

where $t_{i,k}$ is the treatment given on arm k of study i, and $d_{1,c}$ is the relative treatment effect for treatment c compared with treatment 1 (where $d_{1,1} = 0$). Equation (14.7) ensures that the right treatment comparison is picked out for each study arm, and allows each study to have a different reference "arm 1" treatment, $t_{i,1}$. So, a study comparing treatment 2 versus treatment 1 would have $\delta_{i,2} = d_{1,2}$ (because $d_{1,1} = 0$), and a study comparing 4 versus 3 versus 2 would have $\delta_{i,2} = d_{1,3} - d_{1,2}$ and $\delta_{i,3} = d_{1,4} - d_{1,2}$. It is conventional to assume that the treatments are assigned to arms in increasing numerical order to avoid confusion, although this is not strictly necessary for model definition.

Only relative treatment effects compared to treatment 1, $d_{1,c}$, the basic parameters, are estimated and therefore given prior distributions. All other treatment comparisons can be obtained using the consistency equations, which state that:

$$d_{b,c} = d_{1,c} - d_{1,b}. \tag{14.9}$$

The random effects model is the natural extension of the common effect model. For studies with 2 treatment arms we write:

$$\delta_{i,2} \sim \mathrm{N}(d_{1,t_{i,2}} - d_{1,t_{i,1}}, \tau^2) \tag{14.10}$$

where the between-study standard deviation is assumed to be the same across treatment comparisons (the homogenous variance assumption, Lu and Ades, 2004).

Studies with 3 or more treatment arms have correlated relative treatment effects, because they are all relative to the same reference arm 1. Under the homogenous variance assumption, it can be shown that the correlations must be 0.5 (Higgins and Whitehead, 1996). The random effects model then becomes:

$$\begin{pmatrix} \delta_{i,2} \\ \delta_{i,3} \\ \vdots \end{pmatrix} \sim \mathrm{N}\left(\begin{pmatrix} d_{1,t_{i,2}} - d_{1,t_{i,1}} \\ d_{1,t_{i,3}} - d_{1,t_{i,1}} \\ \vdots \end{pmatrix}, \begin{pmatrix} \tau^2 & 0.5\tau^2 & 0.5\tau^2 \\ 0.5\tau^2 & \tau^2 & \vdots \\ 0.5\tau^2 & \dots & \ddots \end{pmatrix} \right).$$

Independent vague Normal priors are given for the study reference treatment (arm 1), (nuisance) parameters, μ_i, and the basic relative effect parameters, $d_{1,c}$ for example

$$\mu_i, d_{1,c} \overset{iid}{\sim} \mathrm{N}(0, 1000)$$

and either a vague uniform prior or an informative prior distribution is given for τ, as for the pairwise case.

14.3.2 Summarising results from NMA

For both the fixed and random effects models, posterior summaries can be obtained for each of the basic parameters $d_{1,c}$ and also for any pairwise comparison $d_{b,c}$ using the consistency Equation (14.9). For the random effects model, these are interpreted as the treatment effects we would expect to see in an "average" study, that is a study in the middle of the distribution of effects (14.10) across studies. An alternative summary is to predict what we would expect to see in a new study population that is exchangeable with the studies included in our meta-analysis, by forming the predictive distribution:

$$\begin{pmatrix} \delta_{new,2} \\ \delta_{new,3} \\ \vdots \end{pmatrix} \sim \mathrm{N}\left(\begin{pmatrix} d_{1,2} \\ d_{1,3} \\ \vdots \end{pmatrix}, \begin{pmatrix} \tau^2 & 0.5\tau^2 & 0.5\tau^2 \\ 0.5\tau^2 & \tau^2 & \vdots \\ 0.5\tau^2 & \dots & \ddots \end{pmatrix} \right).$$

We can think of this as a new study which contains as many treatment arms as there are treatments. Note that the assumption of homogenous variances across all pairwise comparisons induces a correlation of 0.5 between these predicted relative effects, which is captured by sampling from a multivariate Normal distribution (as for multi-arm studies). The predictive estimates will be centred in the same place as the $d_{b,c}$, but with wider credible intervals, reflecting our uncertainty as to where a new study population might lie in the random effects distribution, as well as reflecting parameter uncertainty in the values of $d_{b,c}$ and τ. We can also obtain the shrunken estimates for each comparison made in each study, $\delta_{i,k}$, which are the modeled estimates and will differ from the raw effects observed in each study because the exchangeability model shrinks study effects towards the overall random effect mean, $d_{t_{i,1},t_{i,k}}$, analogous to the pairwise case (Section 14.2.2).

It is often desirable to summarise the results from a NMA in terms of the rankings of the multiple treatments (Caldwell et al., 2005). MCMC simulation makes it straightforward to do so by ranking each treatment at each iteration of the simulation, and then summarising the ranks. We recommend reporting the mean or median rank of each treatment option with a 95% CI (Tan et al., 2014). Some authors also report the proportion of simulations where each treatment was ranked "best", but note that this summary can be very unstable and misleading, due to being strongly influenced by estimates with high levels of uncertainty. A better option is to report not just the proportion of times a treatment is best, but also 2nd, 3rd best etc, as this will give a better impression of the uncertainty in the ranks.

Table 14.4 shows the log-odds ratios and odds ratios for discontinuation in the acute depression in bipolar disorder example for all interventions relative to the reference, placebo in this case. Figure 14.3 displays these log odds ratios in a forest plot. There are 78 possible pairwise comparisons between the 13 treatments. All 78 relative effects and CIs can be derived from the NMA using the consistency equations.

Table 14.5 shows the mean and median ranks with 95% CI for each intervention along with the probability that it is the best intervention. Although the Fluoxetine & Olanzapine combination has a lower mean rank and a tighter CI, Valproate has a probability of being the best treatment which is just over 50%. This reflects the considerable uncertainty in the

TABLE 14.4: Bipolar example: Log-odds ratios (LOR) and odds ratios (OR) for discontinuation. Results are from a random effects model.

	Treatment	LOR for Discontinuation Median	95% CI	OR for Discontinuation* Median	95% CI
1	Placebo	REFERENCE	—	—	—
2	Aripiprazole	0.46	(0.08, 0.84)	1.58	(1.09,2.31)
3	Imipramine	0.30	(−0.58, 1.21)	1.35	(0.56,3.36)
4	Lamotrigine	−0.04	(−0.30, 0.23)	0.96	(0.74,1.26)
5	Lithium	0.03	(−0.52, 0.56)	1.03	(0.59,1.75)
6	Lurasidone	0.15	(−0.25, 0.55)	1.16	(0.78,1.74)
7	Mocolbemide	0.49	(−0.67, 1.66)	1.64	(0.51,5.28)
8	Olanzapine	−0.15	(−0.49, 0.18)	0.86	(0.61,1.20)
9	Paroxetine	−0.04	(−0.51, 0.41)	0.97	(0.60,1.51)
10	Quetiapine	0.03	(−0.19, 0.26)	1.04	(0.82,1.29)
11	Valproate	−0.49	(−1.38, 0.39)	0.61	(0.25,1.48)
12	Ziprasidone	0.37	(0.06, 0.68)	1.44	(1.06,1.96)
13	Fluoxetine & Olanzapine	−0.42	(−0.84, −0.01)	0.66	(0.43,0.99)

*values greater than 1 favour the active treatment compared to Placebo

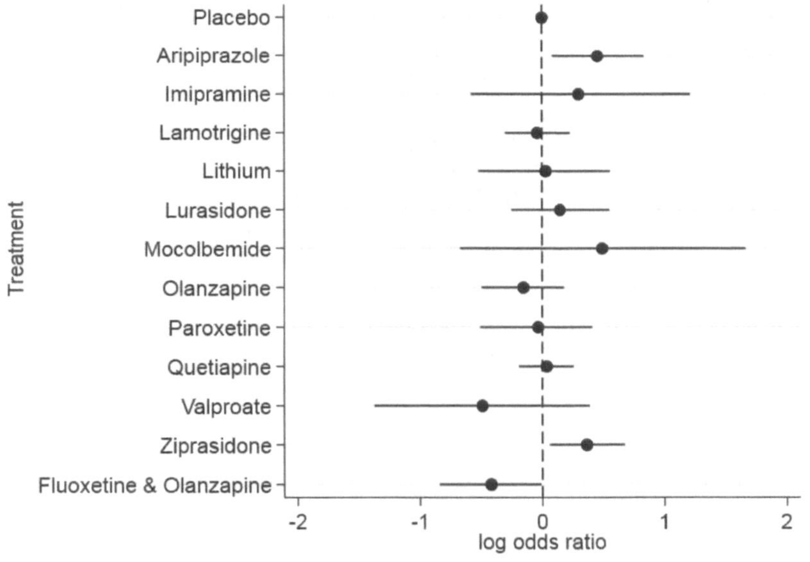

FIGURE 14.3: Bipolar example: Log-odds ratios for discontinuation. Values greater than zero favour placebo (the reference treatment). Results are from a random effects model.

estimates (Figure 14.3) which allow for the possibility that Valproate can be very effective, even better than Fluoxetine & Olanzapine, although it can also be less effective than this combination. Figure 14.4 shows the probability that each intervention is ranked in each of the 13 positions, from best (rank=1) to worst (rank =13). High values on the left hand side represent high probabilities of low ranks and hence indicate an intervention with a high probability of being among the best. Valproate and Fluoxetine & Olanzapine have high probabilities of being ranked 1st or 2nd, as expected.

TABLE 14.5: Bipolar example: Rank statistics and probability of being the best (i.e. ranked 1) of each intervention for the discontinuation outcome. Sorted by mean rank.

Treatment	Mean	Median	95% CI	Pr(best)
Fluoxetine & Olanzapine	2.1	2	(1,6)	34.8%
Valproate	2.8	1	(1,11)	50.8%
Olanzapine	4.3	4	(1,10)	3.0%
Lamotrigine	5.8	6	(2,10)	0.2%
Paroxetine	5.9	6	(1,11)	2.8%
Placebo (pill)	6.4	6	(4,9)	0.0%
Lithium	6.8	7	(1,12)	2.8%
Quetiapine	7.0	7	(3,11)	0.1%
Lurasidone	8.3	9	(3,13)	0.3%
Imipramine	9.1	10	(2,13)	2.2%
Mocolbemide	10.2	12	(1,13)	3.0%
Ziprasidone	10.8	11	(7,13)	0.0%
Aripiprazole	11.4	12	(8,13)	0.0%

14.3.3 Heterogeneity and inconsistency

As for pairwise meta-analysis, model selection can be guided by the posterior mean (residual) deviance which measures fit, inspection of between-studies standard deviation, which indicates evidence of heterogeneity, and DIC, which is a measure that has been proposed to balance model fit and model complexity (Spiegelhalter et al., 2002, 2014). In the Bipolar disorder example the common effects model had a poor fit to the data with a posterior mean of the residual deviance of 70.9, for 64 data points. The random effects model fitted better with posterior mean of the residual deviance of 63.3. The posterior median for the between-study heterogeneity was 0.15 with 95%CI (0.01, 0.32). Although the DIC were comparable across the two models (428.3 and 428.0 for the common and random effects models, respectively), the random effects model was preferred due to its better fit and *a priori* expectation of heterogeneity for this outcome.

As well as assessing heterogeneity by comparing the common effect and random effects model, we also need to assess the consistency assumption. One approach is to fit a model that relaxes the consistency assumption (the inconsistency model, Dias et al., 2013c) and compare that with the model that assumes consistency — see Equations (14.8) and (14.10). The inconsistency model for the common effects model is given by

$$\delta_{i,k} = d_{t_{i,1},t_{i,k}},$$

so that a different treatment effect is estimated for each treatment comparison. The random effects inconsistency model is also changed accordingly:

$$\delta_{i,2} \sim \mathrm{N}(d_{t_{i,1},t_{i,2}}, \tau^2).$$

In the presence of inconsistency, we expect the posterior mean deviance to be reduced for the inconsistency model compared to the consistency model, but a comparison of the DIC can assess whether the extra complexity in the inconsistency model is worthwhile. It is also helpful to inspect the posterior median for the between studies standard deviation, τ. If this is lower under the inconsistency model, it suggests that there is evidence of inconsistency, which manifests as heterogeneity in a consistency model. A plot of each data point's contribution to the deviance under each model is also informative (Dias et al., 2018, 2013c).

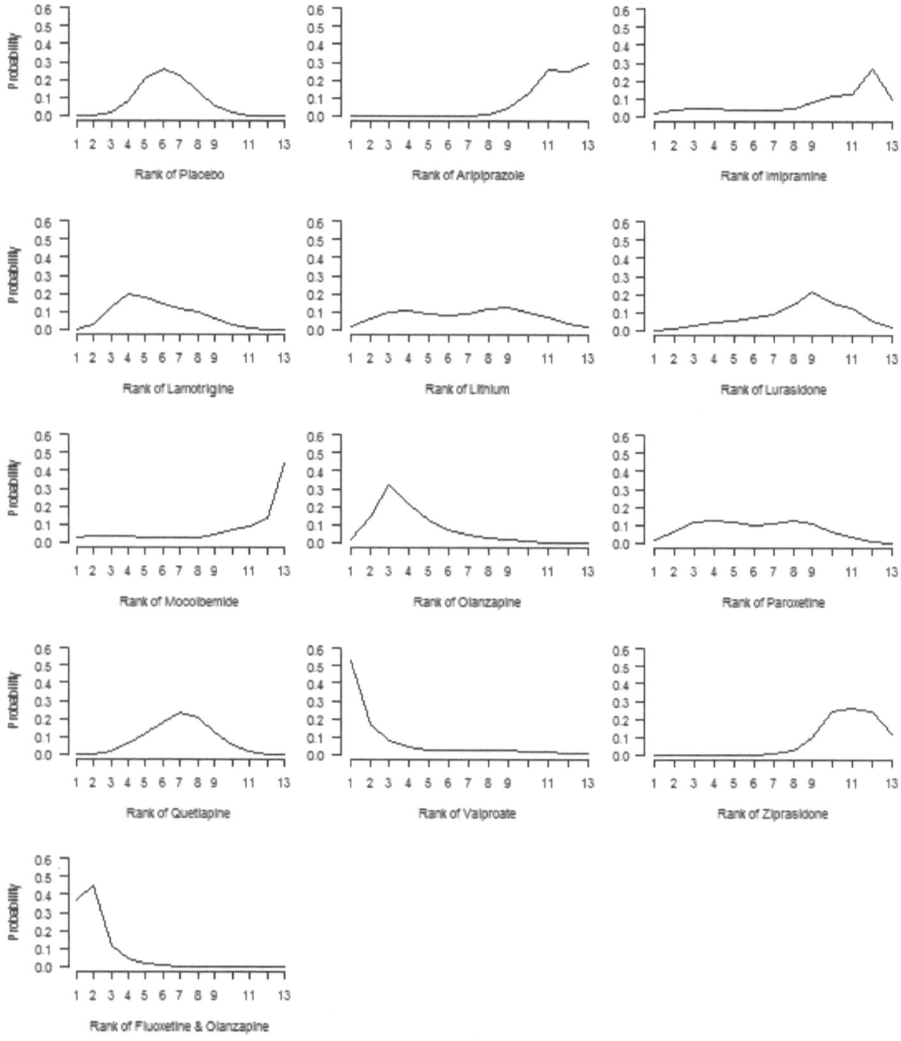

FIGURE 14.4: Bipolar example: Plots of ranking probabilities for each treatment for the discontinuation outcome.

In the Bipolar disorder example, fit slightly improved when a random effects model without the consistency assumption was fitted. The posterior mean of the residual deviance is reduced to 62.1 and DIC is reduced to 425.8. The posterior median of the between-study heterogeneity is also slightly reduced to 0.11 with 95% CI (0.01, 0.29). Figure 14.5 shows the mean of the contribution of each data point to the residual deviance for the random effects models assuming consistency and not assuming consistency. Data points for 3 studies show an improvement in fit when the inconsistency model is fitted. Further inspection of these studies to determine which loops they are involved in can help determine potential causes for inconsistency.

Inconsistency can be further explored using node-splitting models (Dias et al., 2010a), where for a given focal treatment comparison b versus c, the direct evidence from RCTs that compare b versus c head-to-head is "split" from the remaining evidence. The split evidence estimates $d_{b,c}^{direct}$, whereas the remaining evidence estimates $d_{b,c}^{indirect}$, where the between-studies standard deviation is shared across both models (an example of a shared parameter

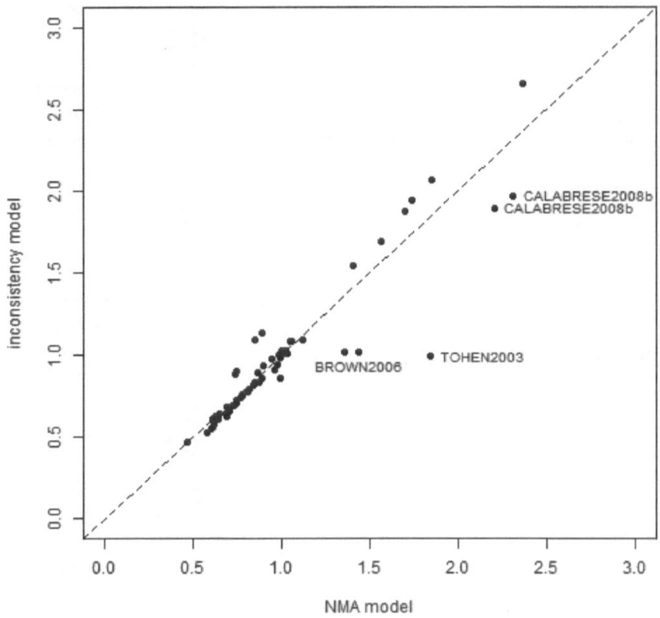

FIGURE 14.5: Bipolar example: Plot of individual data points' contributions to the residual deviance on the NMA model assuming consistency and in the inconsistency model. Studies for which data points have an improved residual deviance in the inconsistency model are noted.

model, Section 14.2.6). Posterior distributions for the direct and indirect estimates can then be compared to assess the existence of inconsistency for the b versus c contrast and a probability of conflict can be calculated (Bayesian P-value, Presanis et al., 2013; Gelman et al., 2014; Spiegelhalter et al., 2004). Node-splitting is computationally intensive because it needs to be run for each focal pair of treatments where it is possible to estimate both direct and indirect treatment effect estimates but it provides a description of potential conflict between direct and indirect evidence for all contrasts where both sources of evidence are pooled.

Table 14.6 shows the results from running node-split models for all nodes that can be split in the Bipolar disorder example. We note that the P-values are smallest for contrasts involving interventions (1,4) and (4,13), which refer to comparisons of Lamotrigine to Placebo and Fluoxetine & Olanzapine to Lamotrigine, respectively (intervention numbers are given in Table 14.4). It should be noted that the studies highlighted in Figure 14.5 also compare these interventions, thus both methods for detecting inconsistency are highlighting potential problems with these comparisons. However, in both cases there is only weak evidence of potential inconsistency.

14.3.4 Network meta-regression and subgroup analysis

As for pairwise meta-analysis, we would like to explain heterogeneity and inconsistency if possible. Subgroup analyses extend naturally to NMA. Meta-regression models can also be specified (Dias et al., 2018, 2013b; Donegan et al., 2012), but for network meta-regression we need to impose the consistency assumption on the regression coefficient, as well as on the treatment effect parameters (Cooper et al., 2009; Donegan et al., 2018, 2017). The network

TABLE 14.6: Bipolar example: Node-split results for discontinuation outcome, including a Bayesian P-value for conflict between direct and indirect evidence. Intervention numbers are as given in Table 14.4.

	Contrasts									
	(1,4)		(1,13)		(4, 13)		(8,13)		(9,10)	
	Median	95%CI	Median	95%CI	Median	95%CI	Median	95%CI	Median	95%CI
Direct	0.059	(-0.21,0.32)	-0.75	(-1.3,-0.19)	-0.063	(-0.56,0.43)	-0.61	(-1.2,-0.047)	-0.088	(-0.62,0.47)
Indirect	-0.73	(-1.5,-0.0023)	-0.0016	(-0.60,0.58)	-0.84	(-1.4,-0.24)	0.31	(-0.46,1.1)	0.63	(-0.40,1.7)
Network	-0.035	(-0.31,0.23)	-0.42	(-0.85,-0.026)	-0.38	(-0.80,0.011)	-0.26	(-0.74,0.20)	0.077	(-0.39,0.58)
SD	0.10	(0.01,0.30)	0.11	(0.01,0.32)	0.10	(0.01,0.30)	0.11	(0.01,0.32)	0.13	(0.01,0.35)
Bayesian p-value	0.046		0.071	0.049		0.055		0.226		

meta-regression model is:

$$g(\theta_{i,k}) = \mu_i + \left(\delta_{i,k} + (\beta_{1,t_{i,k}} - \beta_{1,t_{i,1}})x_i\right) \mathbb{I}_{k \neq 1}, \tag{14.11}$$

where $\beta_{1,c}$ is the additional treatment effect for treatment c compared to treatment 1 for each unit change in covariate x. There is usually insufficient evidence to estimate separate regression coefficients $\beta_{1,c}$ for each treatment, and so some further simplifying assumptions are made (Dias et al., 2018), such as each active treatment has the same (or similar) regression coefficient(s) compared with standard care, treatment 1, i.e. $\beta_{1,c} = \beta$ or $\beta_{1,c} \sim \mathrm{N}(B, \sigma_B^2)$ for $c \neq 1$.

14.4 Bias modeling in pairwise and network meta-analysis

The validity of pooled estimates obtained from pairwise meta-analysis or NMA depends on the validity of the study evidence on which they are based. Meta-analysis suffers from the old adage of "rubbish in rubbish out". The systematic review process used to identify relevant studies should to some extent mitigate this by excluding studies that are not RCTs and therefore excluding observational studies vulnerable to bias when inferring causal effects. However, even RCTs differ in methodological rigour, with some studies at a higher risk of producing biased results than other studies. For example, studies where patients, practitioners and outcome assessors are blinded to the treatment that has been received (e.g. by use of an adequate placebo) have been shown to give less strong treatment effects on average than studies where this isn't the case (Savovic et al., 2012a,b, 2018). Similarly, studies where the person randomising patients to treatment arms is aware of the next treatment allocation tend to give stronger treatment effects than studies where allocation to treatment is adequately concealed (Savovic et al., 2012a,b, 2018). This is a potential source of heterogeneity that should be explored and adjusted for, to avoid drawing conclusions based on results that may be biased.

The meta-regression and network meta-regression models — see (14.6) and (14.11) — can be used to estimate treatment effect modification associated with risk of bias indicators, x_i, as illustrated for pairwise meta-analysis in Section 14.2.4 and for NMA in Dias et al. (2010b). However, there is often very little ability to estimate the regression coefficients given the small number of studies typically included in meta-analyses and even smaller numbers with each combination of risk of bias indicators. A Bayesian approach is useful in this context because external evidence on bias can be used to form prior distributions for the effect modification due to studies at risk of bias in a new meta-analysis, so that the resulting estimates are adjusted for potential bias. Two approaches to use of external data have been proposed, one using evidence-based prior distributions based on analyses of collections of previous meta-analyses, the other using expert elicitations on the extent of bias in the included studies.

14.4.1 Bias adjustment using evidence-based priors

Savovic et al. (2012a,b, 2018) analysed data from collections of over 200 meta-analyses (meta-epidemiological databases), where each study in each meta-analysis was assessed for risk of bias on several indicators of methodological rigour, including random sequence generation, allocation concealment, and double-blinding. They used a model proposed by Welton et al. (2009) that extends the meta-regression model (14.6) to account for bias within and between meta-analyses as follows, extending the notation from Section 14.2.1 to include a meta-analysis indicator, m:

$$\begin{aligned} Y_{i,k,m} \mid \theta_{i,k,m} &\sim f(\theta_{i,k,m}) \\ g(\theta_{i,k,m}) &= \mu_i + (\delta_{i,m} + \beta_{i,m} x_{i,m}) \mathbb{I}_{k \neq 1}, \end{aligned}$$

where $\beta_{i,m}$ is the bias in study i, included in meta-analysis m and associated with risk of bias indicator $x_{i,m}$. Either a common effect or random effects model can be given for the relative treatment effect in studies that are not at risk of bias, $\delta_{i,m}$:

$$\delta_{i,m} = d_m \qquad \text{or} \qquad \delta_{i,m} \sim \mathrm{N}(d_m, \tau_m^2).$$

A multi-level model is given to the bias parameters, $\beta_{i,m}$, so that:

$$\begin{aligned} \beta_{i,m} &\sim \mathrm{N}(b_m, \kappa^2) \\ b_m &\sim \mathrm{N}(b_0, \phi^2), \end{aligned} \tag{14.12}$$

where κ^2 reflects between-study variance in bias within each meta-analysis, and ϕ^2 reflects the between meta-analysis variance in mean bias; b_m is the mean bias in meta-analysis m; and b_0 is the overall bias across meta-analyses.

The bias parameters estimated from the meta-epidemiological evidence can be used to form an informative hierarchical prior for bias in a new meta-analysis, m^* (Welton et al., 2009):

$$\begin{aligned} \beta_{i,m^*} &\sim \mathrm{N}(b_{m^*}, \kappa^2) \\ b_{m^*} &\sim \mathrm{N}(b_0, \phi^2). \end{aligned}$$

This approach adjusts and down-weights the evidence from studies assessed as being at high risk of bias. Savovic et al. (2012a,b, 2018) provide values for b_0, ϕ and κ by outcome type and by risk of bias indicator.

Returning to the chlorhezidine example presented in Section 14.2, we fit the bias-adjustment model with allocation concealment as an indicator of risk of bias. Recall that in Section 14.2.4 we found some evidence that the studies at high or unclear risk of bias due to the approach used to conceal the allocation sequence estimated a stronger treatment effect than the studies with adequate allocation concealment (Ratio of ORs = 0.65, 95% CI 0.39 to 1.03, Table 14.3).

We used estimates reported by Savovic et al. for subjective (patient- or physician-reported) outcomes, to form the following approximate Normal prior distributions for the parameters of the bias model:

$$b_0 \sim \mathrm{N}(-0.16, 0.06^2), \quad \kappa \sim \mathrm{N}(0.20, 0.08^2) \quad \text{and}$$
$$\log(\phi) \sim \mathrm{N}(-2.41, 0.86^2).$$

The resulting bias-adjusted estimate reflecting the predicted bias from the meta-epidemiological literature is 0.72 with 95%CI (0.56, 0.91) and 95%PI (0.45, 1.14). We see that this estimate is a compromise between that from an analysis taking all 18 studies at face value (OR = 0.64, Figure 14.1) and from an analysis restricted to the studies with adequate allocation concealment (OR = 0.78, Table 14.2). The CI is also narrower than that from the subgroup analysis or simple meta-regression, and excludes the null value of 1. Note that this approach relies on the assumption that the study-specific biases in the new meta-analysis are exchangeable with those in the meta-epidemiological data used to form the priors. Savovic et al. (2012a) also report parameter estimates tailored to particular clinical areas, but these estimates are very imprecise. In addition, they explore the impact of adjusting for multiple risk of bias indicators, finding that the effects may be less than additive, although this result is very uncertain due to small numbers of studies with each combination of indicators. Because studies at high risk of bias tend to be smaller studies, a more fruitful approach may be to conduct meta-regression with study size as an effect modifier (Moreno et al., 2011, 2009a,b).

Prior distributions from meta-epidemiological studies can also be applied to NMA; however it becomes necessary to define the direction in which bias is expected to act, especially in studies comparing active treatments, otherwise biases between studies may "cancel out" leading to an underestimate of the mean bias in a meta-analysis (Dias et al., 2010b). Savovic et al. (2012a) excluded trials where it was not clear which direction bias would act. Chaimani et al. (2013) report results from a network meta-epidemiological study, where a collection of network meta-analyses were analysed to estimate bias resulting from indicators of risk of bias. However, they restricted attention to "star-networks" (i.e. those where all treatments have been compared with a common comparator) so that the direction in which bias might act could be assumed to be against the common comparator. They found that imprecise studies were associated with large treatment effects.

14.4.2 Bias adjustment using priors elicited from experts

Turner et al. (2009) proposed a method of bias-adjustment based on magnitude and uncertainty of potential bias elicited from experts. Experts are asked about both internal biases caused by methodological flaws and external biases caused by a lack of generalisability of the included studies to the target parameter of interest for the research question. The method works by first defining the target research question, then describing an idealized version of each available study. Potential internal and external biases are then identified. Opinion on the magnitude and uncertainty for each of these biases is elicited from each assessor by marking ranges on bias elicitation scales that indicate that they believe the bias is twice as likely to lie inside the range than outside it. They are also asked whether the bias is expected to act additively or proportionally. The information given in these ranges is then combined to obtain a bias-adjusted estimate and standard error for each assessor and study. Turner et al. (2009) summarized the assessors' bias-adjusted estimates by taking the median bias-adjusted estimate and the median standard error to represent a "typical" assessor. An alternative approach would be to mathematically pool the estimates across assessors (using for example the linear opinion pool or the logarithmic opinion pool, O'Hagan et al., 2006). The bias-adjusted estimates are then used as inputs to the meta-analysis (or NMA).

This approach has the advantage that it can be used to combine both RCT and observational studies, and also can be used to adjust for external biases as well as internal biases.

It is conceptually simple, however requires considerable time and effort to conduct, experts find it a challenging task to perform, and it is vulnerable to the subjectivity of the experts' beliefs.

14.5 Using meta-analysis to inform study design

The Bayesian paradigm of updating beliefs with the accumulation of new evidence lends itself naturally to the design of new research studies. Where there is existing study evidence that can be summarized by a meta-analysis, a new research study should be designed using information that is available from the existing evidence (Lau et al., 1995). It may be, for example that there is already an over-whelming body of evidence in favour of a new treatment based on a meta-analysis or NMA, and there is therefore no need for a new study. Or there may be uncertainty as to whether a new treatment is effective based on meta-analysis, and a new study will be able to add to the existing evidence to make more certain conclusions. The natural way to express existing information is through a prior distribution, which will be combined with the data observed in the new study to form a posterior distribution. Below we first describe approaches to incorporate prior information in power calculations for the new study. We then discuss different options to form a prior distribution for a new study, based on an existing meta-analysis.

14.5.1 Incorporating prior information in power calculations

Traditional power calculations are derived from a frequentist hypothesis testing framework, and compute the probability of rejecting the null hypothesis at a given significance level (e.g. 0.05) when in fact the null hypothesis is false and the true parameter value is d^* (usually set to a minimally clinically important effect that we would like to be able to detect). Power depends on sample size for the new study, and so sample size can be chosen so that the new study achieves the required level of power.

Two approaches have been proposed to incorporate prior information in power calculations for a new study, both of which assume that the analysis of the new study data will be a Bayesian analysis that combines the prior information with the likelihood, to obtain a posterior distribution for the effect size. Conditional power is computed as the probability of rejecting the null hypothesis if the true parameter value is d^* in the new study, based on the posterior distribution that would be obtained by updating the prior. Conditional power has been proposed in the context of interim analyses within an RCT, where the prior distribution is the data that has accumulated in the RCT at the interim, and the conditional power computation is for the remaining data that will be collected in the RCT. However, the ideas apply equally well to the context of a prior based on a meta-analysis at the start of a new RCT. Rather than setting a value d^* for the alternative hypothesis, Spiegelhalter et al. (2004) suggest computing an average probability of rejecting the null hypothesis, averaged across the prior distribution for the effect size, known as the 'expected power'.

14.5.2 Forming a prior distribution for a new study, based on an existing meta-analysis

Whichever approach is used, we need to decide what summary from the meta-analysis should be used as a prior in the power calculation. If there is no evidence of heterogeneity in the existing meta-analysis, then the posterior distribution for the estimated pooled common effect, d, should be used as a prior for the new study. However, if there is evidence of heterogeneity, then a random effects meta-analysis is appropriate, and there are several options: the random effects mean, d, the predictive distribution, $\delta_{new} \sim \text{N}(d, \tau^2)$, the shrunken estimate for a study i^* considered representative of the new study population, δ_{i^*}, or the entire random effects distribution $\text{N}(d, \tau^2)$, where the new study is expected to be added to the meta-analysis and update our estimates of d and τ (Welton and Ades, 2012; Welton et al., 2015; Jones et al., 2018). We argue that the choice of prior should be based on the interpretation of the heterogeneity that is present in the existing meta-analysis (Jones et al., 2018). It is unlikely that we believe the new study population to be exactly equal to the mean of the previous studies, and so we do not recommend using the random effects mean as a prior. If we believe that the new study population is exchangeable with the previous studies that have been conducted (see Chapter 6), then it is appropriate to use the predictive distribution as the prior for the new study. If we believe that one of the studies (or a sub-set of studies) in the meta-analysis best represents the population in our new study, then the shrunken estimate for that study (or a pooled summary of the sub-set of representative studies) can be used as a prior for the new study. If we can explain aspects of the heterogeneity through sub-group analysis or meta-regression, then we should use the predictive distribution or shrunken estimate for the relevant sub-group or covariate values that we consider relevant for our new study. For example, in the chlorhezidine meta-analysis, assuming we plan to adequately conceal the randomisation sequence in the new study, then we may wish to use the results from the sub-group analysis where allocation concealment is adequate, results from the meta-regression that adjusts for bias due to inadequate/unclear allocation concealment or results from the bias-adjusted meta-analysis (Section 14.4.1).

Finally, if we believe that the heterogeneity seen between studies is due to natural variation that we would see when the intervention is rolled out in practice (e.g. therapist effects), then we would want to update the meta-analysis with the new study results to better estimate the distribution of effects that we would expect to see in practice. Here focus is on the random effects mean of an updated meta-analysis, and on the between-studies standard deviation. Sutton et al. (2007) has extended the expected power calculation to the case where the target for inference is the updated meta-analysis (rather than the posterior distribution for the new study result based on the prior). Similarly, Roloff et al. (2013) have extended the idea of conditional power to the case where the target for inference is the updated meta-analysis.

14.6 Further reading

We end this chapter by briefly describing some further areas where Bayesian methods have been particularly valuable in evidence synthesis and point to key literature for further reading.

For many applications the impact of treatments on survival outcomes (overall survival and progression free survival) are the focal outcomes. Under the proportional hazards assumption, the relative treatment effects can be summarized as hazard ratios, and meta-analysis models can be used for the log-hazard ratios. However, decision models require survival differences to be predicted over a patient's life-time, which depends on (i) extrapolating survival curves beyond the typical follow-up available in RCTs, and (ii) assumptions to be made about the plausibility of the proportional hazards assumption over time. Guyot et al. (2016) propose a method to combine RCT evidence with external evidence from registry data, meta-analysis of related treatments in the same disease area, and expert opinion, to extrapolate treatment benefits into the long-term. The Bayesian approach enables all of these sources of information to be combined to estimate survival benefits over the patient's lifetime.

For interventions that aim to prevent long-term outcomes, it is infeasible to conduct RCTs that follow-up a sufficient number of patients for sufficiently long-periods to have power to detect benefits on the long-term clinical outcomes. For example, interventions to lower blood pressure or reduce cholesterol ultimately aim to reduce cardiovascular events and mortality. Instead, RCTs are powered to detect surrogate outcomes, such as blood pressure or cholesterol levels, which are associated with the long-term clinical outcomes of key interest. While it may be well established that the surrogate and clinical outcomes are associated, a stronger assumption that treatment effect modification on the surrogate outcomes leads to treatment effect modification on the clinical outcome is required. Bayesian multivariate meta-analysis methods have been used to combine information from studies where some studies report surrogate outcomes and other studies report both surrogate and clinical outcomes. This allows the relationship between effect modification on surrogates and clinical outcomes to be estimated, so that the larger body of evidence on the surrogate outcomes can be used to predict the clinical outcomes of interest (Achana et al., 2014; Bujkiewicz et al., 2016, 2013; Daniels and Hughes, 1997; Riley et al., 2007).

In some clinical areas the outcome of interest may be measured using a variety of different scales which all attempt to measure the same underlying construct. For example, there are many different scales that measure depression (HAM-D, BDI, PHQ9, MADRS, etc), and each study may have reported results for one or more of these scales. Bayesian multivariate meta-analysis methods have been developed to combine evidence on all outcomes that are reported, estimating a set of mapping coefficients for the relative treatment effects on one scale into those on another scale (Ades et al., 2015; Lu et al., 2014) so that a single pooled estimate can be obtained on the chosen outcome of interest while still combining evidence from all studies. This approach avoids the need to perform the meta-analysis on a standardized mean difference scale, which is difficult to interpret and use in subsequent analyses (such as cost-effectiveness analysis).

In some cases, it is desirable to combine both RCT and observational evidence (in generalized evidence synthesis, Welton et al., 2012; Prevost et al., 2000). For example, the RCT evidence may be imprecise, and based on small studies at high risk of bias. However, observational evidence is known to suffer from a range of potential biases (Deeks et al., 2003) which we wish to account for. Ibrahim and Chen (2000) have proposed using the observational evidence to form an informative prior for the RCT evidence, but where the likelihood for the observational evidence is raised to a power α (a power-prior). For a value $\alpha = 0$ the observational evidence is totally discounted, and for a value of $\alpha = 1$ the observational evidence is taken at face-value as if it were another RCT. The resulting pooled estimate can be plotted against α as part of a sensitivity analysis to the weight given to the observational evidence. The expert elicitation methods described in Section 14.5 can also be used to form priors for bias adjustment for observational evidence (Turner et al., 2009, and Chapter 6).

Multi-parameter Evidence Synthesis (MPES) models combine evidence from multiple sources that provide information about two or more parameters either directly or indirectly (through a function of parameters, Welton et al., 2012; Ades and Sutton, 2006; Ades et al., 2008). Evidence is combined to estimate a unified model with shared parameters, where all parameters are estimated jointly, which is possible through the specification of a Bayesian model. MPES is particularly valuable when interest is on parameters that are difficult or impossible to measure directly (e.g. prevalence of people who inject drugs), but evidence on functions of those parameters is available (e.g. opioid related mortality). The framework requires a detailed understanding of the data generating process, and how these relate to the underlying model parameters. This allows the assessment of the consistency of the various items of data, to explore robustness of the resulting estimates. MPES methods have been used to estimate the prevalence of HIV (Goubar et al., 2008; Presanis et al., 2012, 2010), prevalence of Hepatitis C (HCV; Sweeting et al., 2008; De Angelis et al., 2009), prevalence of people who inject drugs (Sweeting et al., 2009; Jones et al., 2016), prevalence of toxoplasmosis, and vertical transmission of early onset group B streptococcus (Colbourn et al., 2007a,b).

Bibliography

Achana, F., Cooper, N., Bujkiewicz, S., Hubbard, S., Kendrick, D., Jones, D., and Sutton, A. (2014). Network meta-analysis of multiple outcome measures accounting for borrowing of information across outcomes. *BMC Medical Research Methodology*, 14(1):92.

Ades, A. and Sutton, A. (2006). Multiparameter evidence synthesis in epidemiology and medical decision making: current appoaches. *Journal of the Royal Statistical Society — Series A*, 169(1):5–35.

Ades, A., Welton, N., Caldwell, D., Price, M., Goubar, A., and Lu, G. (2008). Multiparameter evidence synthesis in epidemiology and medical decision-making. *Journal of Health Services Research & Policy*, 13(3_suppl):12–22.

Ades, A. E., Lu, G., Dias, S., Mayo-Wilson, E., and Kounali, D. (2015). Simultaneous synthesis of treatment effects and mapping to a common scale: an alternative to standardisation. *Research Synthesis Methods*, 6:96–107.

Ades, A. E., Lu, G., and Higgins, J. (2005). The interpretation of random effects meta-analysis in decision models. *Medical Decision Making*, 25(6):646–654.

Briggs, A., Claxton, K., and Sculpher, M. (2006). *Decision Modelling for Health Economic Evaluation.* Oxford University Press, Oxford, UK.

Bujkiewicz, S., Thompson, J., Sutton, A., Cooper, N., Harrison, M., Symmons, D., and Abrams, K. (2013). Multivariate meta-analysis of mixed outcomes: a Bayesian approach. *Statistics in Medicine*, 32:3926–3943.

Bujkiewicz, S., Thompson, J. R., Riley, R. D., and Abrams, K. R. (2016). Bayesian meta-analytical methods to incorporate multiple surrogate endpoints in drug development process. *Statistics in Medicine*, 35(7):1063–1089.

Caldwell, D., Ades, A., and Higgins, J. (2005). Simultaneous comparison of multiple treatments: combining direct and indirect evidence. *British Medical Journal*, 331:897–900.

Chaimani, A., Vasiliadis, H., Pandis, N., Schmid, C., Welton, N., and Salanti, G. (2013). Effects of study precision and risk of bias in networks of interventions: a network meta-epidemiological study. *International Journal of Epidemiology*, 42:1120–1131.

Chinn, S. (2000). A simple method for converting an odds ratio to effect size for use in meta-analysis. *Statistics in Medicine*, 19:3127–3131.

Claxton, K. (1999). The irrelevance of inference: a decision-making approach to the stochastic evaluation of heath care technologies. *Journal of Health Economics*, 18(3):341–364.

Claxton, K., Sculpher, M., McCabe, C., Briggs, A., Akehurst, R., Buxton, M., Razier, J., and O'Hagan, A. (2005). Probabilistic sensitivity analysis for NICE Technology Assessment: not an optional extra. *Health Economics*, 14:339–347.

Colbourn, T., Asseburg, C., Bojke, L., Philips, Z., Welton, N., Claxton, K., Ades, A., and Gilbert, R. (2007a). Preventive strategies for group b streptococcal and other bacterial infections in early infancy: cost effectiveness and value of information analyses. *British Medical Journal*, 335:655–661.

Colbourn, T., Asseburg, C., Bojke, L., Phillips, Z., Claxton, K., Ades, A., and Glibert, R. (2007b). Prenatal screening and treatment strategies to prevent group b streptococcal and other bacterial infections in early infancy: cost-effectiveness and expected value of information analysis. *Health Technology Assessment*, 11(29):1–226.

Cooper, N., Sutton, A., Morris, D., Ades, A., and Welton, N. (2009). Addressing between-study heterogeneity and inconsistency in mixed treatment comparisons: Application to stroke prevention treatments in individuals with non-rheumatic atrial fibrillation. *Statistics in Medicine*, 28:1861–1881.

Daniels, M. and Hughes, M. (1997). Meta-analysis for the evaluation of potential surrogate markers. *Statistics in Medicine*, 16:1965–1982.

De Angelis, D., Sweeting, M., Ades, A., Hickman, M., Hope, V., and Ramsay, M. (2009). An evidence synthesis approach to estimating hepatitis C prevalence in England and Wales. *Statistical Methods in Medical Research*, 18:361–379.

Deeks, J., Dinnes, J., D'Amico, R., Sowden, A., Sakarovitch, C., Song, F., Petticrew, M., and Altman, D. G. (2003). Evaluating non-randomised intervention studies. *Health Technology Assessment*, 7(27).

Dias, S., Ades, A. E., Welton, N. J., Jansen, J. P., and Sutton, A. J. (2018). *Network Meta-Analysis for Decision Making.* Statistics in Practice. Wiley.

Dias, S., Sutton, A., Ades, A., and Welton, N. (2013a). Evidence synthesis for decision making 2: A generalized linear modeling framework for pairwise and network meta-analysis of randomized controlled trials. *Medical Decision Making*, 33:607–617.

Dias, S., Sutton, A., Welton, N., and Ades, A. (2013b). Evidence synthesis for decision making 3: Heterogeneity - subgroups, meta-regression, bias and bias-adjustment. *Medical Decision Making*, 33:618–640.

Dias, S., Welton, N., Caldwell, D., and Ades, A. (2010a). Checking consistency in mixed treatment comparison meta-analysis. *Statistics in Medicine*, 29:932–944.

Dias, S., Welton, N., Marinho, V., Salanti, G., Higgins, J., and Ades, A. E. (2010b). Estimation and adjustment of bias in randomised evidence by using mixed treatment comparison meta-analysis. *Journal of the Royal Statistical Society — Series A*, 173(3):613–629.

Dias, S., Welton, N., Sutton, A., and Ades, A. (2011). NICE DSU technical support document 2: A generalised linear modelling framework for pair-wise and network meta-analysis of randomised controlled trials. `http://www.nicedsu.org.uk`.

Dias, S., Welton, N., Sutton, A., Caldwell, D., Lu, G., and Ades, A. (2013c). Evidence synthesis for decision making 4: Inconsistency in networks of evidence based on randomized controlled trials. *Medical Decision Making*, 33:641–656.

Donegan, S., Dias, S., Tudur-Smith, C., Marinho, V., and Welton, N. J. (2018). Graphs of study contributions and covariate distributions for network meta-regression. *Research Synthesis Methods*, 9(2):243–260.

Donegan, S., Welton, N. J., Tudur Smith, C., D'Alessandro, U., and Dias, S. (2017). Network meta-analysis including treatment by covariate interactions: Consistency can vary across covariate values. *Research Synthesis Methods*, 8(4):485–495.

Donegan, S., Williamson, P., D'Alessandro, U., Garner, P., and Tudor Smith, C. (2013). Combining individual patient data and aggregate data in mixed treatment comparison meta-analysis: Individual patient data may be beneficial if only for a subset of trials. *Statistics in Medicine*, 32:914–930.

Donegan, S., Williamson, P., D'Alessandro, U., and Tudor Smith, C. (2012). Assessing the consistency assumption by exploring treatment by covariate interactions in mixed treatment comparison meta-analysis: individual patient-level covariates versus aggregate trial-level covariates. *Statistics in Medicine*, 31:3840–3857.

Egger, M., Davey-Smith, G., and Altman, D. (2001). *Systematic Reviews in Health Care: Meta-analysis in Context*. British Medical Journal publishing group, London, second edition.

Franchini, A., Dias, S., Ades, A., Jansen, J., and Welton, N. (2012). Accounting for correlation in mixed treatment comparisons with multi-arm trials. *Research Synthesis Methods*, 3:142–160.

Gelman, A., Carlin, J., Stern, H., Dunson, D., Vehtari, A., and Rubin, D. (2014). *Bayesian Data Analysis*. Chapman and Hall, 3 edition.

Goubar, A., Ades, A., De Angelis, D., McGarrigle, C., Mercer, C., Tookey, P., Fenton, K., and Gill, O. (2008). Estimates of human immunodeficiency virus prevalence and proportion diagnosed based on Bayesian multiparameter synthesis of surveillance data. *Journal of the Royal Statistical Society — Series A*, 171:541–580.

Guyot, P., Ades, A. E., Beasley, M., Lueza, B., Pignon, J.-P., and Welton, N. J. (2016). Extrapolation of survival curves from cancer trials using external information. *Medical Decision Making*, 37:353–366.

Higgins, J. and Whitehead, A. (1996). Borrowing strength from external trials in a meta-analysis. *Statistics in Medicine*, 15:2733–2749.

Hua, F., Xie, H., Worthington, H., Furness, S., Zhang, Q., and Li, C. (2016). Oral hygiene care for critically ill patients to prevent ventilator-associated pneumonia. *Cochrane Database of Systematic Reviews* , 10:CD008367.

Ibrahim, J. and Chen, M. (2000). Power prior distributions for regression models. *Statistical Science*, 15(1):46–60.

Jones, H., Welton, N., Ades, A., Pierce, M., Davies, W., Coleman, B., Millar, T., and Hickman, M. (2016). Problem drug use prevalence estimation revisited: heterogeneity in capture-recapture and the role of external evidence. *Addiction*, 111:438–447.

Jones HJ, Welton NJ, Sutton AS, Ades AE (2018). Use of a random effects meta-analysis in the design and analysis of a new clinical trial. *Statistics in Medicine*, 37:4665–4679.

Keeney, E., Dawoud, D., and Dias, S. (2018). Different methods for modelling severe hypoglycaemic events: Implications for effectiveness, costs and health utilities. *PharmacoEconomics.*

Lau, J., Schmid, C. H., and Chalmers, T. C. (1995). Cumulative meta-analysis of clinical trials builds evidence for exemplary medical care. *Journal of Clinical Epidemiology*, 48(1):45–57.

Lu, G. and Ades, A. (2004). Combination of direct and indirect evidence in mixed treatment comparisons. *Statistics in Medicine*, 23:3105–3124.

Lu, G. and Ades, A. (2006). Assessing evidence consistency in mixed treatment comparisons. *Journal of the American Statistical Association*, 101:447–459.

Lu, G., Kounali, D., and Ades, A. E. (2014). Simultaneous multi-outcome synthesis and mapping of treatment effects to a common scale. *Value in Health*, 17:280–287.

McCullagh, P. and Nelder, J. (1989). *Generalised Linear Models.* Chapman and Hall, London, 2nd edition.

Moreno, S., Sutton, A., Ades, A., Stanley, T., Abrams, K., Peters, J., and Cooper, N. (2009a). Assessment of regression-based methods to adjust for publication bias through a comprehensive simulation study. *BMC Medical Research Methodology*, 9(2).

Moreno, S. G., Sutton, A. J., Ades, A. E., Cooper, N. J., and Abrams, K. R. (2011). Adjusting for publication biases across similar interventions performed well when compared with gold standard data. *Journal of Clinical Epidemiology*, 64(11):1230–1241.

Moreno, S. G., Sutton, A. J., Turner, E. H., Abrams, K. R., Cooper, N. J., Palmer, T. M., and Ades, A. E. (2009b). Novel methods to deal with publication biases: secondary analysis of antidepressant trials in the fda trial registry database and related journal publications. *British Medical Journal*, 339:b2981.

National Collaborating Centre for Mental Health, National Institute for Health and Care Excellence (2014). The Assessment and Management of Bipolar Disorder in Adults, Children and Young People in Primary and Secondary Care, updated edition.

O'Hagan, A., Buck, C., Alireza Daneshkhah, J., Eiser, R., Garthwaite, P., Jenkinson, D., Oakley, J., and Rakow, T. (2006). *Uncertain Judgements: Eliciting Experts' Probabilities.* Wiley.

Presanis, A., De Angelis, D., Goubar, A., Gill, O., and Ades, A. (2012). Bayesian evidence synthesis for a transmission dynamic model for HIV among men who have sex with men. *Biostatistics*, 12:666–681.

Presanis, A. M., Gill, O. N., Chadborn, T. R., Hill, C., Hope, V., Logan, L., Rice, B. D., Delpech, V. C., Ades, A. E., and De Angelis, D. (2010). Insights into the rise in HIV infections in England and Wales, 2001 to 2008: a Bayesian synthesis of prevalence studies. *Aids*, 24:2849–2858.

Presanis, A. M., Ohlssen, D., Spiegelhalter, D. J., and De Angelis, D. (2013). Conflict diagnostics in directed acyclic graphs, with applications in Bayesian evidence synthesis. *Statistical Science*, 28:376–397.

Prevost, T., Abrams, K., and Jones, D. (2000). Hierarchical models in generalised synthesis of evidence: an example based on studies of breast cancer screening. *Statistics in Medicine*, 19:3359–3376.

Riley, R., Abrams, K., Lambert, P., Sutton, A., and Thompson, J. (2007). An evaluation of bivariate random-effects meta-analysis for the joint synthesis of two correlated outcomes. *Statistics in Medicine*, 26:78–97.

Riley, R., Lambert, P., Staessen, J., Wang, J., Gueyffier, F., and Boutitie, F. (2008). Meta-analysis of continuous outcomes combining individual patient data and aggregate data. *Statistics in Medicine*, 27:1870–1893.

Roloff, V., Higgins, J., and Sutton, A. (2013). Planning future studies based on the conditional power of a meta-analysis. *Statistics in Medicine*, 32:11–24.

Savovic, J., Jones, H., Altman, D., Harris, R., and Juni, P. (2012a). Influence of reported study design characteristics on intervention effect estimates from randomised controlled trials: combined analysis of meta-epidemiological studies. *Health Technology Assessment*, 16(35):81.

Savovic, J., Jones, H., Altman, D. G., Harris, R. J., Juni, P., Pildal, J., Als-Nielsen, B., Balk, E. M., Gluud, C., Gluud, L. L., Ioannidis, J., Schulz, K., Beynon, R., Welton, N., Wood, L., Moher, D., Deeks, J., and Sterne, J. (2012b). Influence of reported study design characteristics on intervention effect estimates from randomized, controlled trials. *Annals of Internal Medicine*, 157:429–438.

Savovic, J., Turner, R., Mawdsley, D., Jones, H., Beynon, R., Higgins, J., and Sterne, J. (2018). Association between risk-of-bias assessments and results of randomized trials in Cochrane reviews: the ROBES meta-epidemiologic study. *American Journal of Epidemiology*, 187(5):1113–1122.

Smith, T., Spiegelhalter, D., and Thomas, A. (1995). Bayesian approaches to random-effects meta-analysis: a comparative study. *Statistics in Medicine*, 14:2685–2699.

Spiegelhalter, D., Abrams, K., and Myles, J. (2004). *Bayesian Approaches to Clinical Trials and Health-Care Evaluation*. Wiley, New York, NY.

Spiegelhalter, D., Best, N., Carlin, B., and van der Linde, A. (2002). Bayesian measures of model complexity and fit. *Journal of the Royal Statistical Society — Series B*, 64(4):583–616.

Spiegelhalter, D., Best, N., Carlin, B., and van der Linde, A. (2014). The deviance information criterion: 12 years on. *Journal of the Royal Statistical Society — Series B*, 76:485–493.

Sutton, A., Abrams, K., Jones, D., Sheldon, T., and Song, F. (2000). *Methods for Meta-Analysis in Medical Research*. Wiley, London.

Sutton, A., Cooper, N., Jones, D., Lambert, P., Thompson, J., and Abrams, K. (2007). Evidence-based sample size calculations based upon updated meta-analysis. *Statistics in Medicine*, 26:2479–2500.

Sweeting, M., De Angelis, D., Ades, A., and Hickman, M. (2009). Estimating the prevalence of ex-injecting drug use in the population. *Statistical Methods in Medical Research*, 18:381–395.

Sweeting, M., De Angelis, D., Hickman, D., and Ades, A. (2008). Estimating HCV prevalence in England and Wales by synthesising evidence from multiple data sources: assessing data conflict and model fit. *Biostatistics*, 9:715–734.

Sweeting, M., Sutton, A., and Lambert, P. (2004). What to add to nothing? Use and avoidance of continuity corrections in meta-analysis of sparse data. *Statistics in Medicine*, 23:1351–1375.

Tan, S. H., Cooper, N. J., Bujkiewicz, S., Welton, N. J., Caldwell, D. M., and Sutton, A. J. (2014). Novel presentational approaches were developed for reporting network meta-analysis. *Journal of Clinical Epidemiology*, 67:672–680.

Turner, R., Davey, J., Clarke, M., Thompson, S., and Higgins, J. (2012). Predicting the extent of heterogeneity in meta-analysis, using empirical data from the Cochrane Database of Systematic Reviews. *International Journal of Epidemiology*, 41:818–827.

Turner, R., Spiegelhalter, D., Smith, G., and Thompson, S. (2009). Bias modelling in evidence synthesis. *Journal of the Royal Statistical Society — Series A*, 172:21–47.

Turner, R. M., Jackson, D., Wei, Y., Thompson, S. G., and Higgins, J. P. T. (2015). Predictive distributions for between-study heterogeneity and simple methods for their application in Bayesian meta-analysis. *Statistics in Medicine*, 34(6):984–998.

Welton, N., Ades, A., Carlin, J., Altman, D., and Sterne, J. (2009). Models for potentially biased evidence in meta-analysis using empirically based priors. *Journal of the Royal Statistical Society — Series A*, 172(1):119–136.

Welton, N. and Ades, A. E. (2012). Research decisions in the face of heterogeneity: what can a new study tell us? *Health Economics*, 21(10):1196–200.

Welton, N., Cooper, N., Ades, A., Lu, G., and Sutton, A. (2008). Mixed treatment comparison with multiple outcomes reported inconsistently across trials: evaluation of antivirals for treatment of influenza a and b. *Statistics in Medicine*, 27:5620–5639.

Welton, N., Sutton, A., Cooper, N., Abrams, K., and Ades, A. (2012). *Evidence Synthesis for Decision Making in Healthcare*. Statistics in Practice. Wiley.

Welton, N., Willis, S., and Ades, A. (2010). Synthesis of survival and disease progression outcomes for health technology assessment of cancer therapies. *Research Synthesis Methods*, 1:239–257.

Welton, N. J., Soares, M. O., Palmer, S., Ades, A. E., Harrison, D., Shankar-Hari, M., and Rowan, K. M. (2015). Accounting for heterogeneity in relative treatment effects for use in cost-effectiveness models and value-of-information analyses. *Medical Decision Making*, 35:608–621.

White, I. (2009). Multivariate random-effects meta-analysis. *Stata Journal*, 9:40–56.

White, I. (2011). Multivariate random-effects meta-regression: Updates to mvmeta. *Stata Journal*, 11:255–270.

White, I. R. (2015). Network meta-analysis. *Stata Journal*, 15(4):951–985.

15

Economic Evaluation and Cost-Effectiveness of Health Care Interventions

Nicky J Welton

University of Bristol, UK

Mark Strong

University of Sheffield, UK

Christopher Jackson

MRC Biostatistics Unit, Cambridge, UK

Gianluca Baio

University College London, UK

Economic evaluation in healthcare comprises a set of analytical tools to combine all relevant evidence on costs and consequences of intervention(s) compared to a control or status quo. The aim is to aid decision-making associated with resource allocation, for example, whether a health service payer should reimburse the provider of a new pharmaceutical product. Recent research has been oriented towards building the health economic evaluation on sound Bayesian decision-theoretic foundations. The aim of this chapter is to provide a review of the background and modeling approaches used in HTA, particularly using a Bayesian approach. In particular, we focus on a brief review of the decision-theoretic framework, before moving to an illustration of concepts from the use of evidence synthesis to inform the modeling to tools such as the Value of Information, which can be used to prioritise and design research, based on the level of current uncertainty in the model inputs.

15.1 Introduction

Broadly speaking, the objective of publicly funded health care systems (e.g. those in the UK, Canada, Australia and many other countries around the world) is to maximise health gains across the general population in specific countries or settings, given finite monetary resources and a limited budget. In this respect, Health technology assessment (HTA) has been defined as a multidisciplinary process that summarizes information about the medical, social, economic and ethical issues related to the use of a health technology in a systematic, transparent, unbiased, robust manner. As part of their HTA system, bodies such as the *National Institute for Health and Care Excellence* (NICE) in the UK provide guidance on decision-making on the basis of *health economic evaluation* (NICE, 2013).

Economic evaluation in healthcare comprises a set of analytical tools to combine all relevant evidence on costs and consequences of intervention(s) compared to a control or status quo. The aim is to aid decision-making associated with resource allocation, for example, whether a health service payer should reimburse the provider of a new pharmaceutical product. Recent research has been oriented towards building the health economic evaluation on sound Bayesian decision-theoretic foundations (O'Hagan and Stevens, 2001; O'Hagan et al., 2001; Spiegelhalter et al., 2004; Baio, 2012), arguably making it a branch of applied statistics (Briggs et al., 2006; Spiegelhalter et al., 2004; Willan and Briggs, 2006).

The focus on decision making here is crucial, because the main output of the analysis is not merely the estimation of relevant population parameters, but rather the identification of the most rational course of action, in the face of uncertain consequences and on the basis of the current evidence. The meaning of "rational decision making" may depend on the jurisdiction or specific setting considered. For instance, in many publicly funded healthcare systems, this coincides with the maximisation of gains across the whole population of interest. For this reason, in settings such as the UK's, NICE has the mandate to recommend whether a new intervention is paid for with tax money and the UK National Health Service is legally obliged to fund and resource medicines and treatments recommended by NICE's technology appraisals. For these reasons, the process of HTA plays a fundamental role within pharmaceutical development.

The aim of this chapter is to provide a review of the background and modeling approaches used in HTA, particularly using a Bayesian approach. The chapter is structured as follows. Firstly in Section 15.2 we introduce the decision theoretic framework utilized in HTA; then in Sections 15.3 and 15.4 we discuss the distinction between HTA based on trial data and those constructed using modeling for long-term outcomes and how this links to availability of data from generalized evidence synthesis and meta-analyses (see Chapter 14). In Section 15.5 we briefly introduce the concept of Value of Information and its use in terms of assessing the impact of uncertainty in the model inputs on the overall decision making process. Finally, in Section 15.6 we summarise some future developments and directions for the field.

15.2 Economic evaluation: A Bayesian decision theoretic analysis

15.2.1 The decision problem

We assume that the decision maker is faced with a set of mutually exclusive decision options, indexed d in the decision space $\mathcal{D}$. In cost-effectiveness analysis, d usually represents a treatment option within some set of competing alternatives in $\mathcal{D}$. Taking an option d will lead to some *consequences* of interest, which in this context are usually the costs, c_d and health effects, e_d associated with decision option d, up until some *time horizon*. The time horizon is often the lifetime of the patient, or the earliest point at which the alternative treatments do not differ in their consequences. Note that e_d and c_d are not individual-level outcomes, but represent average consequences over the population who will be affected by the decision.

For example, a recent NICE clinical guideline presented a model comparing the cost-effectiveness of pharmacological interventions for acute depression in adults with bipolar disorder (NICE, 2014). The decision options d were nine different pharmacological interventions (imipramine, lamotrigine, lithium, moclobemide, olanzapine, paroxetine, quetiapine, valproate semisodium, and the combination of fluoxetine and olanzapine) and "No pharmacological treatment" as the reference comparator. It is recognized that *all* relevant available evidence on the whole set of options $\mathcal{D}$ should be considered when performing the analysis; this usually leads to considering generalized evidence synthesis approaches, e.g. network meta-analysis (NMA; see Chapter 14).

The decision options and identification of relevant evidence will depend on the country or setting under consideration. This is a crucial issue when adapting "global" cost- effectiveness models to specific geographical settings. Patients in different jurisdictions may differ in important characteristics that affect their overall consequences and may even affect the relative efficacy of treatments. It is expected that jurisdiction specific evidence is required to estimate the costs and consequences of patients under standard care in that country. Relative treatment effects tend to be more generalisable across jurisdictions and populations; however care should still be taken to assess whether the studies included in an evidence synthesis are representative of the target population of interest in terms of key factors that may interact with relative treatment effects. Different decision options may be available in different jurisdictions, due to differences in licensing of products. Also, standard care may differ across jurisdictions. NMA allows all treatments to be simultaneously compared, but the results from just those treatments of interest can then be used for decision-making. The advantage of using all the available treatments in the NMA is that evidence from the non-relevant treatments can indirectly contribute to the relative treatment effects for the treatments relevant to the decision. For example, in the case of acute depression discussed in NICE (2014), three pharmacological interventions that were included in the network meta-analysis of the available RCT evidence were excluded from the decision set for the economic evaluation (two because they were not available in the UK setting, and one because it was ineffective compared to placebo and was not considered a viable treatment option).

15.2.2 Utility

In accordance with the precepts of decision theory, if the decision maker wishes to avoid a loss, they will select the option that maximises their utility for the consequences associated with each option (Lindley, 1991; Bernardo and Smith, 1994). The decision maker must therefore define a *utility function* that maps consequences to their value. In many health care systems (e.g. the UK's; NICE, 2013) this utility function is defined to be the net monetary benefit, $\mathcal{U}_d = \lambda e_d - c_d$ where λ (alternatively referred to as k, e.g. Baio, 2012; Baio et al., 2017) is the value to the decision maker, in monetary units, of one unit of health effect. Within the cost-effectiveness analysis paradigm, λ is the *shadow price of the budget constraint*, i.e. the cost per unit health effect for those activities that are *displaced* when a choice is made to adopt an intervention that increases resource use within a fixed budget (Culyer and Chalkidou, 2019).

Often, the health effects are expressed through the *Quality-Adjusted Life Year* (QALY), which combines the time spent in a given health state (e.g. "perfect health") with a preference-based measure that quantifies the "quality" of life associated with that specific health state (Loomes and McKenzie, 1989). Specifically, the QALY $q(T)$ experienced by a person over a period from 0 to T years is $q(T) = \int_0^T u(t)dt$ where $u(t)$ is the health-related quality of life at time t, measured on a scale where $u(t) = 1$ represents full health, and $u(t) = 0$ death. Note that $u(t)$ is often referred to as the "utility", but in this context this refers to the patient's rather than the decision maker's value function.

15.2.3 Estimating costs and benefits

The problem with the formulation above is that the true values of c_d and e_d are almost always unknown. We must therefore estimate them based on current data and/or expert knowledge. One option is to design a study (e.g. a randomized controlled trial) from which we can estimate c_d and e_d directly for all d. This approach is called 'trial-based economic analysis', and we discuss this in Section 15.3 below. Alternatively, we can estimate c_d and e_d *indirectly* via some kind of mathematical or computer *model*. A model expresses our beliefs about the relationship between the unknown c_d and e_d and some vector of input parameters $\boldsymbol{\theta}$ for which we have estimates. The structure of the model encodes our knowledge about disease natural history, clinical pathways, treatment effects, and so on. We discuss this in Section 15.4.

15.2.4 Uncertainty

Whether we estimate c_d and e_d (and therefore our utility) directly in a trial, or indirectly using a model, we are *uncertain* about their true values (where we take 'true' to mean those values we would observe in a perfect study of infinite size). Uncertainty about the true values of c_d and e_d can (but not always) result in *decision uncertainty*. Decision theory tells us that in the face of uncertainty we should choose the option that maximises our *expected* utility (Lindley, 1991; Bernardo and Smith, 1994; Claxton, 1999), where the expectation in this case is taken with reference to the (joint) probability distribution that represents our judgements about c_d and e_d based on *current* evidence. By placing a distribution over the unknown quantities c_d and e_d we are representing uncertainty about our beliefs using probability, and are therefore being Bayesian.

We note that current evidence may be in the form of data characterized by a short follow up or small sample size. It is thus relevant to assess the impact of current uncertainty on the decision making process, particularly where we have the option of delaying a treatment adoption decision in order to gather new data. New data may reduce the chance of a sub-optimal decision, and therefore can have value to the decision maker. We discuss the concept of Value of Information in Section 15.5 below.

In a nutshell, the process of health economic evaluation can be graphically summarized as shown in Figure 15.1. The starting point is a *statistical model* that is used to estimate parameters $\boldsymbol{\theta}$. The estimates from the statistical model are then fed to the economic model, which generates costs and health effects for each decision option. Costs and health effects are then combined in the decision maker's utility function and thus form the basis for the *decision analysis*, which identifies the optimal decision option as that which maximizes expected utility (Lindley, 1991; Bernardo and Smith, 1994).

15.3 Trial-based economic evaluation

In a trial-based economic evaluation, the expected costs and benefits are obtained directly from individual-level data on costs and health effects. Thus in Figure 15.1, the population parameters $\boldsymbol{\theta}$ are identical to the population average costs and benefits required for decision analysis. For example, a typical dataset used in trial-based economic evaluation may look like that presented in Table 15.1.

Notice that, in addition to the "standard" clinical outcome $\boldsymbol{x}$ (possibly measured over a number of follow up points $j = 1, \ldots, J$ for each individual i), which would usually be the

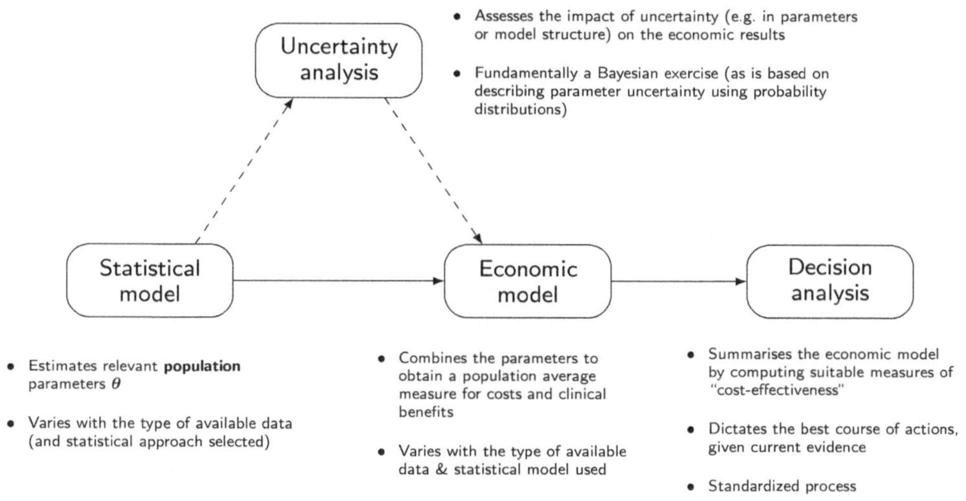

FIGURE 15.1: A graphical representation of the process of health economic evaluation based on cost-effectiveness or cost-utility analysis. Source: Baio et al. (2017)

TABLE 15.1: An example of a typical dataset used in trial-based economic evaluation. The main clinical outcome $\boldsymbol{x}$ may be measured on a number of follow up points and could represent some time-to-event, continuous measurement (e.g. blood pressure) or the occurrence of a clinically relevant event (e.g. myocardial infarction).

		Demographics			**HRQL data**				**Resource use data**				**Clinical outcome**			
ID	**Trt**	Sex	Age	...	u_0	u_1	...	u_J	c_0	c_1	...	c_J	x_0	x_1	...	x_J
1	1	M	23	...	0.32	0.66	...	0.44	103	241	...	80	y_{10}	y_{11}	...	y_{1J}
2	1	M	21	...	0.12	0.16	...	0.38	1 204	1 808	...	877	y_{20}	y_{21}	...	y_{2J}
3	2	F	19	...	0.49	0.55	...	0.88	16	12	...	22	y_{30}	y_{31}	...	y_{3J}
...	...	...	...	...	...	...	...	...	...	...	...	...	...	...	...	...

primary quantity of interest in a trial, the economic evaluation is also concerned with some measure of the individual's utility (health related quality of life), as well as some measure of the costs associated with the use of the relevant resources. Often, the longitudinal cost outcomes c_{ij} and utility outcomes u_{ij} at times $j = 1, \ldots, J$ are aggregated into a single patient-specific outcome c_i and u_i such as the QALY (defined in Section 15.2.2) or total cost. The quantities of interest would then be e_d, the expected QALY and c_d the expected total cost for patients given intervention d, giving a bivariate outcome $y_d = (e_d, c_d)^\top$. This raises interesting statistical challenges. In general, there is a complex structure of relationships linking costs and health effects; there may be strong positive correlation, since effective treatments could be associated with higher unit costs, particularly where benefits have come at the cost of an intensive and lengthy research programme. Conversely, they may be negatively correlated, as more effective treatments may reduce total care pathway costs e.g. by reducing hospitalizations, side effects, etc.

Consequently, an appropriate statistical model for costs and health effects should formally account for this association, e.g. using a bivariate probability distribution. This increases both modeling and computational complexity, particularly because simplifying assumptions such as normality of the underlying joint distribution for costs and effects are usually not valid. This is because costs are typically characterized by a markedly skewed distribution, which is generally due to the presence of a small proportion of individuals incurring large costs. Similarly, clinical outcomes such as the health state preference scores used to form QALYs are usually defined in the bounded interval between 0 and 1.

Observations of individual-level healthcare costs and health-related quality of life are commonly collected as part of clinical trials. Thus it is common to estimate expected costs c_d and health effects e_d (e.g. as quality-adjusted survival) for each treatment over the follow-up period of the trial. These could be simply estimated as the empirical means, with uncertainty quantified through asymptotic normality or bootstrapping (analysing replicate datasets created by sampling with replacement from the data, Hunink et al., 1998). Fully-parametric modeling, however, is often more efficient (O'Hagan and Stevens, 2003) due to the highly non-normal shape of individual cost data, typically right-skewed with excess zeroes.

Thus there have been many applications of Bayesian models for trial-level cost data (Cooper et al., 2003; Nixon and Thompson, 2004) or joint models for cost and effectiveness data (Nixon and Thompson, 2005; Baio, 2014). The framework extends to hierarchical models for multiple centres in cluster randomized trials (Nixon and Thompson, 2005; Grieve et al., 2005), or data from multiple countries (Manca et al., 2007; Willan et al., 2005). Medical cost data also usually comprise multiple components of resource use, such as drugs and hospital admissions, and Bayesian models can make efficient use of partial information in cases where some components are missing (Lambert et al., 2008). The Bayesian approach also extends to averaging over multiple models when the parametric distribution for costs is uncertain (Conigliani and Tancredi, 2009).

The advantages of using Bayesian inference in these examples lie in the accessibility of computational methods for modeling challenging data structures, and the convenient connection to decision analysis, rather than in the explicit use of prior information. However, informative priors have been shown to be useful in these and similar contexts (e.g. McCarron et al., 2013; Spiegelhalter, 2004; Spiegelhalter et al., 2004) to illustrate how initial "scepticism" or "enthusiasm" about the effectiveness of a treatment may be altered by clinical trial evidence.

15.4 Model-based economic evaluation

A model-based health economic evaluation is used instead of a trial-based analysis when a trial alone is insufficient for a decision about whether a treatment is cost-effective. This may be because, for example, there is other relevant evidence available, or follow-up is too short to capture the full course of illness, or the patients recruited for the trial have different characteristics from those seen in the general population, or because the trial does not include all the decision options in the set $\mathcal{D}$ (Buxton et al., 1997).

15.4.1 Constructing a model

An economic model, also called a "cost-effectiveness model", is a representation of beliefs about the mathematical relationship between the costs and health effects associated with each decision option (which we find difficult to estimate directly), and some set of model input parameters (which we find easier to estimate). This is illustrated in Figure 15.1.

We write the model as the function $f(d, \boldsymbol{\theta})$ that relates model input parameters $\boldsymbol{\theta}$ to costs and effects for each decision option d,

$$(e_d, c_d) = f(d, \boldsymbol{\theta}),$$

from which we can compute net monetary benefit, which we take as being the decision maker's utility,

$$\mathcal{U}_d = \lambda e_d - c_d.$$

The optimal decision option is that which maximises expected utility with respect to uncertainty about $\boldsymbol{\theta}$, i.e.

$$d^* = \arg\max_{d \in \mathcal{D}} \mathrm{E}_{\boldsymbol{\theta}}(\mathcal{U}_d).$$

The function $f(d, \boldsymbol{\theta})$ reflects the structure of the underlying model, which in health economic evaluation is often either a decision tree or 'Markov' state-transition model (Briggs et al., 2006), although more complex tools (e.g. individual-level discrete event simulation models; Karnon and Hossein, 2014) are increasingly used. Parameters in the vector $\boldsymbol{\theta}$ typically include costs associated with clinical events or states of health, health state preference measures, epidemiological quantities such as rates of important events, treatment effects and so on. It is unlikely that we will know the true values of $\boldsymbol{\theta}$ with certainty, and we express our beliefs (derived from data and/or expert opinion) via a probability distribution $p(\boldsymbol{\theta})$.

In the guideline for acute depression in adults with bipolar disorder (NICE, 2014), the economic model took the form of a decision tree. A simplified version of the decision tree is displayed in Figure 15.2. Under each treatment decision option, a patient may either discontinue treatment or continue on treatment. For patients who continue on treatment, they may either respond or not, and those that respond may achieve a partial response or a full response. Responders may subsequently relapse, with a probability that depends on whether they had achieved a partial or full response. Patients that relapse may either enter a manic or depressive episode. If patients discontinue treatment or fail to respond, then their subsequent costs and benefits are the same as if they used no pharmacological treatment. The actual model used in the guideline (NICE, 2014) had the added complication that patients who discontinue or fail to respond are given the option of a second-line treatment, where the costs and consequences of the second-line treatment are as for the first-line treatments. The time-horizon of the model was 18 weeks, to capture treatment of the acute depression phase of bipolar disorders, after which long-term pharmacological maintenance treatment would be initiated. The parameters $\boldsymbol{\theta}$ comprise the probabilities of following each path in the tree, and the costs and health effects associated with each outcome, as described in Section 15.4.4.

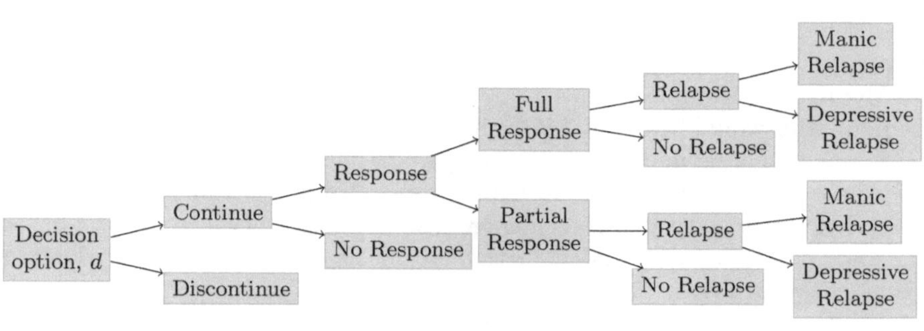

FIGURE 15.2: Decision tree model for depression in adults with bipolar disorder

15.4.2 Probabilistic analysis of health economic models

In health economic practice, the process of quantifying uncertainty about parameters $\boldsymbol{\theta}$ and the consequences of that uncertainty for decision making is usually termed *probabilistic sensitivity analysis* (Baio and Dawid, 2015). Beliefs about the true value of $\boldsymbol{\theta}$ are represented as a joint probability distribution, and the implied distribution of $f(d, \boldsymbol{\theta})$ is then generated using Monte Carlo simulation. Values of $\boldsymbol{\theta}$ are obtained from their distribution, and the corresponding values of $f(d, \boldsymbol{\theta})$ calculated. The expected net benefit $\mathrm{E}_{\boldsymbol{\theta}}(\mathcal{U}_d)$ is then estimated for each d as the empirical mean of the simulated values. Decision uncertainty can be quantified by the probability (with respect to uncertainty about $\boldsymbol{\theta}$) that each treatment d maximises $\mathrm{E}_{\boldsymbol{\theta}}(\mathcal{U}_d)$, thus is the most cost-effective.

This approach is inherently Bayesian, because we are representing uncertainty using the language of probability. This approach is contrasted with "deterministic" modeling, where each input parameter is fixed at a single value, e.g. a point estimate from data. The uncertainty in the estimate would then be ignored, as well as any correlations between input parameters. However, economic models are typically non-linear functions of the input parameters, and so $f(d, \boldsymbol{\theta})$ evaluated at the mean $\bar{\boldsymbol{\theta}} = \mathrm{E}(\boldsymbol{\theta})$ is not usually equal to the expected model output $\mathrm{E}_{\boldsymbol{\theta}}\left[f(d, \boldsymbol{\theta})\right]$. Deterministic models therefore can give biased estimates, and often over-estimate cost-effectiveness — technically this is generally due to the fact that the net benefit function tends to be a concave function in many of the model parameters. Thus, because of Jensen's inequality it is likely that deterministic models tend to generate bias and give overly positive results.

15.4.3 Estimating model input parameters $\boldsymbol{\theta}$

As usually practiced, decision modeling does not use full Bayesian inference from data. However, distributions for $\boldsymbol{\theta}$ are commonly chosen (Briggs et al., 2006) to approximate the posterior that would result from analysing the original data under a vague prior. For example, a log relative risk would be given a normal distribution with mean and variance derived from the published estimate and confidence interval. Any correlations between beliefs about parameters should be represented, for example parameters estimated jointly from the same data, such as relative treatment effects for multiple comparisons in a network meta-analysis (see Chapter 14). For parameters estimated by maximum likelihood, it is common practice to use a multivariate normal distribution defined by the maximum likelihood estimates and their asymptotic covariance matrix. Cholesky decomposition is commonly used to simulate from multivariate normal distributions if the model is implemented in a spreadsheet application (Briggs et al., 2006). Bootstrapping (as in Hunink et al., 1998) is sometimes also used to express parameter uncertainty for health economic modeling, with the bootstrap sample interpreted as an approximate sample from a posterior distribution.

In many cases, Bayesian inference is used *explicitly* to provide inputs to decision models. If we use a Monte Carlo sampling procedure to evaluate the joint posterior distribution of $\boldsymbol{\theta}$ (most commonly this would be by MCMC), then the resulting sample can be used directly as an input into our economic model. Another major strength is the ease with which evidence from multiple sources can be combined, while propagating uncertainties that might result from biases or heterogeneity in the evidence base. In cases where there is limited data, beliefs or "soft" data can be included in the specification of the prior for $\boldsymbol{\theta}$. An elegant example is given by Briggs et al. (2003), in which estimates of the probabilities of a set of events in a health economic model are stabilized by even quite weak priors in the presence of small or zero counts.

15.4.4 Bayesian evidence synthesis in health economic models

Meta-analysis to estimate treatment effectiveness from multiple trials, including network meta-analysis of trials with different comparators, is perhaps the commonest application of Bayesian inference in this context, and is discussed in detail in Chapter 14, as well as in Chapter 9 of Welton et al. (2012). More generally, Bayesian models have been used extensively in situations where there are multiple data sources, not necessarily of the same form, that have some information in common, which is expressed in the form of shared parameters.

For example, in Figure 15.3 we might have datasets X_1, X_2, X_3 representing, respectively, survival for the general population, a registry of people with a specific disease receiving a standard treatment, and a trial of a new treatment compared to a standard treatment in people with the disease (Jackson et al., 2017). X_1 allows us to estimate a baseline expected survival μ , X_2 informs both the baseline survival μ and the hazard ratio α between people with the disease and the general population, while X_3 informs the relative effectiveness β of the new treatment compared to the old one, and might also inform μ and α if the population of X_3 is assumed to be similar to that studied in X_2 (for this reason, in Figure 15.3 the arrows connecting μ and α to X_3 are dashed and not solid).

The health economic model (right dotted box) defines the expected costs and effects under each treatment as a function of parameters $\boldsymbol{\theta} = (\mu, \alpha, \beta)^\top$. There may be multiple studies of the same type; for example dataset X_3 may comprise a meta analysis of RCTs, rather than a single RCT. A common issue arising when populating health economic models is that RCTs only provide outcomes over the relatively short term. Evidence synthesis of registry data sources providing long-term follow-up with short-term RCTs can help extrapolate to the longer term — see, e.g. Chapter 16, Demiris and Sharples (2006); Benaglia et al. (2015); Jackson et al. (2017) and Guyot et al. (2017) for further examples of Bayesian synthesis of longer-term population survival data with shorter-term data from trials.

Given the joint posterior distribution of the parameters $\boldsymbol{\theta}$ informed by the Bayesian evidence synthesis, the posterior distribution of the expected costs and effects $f(d, \boldsymbol{\theta})$ follows as a consequence. For example, if the posterior is described by a set of simulations $r = 1, \ldots, R$ in a Markov Chain Monte Carlo (MCMC) estimation, then each sampled value $\boldsymbol{\theta}_r$ is used in turn as the input to the health economic model, and the sampled values of $f(d, \boldsymbol{\theta}_r)$ form a sample from the posterior distribution of $f(d, \boldsymbol{\theta})$. This approach, where key parameters are estimated from data via Bayesian modeling, and simultaneously used as inputs to a decision model, has been described as "comprehensive decision modeling" (Cooper et al., 2004). This contrasts with the "two stage" approach of explicitly defining priors on $\boldsymbol{\theta}$ based on data, followed by evaluating the decision model, as described in Section 15.4.2 — essentially splitting Figure 15.3 into the two parts illustrated by the dotted lines, each part containing parameters μ, α, β.

In the guideline for acute depression in adults with bipolar disorder, the model depends on various parameters which are estimated from a range of different evidence sources (see Table 21 in NICE, 2014). The probability of treatment discontinuation is estimated by applying log-odds ratios estimated from a network meta-analysis (NMA) of 27 RCTs (described in Table 14.4) to a discontinuation rate on the reference treatment (the predictive distribution from a meta-analysis of placebo arms). However, since discontinuation is not possible on "No pharmacological treatment", discontinuation was interpreted as "no response" for this decision option.

Response conditional on continuation with treatment was estimated from a separate network meta-analysis on a subset of 25 RCTs where this outcome was reported. A separate NMA was conducted because this outcome is conditionally independent of discontinuation.

All the NMAs were estimated using MCMC simulation, and these simulation samples used directly in the economic model to represent joint uncertainty and correlations in these

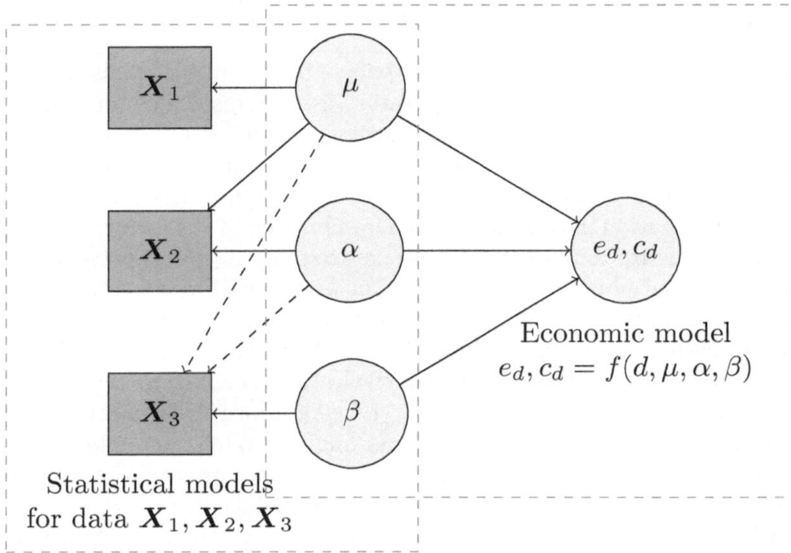

FIGURE 15.3: Multiparameter evidence synthesis and decision modeling.

parameters. This avoids the need to make parametric approximations for the distribution of these parameters.

Other probability parameters in the model are assumed to have a Beta distribution, either estimated directly from a single evidence source or based on expert clinical opinion. Utilities associated with the different health states (no response, full response, partial response, manic relapse, depressive relapse) are given Beta distributions, each estimated from a single evidence source. We note here that a Beta distribution is very often used in these kinds of models as the default approach to describe uncertainty on quantities bounded in the interval $[0-1]$, e.g. probabilities. Of course, this is only *a* possibility and for instance one could use a normal model on the logit scale.

Finally, the number of community mental health team (CMHT) visits and crisis resolution home treatment team (CRHTT) visits are given discrete probabilities, based on expert opinion and a single evidence source. Mean unit costs for CMHT, CRHTT, and hospitalization are given Normal distributions with the "standard deviation" of the distribution representing the standard error of the mean cost. Other parameters, e.g. drug acquisition and lab-testing costs, were assumed known and fixed.

15.4.5 'All models are wrong': Structural uncertainty

All model-based evaluations are, necessarily, conditional on the model. However, 'all models are wrong', (Box, 1976) and this leaves us with a difficult problem. Given that our models are not perfect representations of reality, any prediction that we derive from our model will have an error associated with it. We are almost always uncertain about this 'structural error', and we call this source of uncertainty 'structural uncertainty'. Note that structural uncertainty cannot be 'uncertainty about the model', although this is often how it is described. Models are not uncertain. They are known constructs that we build.

Structural uncertainty is hard to quantify, because it is hard to assess the effect of model imperfection. Various approaches have been proposed in the field of HTA. For example, scenario analysis (Bojke et al., 2009) simply compares results under structural assumptions.

In model averaging (Jackson et al., 2009, 2010) alternative statistical models for the same dataset can be compared according to their fit to data, and their results averaged accordingly. In model discrepancy methods (Strong et al., 2012; Strong and Oakley, 2014) a model is perturbed by adding parameters representing departures from structural assumptions, an approach based on the classic work by Kennedy and O'Hagan (2001) in which model structural error is modelled as a Gaussian process. None of these methods fully addresses the problem of structural uncertainty, and this is an area of ongoing active research.

15.5 Value of information

In HTA, as in all areas of public policy, resource allocation decisions are made under uncertainty. Sometimes we will choose a course of action that turns out to be non-optimal, and consequently we will suffer a loss. If, however, we had perfect information, then we would be able to choose the option that guarantees the maximum benefit. Information therefore has value, and Bayesian decision theory gives us a framework for computing the expected value of new information, given our current uncertainty and the decision problem at hand (Raiffa, 1968).

If we have derived our judgements about the unknown costs and health benefits of a range of competing treatment options using a decision analytic model, then we may be interested in the expected value of learning with certainty some subset of the model input parameters. This quantity is called the *Expected Value of Perfect Information* (EVPI) and can be seen as a sensitivity analysis measure, answering the question: 'for which input parameters is parameter uncertainty resulting in significant decision uncertainty?' (Oakley, 2009).

The EVPI for some subset of parameters (*Expected Value of Partial Perfect Information*, EVPPI) can also be seen as an upper bound on the value of a data collection exercise that will inform judgements about those parameters, i.e. the expected value of a "perfect" study, based on an infinite sample size. This can be of some use, but we are often more interested in the expected value of a *specific* data collection exercise, rather than in its theoretical upper bound. The expected value of a specific data collection study is called the *Expected Value of Sample Information* (EVSI) for that study (Conti and Claxton, 2009).

Given the EVSI for some proposed study and the costs associated with the study we can compute the *Expected Net Benefit of Sampling* (ENBS), which equals the difference between the EVSI and the study costs. If this is positive, then the study is worthwhile, whereas if it is negative it is not. ENBS for a range of study designs (e.g. in terms of different sample sizes) can be computed in order to find the design that maximises the value of the new information relative to the cost of obtaining it (Conti and Claxton, 2009).

Although the Value of Information measures introduced above are useful tools in decision analysis, they have in the past been underused. This is in part due to a historic lack of familiarity within the HTA decision making community, in part due to computational difficulties, and also perhaps a justifiable suspicion about techniques which appear complex and are not fully understood (Welton and Thom, 2015). EVPI and EVSI cannot be calculated analytically except in very restricted settings, and Monte Carlo sampling based approaches can be slow and cumbersome. Recently, a number of fast and easy approximation methods have been published which effectively remove the computational barrier to calculating value of information (Strong et al., 2014, 2015; Madan et al., 2014; Menzies, 2016; Heath et al., 2016).

15.6 Conclusion / outlook

The role of statistical modeling in health economic evaluation has become more and more prominent in the past decades, particularly as the sophistication of the modeling of the underlying clinical and monetary implications of a given intervention has increased. On the one hand, this has contributed to the establishment of robust processes upon which decisions are made (e.g. in terms of adoption and reimbursement of new technologies). On the other hand, this also has implied that the models require solid statistical foundations.

Nevertheless, often the statistical model is still detached from the rest of the economic evaluation — in other words, the "statistical model" block of Figure 15.1 may not be fully integrated with the "economic model" and "decision analysis" blocks; in fact, these are often performed by different researchers/modellers.

The obvious implication is that, at times, there is a mis-alignment between the way in which "clinical" data are analysed and modelled and then used as input to a wider economic model. A full Bayesian approach can then be beneficial, because one module of the bigger model (e.g. the "statistical model" block) can be used in a straightforward way to inform other parts, while propagating uncertainty all the way to the decision making process.

In this chapter, we have presented the two main types of models for economic evaluation, one based on individual level data and trial-based evaluations and the other based on evidence synthesis and decision-analytic modeling. In the case of the former, in many ways a frequentist approach to the underlying statistical model is often still considered as the standard. This is perhaps because the basic statistical analysis is mainly driven by the purely clinical objectives of performing some inference on the intervention effect and the economic evaluation is often only "plugged in" at a later stage. Conversely, by its very nature, decision-analytic modeling is a much more intrinsically Bayesian exercise. Thus, in the latter case, a Bayesian approach is perhaps already the standard, at least for what concerns the statistical model underpinning the decision analysis.

In both cases, however, it is important that the several components of the overall economic model are linked in a principled and coherent way, which a Bayesian approach can often achieve efficiently. In addition, Value of Information methods for sensitivity analysis and prioritising future research explicitly require a Bayesian set-up. This has been arguably the most active research area in the past five to ten years, and the greater use of novel methods in practice promises an ever more Bayesian future.

Bibliography

Baio, G. (2012). *Bayesian Methods in Health Economics.* Chapman Hall, CRC, Boca Raton, FL.

Baio, G. (2014). Bayesian models for cost-effectiveness analysis in the presence of structural zero costs. *Statistics in Medicine*, 33(11):1900–1913.

Baio, G., Berardi, A., and Heath, A. (2017). *Bayesian Cost-Effectiveness Analysis with the R package BCEA.* Springer, New York, NY.

Baio, G. and Dawid, A. P. (2015). Probabilistic sensitivity analysis in health economics. *Statistical Methods in Medical Research*, 24(6):615–634.

Benaglia, T., Jackson, C. H., and Sharples, L. D. (2015). Survival extrapolation in the presence of cause specific hazards. *Statistics in Medicine*, 34(5):796–811.

Bernardo, J. M. and Smith, A. F. M. (1994). *Bayesian Theory*. Wiley, Chichester, UK.

Bojke, L., Claxton, K., Sculpher, M., and Palmer, S. (2009). Characterizing structural uncertainty in decision analytic models: a review and application of methods. *Value in Health*, 12(5):739–749.

Box, G. E. P. (1976). Science and statistics. *Journal of the American Statistical Association*, 71(356):791–799.

Briggs, A., Claxton, K., and Sculpher, M. (2006). *Decision Modeling for Health Economic Evaluation*. Oxford University Press, Oxford, UK.

Briggs, A. H., Ades, A. E., and Price, M. J. (2003). Probabilistic sensitivity analysis for decision trees with multiple branches: use of the Dirichlet distribution in a Bayesian framework. *Medical Decision Making*, 23(4):341–350.

Buxton, M. J., Drummond, M. F., Van Hout, B. A., Prince, R. L., Sheldon, T. A., Szucs, T., and Vray, M. (1997). Modeling in ecomomic evaluation: an unavoidable fact of life. *Health Economics*, 6(3):217–227.

Claxton, K. (1999). The irrelevance of inference: a decision-making approach to the stochastic evaluation of health care technologies. *Journal of Health Economics*, 18(3):341–364.

Conigliani, C. and Tancredi, A. (2009). A Bayesian model averaging approach for cost-effectiveness analyses. *Health Economics*, 18(7):807–821.

Conti, S. and Claxton, K. (2009). Dimensions of design space: A decision-theoretic approach to optimal research design. *Medical Decision Making*, 29(6):643–660.

Cooper, N. J., Sutton, A. J., Abrams, K. R., Turner, D., and Wailoo, A. (2004). Comprehensive decision analytical modeling in economic evaluation: a Bayesian approach. *Health Economics*, 13(3):203–226.

Cooper, N. J., Sutton, A. J., Mugford, M., and Abrams, K. R. (2003). Use of Bayesian Markov chain Monte Carlo methods to model cost-of-illness data. *Medical Decision Making*, 23(1):38–53.

Culyer, A. J. and Chalkidou, K. (2019). Economic evaluation for health investments en route to universal health coverage: Cost-benefit analysis or cost-effectiveness analysis? *Value in Health*, 22(1):99 – 103.

Demiris, N. and Sharples, L. D. (2006). Bayesian evidence synthesis to extrapolate survival estimates in cost-effectiveness studies. *Statistics in Medicine*, 25:1960–1975.

Grieve, R., Nixon, R., Thompson, S. G., and Normand, C. (2005). Using multilevel models for assessing the variability of multinational resource use and cost data. *Health Economics*, 14(2):185–196.

Guyot, P., Ades, A. E., Beasley, M., Lueza, B., Pignon, J.-P., and Welton, N. J. (2017). Extrapolation of survival curves from cancer trials using external information. *Medical Decision Making*, 37(4):353–366.

Heath, A., Manolopoulou, I., and Baio, G. (2016). Estimating the expected value of partial perfect information in health economic evaluations using integrated nested laplace approximation. *Statistics in Medicine*, 35(23):4264–4280.

Hunink, M., Bult, J., De Vries, J., and Weinstein, M. (1998). Uncertainty in decision models analyzing cost-effectiveness: the joint distribution of incremental costs and effectiveness evaluated with a nonparametric bootstrap method. *Medical Decision Making*, 18(3):337–346.

Jackson, C., Stevens, J., Ren, S., Latimer, N., Bojke, L., Manca, A., and Sharples, L. (2017). Extrapolating survival from randomized trials using external data: a review of methods. *Medical Decision Making*, 37(4):377–390.

Jackson, C. H., Sharples, L. D., and Thompson, S. G. (2010). Structural and parameter uncertainty in Bayesian cost-effectiveness models. *Journal of the Royal Statistical Society — Series C*, 59(2):233–253.

Jackson, G. H., Thompson, S. G., and Sharples, L. D. (2009). Accounting for uncertainty in health economic decision models by using model averaging. *Journal of the Royal Statistical Society — Series A*, 172(2):383–404.

Karnon, J. and Hossein, H. A. A. (2014). When to use discrete event simulation (DES) for the economic evaluation of health technologies? A review and critique of the costs and benefits of DES. *PharmacoEconomics*, 32(6):547–558.

Kennedy, M. C. and O'Hagan, A. (2001). Bayesian calibration of computer models. *Journal of the Royal Statistical Society — Series B*, 63(3):425–464.

Lambert, P. C., Billingham, L. J., Cooper, N. J., Sutton, A. J., and Abrams, K. R. (2008). Estimating the cost-effectiveness of an intervention in a clinical trial when partial cost information is available: A Bayesian approach. *Health Economics*, 17(1):67–81.

Lindley, D. V. (1991). *Making Decisions, 2nd Edition*. Wiley.

Loomes, G. and McKenzie, L. (1989). The use of QALYs in health care decision making. *Social Science & Medicine*, 28(4):299 – 308.

Madan, J., Ades, A. E., Price, M., Maitland, K., Jemutai, J., Revill, P., and Welton, N. J. (2014). Strategies for efficient computation of the Expected Value of Partial Perfect Information. *Medical Decision Making*, 34(3):327–342.

Manca, A., Lambert, P. C., Sculpher, M., and Rice, N. (2007). Cost-effectiveness analysis using data from multinational trials: the use of bivariate hierarchical modeling. *Medical Decision Making*, 27(4):471–490.

McCarron, C. E., Pullenayegum, E. M., Thabane, L., Goeree, R., and Tarride, J.-E. (2013). The impact of using informative priors in a Bayesian cost-effectiveness analysis: an application of endovascular versus open surgical repair for abdominal aortic aneurysms in high-risk patients. *Medical Decision Making*, 33(3):437–450.

Menzies, N. A. (2016). An efficient estimator for the Expected Value of Sample Information. *Medical Decision Making*, 36(3):308–320.

NICE (2013). *Guide to the methods of technology appraisal 2013*. National Institute for Health and Care Excellence, London.

NICE (2014). *Bipolar disorder: Assessment and management. Clinical guideline 185*. National Institute for Health and Clinical Excellence, London, UK.

Nixon, R. and Thompson, S. G. (2005). Incorporating covariate adjustment, subgroup analysis and between-centre differences into cost-effectiveness evaluations. *Health Economics*, 14:1217–1229.

Nixon, R. M. and Thompson, S. G. (2004). Parametric modeling of cost data in medical studies. *Statistics in Medicine*, 23:1311–1331.

Oakley, J. E. (2009). Decision-theoretic sensitivity analysis for complex computer models. *Technometrics*, 51(2):121–129.

O'Hagan, A. and Stevens, J. (2001). A framework for cost-effectiveness analysis from clinical trial data. *Health Economics*, 10:303–315.

O'Hagan, A., Stevens, J., and Montmartin, J. (2001). Bayesian cost effectiveness analysis from clinical trial data. *Statistics in Medicine*, 20:733–753.

O'Hagan, A. and Stevens, J. W. (2003). Assessing and comparing costs: how robust are the bootstrap and methods based on asymptotic normality? *Health Economics*, 12(1):33–49.

Raiffa, H. (1968). *Decision Analysis. Introductory Lectures on Choices Under Uncertainty.* Addison-Wesley, Reading, MA.

Spiegelhalter, D., Abrams, K., and Myles, J. (2004). *Bayesian Approaches to Clinical Trials and Health-Care Evaluation.* Wiley, New York, NY.

Spiegelhalter, D. J. (2004). Incorporating Bayesian ideas into health-care evaluation. *Statistical Science*, 19(1):156–174.

Strong, M. and Oakley, J. E. (2014). When is a model good enough? Deriving the Expected Value of Model Improvement via specifying internal model discrepancies. *SIAM/ASA Journal on Uncertainty Quantification*, 2(1):106–125.

Strong, M., Oakley, J. E., and Brennan, A. (2014). Estimating multi-parameter partial Expected Value of Perfect Information from a probabilistic sensitivity analysis sample: a non-parametric regression approach. *Medical Decision Making*, 34(3):311–26.

Strong, M., Oakley, J. E., Brennan, A., and Breeze, P. (2015). Estimating the Expected Value of Sample Information using the probabilistic sensitivity analysis sample: A fast nonparametric regression-based method. *Medical Decision Making*, 35(5):570–583.

Strong, M., Oakley, J. E., and Chilcott, J. (2012). Managing structural uncertainty in health economic decision models: a discrepancy approach. *Journal of the Royal Statistical Society — Series C*, 61(1):25–45.

Welton, N. J., Sutton, A. J., Cooper, N. J., Abrams, K. R., and Ades, A. E. (2012). *Evidence Synthesis for Decision Making in Healthcare.* Wiley.

Welton, N. J. and Thom, H. H. Z. (2015). Value of information. *Medical Decision Making*, 35(5):564–566.

Willan, A. and Briggs, A. (2006). *The Statistical Analysis of Cost-Effectiveness Data.* John Wiley and Sons, Chichester, UK.

Willan, A. R., Pinto, E. M., O'Brien, B. J., Kaul, P., Goeree, R., Lynd, L., and Armstrong, P. W. (2005). Country specific cost comparisons from multinational clinical trials using empirical Bayesian shrinkage estimation: the Canadian ASSENT-3 economic analysis. *Health Economics*, 14(4):327–338.

16

Bayesian Modeling for Economic Evaluation Using "Real-World Evidence"

Gianluca Baio

University College London, UK

This chapter presents an example of the use of Bayesian modeling with "real world evidence". This terminology indicates an increasingly popular body of evidence typically collected in the post-marketing framework and, usually, under observational conditions. Typical examples include population registries, cohort studies, or, more generally "electronic health records". We focus our attention on the case of statistical modeling for economic evaluation of an intervention on the basis of time-to-event outcomes, where the information provided by the available individual level data (e.g. from a Phase III experimental study) is immature and thus benefits from integration with external (population level) sources of information. We present a case study and discuss the advantages of the Bayesian approach.

16.1 Introduction

Generally speaking, we refer to "post-marketing" as the stage of pharmaceutical development after a landmark Phase III study has been conducted and the drug has received approval for marketing. In fact, there may be circumstances where a drug is actually given a license earlier in the development process, for example on the back of a Phase II study or a single-arm trial (Hatswell et al., 2016). In any case, the post-marketing phase seeks to collect and use information from "*real world evidence*" (RWE), i.e. the prescription, consumption, safety and efficacy patterns associated with a given pharmaceutical intervention as observed from data obtained from routine practice.

There are several interesting aspects to the evaluation of pharmaceutical products on the back of post-marketing, or RWE, both from the regulator's and the manufacturer's point of view, which have an impact on the way the statistical analysis is designed and conducted.

Firstly, while it is not impossible that regulators such as the U.S. Food and Drug Administration (FDA) or the European Medicine Agency (EMEA) require further randomized study after a drug has entered a market, post-marketing studies are often based on *observational* evidence. This implies obvious considerations regarding the possibility for bias, e.g. due to self-selection of individuals into different treatment strategies, which becomes embedded in the data collection. In addition, it is possible that there be delays in market entry between major jurisdictions — for example, there is some evidence to suggest that the US market may be more receptive to drugs licensed with non-Phase III evidence (Hatswell et al., 2016; Djulbegovic et al., 2018). In this case, it is possible that other regulators may use the actual post-marketing data from the US to complement experimental evidence before making a decision. This has also relevant implications particularly when the focus of the investigation is in the assessment of the "real world" safety of the drug — a situation often termed "surveillance" or "pharmacovigilance" (for some interesting descriptions of these issues within a Bayesian setting, see Dumouchel, 1999; Ahmed et al., 2009; Madigan et al., 2010; Prieto-Merino et al., 2011).

Secondly, post-marketing data may often be used to construct a wider network of evidence, whose main outcome is the economic evaluation of a set of interventions. In a typical situation, one of the drugs being assessed may be newer and there may be experimental data (perhaps from a Phase III trial) available to quantify its effectiveness, possibly against standard of care or placebo. However, there may be other drugs already existing on the market to target the same disease or condition; as mentioned in Chapter 15, from the economic point of view, it is important to contrast the new option with all the relevant alternatives. For this reason, post-marketing data on the other drugs available can be used to allow for indirect comparisons. RWE can be also used for planning of a clinical development programme (e.g. a Phase III study for a new drug), to inform estimates of treatment effects, again in a network meta-analytic context (Martina et al., 2018). Much of this is addressed in Chapter 14.

Thirdly, a related area in which the use of RWE is particularly important — and, crucially, in which the application of Bayesian methods is pivotal — is the economic evaluation of interventions for which the main clinical outcome is represented by a suitable time-to-event, e.g. oncological drugs. This is interesting because often studies such as those for cancer drugs trials produce relatively immature data, where a large proportion of the sample is subject to censoring (Latimer, 2011). Despite the inherent limited amount of evidence present in these data, the economic evaluation process requires the modellers to *extrapolate* the resulting survival curves over a long-term horizon, in order to assess the economic performance of the interventions being compared.

In this chapter we focus particularly on the last case described above. We present a general framework for the integration of experimental and observational studies (possibly derived by post-marketing evidence, or simply from individual level data sets recording information on ancillary aspects of the model). Firstly, in Section 16.2 we briefly review the main features of data classified as RWE. Then, in Section 16.3, we present the general modeling framework that can be used in the case of time-to-event data and the specific issues encountered when using these kinds of data for economic evaluation. Section 16.4 presents a case study based on the work of Benaglia et al. (2015); this is not meant to be an exhaustive representation of the possibilities associated with Bayesian modeling using RWE, but it is chosen here because it allows to showcase some of the advantages provided by the inbuilt flexibility and modularity of Bayesian analysis. Finally, Section 16.5 provides some general conclusions and outlooks for future research.

16.2 Real World Evidence

Real World Evidence (RWE) is a terminology increasingly often used to describe observational data obtained using Electronic Health Records (EHR). These are collections of large-scale administrative healthcare data (e.g. GP consultation records or hospital admission/mortality records). Such data are reasonably easy to access and represent a relatively inexpensive means of obtaining a large, representative sample of the general population, when compared to specifically-designed epidemiological studies or RCTs. Typically, EHRs are collected for administrative purposes but there is much scope for these data to be used for research, increasingly often under the paradigm of *personalized medicine*. This terminology is used to indicate a model of health care provision based on the customization of medical decisions, treatments, practices, or products being tailored to the individual patient — examples include "big data", including those based on genomic measurements (often termed "biobanks").

The main strengths and challenges of EHRs can be summarized as follows.

16.2.1 Primary care databases

Primary care databases can be generally defined as collections of de-identified individual level data from a network of general practices across a given jurisdiction. Primary care data are often linked to a large number of other health-related data, for example pharmaceutical prescriptions, laboratory exams, mortality, etc., in order to provide a longitudinal and representative population health dataset. They can be summarized as having the following characteristics.

- Cover a large proportion of the general population and are linked longitudinally;
- Data can be modeled at the individual patient, GP practice, regional and/or national level, thus allowing (at least theoretically) for hierarchical structures and levels of information to be accounted for in the analysis;
- Patient self-selection may occur, to some degree; in addition, the level of missing data present can be substantial, for some variables.

16.2.2 Mortality/Hospital admission registries

Population registries are usually compiled and maintained by the national statistical authorities (e.g. the US Census Bureau or the European Union Eurostat and its member states affiliates). Essentially every country has an official statistics office collecting data on the relevant population and often these include health-related measures. Classical examples include mortality counts or hospital admission records (e.g. the Hospital Episodes Statistics data set in the UK, or Medicare in the US). The main features of these types of registry data include the following aspects.

- Cover the whole general population, ensuring statistical power and representativeness;
- Variables such as age, sex, date of event, address and ethnicity are routinely recorded, but typical confounding factors are not, which makes the data less useful at the individual level unless a link with external cohorts/surveys is established;
- Data are often used at a small and consistent geographical level (e.g. Middle Super Output Areas, MSOAs, as defined by the Census in the UK) for disease surveillance and risk assessment. They are generally free from missing data issues.

RWE is increasingly popular in fields such as economic evaluation of health-care interventions, particularly in the case where the underlying evidence upon which not just the statistical, but the entire economic model is built (see Chapter 15) is limited — for example, because of short follow up it does not allow to capture the long term effects of a given intervention/drug.

This is often the case when the main clinical outcome is represented by time-to-event variables. We turn our attention to this case in the following, first by describing the specific issues associated with economic evaluation and the general modeling framework.

16.3 Economic modeling and survival analysis

The use of survival modeling has been discussed in Chapter 10. Here we focus on the specific case of survival analysis as embedded in a wider economic modeling — see Chapter 15 and, among others, Spiegelhalter et al. (2004) and Baio (2012).

While interventions that impact upon survival (e.g. cancer drugs) form a high proportion of the treatments appraised by agencies such as the National Institute for Health and Care Excellence (NICE; Latimer, 2011, 2014), modeling for survival analysis in health economics may be challenging. The main reason is that, in order to quantify accurately the long term economic benefits of a new intervention, it is necessary to estimate the mean survival time (rather than usual summaries, such as the median time). In fact, economic evaluation is concerned with *decision-making*, rather than inference and to do this, we need to estimate the population average benefits of any treatment (i.e. expressed as a function of the mean survival curve). Thus, we usually need to extrapolate the observed survival curves to a (much) longer time horizon than there are data available (see Figure 16.1).

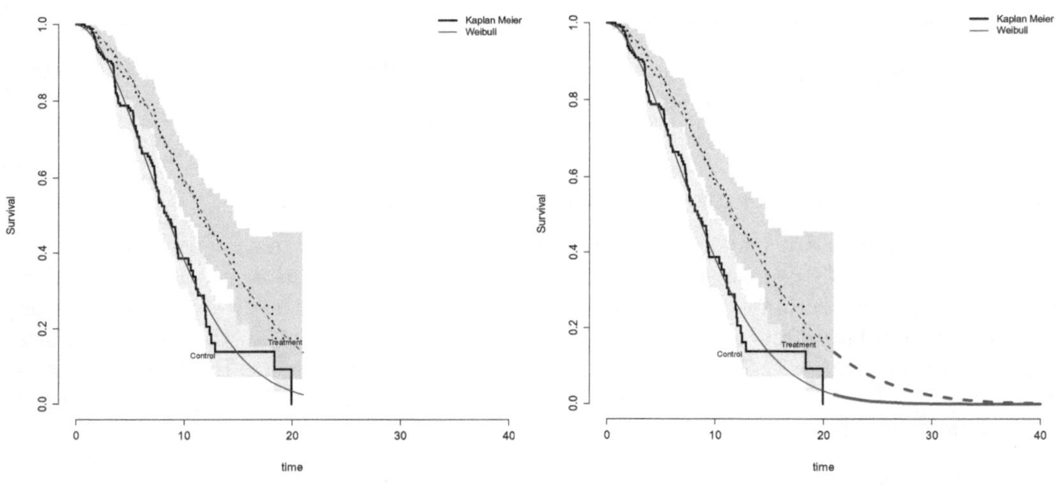

FIGURE 16.1: Survival analysis is generally concerned with determining the *median* time-to-event, as shown in panel (a); in this particular case, the survival curves are presented for two treatment arms. In the controls, the median survival time is 8.33, while it is 11.54 in the active treatment arm. In health economic evaluation, it is necessary to expand the possibly limited time horizon from the experimental data, in order to compute the *mean* time-to-event, e.g. as in panel (b). In this particular analysis, the distance between the two means (9.09 and 10.34 in the control and active treatment) is shorter than in terms of medians.

To this aim, a parametric approach to survival analysis is usually followed and is recommended by NICE technical support document (TSD; Latimer, 2011). This suggests a systematic process in which several parametric models are fitted to the available data in order to select the "best" one, which is then used to produce the relevant output for the economic model, i.e. the most important part of the analytic framework.

16.3.1 General modeling structure

In a study whose main outcome is represented by a time-to-event variable, the observed data consist at least of the pair (t_i, d_i), for individuals $i = 1, \ldots, n$, where: $t_i > 0$ is the observed time at which the event under study occurs; and d_i (for "dummy" variable) is an event indicator, taking value 1 if the event occurs and t_i is indeed observed, or 0 when the ith individual is "censored" (and thus the actual value of t_i is effectively missing). This is usually referred to as "right" censoring and it is usually considered in economic evaluation, although, particularly in the case of RWE, it is possible that individuals are subject to other forms of censoring (for example in the case where the time of the very first measurement might be unknown).

In any case, the observed data are modeled using a suitable probability distribution characterized by a density $f(t \mid \boldsymbol{\theta})$ and defined as a function of a vector of relevant parameters $\boldsymbol{\theta} = (\mu(\boldsymbol{x}), \alpha(\boldsymbol{x}))^\top$. Here we consider: a vector of potential covariates $\boldsymbol{x}$ (e.g. age, sex, trial arm, etc.); a *location* parameter $\mu(\boldsymbol{x})$, which indicates the mean or the scale of the distribution; and a (set of) ancillary parameter(s) $\alpha(\boldsymbol{x})$, which describes its shape or variance. While it is possible for both μ and α to explicitly depend on the covariates $\boldsymbol{x}$, usually the formulation is simplified to assume that these only affect directly the location parameter.

Since $t > 0$, we often model the location parameter using a generalized linear model (GLM)

$$\eta_i = g(\mu_i) = \sum_{j=0}^{J} \beta_j x_{ij}[+\ldots], \tag{16.1}$$

where $g(\cdot)$ is typically the logarithm and $x_{i0} = 1$ for all i, so that β_0 is the intercept — notice however that the choice of the function $g(\cdot)$ depends on the underlying modeling assumptions. Generally speaking, (16.1) can be extended to include additional terms — for instance, we may want to include random effects to account for repeated measurements or clustering as, for example, was done in Chapter 9. We indicate this possibility using the $[+\ldots]$ notation. When using a Bayesian framework, the model needs to be completed by specifying suitable prior distributions for the parameters.

We can use this general framework to complement the information coming from the available individual level data for one of the interventions being assessed, while including in the wider statistical model a number of "modules", which cover other sources of information. By doing so, we may be able to augment the limited evidence (e.g. because of censoring or short follow up) available in the main data set. We show one such example in the next section.

16.4 Case study: Implantable cardioverter defibrillators for the secondary prevention of cardiac arrythmia

Benaglia et al. (2015) consider the case of implantable cardioverter defibrillators for the secondary prevention of cardiac arrhythmia. In particular, following extensive meta-analysis of existing experimental studies, the two interventions being compared to perform a full economic evaluation are: Anti-arrhythmic drugs (AAD; which in this case can be considered as the *reference* treatment); and Implantable cardioverter defibrillators (ICDs; the treatment we wish to evaluate in terms of its economic performance in contrast to the reference). The most interesting aspect of this case study is the use of multiple sources of evidence, including RWE to complement limited information provided by the available time-to-event data.

The main source of data is a UK cohort study consisting of 535 patients implanted with ICDs between 1991 and 2002 (with average age at implant of 60); notice that this data set only includes (partial) information on only one of the two treatments under consideration. In addition, as is often the case (and even more so, in the case of data obtained from relatively small Phase II/III studies of highly innovative drugs), such data provide limited information because the follow up available is not long enough. In the current case, the observed follow up of just over 10 years allows us to produce estimates of the time to event (sudden cardiac death) based on survival curves reaching about 0.37 on the Kaplan-Meier estimates (see Figure 16.2).

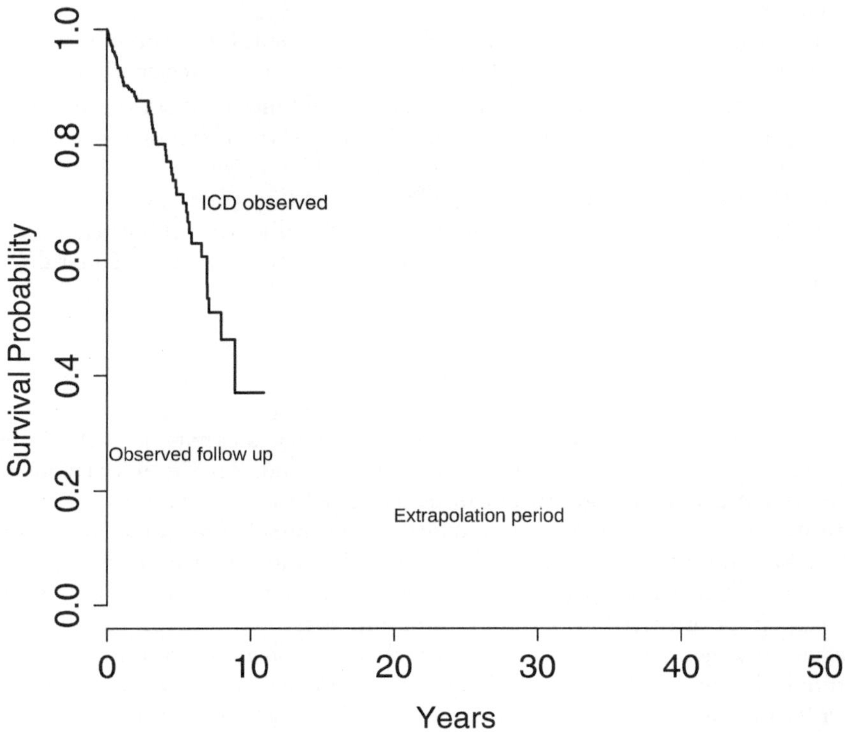

FIGURE 16.2: Kaplan-Meier curve for the observed cohort data on the 535 patients implanted with ICDs. The observed data only reach a survival proportion of about 0.37 over the actual follow up. The $x-$axis covers the actual time horizon required for the economic evaluation (extrapolating over the long term consequences). Adapted from Benaglia et al. (2015)

This means that, although the data may be representative of the overall underlying population, the information available is definitive for only about 60% of the target individuals. For the remaining proportion, we do not have evidence to determine the time at which the event will occur (if it indeed does occur).

For the purposes of the economic evaluation, however, we need to consider two further complications. Firstly, as mentioned above, because of the necessity to extrapolate data over the long term horizon, we typically model data such as those available in this case using parametric models; once the parameters have been estimated based on the observed data, the survival curve can be computed for any required time. However, as happens in this case, a large part of the survival curve will be by necessity based on the extrapolation. In fact, often the underlying data are so "immature" that they do not even reach the median time during the observed follow up (particularly for longer-term outcomes, such as overall survival). Consequently, it is likely that the extrapolation be extremely sensitive to the parametric model chosen to fit the observed data. NICE suggest testing a set of "standard" models, including popular Weibull, Gamma, Gompertz and Log-Normal, but ultimately, the choice over the actual goodness of fit is based on untestable assumptions.

This is where the use of RWE can come handy — particularly when incorporated in a full Bayesian approach. The main idea is that external data can be used to "anchor" the extrapolated curve by adding information, for example, on the general population characteristics. In this particular case, individal level data are also available from an age-sex matched national population registry, produced by the UK statistical authority (Office for National Statistics, ONS). The intuitive rationale behind the use of these data is that the general population is arguably healthier than that considered in the cohort (which is affected by cardiac arrythmia and thus is potentially at greater risk of death). Thus, the general population mortality can act as a sort of upper bound to the survival curve in the cohort. The combination of these two sources of information has the capability of stabilising the inference and the extrapolation from the parametric model of the cohort data.

The easiest way to perform this anchoring is perhaps to assume some form of *proportional hazards* of mortality

$$h_{\text{ICD}}(t) = e^{\gamma} h_{\text{UK}}(t),$$

where $h_{\text{ICD}}(t)$ and $h_{\text{UK}}(t)$ are the hazard function for the ICD and the general UK population, respectively. This would imply that overall mortality in the cohort could be related to overall mortality in the general population by a constant factor e^{γ} (for some parameter γ to be estimated).

However, in a case such as the present, this assumption would be hardly tenable: ICD patients are in fact likely to be perhaps at much greater risk of arrythmia death, because of their very nature. In addition, given that it is likely that the proportion of deaths caused by arrythmia changes over time, this assumption of constant proportionality is almost certain to induce bias over the extrapolation period.

To overcome this issue, Benaglia et al. (2015) build on work presented in Demiris et al. (2015) and use a poly-hazard model for the observed survival times in the cohort data. In a nutshell, poly-hazard models extend the basic set up of a survival model by accounting for the possibility that in fact the observed times are the result of a mixed data generating process, depending on several independent components. For example, we may consider that the occurrence of the event under study depends on M independent causes and that we are willing to model each using a suitable Weibull distribution. Using standard mathematical relationships linking the density of a time-to-event variable to the survival and hazard functions, indicated as $S(t)$ and $h(t)$, respectively (see Chapter 10), we obtain

$$\begin{aligned} f(t_i \mid \boldsymbol{\theta}) &= h(t_i)^{d_i} S(t_i) \\ &= \left[\sum_{m=1}^{M} \alpha_m \mu_{im} t_i^{\alpha_m - 1}\right]^{d_i} \left[\exp\left(-\sum_{m=1}^{M} \mu_{im} t_i^{\alpha_m}\right)\right], \end{aligned}$$

where $\boldsymbol{\theta} = (\boldsymbol{\theta}_1, \ldots, \boldsymbol{\theta}_M)^\top$ and $\boldsymbol{\theta}_m = (\alpha_m, \mu_{im})^\top$ are the shape and scale for the mth component of the mixture. This model is termed a "Poly-Weibull" distribution.

Using population registry mortality data grouped by causes of death (arrhythmia vs. all other causes), we can apply the Poly-Weibull model to effectively assume

$$\begin{aligned} h_{\text{ICD}}(t) &= h^{\text{arr}}_{\text{ICD}}(t) + h^{\text{oth}}_{\text{ICD}}(t) \\ &= e^{\gamma} h^{\text{arr}}_{\text{UK}}(t) + h^{\text{oth}}_{\text{UK}}(t) \\ &= e^{\gamma} \alpha_1 \mu_1 t^{\alpha_1 - 1} + \alpha_2 \mu_2 t^{\alpha_2 - 1} \end{aligned} \tag{16.2}$$

Equation (16.2) encodes the (less restrictive) assumption that it is only mortality for arrythmia that varies differentially between the cohort and the general population, while mortality for all other causes is assumed identical in the two. This makes the symplifying assumption of proportionality in the hazards more tenable.

The way in which the information derived from the registry is combined with the cohort data is the following. The registry data consist of two subsets $(\boldsymbol{t}_1, \boldsymbol{d}_1)$ and $(\boldsymbol{t}_2, \boldsymbol{d}_2)$, indicating the survival times and censoring indicators for those who die for arrythmia (subscript/component 1) and all other causes (subscript/component 2), respectively. We can model these two subsets independently using, e.g. a Weibull model

$$(t_{kj}, d_{kj}) \sim \text{Weibull}(\mu_k, \alpha_k)\mathbb{I}(d_{jk},)$$

for each of the $j = 1, \ldots, J$ individuals included in the registry and for $k = 1, 2$. Here we use the notation $\mathbb{I}(d_{jk},)$ to indicate the potential censoring process — if the jth individual in the registry data dies for other causes, then they will be censored for arrythmia-related mortality and vice-versa. Taking full advantage of the modularity of the Bayesian approach, we model the registry and the cohort data using shared parameters (μ_k, α_k), which will be estimated by explicitly combining the two sources of information.

The second complication to do with the wider objective of the analysis being the full economic evaluation is that we want to estimate the *incremental* benefits of the intervention under investigation (ICD) against the reference (AAD). Thus, it is necessary to include additional evidence into the modeling framework; this comes in the form of aggregated summaries produced by the meta-analysis of published studies. These summaries suggest an estimate for the hazard ratio of ICDs vs. AAD of 0.72 with 95% interval (0.60 — 0.87) for all causes mortality and of 0.50 with 95% interval (0.37 — 0.67) for arrythmia-related mortality.

While this information is obtained from a standard, frequentist analysis, it is possible to combine this information with some fairly general assumptions in order to turn it into an informative distribution capable the current level of uncertainty on the hazard ratio of ICDs vs. AAD. Specifically, Benaglia et al. (2015) assume Normality on the log scale for the hazard ratio of arrhythmia-related mortality and select suitable informative values for the mean and standard deviation (on the log scale) to encode the results of the meta-analysis. Simple computations using statistical software allow us to determine that a $\text{N}(-0.693, 0.148^2)$ produces a distribution such as that shown in Figure 16.3. The picture shows a histogram obtained using 100 000 simulations from the assumed Normal distribution; it is easy to simply exponentiate each of the simulated values and then produce the output shown in Figure 16.3, which depicts the implied distribution for the hazard ratio of ICDs vs. AAD. As it is possible to see, the mean of the distribution is, as requested, around 0.5 and most of the mass is indeed included in the interval (0.37 – 0.67).

We can use this information to build up a model to estimate mortality in the AAD population — one relatively simple way of doing so is to again assume a poly-hazard structure, where all cause mortality is again identical with the age- and sex-matched general population, while the arrhythmia-specific mortality is proportional to the general population. In this case, Benaglia et al. (2015) model

$$h_{\text{AAD}}(t) \quad = \quad e^{\delta+\gamma}\alpha_1\mu_1 t^{\alpha_1 - 1} + \alpha_2\mu_2 t^{\alpha_2 - 1}. \tag{16.3}$$

Equation 16.3 encodes these assumptions as well as the fact that the incremental arrhythmia-related mortality (in comparison to the general population) is described by a combination of two factors. The "baseline" extra log hazard ratio (derived in the ICDs cohort in comparison to the UK population), γ is summed to the log hazard ratio δ, which

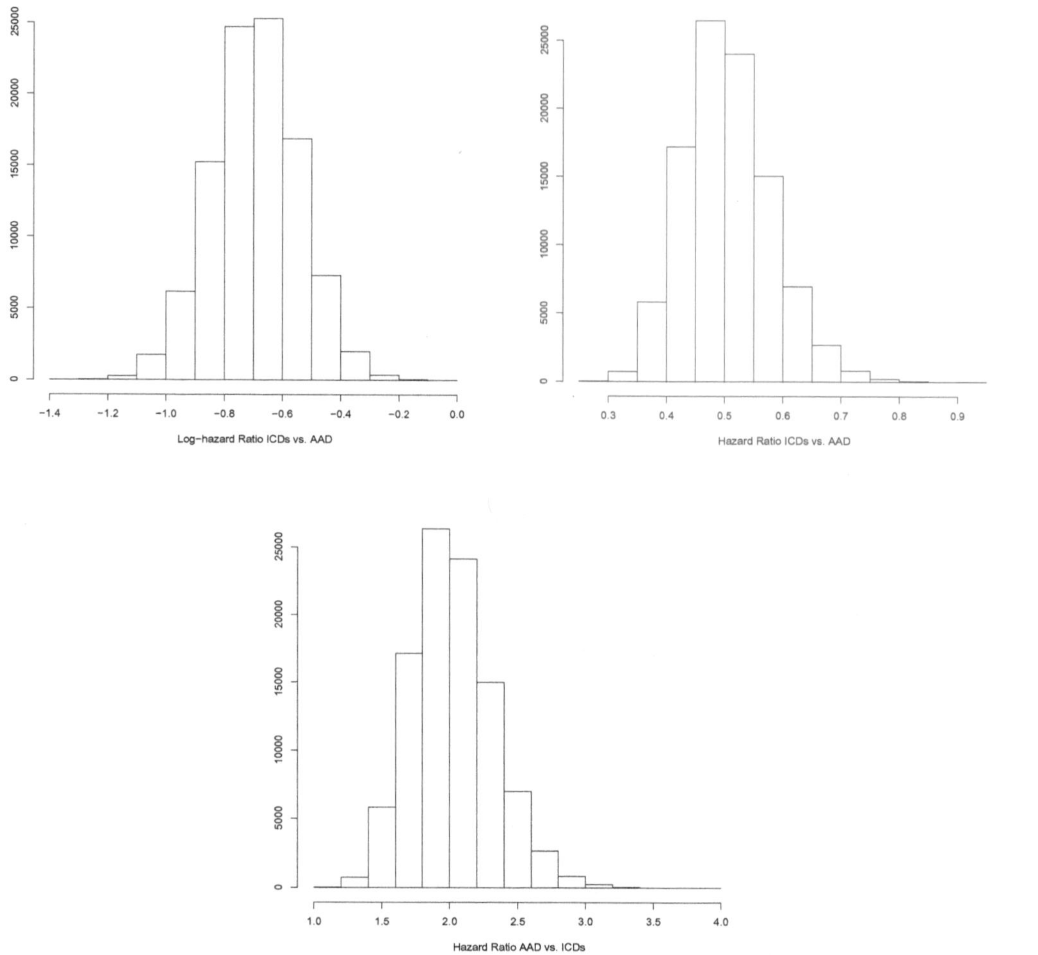

FIGURE 16.3: Panel (a) shows a histogram of a vector of 100,000 simulations from the informative N$(-0.693, 0.148)$; when exponentiated, these values produce the histogram in panel (b), which shows the implied distribution for the hazard ratio of ICDs vs. AAD. Finally, panel (c) shows the histogram of the implied distribution for the hazard ratio of ADD vs. ICDs, obtained by simply exponentiating the inverse of the values simulated and graphed in panel (a).

represents the increase in mortality for AAD vs. ICDs. It is possible to turn the distribution shown in Figure 16.3(a) into one describing the inverse log hazard ratio (i.e. the incremental effect of AAD vs. ICDs), by simply modeling $\delta \sim \text{N}(0.693, 0.148^2)$ — Figure 16.3(c) shows the resulting histogram for 100,000 simulations from this distribution, rescaled to represent the actual hazard ratio of AAD vs. ICDs.

Figure 16.4 shows the results obtained by Benaglia et al. (2015). As it is possible to see, the Poly-Weibull model performs better than the standard Weibull (which would assume a single hazard for all causes of mortality), particularly in the estimation for the AAD "arm". Using a simple Weibull model would artificially inflate the survival curve, thus potentially

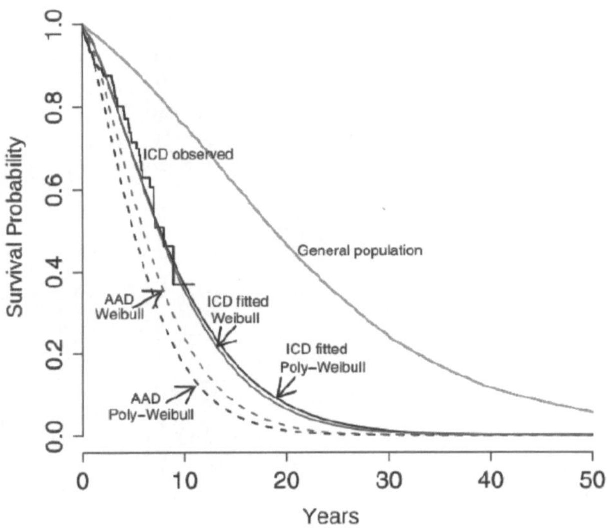

FIGURE 16.4: Survival curves for the two interventions, over a long-term horizon of 50 years. Both the observed individual-level ICD data from the cohort and the aggregated level data for AAD are modeled using a simple Weibull and a Poly-Weibull distribution. The general population (registry) data are also included in the analysis to "anchor" the extrapolation of the survival curves beyond the observed follow up (which is only about 10 years). Adapted from Benaglia et al. (2015)

reducing the benefits of ICDs. The general population survival curve acts as an upper limit, guiding the process of extrapolation beyond the observed follow up — notice that there is no need to extrapolate the registry data, as they are available for the entire population at all ages and thus can be used as a bounded estimate of the arrhythmia-related mortality that might be observed in the ICDs cohort and in the AAD population (which at time 0 are on average 60 years old), if we were able to actually follow them up for further 50 years.

This is interesting because it is related to another element of Bayesian modeling that may be helpful in stabilizing the inference. Given that the age at entry in the observation is, on average, 60, we may reasonably assume an informative prior distribution on the scale parameters used in the Weibull and Poly-Weibull distributions to imply virtually no probability that individuals can survive longer than an other 60 years (i.e. past the time when they would be 120 years old). Benaglia et al. (2015) provide more details on how this has been achieved by setting a Uniform(0, 60) prior on the mean survival time, to then rescale the underlying scale of the Weibull components.

16.5 Conclusions and further developments

Real world evidence is potentially an exciting means to bring external information into analyses based on immature data. The example shown in this chapter has considered a situation in which cohort data are available for a relatively long time horizon, which nonetheless does not allow a full characterisation of the long-term benefits and costs associated with given interventions. This situation is even more prevalent and perhaps important in many experimental studies investigating cancer drugs, one of the most important and researched areas of clinical and pharmaceutical development.

The Bayesian machinery has the advantage of allowing for a principled integration of data sources, which in cases such as this might allow a substantial "regularization" of the resulting inference. Of course, this does not come about by magic — in fact, there are several assumptions that need to be encoded in a complex model, such as the one we have discussed here. Judgements of underlying exchangeability across the (sub-)populations that are investigated in different data (e.g. a trial for the drug under investigation and a population registry for some comparators that are already available on the market) are most likely necessary in order to build and successfully run models such as the one described here. However, as in essentially all Bayesian analyses, these assumptions need to be explicit and the model can be "debugged" in a comprehensive way.

The use of RWE has great potential, particularly when embedded in a wider economic modeling, which is based on the statistical component as the, arguably, most important building block, but that at the same time decisively move forward from the static point of view of finding statistical significance, in favour of a more comprehensive decision-making approach. From the computational point of view, this is also related to innovative methods, such as Hamiltonian Monte Carlo (see Chapter 1), which can be used to produce very efficient estimations in the presence of highly structured models, such as those based on time-to-event and censoring. Research in this area is valuable and in fact ongoing, with recent developments for such models being implemented in software such as `Stan` (see Chapter 1).

Bibliography

Ahmed, I., Haramburu, F., Fourrier-Reglat, A., Thiessard, F., Kreft-Jais, C., Miremont-Salame, G., Begaud, B., and Tubert-Bitter, P. (2009). Bayesian pharmacovigilance signal detection methods revisited in a multiple comparison setting. *Statistics in Medicine*, 28(13):1774–1792.

Baio, G. (2012). *Bayesian Methods in Health Economics*. Chapman Hall, CRC, Boca Raton, FL.

Benaglia, T., Jackson, C. H., and Sharples, L. D. (2015). Survival extrapolation in the presence of cause specific hazards. *Statistics in Medicine*, 34(5):796–811.

Demiris, N., Lunn, D., and Sharples, L. D. (2015). Survival extrapolation using the poly-Weibull model. *Statistical Methods in Medical Research*, 24(2):287–301.

Djulbegovic, B., Glasziou, P., Klocksieben, F. A., Reljic, T., VanDenBergh, M., Mhaskar, R., Ioannidis, J. P. A., and Chalmers, I. (2018). Larger effect sizes in nonrandomized studies are associated with higher rates of EMA licensing approval. *Journal of Clinical Epidemiology*, 98:24–32.

Dumouchel, W. (1999). Bayesian data mining in large frequency tables, with an application to the FDA spontaneous reporting system. *The American Statistician*, 53(3):177–190.

Hatswell, A., Baio, G., Berlin, J., Irs, A., and Freemantle, N. (2016). Regulatory approval of pharmaceuticals without a randomised controlled study: analysis of EMA and FDA approvals 1999–2014. *British Medical Journal Open*, 6(e011666).

Latimer, N. (2011). NICE DSU Technical Support Document 14.

Latimer, N. (2014). Survival analysis for economic evaluations alongside clinical trials—Extrapolation with patient-level data: Inconsistencies, limitations, and a practical guide. *Medical Decision Making*, 33:743–754.

Madigan, D., Ryan, P., Simpson, S., and Zorych, I. (2010). Bayesian methods in pharmacovigilance. In Bernardo, J., Bayarri, M., Berger, J., Dawid, A., Heckerman, D., Smith, A., and West, M., editors, *Bayesian Statistics*. Oxford University Press, 9th edition.

Martina, R., Jenkins, D., Bujkiewicz, S., Dequen, P., and Abrams, K. (2018). The inclusion of real world evidence in clinical development planning. *Trials*, 19(1):468.

Prieto-Merino, D., Quartey, G., Wang, J., and Kim, J. (2011). Why a Bayesian approach to safety analysis in pharmacovigilance is important. *Pharmaceutical Statistics*, 10(6):554–559.

Spiegelhalter, D., Abrams, K., and Myles, J. (2004). *Bayesian Approaches to Clinical Trials and Health-Care Evaluation*. Wiley, New York, NY.

17

Bayesian Benefit-Risk Evaluation in Pharmaceutical Research

Carl Di Casoli

Apellis Pharmaceuticals, US

Yueqin Zhao

Food and Drug Administration, US

Yannis Jemiai

Cytel Inc, US

Pritibha Singh

Novartis Pharmaceuticals Corporation, Switzerland

Maria Costa

Novartis Pharmaceuticals Corporation, Switzerland

Evaluating the benefit-risk trade-off of a new medicinal product or intervention is one of the most complex tasks that sponsors, regulators, payers, physicians, and patients face. Several qualitative frameworks and quantitative methods have been proposed in recent years that try to provide insight into this challenging problem. Bayesian inference, with its coherent approach for integrating different sources of information and uncertainty, and its links to decision theory, provides a natural framework to perform quantitative assessments of the benefit-risk trade-off. This chapter starts by outlining the current state of the art of classical approaches to benefit-risk assessment. It then describes Bayesian methodologies, and how these can be leveraged throughout the life cycle of a medicinal product to support and augment clinical judgment and benefit-risk assessments. Two case studies are chosen to illustrate how the Bayesian approaches are implemented to facilitate decision-making. Gaps and potential new directions that extend the current approaches are also identified.

17.1 Introduction

To gain regulatory approval, a new medicine or intervention needs to demonstrate that its benefits outweigh the risks. This assessment can be one of the most challenging tasks that sponsors, regulators, payers and patients face when making decisions about health-care approaches. How large should the treatment effect be to outweigh specific risks? How should uncertainty be handled? How does the balance of benefits and risks change with new/emerging information? To address these issues, there have been concerted efforts by stakeholders in recent years to develop more structured benefit-risk (BR) approaches with tailored qualitative methods, such as the Pharmaceutical Research and Manufacturers of America Benefit-Risk Action Team (PhRMA BRAT) framework, effects tables, and forest plots (PDUFA V). The PrOACT-URL, developed within the EMA's benefit-risk methodology project, is another such method providing a generic problem setting structure consisting of problem formulation, objectives, alternatives, consequences, trade-off uncertainties, risk attitude and corresponding decision (Hammond et al., 1998). These qualitative frameworks are useful tools to facilitate the BR discussion and to display the elements that contribute to the complete BR profile, but they can be insufficient when available data do not support a clear BR assessment — for example, in scenarios where some endpoints favor the test treatment while others favor the comparator (Colopy et al., 2015). Statistical tools have been developed to quantify the complexity of BR assessments. These methods can provide additional insight into specific questions by, for example, reducing the dimensionality of the problem, making implicit weighting explicit, and by representing uncertainty using meaningful statistical concepts (Coplan et al., 2011). These quantitative approaches are not meant to replace qualitative frameworks and careful clinical judgment, but rather to enhance substantial, consistent, and transparent decision-making by providing a better understanding of stakeholder preferences (weighting) and the impact of uncertainty. Mt-Isa et al. (2016) provide a recent comprehensive review of existing frameworks and methodologies (Mt-Isa et al., 2014, 2016).

It is important to recognize that a BR assessment is not an isolated activity but should be contextualized with existing information on the medicine or intervention of interest. More broadly, it is critical to understand whether, given the accrued evidence and uncertainty, there is support to progress to the next stage of development, for example by estimating the probability that a future Phase III trial will be successful in bringing added value to patients. Sponsors, regulators and payers are likely to include information from previous studies at key decision milestones, even if informally. Quantitative BR techniques can contribute to making this assessment transparent, explicit and robust by explaining what sources of data have been used and why, how they have been integrated and analyzed, and how conclusions were derived. In this context, Bayesian inference naturally supports decision-making with its formal utilization of prior information and repeated updates based on accumulating data. Ashby and Smith (2000) argue that in the context of evidence-based medicine a full Bayesian analysis provides a coherent framework for decision-making. Posterior probabilities can summarize and communicate evidence and uncertainty, which is an essential component of any decision-making framework. In addition, Bayesian inference provides a natural platform for predicting future outcomes of interest. For example, when making decisions at the program level, the ability to quantify the probability of a successful launch based on both efficacy and safety data is clearly desirable. It is important to understand to what extent these two aspects of a medicinal product are dependent on each other, i.e. for an individual patient, the extent to which a beneficial outcome is related to the likelihood of that individual experiencing an adverse event. Bayesian BR methods have been proposed that model this subject-level correlation (Cui et al., 2016; He et al., 2012; He and Fu, 2016).

Finally, the Bayesian updating mechanism based on accumulated evidence allows for the incorporation of external data, expert knowledge or patient insight. This formal inclusion of perspectives from different stakeholders can highlight potential divergences and lead to a more focused dialogue. This approach is a clear example of the "learn and confirm" paradigm introduced by Sheiner (1997) in the late 20th century. In his seminal paper, Sheiner describes how the use of prior information within Bayesian inference naturally supports the learning phase of drug development. The continuously evolving nature of BR assessment, from early phase development to post-market launch and beyond, inherently belongs to Sheiner's "learn and confirm" paradigm, with Bayesian inference being the natural framework to support this process.

17.2 Classical approaches to quantitative benefit-risk

Several classical quantitative approaches have been developed to examine the benefits and risks of a new drug therapy. Many authors have conducted literature reviews summarizing the classical approaches to quantitative BR. Prominent reviews are those of Mt-Isa et al. (IMI-PROTECT Work Package 5, 2013) on behalf of the PROTECT consortium (Pharmacoepidemiological Research on Outcomes of Therapeutics by a European ConsorTium), and Guo et al. (2010). Mt-Isa et al. explore the potential use of eight different quantitative approaches which include: Multi-criteria Decision Analysis (MCDA), Decision Tree, Markov Decision Process (MDP), Benefit-less-Risk Analysis (BLRA), Net Clinical Benefit (NCB), Sarac's Benefit-Risk Assessment Method (SBRAM), Clinical Utility Index (CUI), and Desirability Index (DI). In addition to several qualitative approaches and metric indices, Guo et al. summarize the key features and assessment parameters of 12 quantitative BR assessment techniques. Among these, two approaches are common to those described by Mt-Isa et al. (MCDA and BLRA), while four of the methods described by Guo et al. are classified by Mt-Isa et al. (IMI-PROTECT Work Package 5, 2013) as "Metric Indices" — ratio of Number Needed to Treat to Number Needed to Harm (NNT/NNH), Minimum Clinical Efficacy (MCE)), Maximum Acceptable Risk (MAR), and Quality-adjusted Time Without Symptoms and Toxicity (Q-TWIST). The remaining eight methods contained in Guo et al. that are not included within the Mt-Isa et al. review are: Quantitative Framework for Risk and Benefit Assessment (QFRBA), Relative Value adjusted Number Needed to Treat (RV-NNT), Incremental Net Health Benefit (INHB), Risk-Benefit Plane (RBP) and Risk-Benefit Acceptability Threshold (RBAT), Probabilistic Simulation Methods (PSM) and Monte Carlo Simulation (MCS), and Risk-Benefit Contour (RBC).

All the above classical BR methods have unique advantages and disadvantages specific to the real-life situation under examination. For example, Guo et al. suggest that, if one has a substantial amount of efficacy data, adverse event incidence rates, and patient preference data, then RV-NNT and MCE analyses could potentially be useful. The RV-NNT analysis has a well-described framework involving a simple calculation of NNT and the RV measure which describes patients' preferences for avoiding specific AE's and/or negative clinical outcomes. NNT is defined as the number of patients needed to treat to benefit one more patient, compared with a control treatment. Suppose that the probability of a patient responding to the test and control treatments are p_1 and p_2, respectively. Then NNT $= 1/(p_2 - p_1)$, the inverse of the event rate difference, is a number between 1 and ∞, where lower values of NNT represent more effective treatments. Interpreting the NNT statistic correctly can be challenging. If $p_2 > p_1$ the NNT is the average number of typical patients which need to be treated via treatment 2 to achieve one additional positive response over treatment 1. A negative NNT represents a poorer drug outcome, and should be interpreted as "the number needed to harm" (NNH). Although used routinely in medical practice, due to their apparent simplicity, the NNT and NNH approach has several limitations. By definition, there is no value of NNT (or NNH) corresponding to the "no difference" scenario. In addition, although confidence intervals for NNT can, in principle, be derived from those of $p_2 - p_1$, these seldom give sensible results, particularly when data is sparse (Hutton, 2009).

To account for patient preferences, both NNT and NNH have been revised to incorporate the relative utility values from patients. This metric is called the relative value (RV) and represents specific outcomes regarding patients' preferences. It can be expressed as

$$\text{RV} = \frac{(1 - \text{utility of adverse event})}{(\text{utility of improvement using a specific treatment})},$$

and an RV value of 1 signifies a state of perfect health. Both NNH and NNT can be adjusted for RV, enabling one to derive a BR ratio (RV – NNH / NNT) between treatment and control groups, where a ratio greater than 1 represents a favorable BR profile for the treatment group. Although NNH and NNT can be extended to multiple benefits and risks they are more commonly implemented for the situation where one is considering BR assessment for a single benefit and a single risk (Jiang and Xia, 2014).

The minimal clinical efficacy (MCE) can be expressed as the required minimum clinical efficacy by the experimental treatment of interest when comparing to a standard, comparator treatment after considering the comparator treatment's efficacy, the safety profiles of both the comparator treatment and the experimental treatment of interest, as well as the risk of the disease of interest associated with no treatment. This implies that, in addition to accounting for both the benefits and risks of the experimental and standard treatments, MCE also considers the natural characteristics of the disease of interest within the general population, which is represented by an untreated group (Holden et al., 2003). The benefit can be represented by the efficacy versus harm difference; these are expressed on a 0 to 1 probability scale by applying both the reductions in relative risks (treatment benefits) and increases in relative risks (harms) to probabilities as observed in the groups with no treatment (Holden et al.). If the risk difference is lower than the efficacy difference, then one can conclude that the new, experimental treatment is justified over the standard treatment. The MCE framework allows for easy communication of the BR profile to all relevant stakeholders involved in the design and conduct of a given clinical trial. However, when data are sparse, conclusions drawn from MCE analyses can be unreliable. In addition, with MCE it is not possible to provide estimates regarding the uncertainty for the benefit and harm comparison metric; that is, only a single point estimate is produced. Therefore, constructing confidence intervals for an MCE analysis is not possible. These examples illustrate some of the problems encountered when applying classical inference in the context of BR.

The variety of quantitative and semi-quantitative methods proposed for BR assessment highlights the challenging nature of this stage of drug development. To date the number of available examples where these methods have been applied prospectively in clinical trials is sparse. However, one method that has received considerable attention in the literature and by regulatory agencies is MCDA and its extensions such as Stochastic Multicriteria Acceptability Analysis (SMAA, Saint-Hilary et al., 2017). In what follows, we will focus on the classical inference approach to MCDA. Readers interested in the details of the other methods are referred to Guo et al.

17.2.1 Multi-criteria decision analysis

Multi-criteria Decision Analysis (MCDA) is a framework based on statistical decision theory which allows one to break down a high dimensional problem into individual components and deal with multiple, potentially conflicting, objectives. In the context of BR, the components represent the individual benefits and risks, and the output is a weighted BR score which defines the BR trade-off for the intervention under consideration (Mussen et al., 2007). Although the MCDA framework does not constrain the user to a frequentist approach, it has primarily been implemented as such in the statistical and clinical literature and is the focus of this section. Later in this chapter, we discuss a Bayesian approach to the MCDA framework.

In the MCDA approach, the benefit and risk categories are typically chosen using one of the structured qualitative frameworks, such as the PrOACT-URL described earlier, and represented through a value tree as shown in Figure 17.1 (Mt-Isa et al. IMI-PROTECT Work Package 5). In this example, the favourable effects (the benefits) include the two primary efficacy endpoints of interest, the American College of Rheumatology score (ACR) and the modified Total Sharp Score. ACR is a dichotomous variable with either a positive or negative outcome, corresponding to responders and non-responders, respectively. It measures improvement in tender or swollen joint counts in at least three of the following parameters: patient assessment, physician assessment, pain scale, disability / functional questionnaire, and acute phase reactant, e.g. Erythrocyte Sedimentation Rate (ESR) or C-Reactive Protein (CRP). ACR XX (where $XX = 20, 50$, or 70 in Figure 17.1) has a positive outcome if $XX\%$ improvement in tender or swollen joint counts is achieved. The psoriatic arthritis (PsA) score was split into two components: an erosion score ranging from 0-270, and a joint space narrowing score ranging from 0-200, with higher numbers representing worse outcomes; hence, the modified Total Sharp Score (mTSS) may vary between 0 and 470 (Wassenberg, 2015). The unfavourable effects include adverse events (AEs), which are specified as infections and serious adverse events (SAEs), in addition to deaths, tuberculosis and malignancies.

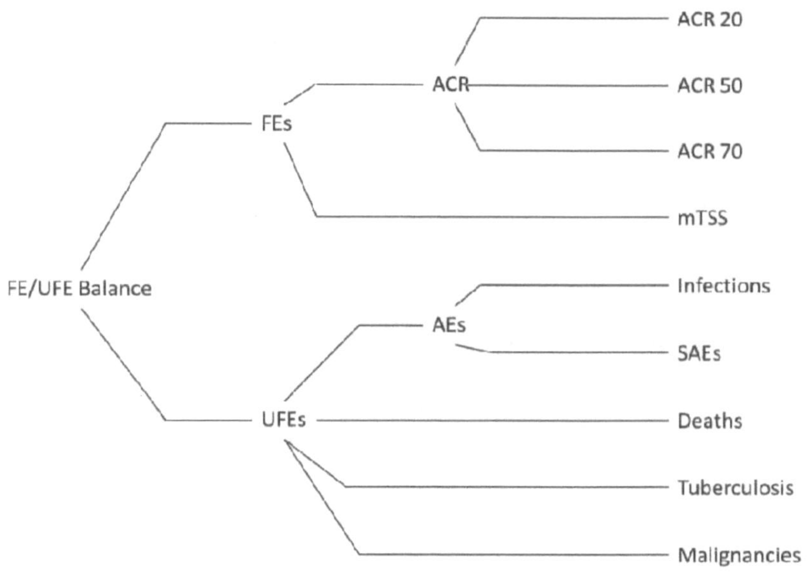

FIGURE 17.1: Value Tree example for drug X used in combination with Methotrexate for adult lupus. This figure was adapted from (Mt-Isa et al., 2012).

The next step requires a pre-specified utility function and a weight for each outcome (see also Chapter 15, for a discussion of a decision-theoretic approach to the economic evaluation of healthcare interventions). The utility function maps the observed measure to a subjective measure of value between 0 (the worst-case scenario) and 1 (the best-case scenario). Weights must be elicited to allow calculation of the overall utility for each treatment as a weighted sum of the utilities for all outcomes. For illustration, consider the scenario where the team wishes to examine the performance of a new drug and comparator in a BR assessment using MCDA. Define the response in a benefit criterion of interest as y, where a represents the worst possible value, b represents the best possible value, and $U(\cdot)$ represents an arbitrary utility function:

$$U(y) = \frac{y-a}{b-a} \times 100, \qquad a \leq y \leq b.$$

The range for the response in the benefit criteria in the transformed space is between 0 and 1 (where 0 is the worst, and 1 is the best). The performance of the drug and comparator under each of the risk criteria is assessed in a similar fashion. Define the response in a risk criterion of interest as z, where c represents the best possible value and d represents the worst possible value:

$$U(z) = \frac{z-c}{d-c} \times 100, \qquad c \leq z \leq d.$$

Note that the utility function can have a different functional form, for example quadratic, piecewise linear, and others, with the exact shape being context specific. Once the utility function is chosen, the next step is to develop a set of weights for the criteria based on their relative importance. The weight of a criterion should reflect both the observed range of responses and how much that difference matters. A decision conference is typically set up to select appropriate utility functions and weights based on input from multiple stakeholders, which can include patients and payers.

To build the MCDA score itself, suppose that one has m alternatives (for example, different treatments) and n benefit criteria defined such that higher values represent better outcomes. Let w_j represent the corresponding importance weight of criterion C_j and u_{ij} represent the performance value, or utility score, of alternative A_i when evaluated in terms of criterion C_j. The final MCDA score can be represented as the sum of the weighted utility scores as follows:

$$A_i^{MCDA} = \sum_{j=1}^{n} w_j u_{ij}, \qquad \text{for } i = 1, \ldots, m.$$

The goal is to choose the alternative that yields the highest MCDA score. This MCDA approach can be repeated when all the criteria are risk measures; in this case, the goal is to choose the alternative that yields the lowest possible score. An overall MCDA score comprising both benefits and risks can be calculated as the difference between the weighted sum of the transformed benefits versus the weighted sum of the transformed risks. A positive score indicates that, for alternative A_i, the benefits outweigh the risks. This overall score can thus be used to rank the different alternatives, with the best choice being that corresponding to the highest overall MCDA score. Note that the above is based on the arithmetic mean which is employed prevalently in the literature. However, since the utilities are mostly contained in an interval ranging from 0 to 1, the geometric mean may be preferable in certain scenarios. For example, if one criteria has a utility of 0 (e.g. death) then the arithmetic mean suggests that this could have some benefit if the other criteria are non-null; that is, the impact of the event "death" could be offset by the efficacy which is clearly undesirable. However, when using the product, or geometric mean, the overall score remains 0, which is more consistent.

The subjective nature of the choice of weights and utility functions means that sensitivity analyses should be conducted to understand how the results depend on these choices. Lastly, one of the main drawbacks of classical MCDA is the lack of a standard probabilistic method to quantify and/or propagate uncertainty, as point estimates of the treatment effects without 95% confidence intervals are typically used (Waddingham et al., 2016).

17.3 Bayesian approaches to quantitative benefit-risk

Efficient decision-making requires several types of information: accumulating information on benefits and risks, possible consequences of alternative decisions, and external or subjective information on the relative importance of possible consequences (Berger, 1993). Bayesian inference provides a framework to formally and coherently utilize prior information and repeatedly update decisions based on accumulating knowledge, which naturally supports decision theory (Ashby and Smith, 2000). It also provides a logical foundation for handling uncertainty, as well as a clear framework for making predictions about "future" outcomes of interest, thus enabling inference from the population to the patient level. In addition, the Bayesian updating mechanism allows for the incorporation of opinions from different stakeholders, which can lead to a more focused dialogue (Ashby and Smith, 2000). The advantages of Bayesian approaches for decision-making in the context of BR have been demonstrated across different phases of drug development. This section provides a summary of current methods.

One area that has received considerable attention is the use of Bayesian methods for sequential dose selection, most of which make extensive use of the updating mechanism inherent to the Bayesian framework. Assuming linear dose-responses for both toxicity and efficacy as measured by binary outcomes, Braun developed a bivariate distribution on the log-odds scale, with the association between the two outcomes modeled as a function of their odds ratio (Braun, 2002). Fixed target thresholds for efficacy and toxicity were defined using various decision-making metrics, for example reaching the optimal dose or stopping the trial early for failure to identify the maximum tolerated dose. The use of a prior distribution allows for a sensible dose allocation at the early stages of the trial when data is sparse. The prior offers direction to dose assignment when only a few subjects are present and is vague enough that its impact decreases as data accrues. Thomann (2015) generalized this method to non-linear dose-response models. Thall and Cook (2004) extended the approach of Braun by providing an algorithm for eliciting subjective prior distributions, and by using efficacy-toxicity trade-off contours rather than fixed target thresholds.

Graham et al. (2002) proposed a non-linear Bayesian hierarchical model for decision-making at the end of a dose-response trial using utility functions. This method can include different response types (e.g. count and categorical data) when defining the utility function representing the BR trade-off. In addition, this model allows one to drill down to different sources of variability, including within-subject variability. It also provides a natural framework for predicting the utility of specific dosing regimens for a future patient. Furthermore, this Bayesian hierarchical model has the flexibility to incorporate expert knowledge through utility functions and to use information from previous clinical trials through prior distributions.

He et al. (2012) developed and explored a Bayesian joint modelling and joint evaluation framework for BR assessment using single efficacy and safety outcomes. By comparing the posterior estimates for the effect sizes against clinically relevant efficacy and safety thresholds, the proposed joint model can derive the posterior probability of success for the intervention of interest. The Bayesian framework allows for easy predictions of success for the next stage of development. He and Fu (2016) later extended this method to model multiple efficacy and safety outcomes.

Bayesian inference has also been applied to well-known BR measures such as NCB. Shaffer and Watterberg (2006) built a bivariate model for binary efficacy and safety outcomes, and derived confidence regions for the difference in risk and benefit using a Normal approximation. The use of Bayesian inference allowed quantification of uncertainty through probability distributions and the use of posterior probabilities to represent the strength of evidence.

Sutton et al. (2005) extended Bayesian BR assessment to a post-marketing setting that integrates evidence from both randomized controlled trials and observational studies. They developed a NCB model and used Bayesian inference to propagate uncertainty and derive posterior probabilities of desired outcomes which were then used to support decision-making.

To date there are no publicly available examples of the application, in a prospective manner, of the Bayesian BR methods described above. However, as regulatory experience with Bayesian approaches to clinical trial design increases (see, for example, Chapters 6 and 9), it is likely that this will extend to the area of quantitative BR assessment.

The next two sections provide more in-depth reviews of two specific Bayesian BR approaches, a Bayesian MCDA model, and a Bayesian approach for longitudinal BR assessment. The first method serves to highlight how Bayesian inference provides a coherent framework for decision-making by quantifying uncertainty through probability models, and the second method to illustrate how the repeated updating mechanism based on accumulating knowledge inherent to the Bayesian framework supports decision-making. These methods will be illustrated through real data examples.

17.3.1 Bayesian multi-criteria decision analysis

As described in Section 17.2, there is no well-established method for propagating uncertainty of treatment effect data through a classical MCDA model, and therefore it is not clear how to quantify the variability in the BR trade-off. Bayesian statistics provides a coherent framework to handle and characterize uncertainty, and this makes it a natural fit to express uncertainty in an MCDA setting. Waddingham et al. (2016) developed a Bayesian extension to MCDA that includes an additional step where a probability model for individual outcomes and prior distributions for model parameters are defined. Markov chain Monte Carlo (MCMC) simulations are then used to estimate the posterior distribution of the overall BR score. Bayesian inference was thus used to strengthen the MCDA framework through a structured quantification of uncertainty.

Waddingham et al. (2016) illustrated this Bayesian approach to MCDA with the natalizumab example for relapsing-remitting multiple sclerosis. The objective of the MCDA analysis was to compare the BR profile of three active treatments: natalizumab, interferon-beta and glatiramer acetate. The key safety endpoints included were progressive multifocal leukoencephalopathy (PML), seizures, congenital abnormalities, herpes reactivation, hypersensitivity reactions, flu-like reactions, transaminase elevation and infusion/injection site reactions. The key efficacy endpoints were disability progression, relapses and treatment convenience. These efficacy and safety endpoints constitute the key benefit and risk outcomes. The authors used data from three clinical trials (for most efficacy and safety endpoints) and post-marketing studies (for PML incidence, since no clinical trial data were available).

Waddingham et al. (2016) illustrated this Bayesian approach to MCDA with the natalizumab example for relapsing-remitting multiple sclerosis. The objective of the MCDA analysis was to compare the BR profile of three active treatments: natalizumab, interferon-beta and glatiramer acetate. The key safety endpoints included were progressive multifocal leukoencephalopathy (PML), seizures, congenital abnormalities, herpes reactivation, hypersensitivity reactions, flu-like reactions, transaminase elevation and infusion/injection site reactions. The key efficacy endpoints were disability progression, relapses and treatment convenience. These efficacy and safety endpoints constitute the key benefit and risk outcomes. The authors used data from three clinical trials (for most efficacy and safety endpoints) and post-marketing studies (for PML incidence, since no clinical trial data were available).

TABLE 17.1: Risks, benefits, measures, utility functions and weights for the natalizumab case study

Endpoint	Measure	Utility Function	Weight
Risks:			
PML	prop. with event in 2 years	1−proportion	0.538
Seizures	prop. with event in 2 years	1−proportion	0.054
Congenital abnormalities	prop. with event in 2 years	1−proportion	0.054
Herpes reactivation	prop. with event in 2 years	1−proportion	0.064
Hypersensitivity reactions	prop. with event in 2 years	1−proportion	0.011
Flu-like reactions	prop. with event in 2 years	1−proportion	0.011
Transaminases elevation	prop. with event in 2 years	1−proportion	0.107
Infusion/injection reactions	prop. with event in 2 years	1−proportion	0.027
Benefits:			
Disability progression	prop. progressing in 2 years	1−proportion	0.054
Relapses	2-year relapse rate	1−0.5×rate	0.075
Convenience	Route of administration	1 (daily oral)	0.005
		0.7 (monthly infusion)	
		0.5 (weekly intramuscular)	
		0 (daily subcutaneous)	

Various Bayesian models were used to implement a probabilistic assessment of the BR balance. Binary outcomes such as PML, seizures, congenital abnormalities, herpes reactivation, hypersensitivity reactions, flu-like reactions, transaminase elevation and infusion/injection site reactions, were modelled assuming a Binomial distribution. If $X_{ij,k}$ is the number of patients who experience outcome k in arm j of trial i, then $X_{ij,k} \sim \text{Bin}(\pi_{ij,k}, n_{ij,k})$, where $n_{ij,k}$ is the total number of patients in trial arm j and $\pi_{ij,k}$ is the underlying risk for the outcome k. Let $\mu_{ik} = \left[\text{logit}(\pi_{i1k}) + \text{logit}(\pi_{i2k})\right]/2$ for the mean proportion over both arms in the log-odds scale, and $\delta_{ik} = \left[\text{logit}(\pi_{i1k}) - \text{logit}(\pi_{i2k})\right]/2$ for the log odds ratio.

The 10th outcome in Table 17.1, relapses, was modelled as a Poisson distributed variable. If $X_{ij,10}$ is the number of patients who experience relapse in arm j of trial i, then $X_{ij,10} \sim \text{Poisson}(n_{ij,10}\pi_{ij,10})$, where $n_{ij,10}$ is the total patient-years of exposure in trial arm j, and $\pi_{ij,10}$ is the underlying event rate. Let $\mu_{i,10} = \left[\log(\pi_{i1,10}) + \log(\pi_{i2,10})\right]/2$ be the mean log relapse rate over both arms, and $\delta_{i,10} = \left[\log(\pi_{i1,10}) - \log(\pi_{i2,10})\right]/2$ the log rate ratio. The utility associated with route of administration was modelled deterministically. The authors assumed a common prior across all treatments i and outcomes k, $\delta_{ik} \sim \text{N}(d, \sigma^2)$, with hyperpriors $d \sim \text{Uniform}(-1, 1)$ and $1/\sigma^2 = \tau \sim \text{Gamma}(3, 1)$. The prior for μ was specified as $\mu_{ik} \sim \text{N}(0, 4)$, where 4 is the variance.

The total Bayesian MCDA score was defined as the weighted sum of the utility functions in Table 17.1. The empirical estimates of δ and μ were calculated from the data, using pre-specified formulae. For binary outcomes the authors used, $\widehat{\delta}_{ik} = \log\left(\frac{x_{i2k}+\frac{1}{2}}{n_{i2k}-x_{i2k}+\frac{1}{2}}\right) - \log\left(\frac{x_{i1k}+\frac{1}{2}}{n_{i1k}-x_{i1k}+\frac{1}{2}}\right)$ and $\widehat{\mu}_{ik} = \log\left(\frac{x_{i2k}+\frac{1}{2}}{n_{i2k}-x_{i2k}+\frac{1}{2}}\right) + \log\left(\frac{x_{i1k}+\frac{1}{2}}{n_{i1k}-x_{i1k}+\frac{1}{2}}\right)$. The formulæ for relapse rate are $\widehat{\delta}_{ik} = \log\left(\frac{x_{i2k}+\frac{1}{2}}{n_{i2k}+\frac{1}{2}}\right) - \log\left(\frac{x_{i1k}+\frac{1}{2}}{n_{i1k}+\frac{1}{2}}\right)$ and $\widehat{\mu}_{ik} = \log\left(\frac{x_{i2k}+\frac{1}{2}}{n_{i2k}+\frac{1}{2}}\right) + \log\left(\frac{x_{i1k}+\frac{1}{2}}{n_{i1k}+\frac{1}{2}}\right)$.

Using MCMC simulation, the posterior distributions of the overall MCDA scores of interest (in absolute terms and relative to natalizumab) were derived and are summarized in Table 17.2, along with the rank 1 acceptability index (ranks based on the proportion of simulations in which the specific treatment had the highest overall utility, or BR score).

The highest overall median MCDA score was 0.957 for natalizumab, with 95% credible interval (0.954, 0.961). The rank 1 acceptability index for natalizumab was 1.0. The results

TABLE 17.2: Risks, benefits, measures, utility functions and weights for the natalizumab case study

Treatment	MCDA score overall	Relative to Natalizumab	Probability of rank 1, 2, 3, 4			
Placebo	0.923 (0.919, 0.928)	0.034 (0.029, 0.040)	0	0	0.12	0.88
Natalizumab	0.957 (0.954, 0.961)	0.000 (0.000, 0.000)	1	0	0	0
BI	0.931 (0.919, 0.942)	0.026 (0.015, 0.039)	0	0.39	0.53	0.08
GA	0.933 (0.920, 0.944)	0.024 (0.013, 0.038)	0	0.6	0.35	0.05

Results are medians (95% credible intervals). BI, beta-interferon; GA, glatiramer acetate.

show that natalizumab has the highest MCDA score, among all four treatments included in the analysis. By using the Bayesian approach in an MCDA model, the uncertainty in the data is propagated, the variability of the BR trade-off is quantified, and the decision-making process becomes more transparent, robust and interpretable.

The specific disease under consideration will determine not only the measures to be included but also the weights and utilities. For example, whereas in a migraine setting the clinical team may give higher weight to risk measures, in an oncology setting these may not be deemed as relevant compared to the potential benefits. The structured approach to these discussions inherent to Bayesian MCDA is invaluable. Extensions to the Bayesian MCDA methods of Waddingham et al. (2016) have been proposed in the literature. To conduct a sensitivity analysis regarding the selection of weights, approaches like stochastic multi-criteria analysis (SMAA) could be used (Tervonen et al., 2011). However, the additional flexibility can lead to variability levels that hinder decision-making rather than supporting it (Saint-Hilary et al., 2017; Waddingham et al., 2016).

17.3.2 Bayesian approaches for longitudinal benefit-risk assessment

In clinical trials, it is typically the case that patients are followed for multiple visits. Zhao et al. (2014) proposed a Bayesian model for longitudinal BR assessment in this setting. The model is based on Chuang-Stein's BR outcome categories, and assumes that subject-level outcomes can be classified into five mutually exclusive groups: benefit, benefit with AE, no benefit with no AE, no benefit but with AE, and withdrawal (Chuang-Stein et al., 1991).

Denote the number of patients that fall into each of the five BR categories at visit $t = t_m$ by $\boldsymbol{n_m} = (n_{1m}, \dots, n_{5m})$. Assume that $\boldsymbol{n_m}$ follows a Multinomial distribution, $\boldsymbol{n_m} \mid \boldsymbol{p} \sim \text{Mult}\left(\boldsymbol{n_{.m}}, \boldsymbol{p}\right)$, $m = 1, \dots M$, where $\boldsymbol{p} = (p_1, \dots, p_5)$, $0 < p_i < 1$, $\sum_{i=1}^{5} p_i = 1$, and $\boldsymbol{n_{.m}} = \sum_{i=1}^{5} n_{im}$. In the scenario where there are two arms in the clinical trial, treatment and control, let $\boldsymbol{p_d} = (p_{1,d}, \dots, p_{5,d})$, $d \in \{T = Treatment,\ C = Control\}$. Chuang-Stein et al. (1991) defined a set of three global benefit-risk (GBR) scores that can be used to evaluate a new medicine:

$$\text{Linear Score} = \sum_{i=1}^{2} w_i p_{i,d} - \sum_{i=3}^{5} w_i p_{i,d},$$

$$\text{Ratio Score} = \frac{\left(\sum_{i=1}^{2} w_i p_{i,d}\right)^e}{\sum_{i=3}^{5} w_i p_{i,d}}$$

where $w_i > 0$, $i = 1, \ldots, 5$ are the pre-specified weights and the nonnegative exponent e reflects the relative importance of benefit to risk in constructing the ratio BR score. For the pre-specified weights, they used $w_1 = 2$, $w_2 = 1$, $w_3 = 0$, $w_4 = 1$, and $w_5 = 2$ for easy illustration, considering "Benefit with no AEs" has a higher weight than "Benefit with AEs" in terms of benefit; and "Withdrawal" has a higher weight than "No benefit with AE" in terms of risk. Based on the global scores, the benefit-risk (BR) difference between treatment and control can be measured as follows:

$$\begin{aligned}
\text{BR Linear} &= \left(\sum_{i=1}^{2} w_i p_{i,T} - \sum_{i=3}^{5} w_i p_{i,T}\right) - \left(\sum_{i=1}^{2} w_i p_{i,C} - \sum_{i=3}^{5} w_i p_{i,C}\right), \\
\text{BR Ratio} &= \log\left(\frac{\left(\sum_{i=1}^{2} w_i p_{i,T}\right)^e}{\sum_{i=3}^{5} w_i p_{i,T}}\right) - \log\left(\frac{\left(\sum_{i=1}^{2} w_i p_{i,C}\right)^e}{\sum_{i=3}^{5} w_i p_{i,C}}\right), \\
\text{BR Cmp Ratio} &= \log\left(\frac{w_i p_{i,T}}{w_t p_{5,T}}\left[\frac{w_2 p_{2,T}}{w_3 p_{3,T} + w_4 p_{4,T}}\right]^f\right) - \\
&\quad \log\left(\frac{w_i p_{i,C}}{w_t p_{5,C}}\left[\frac{w_2 p_{2,C}}{w_3 p_{3,C} + w_4 p_{4,C}}\right]^f\right).
\end{aligned}$$

Note that the nonnegative exponent f is used to give a different weight to different benefit or risk categories in constructing the composite ratio score. While the linear BR measure is a weighted sum of the probability that a patient falls into each of the five BR groups, and it is convenient when comparing two treatments, the ratio BR measure compares benefits and risks by weighting their relative magnitudes, and can be applied in the absence of a comparator arm. The authors used a Dirichlet distribution as the prior for the probability of the five categories at first visit, $p \sim \text{Dirichlet}(\boldsymbol{\alpha})$, where $\boldsymbol{\alpha} = (\alpha_1, \ldots, \alpha_5)$, $\alpha_i > 0$, and $\sum_{i=1}^{5} \alpha_i < \infty$. Using the updated posterior distributions from previous visits as priors for subsequent visits, the posterior distributions of the BR measures at each visit were recursively obtained through MCMC simulations. The posterior median and 95% credible intervals were then used to represent the BR profile over time. A non-informative power prior of the form $a_0 \sim \text{Beta}(1, 1)$ can be implemented to discount information from previous visits (for more details on the use of power priors see Chapters 6, 12 and 13). In cases when informative priors could be estimated from historical data or expert opinions, an informative prior could also be used. This method does not take the whole longitudinal profiles at once; instead it updates the posterior for each visit using the accumulated information prior to that visit. Even though the model is based on Chuang-Stein's five BR categories, it can be easily extended to include additional outcome categories as needed. Cui et al. (2016) further extended this methodology to account for the subject-level dependency between visits.

Zhao et al. (2014) applied the longitudinal Bayesian BR score method to data from a clinical trial assessing the BR profile of Hydromorphone, a treatment for pain. In this two-arm study, 268 patients were randomly assigned to receive Hydromorphone or control, and each patient was followed for eight visits. Their outcomes were evaluated by medical doctors and assigned to one of the five BR categories, "Benefit", "Benefit with AEs", "No benefit with no AEs", "No benefit with AE" and "Withdrawal", arranged from the most to the least desirable. Figure 17.2 represents the distribution of BR categories.

Zhao et al. (2014) recursively derived the posterior distributions of cell-probabilities using MCMC simulation, as data from the eight visits became available.

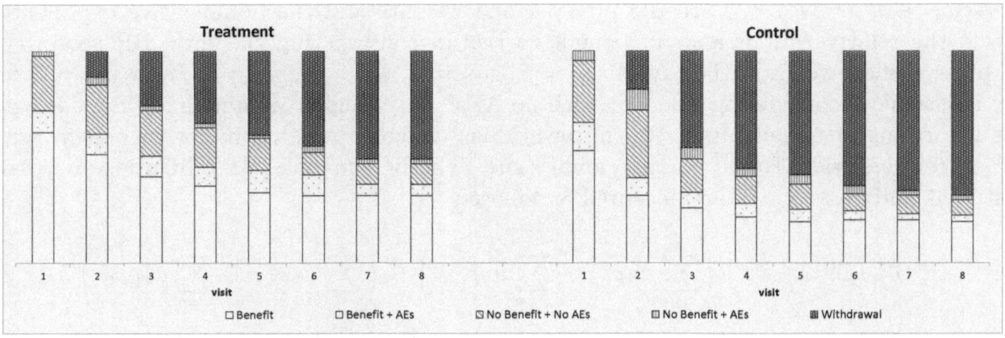

FIGURE 17.2: Hydromorphone case study: The frequency distribution of the five BR categories (this figure was reproduced with the author's permission.)

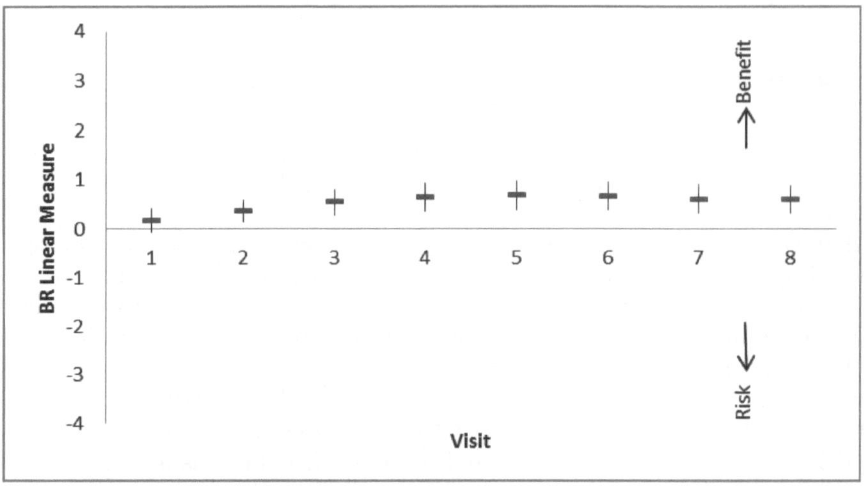

FIGURE 17.3: Hydromorphone case study: The longitudinal posterior summaries for the linear BR measure. The dashes (–) mark the means, and the strikes (|) represent the width of the 95% credible intervals. Values above zero favor Hydromorphone against the control (this figure was reproduced with the author's permission).

Figure 17.3 depicts the longitudinal BR assessment results using the linear BR measure. The 95% credible intervals for the linear BR measure contain zero at visit 1 and exceed zero for the rest of the visits. This shows that the benefits of Hydromorphone outweigh the risks after visit 1, compared to control. This Bayesian approach to the longitudinal assessment of BR maximizes the use of all available evidence, including historical data, recursively updates the BR profiles as information accrues, and provides a natural mechanism for making inferences at different stages of development. This example illustrates how the continuously evolving nature of Bayesian methodology makes it a natural tool to support BR assessment.

17.4 Outlook for Bayesian benefit-risk

This chapter has described how Bayesian inference can be a useful framework to support decision-making when performing quantitative BR assessments. In addition to the methods above, there is scope for further developments in the application of the Bayesian framework to other BR areas.

One such area is personalized medicine, where the objective is to understand which subgroups of patients are likely to have the most positive BR profile, and which the least. Thomas and Bornkamp (2016) outline a Bayesian approach that identifies subgroups based on adjusted posterior treatment effects for efficacy responses using ideas from model selection to minimize bias. Extending this approach to adjust for safety responses could help identify the patient subgroup with the smallest separation between active drug and comparator and thus derive subgroup specific BR scores from the joint adjusted posterior treatment effects. Still in personalized medicine, there is increased awareness of the importance of accounting for patient preferences. MCDA can aid preference-based personalized medicine by combining patient preferences, represented by the choice of outcomes and corresponding weights, and clinical data.

As mentioned earlier, uncertainty is inherent to BR assessments. For example, the uncertainty present in the clinical data can have a substantial impact on the overall BR profiles. It is important, therefore, to understand the impact that different sources of uncertainty could have on the BR assessment to explore the limits of the evidence generated. Furthermore, within a clinical development program it is crucial to assess how uncertainty in the data influences the BR profile to minimize late stage attrition. For example, given the selected weights and utilities, the Bayesian approach can be utilized to better understand how many occurrences of type X would need to be observed to change the BR conclusions. Within MCDA, the following different types of uncertainties should be accounted for: uncertainty in weights assigned to the criteria identified for decision-making and the corresponding utility functions, uncertainty due to the variability in the clinical data, and uncertainty due to different data sources, for example when efficacy and safety populations do not coincide. MCDA could be extended with probabilistic models to address the latter. Chuang-Stein et al. (2016) discuss examining data from different sources with the aim of providing a BR assessment at the clinical development program level. Bayesian approaches to propagate uncertainty due to different data sources through the inference mechanism could aid in the BR assessment.

Another area where Bayesian approaches could be useful is to support the physician's clinical decision-making by providing predictive statements on the BR profile of future patients, given a set of characteristics or covariates. In the case of rare events, a physician may find it challenging to quantify a particularly rare safety risk. Bayesian approaches can guide these discussions, for example by quantifying the rare nature of the event with a probability, conditional on the knowledge that the event is rare as represented via the prior distribution. Data for rare events will inherently have limitations; however it is important to assess whether a change in safety management is required based on the new data accrued. Hence, calculating the probability of the rare event occurring is crucial and several authors have explored the impact of using informative priors or Bayesian hierarchical models (Winkler et al., 2002; Chen and McGee, 2016). They found that results could be misleading when trying to be non-informative, especially when it is not the event rate but a function of the event rate that is the quantity of interest. Bayesian approaches for rare and orphan diseases are discussed in detail in Chapter 12.

17.5 Discussion

Bayesian approaches to BR have been shown to provide intuitive and direct probabilistic statements that can be used to assess the chances of success in clinical trial development. This information can then be employed by the relevant stakeholders to make decisions on key questions that typically arise in drug development. For example, the choice of optimal dose to carry forward into the next trial, the choice of subgroups with optimal BR profile when planning a large scale late-phase trial, understanding how to quantify variability and uncertainty from a variety of data sources, or whether a drug should continue to regulatory or health technology assessment (HTA) submission. There is also potential for developing these ideas into relatively new areas such as personalized medicine or subgroup analysis, and for extensions of more established approaches such as MCDA.

Despite the demonstrated ability of Bayesian approaches to bring clarity and robustness into BR discussions, there is still resistance among many stakeholders who tend to resort to simple summary statistics rather than a quantitative, and more specifically, a Bayesian BR approach. Statisticians and other quantitative scientists can play a major role in educating the clinical community on the importance and added value of quantitative approaches to BR assessment, and how Bayesian inference can help address some of the shortcomings. More broadly, a multidisciplinary effort among quantitative scientists, clinicians, and others, is imperative to influence the development of Bayesian BR strategies that can adequately support all different phases of clinical trial development and beyond (e.g. marketing, HTA payers, etc.). To do this, it will be important to a) at the design stage ensure that the research BR question of interest is clearly formulated such that the relevant data is collected to address it, and b) build resource and capability among quantitative scientists such that, if relevant, more complex, quantitative methodologies can be applied.

As the field of Bayesian BR evolves, it will be important for stakeholders to share case studies and their own personal experiences with quantitative BR approaches. In addition, it is critical to continue to promote an open dialogue and engage with experts in the field through conferences, workshops, publications, etc. The result should be more focused and robust discussions leading to cost-effective, efficient study designs which provide added value for the patients.

Bibliography

Ashby, D. and Smith, A. F. (2000). Evidence-based medicine as Bayesian decision-making. *Statistics in Medicine*, 19(23):3291–3305.

Berger, J. (1993). *Statistical Decision Theory and Bayesian Analysis.* Springer-Verlag, 3rd edition.

Braun, T. M. (2002). The bivariate continual reassessment method. Extending the CRM to phase I trials of two competing outcomes. *Controlled Clinical Trials*, 23(3):240–256.

Chen, Z. and McGee, M. (2016). A Bayesian approach to zero-numerator problems using hierarchical models. *Journal of Data Science*, 6:261–268.

Chuang-Stein, C., Mohberg, N. R., and Sinkula, M. S. (1991). Three measures for simultaneously evaluating benefits and risks using categorical data from clinical trials. *Statistics in Medicine*, 10(9):1349–1359.

Chuang-Stein, C., Quartey, G., and He, W. (2016). Sources of data to enable benefit-risk assessment. In Jiang, Q. and He, W., editors, *Benefit-Risk Assessment Methods in Drug Development: Bridging Qualitative and Quantitative Assessments*. CRC Press.

Colopy, M. W., Damaraju, C. V., He, W., Jiang, Q., Levitan, B. S., Ruan, S., and Yuan, Z. (2015). Benefit-risk evaluation and decision making: Some practical insights. *Therapeutic Innovation & Regulatory Science*, 49(3):425–433.

Coplan, P. M., Noel, R. A., Levitan, B. S., Ferguson, J., and Mussen, F. (2011). Development of a framework for enhancing the transparency, reproducibility and communication of the benefit-risk balance of medicines. *Clinical Pharmacology and Therapeutics*, 89(2):312–315.

Cui, S., Zhao, Y., and Tiwary, R. (2016). Bayesian approach to personalized benefit-risk assessment. *Statistics in Biopharmaceutical Research*, 8:316–324.

Graham, G., Gupta, S., and Aarons, L. (2002). Determination of an optimal dosage regimen using a Bayesian decision analysis of efficacy and adverse effect data. *Journal of Pharmacokinetics and Pharmacodynamics*, 29(1):67–88.

Guo, J. J., Pandey, S., Doyle, J., Bian, B., Lis, Y., and Raisch, D. W. (2010). A review of quantitative risk-benefit methodologies for assessing drug safety and efficacy-report of the ISPOR risk-benefit management working group. *Value in Health*, 13(5):657–666.

Hammond, J. S., Keeney, R. L., and Raiffa, H. (1998). *Smart Choices: A Practical Guide to Making Better Decisions*. Boston: Harvard Business School Press.

He, W., Cao, X., and Xu, L. (2012). A framework for joint modeling and joint assessment of efficacy and safety endpoints for probability of success evaluation and optimal dose selection. *Statistics in Medicine*, 31(5):401–419.

He, W. and Fu, B. (2016). Benefit-risk evaluation using a framework of joint modeling and joint evaluations of multiple efficacy and safety endpoints. In Jiang, Q. and He, W., editors, *Benefit-Risk Assessment Methods in Drug Development: Bridging Qualitative and Quantitative Assessments*. CRC Press.

Holden, W., Juhaeri, J., and Dai, W. (2003). Benefit-risk analysis: examples using quantitative methods. *Pharmacoepidemiology and Drug Safety*, 12:693–697.

Hutton, J. (2009). Number needed to treat and number needed to harm are not the best way to report and assess the results of randomised clinical trials. *British Journal of Haematology*, 146:27–30.

Jiang, Q. and Xia, H. (2014). *Quantitative Evaluation of Safety in Drug Development: Design, Analysis, and Reporting*. CRC Press.

Mt-Isa, S., Wang, N., Hallgreen, C. et al. (2012). On behalf of PROTECT Work Package 5 participants, Review of methodologies for benefit and risk assessment of medication, Version 4, 14 Feb 2012. http://protectbenefitrisk.eu/documents/Shahruletal ReviewofmethodologiesforbenefitandriskassessmentofmedicationMay2013.pdf.

Mt-Isa, S., Hallgreen, C. E., Wang, N., Callreus, T., Genov, G., Hirsch, I., Hobbiger, S. F., Hockley, K. S., Luciani, D., Phillips, L. D., Quartey, G., Sarac, S. B., Stoeckert, I., Tzoulaki, I., Micaleff, A., Ashby, D.; IMI-PROTECT benefit-risk participants. (2014). Balancing benefit and risk of medicines: a systematic review and classification of available methodologies. *Pharmacoepidemiology and Drug Safety*, 23(7):667–678.

Mt-Isa, S., Ouwens, M., Robert, V., Gebel, M., Schacht, A., and Hirsch, I. (2016). Structured Benefit-risk assessment: a review of key publications and initiatives on frameworks and methodologies. *Pharmaceutical Statistics*, 15(4):324–332.

Mussen, F., Salek, S., and Walker, S. (2007). A quantitative approach to benefit-risk assessment of medicines - part 1: the development of a new model using multi-criteria decision analysis. *Pharmacoepidemiology and Drug Safety*, 16 Suppl 1:S2–S15.

Saint-Hilary, G., Cadour, S., Robert, V., and Gasparini, M. (2017). A simple way to unify multicriteria decision analysis (MCDA) and stochastic multicriteria acceptability analysis (SMAA) using a Dirichlet distribution in benefit-risk assessment. *Biometrical Journal*, 59(3):567–578.

Shaffer, M. L. and Watterberg, K. L. (2006). Joint distribution approaches to simultaneously quantifying benefit and risk. *BMC Medical Research Methodology*, 6:48.

Sheiner, L. B. (1997). Learning versus confirming in clinical drug development. *Clinical Pharmacology and Therapeutics*, 61(3):275–291.

Sutton, A. J., Cooper, N. J., Abrams, K. R., Lambert, P. C., and Jones, D. R. (2005). A Bayesian approach to evaluating net clinical benefit allowed for parameter uncertainty. *Journal of Clinical Epidemiology*, 58(1):26–40.

Tervonen, T., van Valkenhoef, G., Buskens, E., Hillege, H. L., and Postmus, D. (2011). A stochastic multicriteria model for evidence-based decision making in drug benefit-risk analysis. *Statistics in Medicine*, 30(12):1419–1428.

Thall, P. F. and Cook, J. D. (2004). Dose-finding based on efficacy-toxicity trade-offs. *Biometrics*, 60(3):684–693.

Thomann, M. (2015). The flexible bivariate continual reassessment method. PhD thesis, University of Iowa.

Thomas, M. and Bornkamp, B. (2016). Comparing approaches to treatment effect estimation for subgroups in early phase clinical trials. *Statistics in Biopharmaceutical Research*, 9:160–171.

Waddingham, E., Mt-Isa, S., Nixon, R., and Ashby, D. (2016). A Bayesian approach to probabilistic sensitivity analysis in structured benefit-risk assessment. *Biometrical Journal*, 58(1):28–42.

Wassenberg, S. (2015). Radiographic scoring methods in psoriatic arthritis. *Clinical and Experimental Rheumatology*, 33(5 Suppl 93):S55–59.

Winkler, R. L., Smith, J. E., and Fryback, D. G. (2002). The role of informative priors in zero-numerator problems. *The American Statistician*, 56(1):1–4.

Zhao, Y., Zalkikar, J., Tiwari, R., and LaVange, L. (2014). A Bayesian approach for benefit-risk assessment. *Statistics in Biopharmaceutical Research*, 6:326–337.

Part IV

Product development and manufacturing

18

Product Development and Manufacturing

Bruno Boulanger
Pharmalex, Belgium

Timothy Mutsvari
Pharmalex, Belgium

This chapter gives first an overview of the common problems that need to be addressed during the development of new drug products. It covers topics such as i) the development of robust processes as required by the quality by design regulation, ii) the qualification and the control of the processes, iii) the development, validation and control of the measurement systems used to evaluate the drug products and iv) common quality evaluations of batches of drug products produced such as the stability, the content uniformity and the dissolution. To describe the very objectives that need to be addressed in manufacturing, the problem of comparability of two processes and analytical similarity are addressed from a Bayesian perspective. It is a very illustrative example since it allows us to cover topics key in quality, i.e. the setting of the quality specifications for individual batches of drug products and the predictive probability that the new process will produce each future batch within the specifications. The use of the posterior predictive distribution to address both questions is proposed since the decision is about future individual batches or units. The posterior distribution of the parameters has little direct interest in manufacturing as opposed to the clinical setting, since the decision is not about the drug product per se, but rather about the capability of the process to produce individual batches of the drug product within the specifications defining the quality.

18.1 Introduction

When a new treatment opportunity (drug product and the related putative mechanism of action) has been discovered, it requires further development through extensive and lengthy clinical development phases to verify and confirm that it can potentially be beneficial for the patients suffering from the envisioned indication. The clinical development has as objectives to address conditions of optimal use if the new treatment appears to be effective. Among these conditions of use one can cite dose, formulation, route of administration, regimen, duration, diagnostic criteria, phenotype/genotype and age of the patients. The list is not exhaustive and can be specific depending on the nature of the drug product and the disease. In about 10% of the cases, new treatments that enter into clinical development are finally approved by regulatory authorities and can, potentially, be commercialized, and so be manufactured.

Therefore, in parallel to this clinical development the drug product itself has to be developed and its profile should be optimized to cope with the evolving and changing requirements provided during the clinical development (Burdick et al., 2017). Among the attributes of the drug product that must be adapted are for example the doses, the formulations, the dissolution or diffusion profile, the stability, etc. Once the drug product overall profile appears to be defined, the Phase III clinical trials aim at confirming that the nearly final product achieves its promises for the population of patients retained. But before entering the confirmatory phases, a manufacturing process, preferably at real large scale, i.e. at commercial scale, has to be developed and qualified. The whole purpose is to ensure that the process will be capable of producing in the future batches of the drug product whose quality remain constant over time and consistent with the quality attributes (QAs) defined by the Target Product Profile (TPP), i.e. the formal requirements. These Process Validation steps are described in the 2011 FDA Guidance for Industry Process Validation: General Principles and Practices (U.S. Food and Drug Administration, 2011). The biopharmaceutical manufacturing processes are considered in three stages: Process Development and Design (Stage 1), Process Performance Qualification (PPQ, Stage 2), and Continued Process Verification (CPV, Stage 3). The problems that need to be addressed in Stage 1 are covered in Chapter 19 and described also in Peterson and Altan (2016). The global aim of the development and design stage from a statistical perspective is to ensure that in the future the quality of the drug product will remain within some limits unaffected by reasonable or normal variations that could be encountered in the (critical) process parameters (CPP). For example, from one production batch to another, small changes in temperature or pH will occur but it should not impact the quality of the product. The robustness of the process with respect to changes in CPP is usually considered as the consequence of a proactive design strategy described in the ICH-Q8 (International Conference on Harmonization, 2009) regulation under the generic name "Quality by Design" (Peterson, 2010). The Stage 2 of the process qualification, PPQ, has as its purpose to demonstrate with a limited number of so-called validation batches that the drug product is indeed within the specifications. Finally, the Stage 3, CPV, is the quality control strategies that the producer has to set up to continuously verify the quality of the products, prevent potential drift in the manufacturing process over time and preferably take actions as knowledge accumulates to improve the quality. The PPQ and CPV stages are covered in Chapters 20 and 24. The development of such a manufacturing line requires several years of experiments and major investments that should start well before the confirmatory trials being envisaged, in other words before knowing if the product will ever be approved for commercialisation.

The development of a process to manufacture a drug product also requires the development and validation of a wide variety of measurements systems, analytical procedures and bioassays that will be able to quantify reliably the QAs of the drug products. The Bayesian approaches to ensure the measures can be trusted to make the decision are described in Chapter 20 on validation of analytical procedures and regulated by International Conference on Harmonization (2005). Among the procedures usually performed for the tablets, there is the evaluation of the speed or profile of dissolution since a dissolution that is too rapid or too slow may affect the global exposure to the drug and therefore its efficacy and safety profile. Changes in the dissolution profile depend by nature on the manufacturing process itself and not the active ingredient. The methodologies to demonstrate that the dissolution profiles are comparable is addressed in Chapters 19, 22 and 24. An additional mandatory evaluation is the so-called content uniformity test whose purpose is to give assurance that individual units (e.g. a tablet) within each batch are also within specification limits defined by the TPP. This issue is addressed in Chapters 20 and 22.

Finally, it is not only required that the drug product should be within the specifications at the time of the release of the material, usually right after manufacturing, but the producer has also to ensure that each batch of the product will also remain within the same specifications during the whole period the product is on the market, meaning up to the end of the shelf-life or expiry date. The evaluation of the shelf-life of a product and the computation of the expiry date, as well as the strategies to ensure each batch of product will remain within the specifications are covered in Chapter 21 on design and analysis of stability data. Having such a shelf-life defined requires long term stability studies, usually up to two or three years, to be conducted on the final drug product before the product is approved (ICH, 2003a,b; Yang and Zhang, 2012). Once again, this type of long-term studies has to be carefully planned well in advance to avoid costly delays in the authorization for marketing.

After approval and commercialisation, if a major change in the manufacturing process is made, more or less extensive qualification and control studies are needed to ensure the "test" drug product is still comparable with the original "reference" approved manufactured drug product. This so-called comparability study is required for the drug product to be authorized again. The comparability study can be more or less extensive and complicated depending upon whether the drug is a synthetic compound or a biological product such as a vaccine or a monoclonal antibody. There are usually many more QAs required to characterize a biological drug product than are needed for a synthetic drug product.

When a drug product is out of patent, then other companies can attempt to manufacture a generic or copy of the original drug product. When the reference product is a synthetic drug then there are ways to ensure that the test active ingredient is the same as the reference active ingredient. In that case, then a rather limited number of evaluations are required on the drug product and its manufacturing process to ensure it will provide an equivalent efficacy and safety. In that case, dissolution tests and pharmacokinetic studies are key for success to avoid having to conduct full clinical trials. These are known as the bioequivalent studies.

However, if the drug product is a biological product, as opposed to a chemical entity, then there is no unambiguous way to ensure the test product is of the same nature as the reference biological product. A rather extensive list of QAs, usually more than fifty, have to be measured with low uncertainty to compare the new test drug product to the reference product. This investigation is also known as the analytical biosimilarity assessment (U.S. Food and Drug Administration, 2019; European Medicine Agency, 2017). The comparability and the analytical biosimilarity will be developed in Sections 18.3 and 18.4 from a Bayesian perspective.

18.2 What is the question in manufacturing?

From a statistical and decision-making perspective, the very question that should be addressed in manufacturing is fundamentally different from the central question in clinical research as commonly accepted today. In clinical research the aim is to obtain estimates or posterior distributions of the parameter(s) in relation to the efficacy or the safety, to make a decision about the drug product itself. In manufacturing, the focus is on the predictive probability that each individual future batch, unit, stability result or measurement will fall within the specifications or acceptance limits given the past information and data available. Estimating the mean and variance of a manufacturing process is of limited interest while it is the question in clinical research to estimate the efficacy (safety) of a new treatment strategy. When the qualification of a manufacturing process is envisaged, it is important to realise that a patient will never receive a "manufacturing process" as it is, but will rather receive one or several units (e.g. tablets) from one or fewer of the future batches that will be produced. Therefore, from a patient perspective, that also should be the regulatory perspective, it is the (predictive) probability of each unit to be within the specifications that matters. This ability to produce within the specifications is also known generically as the capability of a process. This could become a rather tricky problem to address if the stockpiling of uncertainties is considered: manufacturing process variability, unit-to-unit variability within each batch and uncertainty of the many measurements of each unit in various conditions over time. The objective is multivariate by nature.

The Bayesian frame and in particular the joint posterior predictive distribution precisely addresses this question about future individual values (batches, units, dissolution, stability, measurements) given past data and information. The focus on the future individual values instead of the parameters of the model is the fundamental difference between manufacturing and clinical development and qualification.

This gives some insights about the very nature of Bayesian statistics in manufacturing. The particular question of process comparability and the analytical similarity studies will be developed in the next sections as examples of applications of Bayesian thinking to manufacturing.

18.3 Bayesian statistics for comparability and analytical similarity

18.3.1 Small molecule versus biological

Biological drug products are defined by the process while for a small molecule can be identified by its structure in an unambiguous way, ensuring the mechanism of action (MOA) will be the same. Biological drug products should be characterized by a large number of quality attributes (QA) and therefore the future capability in several dimensions of the new process, not only the central locations, should be integrated as part of the assessment. For generic small molecules the problem reduces in assessing that the new process is capable of making the drug product based on a more limited number of QA, a critical one being the dissolution and therefore the efficacy. In a comparability study, for biological drug products or small molecules, it is the process and in particular its capability that should be evaluated; i.e. the risk of producing batches outside defendable limits is key in the evaluation. It is not the new drug product per se that is evaluated since that is not really relevant.

18.3.2 Defining acceptance limits and specifications

The capability of a new process requires having specifications or acceptance limits, existing or to be defined. For comparisons pre-post change (comparability study) the previous specifications or the previous control limits could be used for evaluating the current and future capability of the new process. For biosimilar products, there are no pre-defined specifications or control limits and these have to be built and defended using a limited amount of material. The difference with generic small molecules is that the specifications are often predefined (pharmacopeia) or imposed by various regulations and therefore agreed (e.g. $f_2 > 50$ in dissolution, see chapter 23).

The proposed objective is to evaluate the patient's risk, therefore the limits to be used or defended should apply to the individual batches and not depend on the parameters to be estimated such as the mean or the variance. Those parameters are nevertheless key, but intermediate, to compute the patient's risk in the future. Indeed, a patient will never receive a mean batch and even less a variance of a process.

18.3.3 Manufacture limits or clinically justified limits

In the comparison pre/post change, it is clearly the manufacture limits (specifications, control limits) that should be used. Those limits are intrinsically proven as clinically defendable. The drug product is already marketed and was approved originally based on this manufacturing process. For biosimilar drug products, the new acceptance limits should be clinically justified while having no history in clinic on patients. The strategy is then to assay a more or less extended number of independent batches of reference product on the market. Those reference batches considered as clinically acceptable since they are on the market and within the original specifications of the drug product. The key question is then how to derive clinically relevant fixed limits based on a reduced number of batches of reference products, i.e. with uncertainty, to ensure that the patient risk is controlled.

18.3.4 Acceptance limits for individual batches

For analytical biosimilarity as well in comparability studies for biological drug product, the acceptance limits should be defined for the individual batches and not on the parameters (mean, variance) as in bioequivalence studies. Assessing the identity of the product and the capability of the process is by practice split into two separate steps for small molecules. This is the current practice that remains nevertheless questionable today. This reasoning does not apply for biologicals, since as mentioned above, it is the process itself that defines the drug product.

The proposal is to use the posterior predictive interval to define acceptance limits based on results obtain with reference drug product. This approach is more statistically sound than using min-max or using the mean ± a multiple of the SD, as proposed by the U.S. Food and Drug Administration (2019). Of course, there is a minimal number of samples needed to compute a prediction interval that is not too wide and remains clinically relevant.

18.3.5 Future batches and patient risk

Having acceptance limits being defined, computed or pre-existing, the key question is the statistical way to make an inference and a decision about the test drug product. It is the future capability of the test process that should be evaluated, therefore the posterior predictive distribution should then be considered and the predictive probability to be within the acceptance limits. The predictive distribution allows us to evaluate the future capability of the test process. If the predictive probability or capability is greater than a minimal probability or quality criterion, then the test process is declared comparable or analytically biosimilar for the QA considered. Note that the predictive distribution includes or propagates by definition the uncertainty about the performance parameters estimates (mean, variance) in other words the uncertainty about the capability of the process.

18.4 Bayesian approach to comparability and biosimilarity

18.4.1 Defining acceptance limits

In the case of a pre-post change comparison, or comparability study, the acceptance limits $[L_r, U_r]$ for the reference are already available, determined and part of the approval. These should then not be evaluated and defended.

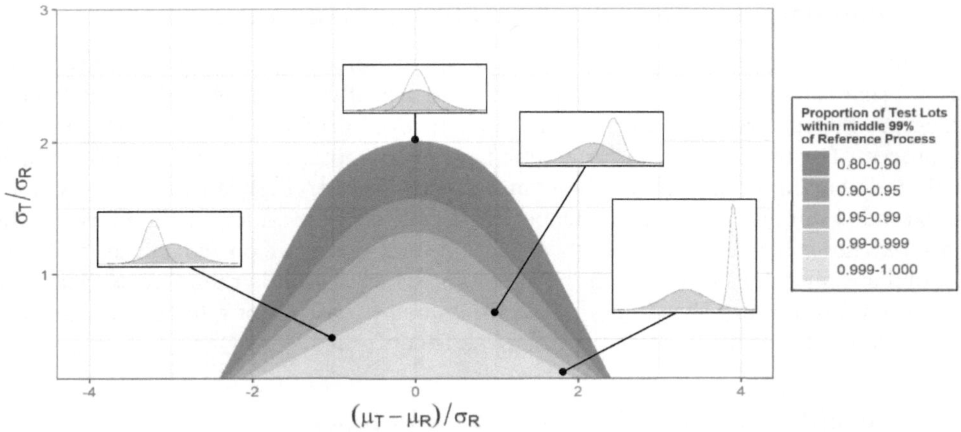

FIGURE 18.1: True region of acceptance of biosimilar test processes as a function of the proportion of test batches within the 99% prediction interval of the reference.

When it is a biosimilar product then the limits have to be evaluated. Suppose we have a reference process with distribution $\mathrm{N}(\mu_r, \sigma_r^2)$ and $x_r = (x_{r1}, \ldots, x_{rn})^T$ being a sample from reference drug product. The posterior predictive distribution with unknown mean and variance is given by:

$$p\left(\tilde{x}_r \mid \boldsymbol{x}_r\right) = \int\int p\left(\tilde{x}_r \mid \mu_r, \sigma_r^2\right) p(\mu_r, \sigma_r^2 \mid \boldsymbol{x}_r) d\mu_r d\sigma_r^2. \tag{18.1}$$

The acceptance limits $[L_r, U_r]$ are computed as the two-sided $\beta\%$ quantiles or the $\beta\%$ HPD interval of the reference predictive distribution. Using $\beta = 99$ is a common practice and recommendation. In the case of a biosimilar product requiring that the acceptance limits being evaluated based on samples from the reference, the true region of acceptance for the test process is shown in Figure 18.1.

A good decision rule about biosimilarity would mostly accept the test process if inside the 0.99–1.0 region and reject it if outside 0.8 region.

For example assume that 10 independent reference batches have been determined for specific QAs:

$$\boldsymbol{x}_r = (100.7, 100.6, 100.6, 101.9, 101.4, 100.7, 100.3, 99.9, 100.4, 101.1)^T.$$

The acceptance limits are defined as the 95% quantile range: $[L_r, U_r] = [99.94, 101.58]$. Note that if non-informative prior distributions are considered, as is usually the case, this turns out to be a t distribution given by:

$$p\left(\tilde{x}_r \mid \boldsymbol{x}_r\right) = t_{n-1}\left(\bar{x}_r, s^2\left(1 + \frac{1}{n}\right)\right).$$

Therefore the $\beta\%$ quantiles interval of this distribution is numerically equal to the β-expectation tolerance interval as defined by Mee (1984), but with different interpretation (Hamada, 2004). For the data of the reference batches we have $p\left(\tilde{x}_r \mid \boldsymbol{x}_r\right) \sim t_9\left(100.72, 0.82\right)$.

The predictive distribution can be generalized for given specific prior distributions, e.g. $\mu|\sigma^2 \sim N(\mu_0, \sigma^2/\kappa_0)$, $\sigma^2 \sim Inv - \chi^2(\nu_0, \sigma_0^2)$, the resulting posterior predictive distribution is a t-distribution $t_{\bar{\nu}}\left(\bar{x}, s^2\left(1+\frac{1}{\kappa_0+n}\right)\right)$, where $\bar{\nu} = \nu_0 + n$, κ_0 and ν_0 are 'prior sample size' which influences the informativeness of the prior distributions for the mean and variance, respectively (Lesaffre and Lawson (2012); Gelman, Carlin, Stern and Rubin (2003)). In the case of informative prior, there is no more numerical equivalence with the β-expectation tolerance interval and the Bayesian posterior predictive distribution has to be considered.

18.4.2 Assessing comparability and analytical similarity

Suppose we have a test process with distribution $N(\mu_t, \sigma_t^2)$ and $\boldsymbol{x}_t = (x_{t1}, \ldots, x_{tn})^T$ is a sample from test drug product. The posterior predictive distribution is derived as in Equation (18.1). The biosimilarity assessment proceeds by integrating the predictive over the acceptance range, i.e.:

$$\Pr(\text{Biosimilarity} \mid \text{Data}) = \int_{L_r}^{U_r} p\left(\tilde{x}_t \mid \boldsymbol{x}_t\right).$$

If non-informative priors are considered, then the probability of being biosimilar can equivalently be computed as follows:

$$\Pr\left(\text{Biosimilarity} \mid \text{Data}\right) = \Pr\left(L_r \leq t_{n-1}\left(\bar{x}_t, s_t^2\left(1+\frac{1}{n}\right)\right) \leq U_r\right).$$

Biosimilarity is concluded if $\Pr\left(\text{Biosimilarity} \mid \text{Data}\right) \geq \pi$, the required quality level, usually 0.9.

Assume samples of observations from the biosimilar test product:

$$\boldsymbol{x}_t = (99.6, 99.6, 100.4, 102.1, 101.2, 100.9, 100.7, 101.3, 101.6, 99.8)^T.$$

Then, $\Pr\left(\text{Biosimilarity} \mid \text{Data}\right) = 0.97 > 0.9$ and therefore the new test product is declared as biosimilar for this quality attribute.

Figure 18.2 illustrates the Biosimilarity assessment using the predictive probability of the test product being within the 99% prediction interval of the reference product.

18.4.3 Operating characteristics

As shown in Figure 18.1, the region of biosimilar test processes is represented by the rounded triangle and a perfect decision rule should overlap the regions. In Figure 18.3, represented are the regions of acceptance as a function of the predictive probability ranging from 0.05 to 0.99 and for various sample size of the test product: 5, 10 or 15. Similar number of batches have been considered for the reference.

As can be seen on Figure 18.3, there is very little chance to accept biosimilarity outside the true region of biosimilarity and therefore the decision rule proposed is achieving its objective.

18.5 Conclusions

Most of the decision-making process in manufacturing of biopharmaceutical products is based on the future individual batches, units or measurements given the data observed in

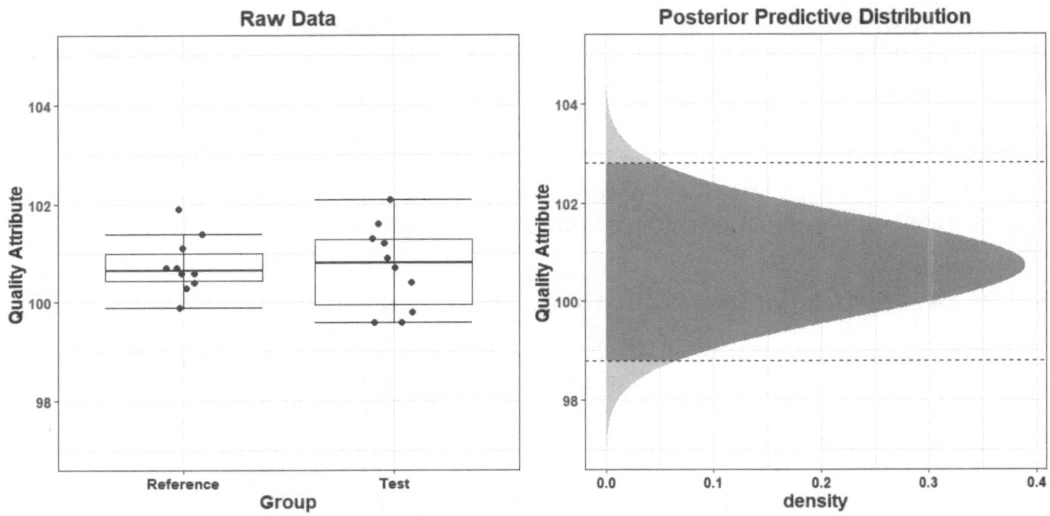

FIGURE 18.2: Illustration of Biosimilarity assessment data observed and the posterior predictive distribution.

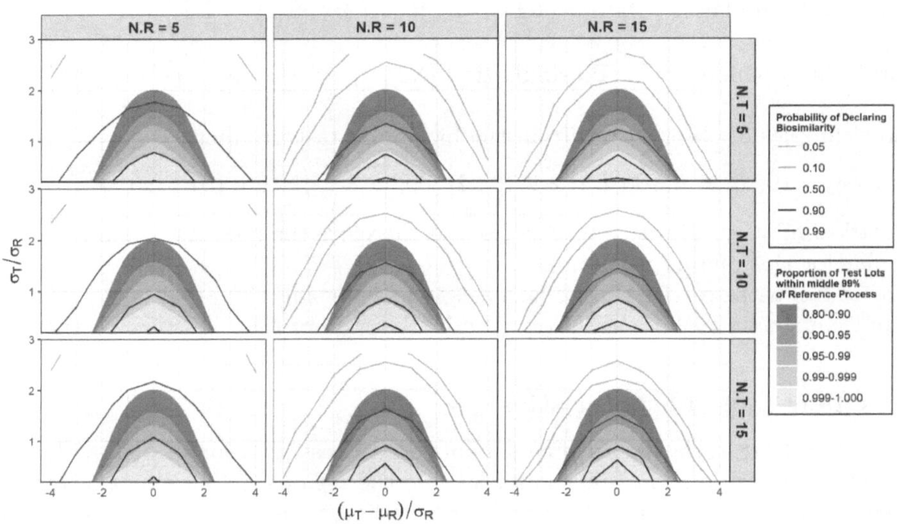

FIGURE 18.3: Operating Characteristics of Biosimilarity decision based assuming 5, 10 or 15 batches for both reference and test batches as a function of the probability to declare biosimilarity.

recent studies. At large most are capability-related questions and therefore the posterior predictive distribution is the appropriate Bayesian approach that should be considered either to compute a predictive probability or an interval. This is the main difference with other areas such as clinical development whose focus is on the parameters. Also, since most of the questions to be addressed in manufacturing are of the "equivalence" or "comparable" type, then using acceptance limits based on individual values (batches, units, ...) is easier to justify and obtain. In addition, dealing with the posterior predictive distribution, it is straightforward to compute the predictive probability to be within some specifications or acceptance limits instead of working with the cumbersome interval hypothesis testing as applied for bioequivalence and whose region of acceptance is a matter of debate.

Bibliography

Burdick, R. K., LeBlond, D. J., Pfahler, L. B., Quiroz, J., Sidor, L., Vukovinsky, K., and Zhang, L. (2017). *Statistical Applications for Chemistry, Manufacturing and Controls (CMC) in the Pharmaceutical Industry*. Springer, Cham, Switzerland.

European Medicine Agency (2017). Statistical methodology for the comparative assessment of quality attributes in drug development. Draft reflection paper. `https://tinyurl.com/y2ltzf5v`; accessed March 31, 2020.

Gelman, A., Carlin, J. B., Stern, S.H., and Rubin, B. D. (2004). Bayesian Data Analysis (2nd ed.). Chapman and Hall/CRC.

Hamada, M. E. (2004). Bayesian prediction intervals and their relationship to tolerance intervals. *Technometrics*, 46:425–459.

ICH (2003a). ICH Harmonised tripartite guidelines. Evaluation for Stability data, Q1E. `https://tinyurl.com/y68pnxed`; accessed March 31, 2020.

ICH (2003b). ICH Harmonised tripartite guidelines. Stability testing of new drug substances and products Q1A(R2). `https://tinyurl.com/y4jk554x`; accessed March 31, 2020.

International Conference on Harmonization (2005). Validation of Analytical Procedures: Text and Methodology Q2(R1).

International Conference on Harmonization (2009). Pharmaceutical Development Q8(R2).

Lesaffre, E. and Lawson, A. B. (2012). Bayesian Biostatistics. John Wiley & Sons. New York. ISBN: 978-0-470-01823-1.

Mee, R. W. (1984). β-expectation and β-content tolerance limits for balanced one-way anova random model. *Technometrics*, 26(3):251–254.

Peterson, J. (2010). What your ICH Q8 design space needs: A multivariate predictive distribution. *Pharma Manufacturing.com*, 8(10):23–28.

Peterson, J. and Altan, S. (2016). Overview of drug development and statistical tools for manufacturing and testing. In Check, N. T., editor, *Nonclinical Statistics for Pharmaceutical and Biotechnology Industries*. Springer, New York, NY.

U.S. Food and Drug Administration (2011). Guidance for Industry Process Validation: General Principles and Practices. U.S. Department of Health and Human Services, FDA. Center of Drug Evaluation and Research (CDER): Rockville, Maryland. `https://www.fda.gov/downloads/drugs/guidances/ucm070336.pdf`; accessed March 31, 2020.

U.S. Food and Drug Administration (2019). Development of Therapeutic Protein Biosimilars: Comparative Analytical Assessment and Other Quality-Related Considerations. Guidance for Industry. U.S. Department of Health and Human Services, FDA. Center of Drug Evaluation and Research (CDER): Rockville, Maryland. `https://www.fda.gov/media/125484/download`; accessed March 31, 2020.

Yang, H. and Zhang, L. (2012). Evaluation of statistical methods for estimating shelf-life of drug products: A unified and risks-based approach. *Journal of Validation Technology*, pages 67–74.

19

Process Development and Validation

John J. Peterson

GlaxoSmithKline Pharmaceuticals, US

Bayesian statistical methodology has two useful characteristics. It can make use of prior information, and most statisticians know this. Perhaps just as important though is that the Bayesian approach is very flexible for modeling complex (manufacturing or assay) processes or complex quantifications of such a process. In the act of such modeling, the Bayesian method also accounts for the uncertainties of the unknown model parameters. In addition, since posterior probabilities of events of interest can typically be quantified in a straightforward manner, Bayesian methods are also very useful and natural for risk quantification, an important aspect of quality-by-design. This chapter will review two important aspects of process development and validation. One development aspect to be reviewed is that of "design space" as defined in the International Conference on Harmonization Q8 regulatory guidance. The other aspect to be assessed (during late development or early validation), is the assessment of measurement system or assay robustness. An assay is robust if it is insensitive to small deviations in its basic operating factors. This chapter will also show that realistic, natural quality criteria may exist in complex quantitative forms. The flexibility of the Bayesian approach nonetheless adapts in a straightforward manner to these complexities.

19.1 Introduction

Bayesian statistical methodology has two useful characteristics. It can make use of prior information, and most statisticians know this. Perhaps just as important though is that the Bayesian approach is very flexible for modeling complex (manufacturing or assay) processes or complex quantifications of a such a process. In the act of such modeling, the Bayesian method also accounts for the uncertainties of the unknown model parameters. In addition, since posterior probabilities of events of interest can typically be quantified in a straightforward manner, Bayesian methods are also very useful and natural for risk quantification, an important aspect of *quality-by-design* (QbD) (Rathore, 2009).

This chapter will review two important aspects of *process development and validation.* One development aspect to be reviewed is that of *design space* as defined in the International Conference on Harmonization (ICH) Q8 regulatory guidance (ICH, 2009). The other aspect to be assessed (during late development or early validation), is the assessment of measurement system or assay robustness. An *assay is robust* if it is insensitive to small deviations in its basic operating factors (typically mechanical or chemical factors, such as flow of the mobile phase or pH of the buffer).

The issues of process development and process validation come under the broader pharmaceutical development and manufacturing regulatory area known as *chemistry and manufacturing control (CMC)*. The CMC area has three basic parts to its lifecycle: (i) process design, (ii) process qualification, and (iii) process monitoring and continuous process verification. All three stages of the *CMC lifecycle approach* are discussed in detail in Burdick et al. (2017). Further reviews of CMC statistics can also be found in Peterson et al. (2009b) and Peterson and Altan (2016). Yang (2017) and Coffey and Yang (2018) review CMC statistics from the biopharmaceutical perspective. For the sake of space and simplicity of exposition, this chapter will only focus on the CMC topics of design space and assay robustness. However, these two areas are very useful for illustrating the advantages of the Bayesian approach to pharmaceutical process and assay development and validation.

QbD (Juran, 1992) has been espoused by the U.S. Food and Drug Administration as a recommended approach to pharmaceutical manufacturing (Moore, 2012). QbD espouses that quality should be designed into a product from the beginning, and that increased testing does not necessarily improve product quality (Yu et al., 2014).

It is possible to incorporate the Bayesian approach into the QbD paradigm in a straightforward, two-step way. The first step is to quantitatively define a quality criterion for the manufacturing process at hand. For example, for tablet dissolution, it could involve meeting lower and upper specification limits, over various time points, on the percent dissolved (Novick et al., 2015). After a quality criterion is agreed to, then using the Bayesian approach one can compute, following suitable data acquisition, the posterior probability of the quality criterion being met. Due to the flexibility of the Bayesian approach it is often easier to make statistical inferences about a natural pharmaceutical quality criterion than using a frequentist approach. This basic concept is illustrated in the following sections on ICH Q8 Design Space (19.2) and Assay Robustness (19.3).

19.2 ICH Q8 design space

The ICH Q8 guidance document on pharmaceutical development proposes the notion of a design space. ICH Q8 formally defines a design space as "The multidimensional combination and interaction of input variables (e.g. material attributes) and process parameters that have been demonstrated to provide assurance of quality." (ICH, 2009). A design space would be typically associated with some part of the manufacturing process. The ICH Q8 guidance states that pharmaceutical manufacturers can change manufacturing conditions (without formal regulatory approval) as long as those operating conditions are within an approved design space. The design space construction problem is challenging in that most pharmaceutical processes have several quality characteristics that must be simultaneously met. Therefore the demonstration to provide assurance of quality, as required by the design space definition, typically requires a multivariate risk quantification.

19.2.1 Design space development using classical frequentist methods

As also noticed by Dispas et al. (2018), many papers on ICH Q8 design space development have relied upon classical *response surface methodology*, see for example: am Ende et al. (2007); Kamm (2007); Harms et al. (2008) and LePore and Spavins (2008). The thinking here is that a well-modeled (mean) response surface can be used to calibrate a design space, i.e. determine the limits, or combinations, of process parameters that have been demonstrated to provide assurance of quality. This thinking is flawed from a risk, i.e. *assurance of quality*, perspective because classical response surface methodology focuses mostly on the mean response surface, which does not do a good job of risk quantification (e.g. assessment of the joint probability of meeting process specifications). This is particularly true for response surface methodology involving multiple response variables or *Critical Quality Attributes (CQA's)*. Section 19.2.2 will show how the Bayesian approach to design space can establish a straightforward solution to this problem.

The classical frequentist approach to design space construction, involving multiple quality characteristics, often employs the *overlapping means approach* to multiple response surface optimization (Lind et al., 1960). While this approach is easy to understand, and can be simple to execute using certain point-and-click statistical packages (such as JMP® or Design Expert®), it can produce a design space that is far too large, possibly harboring process operating conditions that have high probability of failure (Peterson and Lief, 2010).

The overlapping means approach to design space plots the overlapping mean response surfaces and shades in those points where the predicted process mean responses simultaneously meet their respective specification limits. To statistically define an overlapping means design space, proceed as follows. Let $\boldsymbol{Y}$ be a vector of future quality response variables (e.g. tablet disintegration time, tablet friability, tablet hardness, etc.) and let $\boldsymbol{x}$ be a vector of process operating factors (e.g. compression force, water quantity, proportion of excipient A, etc.). Furthermore, let S denote a multidimensional specification region for the pharmaceutical manufacturing process for which the design space will be created. Typically, the set S will have the form: $[LSL_1, USL_1] \times [LSL_2, USL_2] \times \ldots \times [LSL_r, USL_r]$, for r different response variables. Here, the acronym LSL represents the lower specification limit, while USL represents the upper specification limit. The overlapping means approach to design space is defined by $DS_{OLM} = \{\boldsymbol{x} : \widehat{\boldsymbol{Y}}(\boldsymbol{x}) \in \mathcal{S}\}$, where $\widehat{\boldsymbol{Y}}(\boldsymbol{x}) = \left(\widehat{Y}_1(\boldsymbol{x}), \ldots, \widehat{Y}_r(\boldsymbol{x})\right)^\top$ is the predicted vector of (mean) process responses. Actual examples of such specification intervals can be found in Sections 19.2.2 and 19.3.2.

Peterson and Lief (2010) employ six different real examples to show that the overlapping means approach to design space produced regions that had process conditions with poor assurance for jointly meeting quality specifications in the future, between 11 and 34 percent! As it turns out, it is possible for a multivariate distribution, even a symmetric one, to have all of its means within the respective process specification limits, but only a small proportion of the distribution within the specification region. This risk increases with the number of quality attributes (Peterson and Lief, 2010). A pharmaceutical process capable of producing good quality product should meet all of its manufacturing specification limits in a reliable fashion. This is why the ICH Q8 design space definition contains the phrase, "...process parameters that have been demonstrated to provide assurance of quality."

In situations where there is only one quality response variable, the classical frequentist approach can be modified to better address the ICH Q8 design space definition relating to assurance of quality. With only one response variable, one can place prediction limits around the response surface, and use such limits to calibrate a design space that will provide assurance of quality for a future response. For example, using the response surface and associated 95% prediction intervals one could determine the set of operating conditions such that (for a given point in the design space) a future response will be expected to be within the specification limits at least 95% of the time. This is done by selecting only those points for the design space that are associated with 95% prediction intervals that are within the specification limits. Clearly, such a frequentist prediction approach is more difficult for a process with multiple responses.

19.2.2 Bayesian approach to design space

A Bayesian approach to the design space problem has been put forth by Peterson (2008). Since one can quantify assurance with a probability measure (see e.g. also in Chapter 1), a Bayesian approach to design space construction can be naturally expressed as:

$$\{\boldsymbol{x} : \Pr(\boldsymbol{Y} \in \mathcal{S} \mid \boldsymbol{x}, \text{data}) \geq R\}, \tag{19.1}$$

where R is a pre-specified reliability level, $\boldsymbol{Y}$ is a vector of future CQA's, and $\boldsymbol{x}$ is a vector of specific manufacturing operating conditions. Here, $\mathcal{S}$ is a specification region and data refers to the data from the experimental design used to develop the design space in (19.1). The probability expression in (19.1) is based upon the posterior predictive distribution for a (univariate or multivariate) response surface model. Curiously, the ICH Q8 guidance document is silent on how much assurance of quality a pharmaceutical process should have, i.e. R.

Peterson and Lief (2010) show a real-life example where the overlapping means approach to design space is compared to the Bayesian approach in (19.1). The example involves an experiment to formulate a pharmaceutical tablet. Here, six factors were studied with regard to their influence on three tablet critical quality responses (or attributes), namely: dissolution time, friability (i.e. tendency to break or crumble), and hardness. The six process factors studied were: quantity of water, rate of water addition, wet massing time, main compression force, main compression/precompression ratio, and speed. The three quality responses (and their specifications) were: y_1 = tablet disintegration time (at most 15 min.) , y_2 = friability (at most 0.8%), and y_3 = hardness (8 to 14kp). Three granulation factors were studied: x_1 = quantity of water added, x_2 = rate of water addition, x_3 = wet massing time, while the three compression factors utilized were: x_4 = main compression force, x_5 = main compression/precompresion ratio, and x_6 = speed.

Figure 19.1 shows both the overlapping means design space in gray and the Bayesian design space (with reliability equal to 0.8) as a black oval. The speed factor had no apparent effect and was not included in the final model, while the main compression/precompression ratio had only a small effect. This factor was fixed at its center point for purposes of displaying the design space in Figure 19.1.

The set described in (19.1) can be high dimensional and not of a regular shape (e.g. a hyper-rectangle). As such, some design spaces may be difficult to view graphically. For dimensions of four or less, panel-type (i.e. lattice) plots can be used. For higher dimensional design spaces, Peterson (2008) recommended use of read-only, sortable spreadsheets (containing the design space) as a way to move around within a design space in an intelligent fashion.

It is also useful to note that applying the Bayesian approaches of Peterson (2004) and Peterson et al. (2009a) to design space development does allow one to forecast the effects of additional data on expanding the design space by reducing model parameter uncertainty. For the Bayesian approach to design space, as in Peterson (2008), the design space depends directly upon the posterior predictive distribution of the CQA's. As it turns out, for the classical multivariate regression model (Timm, 2002, pages 186–192) or the seemingly unrelated regressions model (Timm, 2002, pages 311–318), the posterior predictive distribution depends upon the design matrix and a number of degrees of freedom related to the number of observations (Peterson, 2004; Peterson et al., 2009a). Furthermore, if one assumes that the regression model parameter and covariance matrix estimates will be similar with future data augmentation, one can then forecast the effects of reduction of variation in the posterior predictive distribution that one would obtain by adding additional observations at specified operating conditions. This reduction in variation induces a forecasted increase

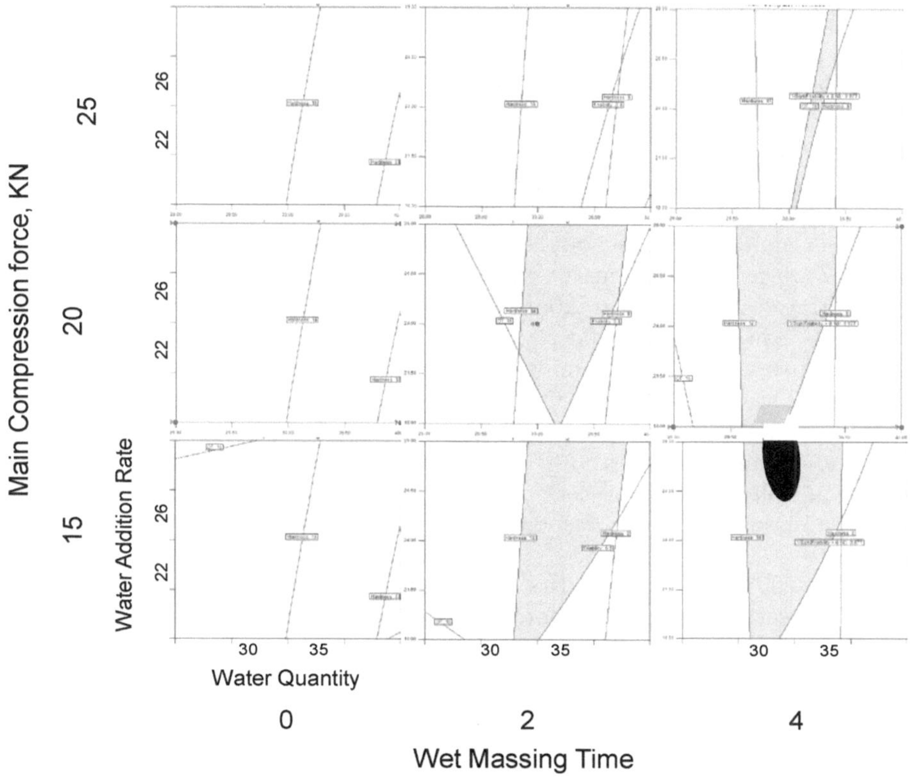

FIGURE 19.1: Overlapping means design space and Bayesian design space. The gray regions represent the OMR DS. The black region represents the Bayesian posterior predictive DS with reliability value R=0.8.

in the design space that one can compute. This approach should certainly be considered if the design space is small and based upon a small amount of data.

The design space also needs to consider the issue of scale-up with regard to a process that has been optimized at laboratory or pilot-plant scale. Unfortunately, it may be too costly to execute a full response surface design at the manufacturing scale. Maeda et al. (2012) consider the use of Bayesian methodology along with a *scale-up strategy* to develop a design space for manufacturing scale. They employ the *scale-up model*:

$$\boldsymbol{Y}_{FS} = \boldsymbol{a} + \boldsymbol{b} \times \boldsymbol{f}_{SS}(\boldsymbol{x}; \boldsymbol{\beta}) + \varepsilon, \tag{19.2}$$

where $\boldsymbol{Y}_{FS}$ is the vector of process responses at full scale (manufacturing), $f_{SS}(\boldsymbol{x}; \boldsymbol{\beta})$ is the (vector-valued) response surface function at small scale, and ε is a residual error vector. Here, $\boldsymbol{a}$ is an additive scale change vector and $\boldsymbol{b}$ is a multiplicative scale change vector — the multiplicative operator in (19.2) is elementwise. The response surface function f_{SS} is assumed known, except for the unknown model parameter vector, $\boldsymbol{\beta}$. This assumption implies that the underlying response surface at the full scale has basically the same shape as that of the underlying response surface at small scale. Fortunately, the model in (19.2) does not require a lot of data at the manufacturing level. This is because only two parameters (per CQA), $\boldsymbol{a}$ and $\boldsymbol{b}$, need to be estimated by manufacturing plant data. The example in Maeda et al. (2012) only uses five data points at the manufacturing level. Some further publications making use of the Bayesian approach to design space are: Stockdale and Cheng (2009); Kriera et al. (2011); Lebrun et al. (2012); Hubert et al. (2014); Bano et al. (2018); Dispas et al. (2018) and Gonzalez et al. (2019).

It is also useful to note that the posterior predictive probability in (19.1), when considered as a function of $\boldsymbol{x}$, as in $p(\boldsymbol{x}) = \Pr(\boldsymbol{Y} \in \mathcal{S} \mid \boldsymbol{x}, \text{data})$, can be used as a type of desirability function for process optimization (Peterson, 2004). Miro-Quesada et al. (2004) have shown that minor modifications to the process optimization approach of Peterson (2004) can be done to perform multiple-response process optimization in the presence of noise variables. Noise variables are process parameters which have a certain degree of random variation at the manufacturing scale, but not at laboratory scale. Therefore, such process parameters are measured and used in experimental designs at the laboratory scale, but QbD risk is assessed at the manufacturing scale by assuming the noise variables will propagate their influence randomly there. The results of Miro-Quesada et al. (2004) allow one to generalize the approach in (19.1) to create a Bayesian design space for a process that contains noise variables. (See the second example in Peterson (2008) for details.) In fact, the Bayesian probabilistic approach to multiple response process optimization discussed in this paragraph has been mentioned as a major advance in response surface techniques (Colosimo and Del Castillo, 2007, Preface).

Del Castillo (2007, Chapter 12) lists several advantages of the Bayesian predictive approach over the overlapping means approach for process optimization (and by implication design space):

(i) It considers the uncertainty of all of the unknown model parameters;

(ii) It allows, of course, for the incorporation of prior information;

(iii) It considers correlation among multiple responses;

(iv) It provides a quantitative measure of uncertainty (i.e. probability) for a process operation condition or a minimum probability for a (sweet spot) operating region;

(v) It allows for a pre-posterior analysis to determine if further experimentation is needed.

Further details can be found in Peterson (2004); Peterson et al. (2009a) and Del Castillo (2007, Chapter 12).

19.3 Assay robustness

A pharmaceutical assay is considered *robust* if it is insensitive to small deviations from its operation set point. Robustness provides an indication of the ability of the assay to perform under typical usage. Robustness measures the effect of deliberate changes in assay factors (e.g. incubation time, temperature, sample preparation, buffer pH) that can be controlled according to the assay protocol. An assessment of assay robustness is typically an expected part of an assay validation that needs to be done to satisfy regulatory requirements; see for example the ICH Q2 regulatory guidance on validation of analytical procedures (ICH, 2005). ICH Q2 states: "The evaluation of robustness should be considered during the development phase and depends on the type of procedure under study. It should show the reliability of an analysis with respect to deliberate variations in method parameters." A key word in the preceding sentence is reliability. Analogous to ICH Q8 design space, if an assay has multiple quality responses that must be assessed, then a Bayesian approach allows for a more natural and straightforward solution than a classical frequentist testing or interval approach.

19.3.1 Classical approach to assay robustness

The classical frequentist approach to assessment of assay robustness is described in Vander Heyden et al. (2001). The basic strategy is to run a screening experimental design such as a *Plackett-Burman* (Plackett and Burman, 1946) or *fractional factorial design* (Del Castillo, 2007) using assay operational factors described in the assay protocol. The factor level extremes used in the design are typically relatively small and based upon variation that could occur in practice. One then executes the analysis of variance(s) using the data from the experimental design. Often, there will be more than one response variable needed to properly ascertain assay robustness. For example, Vander Heyden et al. (2001) show an example where there are six assay response variables used to assess robustness, which are the active substance amount, along with two related compounds in the tablets and three chromatographic responses.

If any effects from the analysis of variance on any of the response variables are statistically significant, then some doubt is cast upon the robustness of the assay. However, it may be the case that (e.g. due to small assay variation) a statistically significant effect is small enough to be not practically significant. From a frequentist's perspective, it appears that some experimenters do not worry about the issue of multiplicity or P-value adjustment. Formal assessment of the Type II error rate or the computation of power for hypothesis tests also do not appear to be part of the typical approach to classical frequentist assessment of assay robustness.

19.3.2 Bayesian approach to assay robustness

Peterson and Yahyah (2009) proposed a Bayesian predictive method for assessing assay robustness based upon the notion of a Bayesian design space in (19.1). In robustness testing, only small deviations from the operating set point are assessed. These small deviations map out a *robustness region* (typically a hyper-rectangle). See below for an example. As such, it is often assumed that a linear (or a simple second-order model, e.g. only some pairwise interactions) would provide an adequate approximation of a response surface about the robustness region. For such a model, one could easily apply the Bayesian design space concept in (19.1) to assess robustness.

Suppose that one has used a Plackett-Burman or a fractional factorial design with which to conduct the robustness experiment. Using the resulting prediction models (over the small robustness region) as a response surface model, one could compute the design space as in (19.1) and compare this to the a priori determined robustness region. If the robustness region is a subset of the robustness design space, for a pre-specified reliability level R, then the assay (or process) can be considered rugged, with a reliability of at least R. (Note that even though these designs are typically used for factor screening, in robustness assessment they may be practically employed as response surface designs due to the fact that only small deviations from the target conditions are used in the design.)

Peterson and Yahyah (2009) show that the standard frequentist approach outlined in Vander Heyden et al. (2001) has serious flaws due to the fact that it bases predictions on means of various response types (e.g. percent recovery, resolution, tailing, etc.) rather than the joint predictive distributions for those response types.

Vander Heyden et al. (2001) discuss a robustness study of a High-Performance Analytical method and assay Liquid Chromatographic (HPLC) assay for the identification of an active substance (main compound or MC), the detection of two related compounds (RC1 and RC2)

TABLE 19.1: Response types and system suitability specifications for the HPLC assay robustness experiment.

Response	Response Description	System Suitability Limits
y_1	Percent recovery for main compound	95%-105%
y_2	Percent recovery for residual compound 1	95%-105%
y_3	Percent recovery for residual compound 2	95%-105%
y_4	Resolution (of the critical peak)	not less than 4.40
y_5	Capacity factor	not less than 2.57
y_6	Tailing factor	not greater than 1.62

in tablets, and three chromatographic variables (resolution of the critical peak, capacity, and tailing). See Table 19.1 for the corresponding quality response specifications.

The factors used in this study (in $\pm$ coded form) were: x_1 = pH (of the buffer), x_2 = column type (one of two types), x_3 = column temperature, x_4 = percent of solvent at the start of the gradient, x_5 = percent of solvent at the end of the gradient, x_6 = flow of the mobile phase, x_7 = wavelength of the detector, and x_8 = buffer concentration. Hence (in coded form) the robustness experimental design region is $[-1, 1]^8$. The quality responses employed relative to system suitability limits are listed in Table 19.1. As per Vander Heyden et al. (2001), first-order linear regression models were fitted for each of the six response types.

This assay was considered robust by Vander Heyden et al. (2001). However, a Bayesian analysis by Peterson and Yahyah (2009), using a non-informative prior, shows that the posterior predictive probability of meeting all specifications (within the robustness testing limits) is only 0.310 for one column type and only 0.813 for the second column type. Thus, over the region of robustness assessment if we desired a reliability of 0.90 or 0.95, then clearly the assay in question is not robust.

Inferences on mean response variables cannot be used to quantify the probability of a future run of the assay to meet all specifications with reliability, R. Because a robustness study may well involve more than one quality response type, something needs to be done to adjust for the multiplicity effect of making inferences on more than one response variable. The (frequentist) approach of Vander Heyden et al. (2001) does not address this multiplicity issue, although it could be addressed with common multiplicity adjustment techniques. The Bayesian approach of Peterson and Yahyah (2009) makes a natural adjustment for multiplicity through the joint posterior probability that these multiple quality responses all meet their specification limits. Of course, marginal probabilities of meeting specification for individual quality responses can be computed as well.

19.4 Challenges for the Bayesian approach

Due to the flexibility of the Bayesian approach it is often easier to make statistical inference about natural pharmaceutical quality criteria than using a frequentist approach. However, for practical reasons, some challenges remain for utilization of the Bayesian approach to pharmaceutical QbD. First, it may be difficult to get all parties (different pharmaceutical companies and different regulatory bodies) to agree on a common quality criterion or statistical method to use. This may even be true despite the existence of a previous (frequentist) statistical approach that has clear flaws relative to documented regulatory requirements.

See for example Stroup and Quinlan (2016, Chapter 22), where they point out serious flaws in established statistical (frequentist) methodology for drug shelf-life determination. Sometimes there is considerable inertia surrounding industry and regulatory agencies to change established quantitative approaches to decision making, almost all of which are frequentist in nature.

Second, the Bayesian approach appears to find support among non-statisticians usually when there is clearly useful prior information readily available. Historical prior information has been used in the medical device area and in clinical or animal studies involving placebo or control information, respectively. But, in pharmaceutical product development and manufacturing, historical prior information appears to be less available, in part due to the variety of different physical and chemical properties among novel compounds. However, the viewpoint of Bayesian inference primarily for the utilization of prior information can be overly restrictive. The flexibility of the Bayesian approach, particularly for complex multivariate models, is well suited for making natural and easy-to-understand quantitative inferences with or without a strong amount of prior information. The Bayesian approaches to ICH Q8 design space and assay robustness are important examples that do not require strong degrees of prior information.

In addition, there are some other, lower-level, issues that slow the utilization of Bayesian statistics in pharmaceutical product development and manufacturing, such as sparsity of point-and-click software, possible fear of acceptance by regulators, or simply lack of Bayesian computational skills among some statistical staff. However, these challenges can be overcome in due time, provided scientists and statisticians place greater value on QbD in pharmaceutical manufacturing and the efficacious role that Bayesian statistical inference can play in achieving that goal. As stated in the Introduction, the Bayesian approach is very flexible for modeling complex pharmaceutical processes. There is evidence that increasing technological sophistication in manufacturing is finding its way into the pharmaceutical industry, and affecting the need for more sophisticated data structures and quantification of quality measures (Peterson et al., 2019). It is hoped that Bayesian approaches to QbD for pharmaceutical manufacturing will find greater utilization to address these changing needs.

Bibliography

am Ende, D., Bronk, K. S., Mustakis, J., O'Connor, G., Santa Maria, C. L., Nosal, R., and Watson, T. J. N. (2007). API quality by design example from the Torcetrapib manufacturing process. *Journal of Pharmaceutical Innovation*, 2:71–86.

Bano, G., Facco, P., Bezzo, F., and Barolo, M. (2018). Probabilistic design space determination in pharmaceutical product development: A Bayesian/latent variable approach. *American Institute of Chemical Engineers Journal*, 64(7):2438–2449.

Burdick, R. K., LeBlond, D. J., Pfahler, L. B., Quiroz, J., Sidor, L., Vukovinsky, K., and Zhang, L. (2017). *Statistical Applications for Chemistry, Manufacturing and Controls (CMC) in the Pharmaceutical Industry.* Springer, Cham, Switzerland.

Coffey, T. and Yang, H. (2018). *Statistics for Biotechnology Process Development.* Chapman & Hall/CRC, Boca Raton, FL.

Colosimo, B. M. and Del Castillo, E. (2007). *Bayesian Process Monitoring, Control, and Optimization.* Chapman & Hall/CRC, Boca Raton, FL.

Del Castillo, E. (2007). *Process Optimization – A Statistical Approach*. Springer, New York, NY.

Dispas, A., T., A. H., Lebrun, P., Hubert, P., and Hubert, C. (2018). Quality by Design approach for the analysis of impurities in pharmaceutical drug products and drug substances. *Trends in Analytical Chemistry*, 101:24–33.

Gonzalez, F. L., Tabora, J. E., Huang, E. C., Wisniewski, S. R., Carrasquillo-Flores, R., Razler, T., and Mack, B. (2019). Development and implementation of a quality control strategy for an atropisomer impurity grounded in a risk-based probabilistic design space. *Organic Process Research and Development*, 23:211–219.

Harms, J., Wang, X., Kim, T., Yang, X., and Rathore, A. S. (2008). Defining product design space for biotech products: Case study of pichia pastoris fermentation. *Organic Process Research and Development*, 24:655–662.

Hubert, C., Lebrun, P., Houari, S., Ziemons, E., Rozet, E., and Hubert, P. (2014). Improvement of a stability-indicating method by quality-by-design versus quality-by-testing: A case of a learning process. *Journal of Pharmaceutical and Biomedical Analysis*, 88:401–409.

ICH (2005). ICH Harmonised Tripartite Guidelines: Validation of Analytical Procedures, Text and Methodology, Q2(R1). `https://tinyurl.com/y2vkh4gv`; accessed March 31, 2020.

ICH (2009). ICH Harmonised Tripartite Guideline: Pharmaceutical Development, Q8(R2). `https://tinyurl.com/yxhc572e`; accessed March 31, 2020.

Juran, J. M. (1992). *Quality by Design — The New Steps for Planning Quality into Goods and Services*. The Free Press, New York, NY.

Kamm, J. (2007). Can you win the space race? *Pharmaceutical Manufacturing*, 6(5). `"http://www.pharmamanufacturing.com/articles/2007/091.html"`.

Kriera, F., Brion, M., Debrus, B., Lebrun, P., Driesen, A., Eric Ziemons, E., Evrard, B., and Hubert, P. (2011). Optimisation and validation of a fast HPLC method for the quantification of sulindac and its related impurities. *Journal of Pharmaceutical and Biomedical Analysis*, 54:694–700.

Lebrun, P., F., K., Mantanus, J., Grohganz, H., Yang, M., Rozet, E., B., B., Evrard, B., J., R., and Hubert, P. (2012). Design space approach in the optimization of the spray-drying process. *European Journal of Pharmaceutics and Biopharmaceutics*, 80:226–234.

LePore, J. and Spavins, J. (2008). PQLI design space. *Journal of Pharmaceutical Innovation*, 3:79–87.

Lind, E. E., Goldin, J., and Hickman, J. B. (1960). Fitting yield and cost to response surfaces. *Chemical Engineering Progress*, 56:62–68.

Maeda, J., Suzuki, T., and Takayama, K. (2012). Novel method for constructing a large-scale design space in lubrication process by using Bayesian estimation based on the reliability of a scale-up rule. *Chemical and Pharmaceutical Bulletin*, 60(9):1155–1163.

Miro-Quesada, G., del Castillo, E., and Peterson, J. (2004). A Bayesian approach for multiple response surface optimization in the presence of noise variables. *Journal of Applied Statistics*, 31:251–270.

Moore, C. M. V. (2012). Quality by design – FDA lessons learned and challenges for international harmonization. Presentation at International Conference on Drug Development, February 28th, Austin, TX.

Novick, S. J., Shen, Y., Yang, H., Peterson, J. J., LeBlond, D., and Altan, S. (2015). Dissolution curve comparisons through the F2 parameter, a Bayesian extension of the f2 statistic. *Journal of Biopharmaceutical Statistics*, 25(2):351–371.

Peterson, J., Miro-Quesada, G., and del Castillo, E. (2009a). A Bayesian reliability approach to multiple response optimization with seemingly unrelated regression models. *Journal of Quality Technology and Quantitative Management*, 6(4):353–369.

Peterson, J. J. (2004). A posterior predictive approach to multiple response surface optimization. *Journal of Quality Technology*, 36:139–153.

Peterson, J. J. (2008). A Bayesian approach to the ICH Q8 definition of design space. *Journal of Biopharmaceutical Statistics*, 18:959–975.

Peterson, J. J. and Altan, S. (2016). Overview of drug development and statistical tools for manufacturing and testing (Chapter 5). In Zhang, L., Kuhn, M., and Peers, I., editors, *Nonclinical Statistics for Pharmaceutical and Biotechnology Industries*. Springer, New York, NY.

Peterson, J. J., Kramer, T. T., Hofer, J. D., and Atkins, G. (2019). Opportunities and challenges for statisticians in advanced pharmaceutical manufacturing. *Statistics in Biopharmaceutical Research*, 11:152–161.

Peterson, J. J. and Lief, K. (2010). The ICH Q8 definition of design space: A comparison of the overlapping means and the Bayesian predictive approaches. *Statistics in Biopharmaceutical Research*, 2:249–259.

Peterson, J. J., Snee, R. D., McAllister, P., Schofield, T. L., and Carella, A. J. (2009b). Statistics in the pharmaceutical development and manufacturing (with discussion). *Journal of Quality Technology*, 41:111–147.

Peterson, J. J. and Yahyah, M. (2009). A Bayesian design space approach to robustness and system suitability for pharmaceutical assays and other processes. *Statistics in Biopharmaceutical Research*, 1(4):441–449.

Plackett, R. L. and Burman, J. P. (1946). The design of optimum multifactorial experiments. *Biometrika*, 33:305–325.

Rathore, A. S. (2009). Roadmap for implementation of quality by design (QbD) for biotechnology products. *Trends in Biotechnology*, 27(9):546–553.

Stockdale, G. W. and Cheng, A. (2009). Finding design space and a reliable operating region using a multivariate Bayesian approach with experimental design. *Quality Technology and Quantitative Management*, 6(4):391–408.

Stroup, W. and Quinlan, M. (2016). Statistical considerations for stability and the estimation of shelf life. In Zhang, L., editor, *Nonclinical Statistics for Pharmaceutical and Biotechnology Industries*, pages 575–604. Springer International Publishing, Cham, Switzerland.

Timm, N. H. (2002). *Applied Multivariate Analysis*. Springer-Verlag, New York, NY.

Vander Heyden, Y., Nijhuis, A., Smeyers-Verbeke, J., Vandeginste, B. G. M., and Massart, D. L. (2001). Guidance for robustness/ruggedness tests in methods validation. *Journal of Pharmaceutical and Biomedical Analysis*, 24:723–753.

Yang, H. (2017). *Emerging Non-clinical Biostatistics in Biopharmaceutical Development and Manufacturing.* Chapman & Hall/CRC, Boca Raton, FL.

Yu, L. X., Amidon, G., Khan, M. A., Hoag, S. W., Pollo, J., Raju, G. K., and Woodcock, J. (2014). Guidance for robustness/ruggedness tests in methods validation. *American Association of Pharmaceutical Scientists Journal*, 16(4):771–783.

20

Analytical Method and Assay

Pierre Lebrun
PharmaLex, Belgium

Eric Rozet
PharmaLex, Belgium

Spanning the complete drug development process, from early discovery to clinical trial and manufacturing, measurements are legion. Analytical methods and assays are these central pieces that allow obtaining the analytical results on which all the decisions are taken: a batch release, the drug efficacy, some toxicology issues, the drug stability and the drug shelf-life, ... the list is endless. Without these results, nobody would be able to characterize the drug product and its intermediates during manufacturing.

A measurement is of particular statistical interest, for there exists no measurement without uncertainty. Uncertainty can be very small, nearly imperceptible, or incredibly large due to the biological nature of the assay. What is important is that this uncertainty exists and cannot be removed. Instead, the skilled statistician will be able to cope with it and translate its impact to the important decisions about the drug and its manufacturing process. Indeed, if the impact of measurement uncertainty can affect the results of an expensive clinical trial, it is better to plan and see how assay understanding and tools like replication can help avoid the risk of failure.

Scientists are now invited to better describe their performance objective in terms of results' reliability, through the Analytical Target Profile. Throughout the lifecycle of the assay, science-based developments using designed experiments, an appropriate control strategy and fit-for-purpose method validation are more and more the common strategies to be applied.

This chapter aims at explaining these strategies. First, it is shown how an analytical method or an assay can be developed following the best practice of the industry — namely, the Analytical Quality by Design — to ensure a high reliability of the results obtained. Then, it illustrates how the measurement error (also known as total error) can be used to better predict the impact of the uncertainty during routine use, but also during activities like assay transfer between sites.

20.1 Introduction

During the drug development process, analytical methods and assays are everywhere: from early discovery of compounds to the expensive clinical trials, and to the large-scale manufacturing of the drug product, there is a need to characterize the *active pharmaceutical ingredients* (API), the excipients, the various possible impurities of the drug product or any of its intermediates. Careful characterization is mandatory at all stages. Here are two obvious situations where measurements are central in decision making: for release of new drug product lots and assessment of drug product used in clinical trials.

For a lot release, the drug manufacturer needs to measure the drug product and verify its adequacy with quality attributes specifications. If the result is within specifications, the product is released; otherwise, it is withdrawn. But now, what would happen if the measurement is not "accurate"? In this case, sometimes the manufacturer would withdraw good lots (out of specification due to the measurement), and sometimes, a bad lot would be released (the measurement would be good "by chance"). This might be harmful for the patients and for the manufacturer's credibility. Second example: the results of a clinical trial would strongly depend upon the dose(s) administrated to patient. So, what if this dose was not well characterized and the drug provided to patients is not the one scientists and doctors expected? What about the dose/response modeling, etc.? Thus, the analytical methods and assays must be precisely defined systems that allow making all these measurements to obtain accurate results, i.e. precise and non-biased information on the drug.

It is crucial to understand the substantial differences in the definition of three main validation characteristics. The first one is *Precision of the analytical procedure* that is defined as "The precision of an analytical procedure expresses the closeness of agreement (degree of scatter) between a series of measurements obtained from multiple sampling of the same homogeneous sample under the prescribed conditions" (ICH Q2(R1), 2005; Joint Committee for Guides in Metrology, 2018). It is related to random errors of the analytical procedure and is measured by variances, standard deviations or relative standard deviations (RSD). The second one is *Trueness of the analytical procedure*: "Closeness of agreement between the average of an infinite number of replicate measured quantity values and a reference quantity value" (Joint Committee for Guides in Metrology, 2018). Trueness is related to systematic error of the analytical procedure and can be measured by biases, relative biases or mean recoveries. The last one is *Accuracy of the measurements*. It is defined by: "The accuracy of an analytical procedure expresses the closeness of agreement between the value which is accepted either as a conventional true value or an accepted reference value and the value found" (ICH Q2(R1), 2005; Joint Committee for Guides in Metrology, 2018). It relates to the total error of the measurements or results, i.e. the combination of systematic and random errors. It is acknowledged that confusion exists between Trueness and Accuracy, especially in the pharmaceutical world although clear distinctions arise from their definitions.

Types of measurements are multiple, from basic ones, e.g. weighing, visual appearance, hardness, friability, color, density, etc.; to more complex ones, for instance concentration of API, of impurities, characterization of excipients, etc.; to even biological activity such as in-vitro or in-vivo efficacy and toxicity, etc. The enthusiastic reader is invited to go back and forth in this book, across all chapters, and identify all those measurements and drug characterizations, used in every single paragraph ....

This present chapter aims at presenting what is a "good" measurement, what statistics can bring to describe measurement uncertainty, and how analytical methods and assays can be developed in order to achieve this desired high quality in order to be fit for their very purpose: to provide unbiased, precise i.e. accurate results at each single measure that is made.

The general aim in the pharmaceutical industry is to switch from the outdated *Quality by Testing* (QbT) to the up-to-date *Quality by Design* (QbD) paradigm. Product quality is identified in QbT mainly by end product testing and restricting flexibility in the manufacturing process. However, pharmaceutical product development requires a more scientific, risk-based, proactive approach with established feed-forward and feed-back control strategies. Implementation of QbD paradigm leads to profitable product development and timely regulatory approval by these key areas: *Analytical target profile, risk assessment, design space, control strategy* and *product lifecycle management.* When QbD is properly executed, it brings an incredible advantage of being robust to manufacturing conditions that are –and will never be– perfectly controlled. Whenever a manufacturer operates within the design space of its processes, the quality of the product would be guaranteed.

The International Council for Harmonisation of Technical Requirements for Pharmaceuticals for Human Use (ICH) brings together the pharmaceutical industry and medicines regulatory authorities of Europe, Japan and the United States. It defines quality as "the suitability of either a drug substance or drug product for its intended use" and has published guidance for the pharmaceutical industry that defines the concept and application of QbD: "A systematic approach to development that begins with predefined objectives and emphasizes product and process understanding and process control, based on sound science and quality risk management." To this end, QbD concepts are well defined in the ICH guidelines Q8(R2): Pharmaceutical development; Q9: Quality risk management; and Q10: Pharmaceutical quality system (ICH Q8, 2009; ICH Q9, 2005; ICH Q10, 2008), furthermore, FDA's cGMP for the 21st Century (U.S. Food and Drug Administration, 2009), and Process Analytical Technology (PAT) (U.S. Food and Drug Administration, 2004) guidance support the implementation of QbD concepts.

The fundamental idea in QbD is that product quality results from the knowledge of what needs to be achieved (summarized in the *Quality Target Product Profile, (QTPP)*), appropriate design, demonstrated control of formulation and manufacturing process. As a consequence, the concept and application of the QbD paradigm has been an emerging topic in the early 2000's in the pharmaceutical industry, and a literature review reveals its implementation and importance nowadays (Rozet et al., 2013; Lebrun et al., 2012).

To match what can be found in all previous citations and in this chapter, the reader may substitute throughout the references the words "product" and "process" by "analytical result" and "assay", respectively. It would be sufficient to demonstrate that ICH Q8-9-10 are directly applicable to measurements systems, and not only to (pharmaceutical) processes. This parallelism between process/product and assay/result is quite logical and intuitive, as an assay is simply a process used to obtain a measurement or result.

20.2 Analytical quality by design

The concept of QbD applied to analytical method and assay is defined as *analytical quality by design* (AQbD Rozet et al., 2013). AQbD is based on implementation of method performance and scope, which comprehend the product file in the form of *analytical target profile* (ATP) and *critical quality attributes.* Depending on the target measurement, a suitable selection of analytical technique, risk assessment process, method development using *design of experiments* (DoE), *analytical design space* (DS), control strategy and method validation can be defined (Rozet et al., 2013, see also Figure 20.1).

AQbD enhances method understanding and robustness, aligning method with process. This results in a better understanding of the analytical result and the different sources of variability. Robustness of operation assesses the quality of the analytical results by evaluating the impact of different assets of AQbD, such as repeatability and reproducibility, analytical transfer, validation and routine procedures among others.

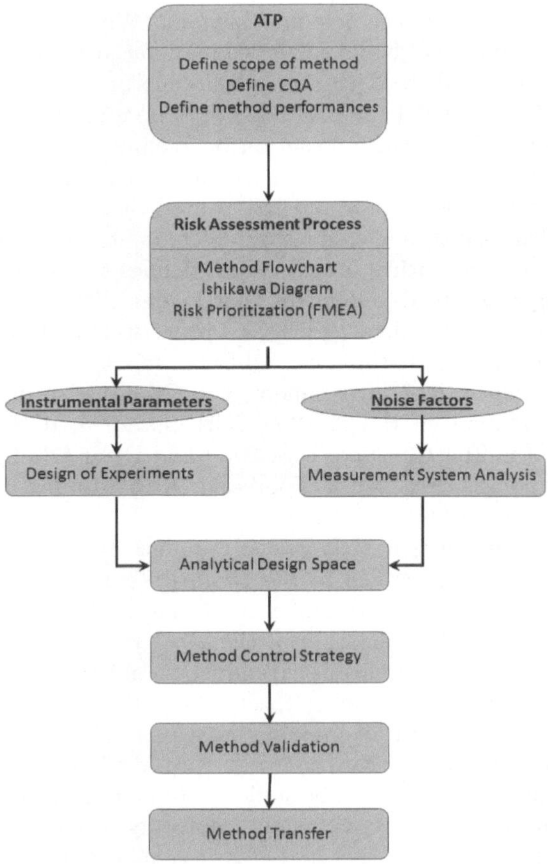

FIGURE 20.1: Schematic procedure for Analytical Quality by Design.

20.2.1 Analytical target profile

When using AQbD, the objectives of the analytical methods and assays development are defined by the *Analytical Target Profile*, analogous to the *Quality Target Product Profile* for QbD. The implementation of an ATP provides the requirements on the analytical result, summarizing the objectives in terms of *Critical Quality Attributes.* The importance of the implementation of ATP in pharmaceutical processes is pointed out in numerous peer-reviewed publications (Schweitzer et al., 2010; Nethercote et al., 2010; Borman et al., 2010; Rozet et al., 2012). ATP thus describes the minimal performance the analytical method must achieve. For instance, the error of measurement must be smaller than 10%, with a range of dosing from 20 to 250 mg. Or, in a defined ATP for a drug product assay, the procedure must be able to accurately quantify the API in film coated tablets over the range of 90 - 110% of the nominal concentration with such accuracy that measurements fall within $\pm$ 2.0% of the true value, with 0.95 probability (Hanna-Brown et al., 2014). It is generally convenient to use an ATP that describes method performance criteria based on a probability of result within a given range from the "true value", as it is aligned with the statistical reality that measurements are always observed with some uncertainty (Rozet et al., 2011).

20.2.2 Critical quality attributes

The *critical quality attributes* of the analytical procedure are the responses that are measured to judge its quality (Rozet et al., 2015). ICH guideline Q8(R2) defines critical quality attributes (CQAs) as "a physical, chemical, biological or microbiological property or characteristic that should be within an appropriate limit, range, or distribution to ensure the desired product quality" (ICH Q8, 2009). For instance, for chromatographic analytical procedures, the CQAs can be related to the method selectivity, such as the resolution (RS) or separation (S) criteria (Lebrun et al., 2012). Other CQAs can be the run time of the analysis, signal-to-noise ratio, the precision and the trueness of the analytical procedure, the lower limit of quantification (LOQ), or the width of the dosing range of the analytical method. A crucial CQA for any quantitative assay is the accuracy of the results obtained.

Based on the ATP, a risk assessment is generally done: what are the CQA that are the most critical and the ones that will not impact the intended purpose of the method (e.g. the release of a good drug product or the withdrawal of a bad one)? This risk assessment can be achieved using for instance the *Failure Mode and Effects Analysis* (FMEA; Rausand and Hoyland, 2004).

20.2.3 Design of experiments

Design of experiments is an excellent methodology to analyze and evaluate the effect of a set of *critical method parameters* (CMPs) on *critical quality attributes* (Montgomery, 2009). ICH guideline Q8(R2) defines DoE as a "structured, organized method for determining the relationship between factors affecting a process and the output of that process" (ICH Q8, 2009). DoE provides the flexibility in the experimental strategy (setting of operating conditions) to lay out the expected method performance and method response defined by the combinations of CMPs to produce results in concordance with the defined ATP.

Once an analytical method is selected, analytical experts can create DoE to optimize it, and usually, the data collected is analyzed using statistical models – e.g. using Bayesian analysis (see Section 20.2.5). It is paramount to confirm the statistical model quality, whenever possible using a scientific rationale in terms of understanding of the assay/method. It is noted that selecting a model based on the statistical significance of its parameters is not advised. A better option that has been found valuable is to select effects that potentially make a CQA move significantly in the range of its specification limits (even if the effect seems only partially "statistically significant" e.g. due to noisy estimate), instead of selecting very "significant" parameters (with, say, a P-value < 0.05), but for which the CQA might stay comfortably within the specification limits, as illustrated in Figure 20.2 (Lebrun et al., 2018). Avoiding a P-value based decision is seen here as critical, if not mandatory, and hopefully this can be helped using Bayesian analysis, that can easily translate parameter uncertainty into their impact on model response. This also dictates strongly how an adequate tool has to be developed, for the analysis of such results, as discussed in the next section.

20.2.4 Design space

The *design space* (DS) has been defined in ICH Q8(R2) as the "the multidimensional combination and interaction of input variables (e.g. material attributes) and *process parameters* (PPs) that have been demonstrated to provide assurance of quality" for the product or processes involved in pharmaceutical development (ICH Q8, 2009). Parallelism with the analytical world can be made again to understand the concept of an "analytical" design space. As shown in Figure 20.1, DS is a key component for the development of analytical procedure

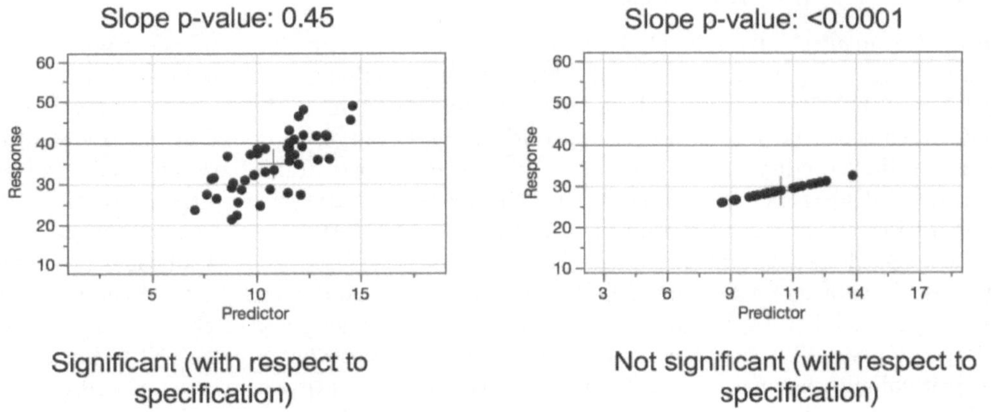

FIGURE 20.2: Illustration of model parameter selection beyond the P-value. Horizontal plain line: Upper specification limit (40). Left: A non-statistically significant factor (P-value > 0.05) with a strong effect on a CQA. This may not be picked by a stepwise parameter selection. Right: A very statistically significant factor (P-value < 0.05) with low to no effect on the CQA. This would be picked by stepwise analysis. Notice that the depicted P-values are not accurate and are indicated for illustration only.

using AQbD. DS can be seen as the sufficient information and knowledge gathered during development studies to provide a scientific rationale for the design and maintenance of the assay for a pharmaceutical product (Yu, 2008).

The DS is a region of reliable robustness identified in the knowledge space (also called experimental domain χ). DS should be defined in a risk-based framework to provide the appropriate criteria of quality. As a result, DS is a part of the experimental domain where the quality can be guaranteed. Formally, DS is defined as:

$$\text{DS} = \{\boldsymbol{x}_0 \in \boldsymbol{\chi} \mid \Pr(\mathbf{CQA's} \in \boldsymbol{\Lambda} \mid \boldsymbol{x}_0, \boldsymbol{\Theta}, \mathbf{data}) \geq \pi\}. \tag{20.1}$$

In other words, DS is a region of the experimental domain χ, where the predictive posterior probability that the CQA's are within specifications Λ, is higher than a specified quality level π, given the data and the model parameters $\boldsymbol{\Theta}$, that include the uncertainty estimated by the statistical model. Predictive probability is central when dealing with concepts such as DS, as it allows the quantification of the guarantees that specifications will be met in the future runs of the assay, given today's information. Specifications Λ express the minimal satisfying qualities that the experimenters want to obtain on the CQA's (e.g. Run time < 10 mins, Trueness $< 5\%$, etc.).

20.2.5 Bayesian analysis

While conceptually meaningful and relevant to ensure the future quality of analytical results, the AQbD paradigm poses several challenges from a statistical standpoint and requires a methodological shift from traditional statistical practices. Indeed, demonstrating robustness for the analytical results that will be provided tomorrow (e.g. during routine) implies the necessity to make predictions about the future quality given the past evidence and data. It appears that the framework of Bayesian statistics is particularly well-suited for this type of computation. Evaluating the predictive probability of success of jointly meeting each set of specifications of the ATP, given the assumed underlying model and high dependencies between measurements, is a challenge that may prove cumbersome or even impossible using the better-known frequentist statistics.

To identify the DS using Bayesian analysis, the predictive probability of success is central (Lebrun et al., 2012). It is simply computed based on a (sampled) posterior predictive distribution of the CQA. A fine grid is created over the CPP on the experimental domain χ. Within each point of the grid, the predictive probabilities are computed, according to the following sequence (see Figure 20.3 for illustration):

1. Draw, say, 10,000 samples from the predictive distribution, including back-transformation to the original scale of the response(s). An example of predictive distribution is provided in the next sections.
2. The probability of success is computed as follows: for the 10,000 posterior samples, calculate the proportion of them that satisfies the specifications (jointly, if the distribution is multivariate with multiple CQA's. Figure 20.3: crosses). This proportion is the MCMC estimate of the probability of success of achieving the ATP or part of the ATP.

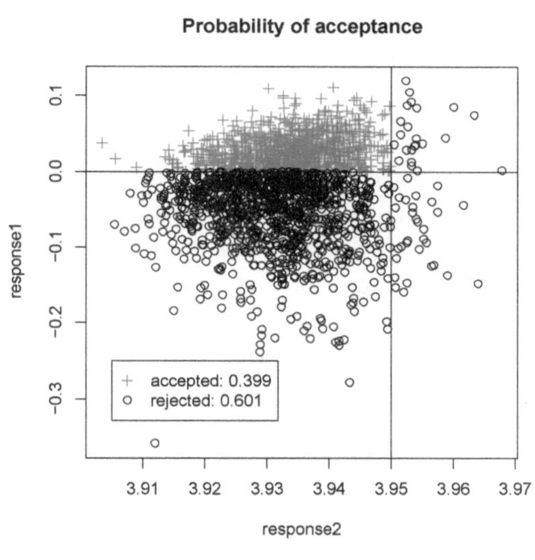

FIGURE 20.3: Computation of the predictive probability of success as the proportion of posterior samples lying within acceptance limits (crosses), for two CQA's: Response1 and response2.

20.3 Assay development

There are numerous scientific publications in the literature reporting the application of Bayesian statistical models for the development of high performance liquid chromatography (HPLC) assay, including optimization and robustness assessment (Rozet et al., 2013, 2015;

Deidda et al., 2018; Borman et al., 2010). In this regard, take as example the study of (Lebrun et al., 2012), which describes the mathematical foundations on how to derive this predictive distribution and how it is applied to compute the assay Design Space for CQA related to chromatographic quality of elution (e.g. critical resolution and separation, run time, etc.). Interestingly, there are not any huge differences from what can be found for similar topics applied to process development, as found in numerous examples of applications (Peterson, 2004, 2008; Peterson and Yahyah, 2009; Peterson and Lief, 2010).

In conclusion, although the previous methodology has been widely illustrated on HPLC system developments, this methodology is applicable with minor changes to any type of assays, including other separative techniques such as super critical fluid chromatography (Dispas et al., 2017), gas chromatography, capillary electrophoresis (Lamalle et al., 2012), potentially coupled with an advanced detector such as mass spectrometer (Hubert et al., 2015), etc., but also the non-separative biological potency assay (ELISA, qPCR, QPA, etc.; Yarovoi et al., 2013; Verch, 2014).

20.3.1 HPLC method development

The high-performance liquid chromatography (HPLC) method is a technique used to separate compounds of interest (e.g. API and impurities). Compounds are transported using a liquid solvent (the mobile phase), by creating affinities between them and a solid phase. This latter is generally a column containing solid adsorbent particles (e.g. silica or polymers) with various nature, allowing the fine tuning of affinities between the mobile and solid phases. During the time the compounds and the mobile phase are percolating through the solid phase, the formers are being physically separated, allowing further analysis, such as detection, quantitation, or extraction of purified material in the case of preparative chromatography. Visualization of this separation process is made through a chromatogram, generally consisting of a graph of the absorption of UV/visible light vs. the time peaks/compounds go out of the solid phase (time referred as elution time). Each peak thus shows the presence of some compounds absorbing some light wavelength (see Figure 20.5). When peaks are well separated, the chromatogram shows that compounds are physically well separated.

Bayesian models for statistical evaluation can be implemented for HPLC method development. Multivariate models are created for the chromatographic behavior of all peaks of the chromatogram at three time points of interest: start of the peak, apex of the peak (called retention time) and end of the peak (Lebrun et al., 2012). In addition, compounds with similar properties and chemical structure can also have their peaks assumed correlated.

Multivariate multiple linear regression (MMLR) is adopted to account for the correlations that can be observed between responses. The strength of this model among other statistical models is that MMLR offers the advantage of simplicity for the identification of its predictive distribution. Notably, MMLR fits for every response jointly ($\boldsymbol{Y}$). The following model can be applied:

$$\boldsymbol{Y} = \boldsymbol{X}\boldsymbol{B} + \boldsymbol{E},$$

with ε_n, the nth line of $\boldsymbol{E}$, assumed to follow a multivariate Normal distribution, $\varepsilon_n \sim \mathrm{N}(\boldsymbol{O}, \boldsymbol{\Sigma})$, $(n = 1, \ldots, N)$, with N the number of experiments. $\boldsymbol{X}$ is then the $(N \times F)$ centered and reduced design matrix and $\boldsymbol{B}$ is the $(F \times M)$ matrix containing the F effects for each of the M responses. The modeled effects have been chosen so that the model has the best properties for every response, jointly. $\boldsymbol{\Sigma}$ is the covariance matrix of the residuals.

In order to account for the variability of the parameters $\boldsymbol{B}$ and $\boldsymbol{\Sigma}$, a predictive density of new predicted responses can be obtained in the Bayesian framework, considering the non-informative prior distribution $p(\boldsymbol{B}, \boldsymbol{\Sigma}) \propto |\boldsymbol{\Sigma}|^{-(M+1)/2}$ (Lebrun et al., 2012; Geisser, 1965; Box and Tiao, 1973). In this context, the predictive posterior density of a new predicted

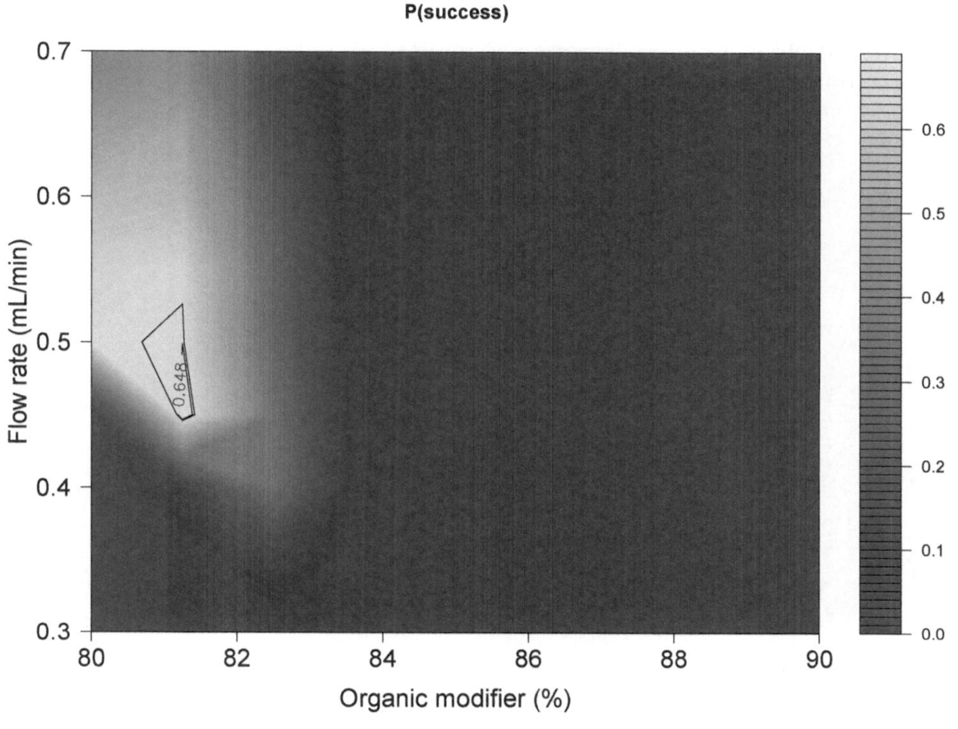

FIGURE 20.4: Probability plot obtained for the optimization of a chromatographic method showing the design space (whiter area) at 64% probability level over two HPLC factors: The proportion of Organic Modifier in the mobile phase and the Flow rate of the mobile phase through the column.

set of responses $(\widetilde{\boldsymbol{y}} \mid \boldsymbol{X} = \boldsymbol{x}_0, \textbf{data})$ at a new operating condition $\boldsymbol{x}_0 \in \chi$, is identified as a multivariate t-distribution T_m, defined as follows

$$(\widetilde{\boldsymbol{y}} \mid \boldsymbol{X} = \boldsymbol{x}_0, \textbf{data}) \sim T_m \left(\boldsymbol{x}_0 \widehat{\boldsymbol{B}}, \frac{\boldsymbol{A}}{\nu} \left(\mathbf{1} + \boldsymbol{x}_0 (\boldsymbol{X}^\top \boldsymbol{X})^{-1} \boldsymbol{x}_0^\top \right), \nu \right), \tag{20.2}$$

where $\widehat{\boldsymbol{B}}$ is the least squares estimate of $\boldsymbol{B}$, $\widehat{\boldsymbol{B}} = (\boldsymbol{X}^\top \boldsymbol{X})^{-1} \boldsymbol{X}^\top \boldsymbol{Y}$, and $\boldsymbol{A} = (\boldsymbol{Y} - \boldsymbol{X}\widehat{\boldsymbol{B}})^\top (\boldsymbol{Y} - \boldsymbol{X}\widehat{\boldsymbol{B}})$ is a scale matrix with $\nu = N - (M + F) + 1$ being the degrees of freedom. Note that the predictive distribution under proper and configurable priors is also identified as a t distribution, although parameterization is slightly more complex. However, this means an advantage to be able to easily incorporate information from previous experiments and to smoothly implement a valuable Bayesian update mechanism.

The use of this predictive distribution allows the prediction of chromatograms from the seminal work of Dewé et al. (2004), as well as their uncertainty. Predictive probability maps, as illustrated in Figure 20.4, can be derived to fulfill one or several pre-specified goals, such as having a minimum separation of peaks of at least one minute and having a maximum elution time lower than, for example, 15 minutes. Figure 20.5 shows the predicted chromatogram obtained at the optimal operating condition together with its uncertainty region. As can be seen the observed chromatogram at the same operating condition is fully in line with the prediction. Even after geometric transfer of the HPLC method to Ultra High Performance Liquid Chromatography (UHPLC) equipment to reduce analysis time, the observed chromatogram shown on Figure 20.5 is coherent with the prediction, illustrating the robustness and the high value of the methodology.

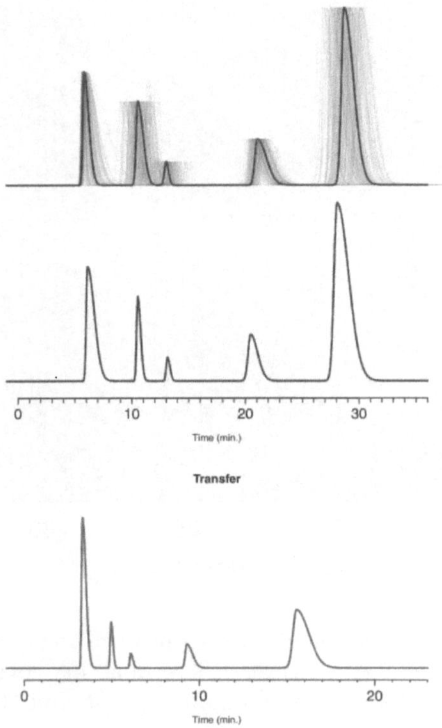

FIGURE 20.5: Top: Predicted chromatogram with uncertainty region, at the optimal condition. Middle: Observed chromatogram at the same experimental condition. Bottom: Chromatogram observed after geometric transfer to UHPLC equipment to reduce analysis time, illustrating the high robustness of the methodology.

20.3.2 ELISA assay development

Ligand-binding assays, in particular ELISA, are widely used to quantify proteins. The mechanism of detection is based on biology by opposition as for chromatographic methods relying on physico-chemical properties. Quantification of the amount of analyte existing in samples is usually performed by relating the signal of the assay (optical density) to concentration of a standard sample, namely a calibration curve. Typical models used to fit the standard curve are non-linear, such as 4 or 5-parameter logistic functions (see Figure 20.6). Numerous assay parameters can be tuned to optimize such assays such as the nature of enzymes, volumes of products, different incubation times, etc. (Yarovoi et al., 2013; Verch, 2014). Each combination of these parameters will influence the shape of the calibration curve and hence alter the predicted concentration of analyte. The final aim of such assays is to be able to provide accurate analytical results. This is generally translated in an operational way by requiring having results with less than $\lambda\%$ total error, e.g. 30%. To this end, the path to optimization is to select the ranges of the assay parameters that will reach high probability to provide accurate results.

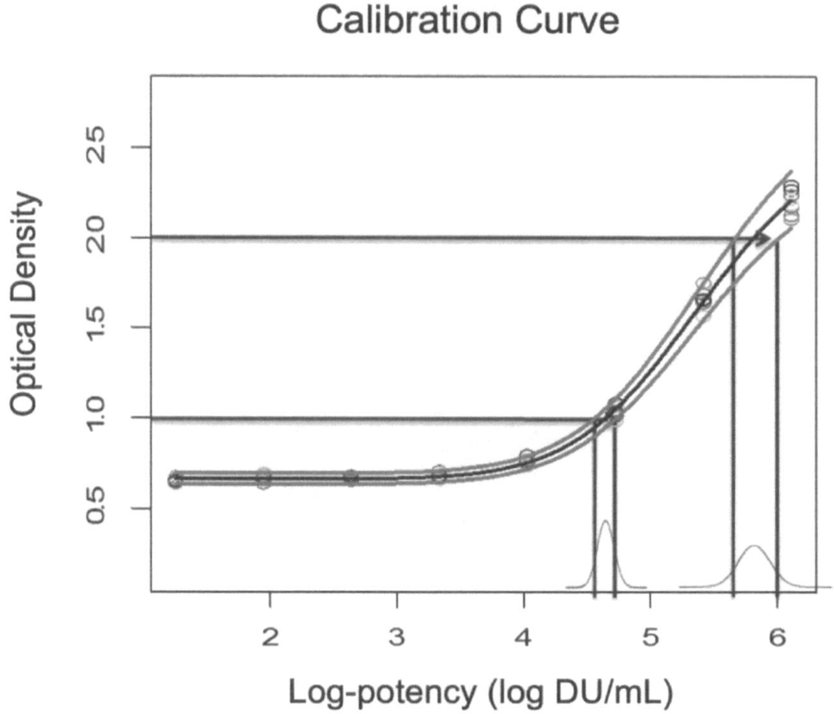

FIGURE 20.6: Example of a calibration curve for ELISA showing the predicted results with their posterior distribution (DU: D-Antigen units).

Using an appropriate Design of Experiments to collect data, parameters of the non-linear calibration curves can be expressed as a function of the assay parameters and the predictive distribution of analyte concentration/potency is obtained by exploring the knowledge space using the fitted Bayesian model.

For each combination of the assay parameters (i.e. for each calibration curve), the predictive probability to have analytical results with less than $\lambda\%$ total error (e.g. 30% over the potency range studied) can be obtained and used to select the most or the set of the most optimal conditions for the ELISA (Figure 20.7).

20.4 Analytical validation and transfer

The next step in the life cycle of analytical methods is the demonstration that the analytical procedure is fit for its intended purpose described in the ATP (Nethercote and Ermer, 2012). This exercise is called *analytical validation*, or, referring to the QbD terminology, "assay performance qualification" (of Process Performance Qualification — PPQ; ICH Q2(R1), 2005; U.S. Food and Drug Administration, 2011). Hence, the final aim of a given quantitative analytical procedure is to provide analytical results of adequate quality in order to make

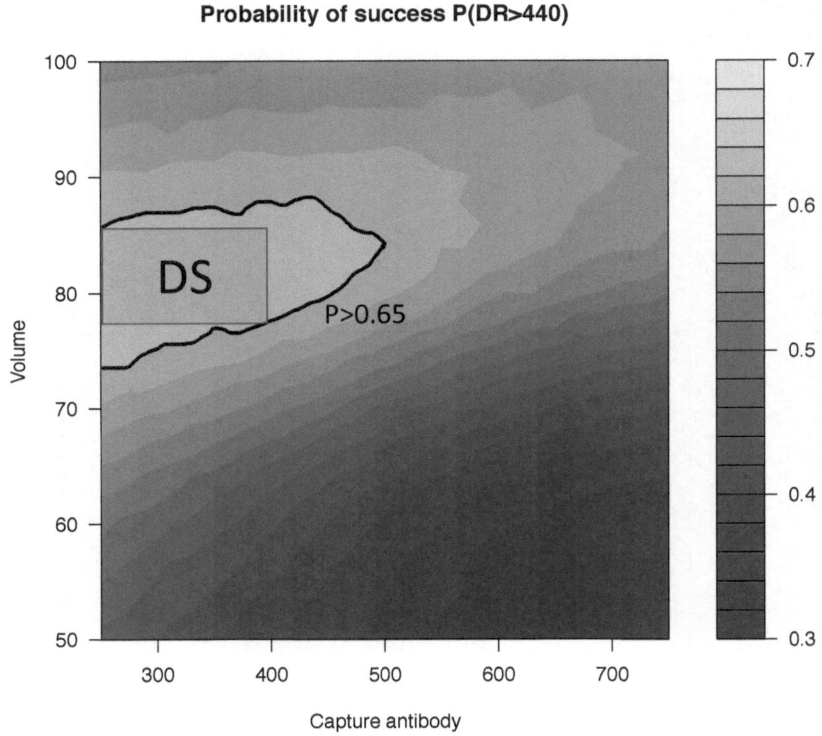

FIGURE 20.7: Probability plot for the optimization of an ELISA assay, showing the probability of having a valid Dosing Range (DR) of at least 440 ng/ml for two method parameters: Volume and concentration of capture antibody (CaptureA).

reliable decisions with them. It implies that the CQAs for quantitative procedures should be related to the reliability of analytical results, i.e. the accuracy (combination of bias and precision) of the results obtained by the procedure is the key CQA. The ATP should work towards this end, and provide objective acceptance criteria, ideally related to the product the assay will characterize.

The validation phase of any quantitative analytical procedure is therefore in line with the AQbD framework. The CQA that should be monitored during analytical procedure validation is the prediction of the ability of the analytical procedure to provide accurate results over a defined range of concentration or activity. Another type of validation experiment is the transfer of an analytical method or assay from one laboratory (the reference assay) to another (the new assay). The principle for the experimenter is the same. The aim is to show that the analytical results that will be provided by the new assay will be of adequate quality and aligned to the reference measurement on similar product.

20.4.1 Critical assay parameters in analytical procedure validation

Firstly, the main factor that has to be included in analytical procedure validation is the concentration/amount/potency range over which the procedure is intended to characterize the analyte(s) or biological product. This range is a fixed factor and it is covered by several samples called validation standards (or quality control samples) of known concentration/amount/potency. In addition, the main sources of variability that will be encountered during the future routine of the procedure must be included in the validation design as random factors, such as operators, equipment, reagent batches or days. The combination of these sources of variability is generally called "runs" or "series".

20.4.2 Experimental designs for analytical procedure validation

ICH Q8(R2) and FDA Process Validation guidelines highly promote the use of adequate design of experiments when developing pharmaceutical processes (ICH Q8, 2009; U.S. Food and Drug Administration, 2011). The main designs used in analytical procedure validation are nested designs or (fractional) factorial designs or their combination (Hubert et al., 2004, 2006, 2007). These designs are used to estimate variance components as they will occur in future runs of the assay. The use of as many possible levels of each factor is recommended to have precise estimations (e.g. 2 or 3 technicians operating during 3 or 4 days). Nonetheless, the different sources of variation included in the analytical procedure validation are generally combined into "series" or "runs" to mimic the way analytical procedures are effectively routinely employed.

The statistical model widely used in analytical procedure validation is a linear mixed model also called hierarchical linear model including runs (or series) as a factor performed for each of the ith concentration levels of the validation standards. Define J as the number of runs and assume that K replicates are performed in each run. As a result, the validation experiments can be defined for each of the ith concentration levels studied by the following model:

$$X_{ijk} = \mu_i + \alpha_{ij} + \varepsilon_{ijk}, \quad \alpha_{ij} \sim \mathrm{N}(0, \sigma^2_{\alpha,i}), \quad \varepsilon_{ijk} \sim \mathrm{N}(0, \sigma^2_{\varepsilon,i}), \tag{20.3}$$

where μ_i is the overall mean of the ith concentration level studied of the validation standard, $\mu_i + \alpha_{ij}$ is the mean in run $j = 1, \ldots, J$, ε_{ijk} is the residual error of the kth replicate $(k = 1, \ldots, K)$ of the jth run, $\sigma^2_{\alpha,i}$ is the run-to-run variance, and $\sigma^2_{\varepsilon,i}$ is the within-run or repeatability variance, both for the ith concentration level.

The overall variability of the analytical method is measured by the intermediate precision variance $\sigma^2_{IP,i} = \sigma^2_{\alpha,i} + \sigma^2_{\varepsilon,i}$. The resolution of the model in the frequentist statistical framework is well known, and it is described in various studies performed by Mee (1984). To adjust this model in the Bayesian setting, weakly informative priors for the model parameters can be used (Wolfinger, 1998):

$$\begin{aligned} \mu_i &\sim \mathrm{N}(0, 10,000), \\ \sigma^2_{\varepsilon,i} &\sim \text{Inv-Gamma}(0.0001, 0.0001), \\ \sigma^2_{\alpha,i} &\sim \text{Inv-Gamma}(0.0001, 0.0001). \end{aligned} \tag{20.4}$$

Therefore, two options can be used to evaluate and validate the success of the analytical method (Figures 20.8 and 20.9).

1. Determination of prediction interval defined for a pre-specified probability beta (0.90 or 0.95) (Hamada et al., 2004; U.S. Food and Drug Administration, 2011). If this predictive interval falls within the acceptance criteria for each concentration level i, the analytical method can be considered validated over the full range of the studied concentrations. (Figure 20.8).
2. Estimation of the predictive posterior probability (see Section 20.2.5) to observe future results within the acceptance criteria previously chosen at each ith concentration level of the validation standards (Rozet et al., 2011, 2015). If the prob-

ability is greater than a pre-specified probability level, the analytical method is valid over that range of concentrations (Figure 20.9).

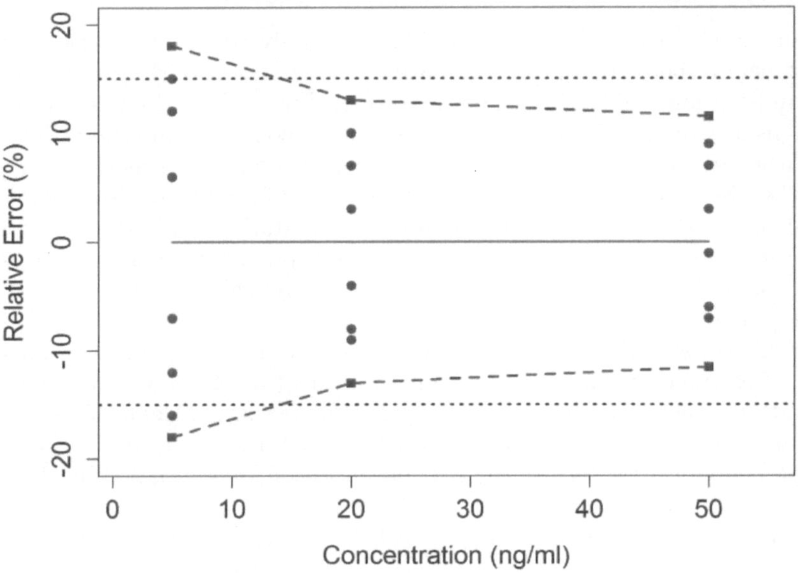

FIGURE 20.8: Accuracy Profile: Illustration using a 95% prediction interval (Long-dashed lines) of the analytical procedure results when the simple linear model is chosen as response function. Acceptance limits (dotted black) are set at ± 20%. The plain horizontal line is the relative bias. The valid dosing range is defined as the concentration range where the 95% prediction interval is fully included within the acceptance limits.

20.4.3 Design space and analytical procedure validation

Similar to the probability profile of Figure 20.9, the analytical procedure validation can be used to define a DS as the range of concentration i where it has been demonstrated that the procedure provides assurance of quality results (Rozet et al., 2013, 2011):

$$\pi_i = \Pr(-\lambda < X_i - \mu_{Ti} < \lambda). \tag{20.5}$$

The objective of the validation phase can be summarized to evaluate the range of concentration where the predictive probability π_i that each future result will fall within predefined acceptance limits (λ) is greater than or equal to a minimum claimed level π_{min}. Thus, as the predictive probability π_i needs to be estimated, all the uncertainty sources have to be included in its estimation when comparing it to a minimal satisfactory, π_{min}. This is an important issue to account since it has no exact small sample solution in frequentist statistics but it can be easily tackled with Bayesian modeling. Therefore, the DS is the range of concentration over which this predictive probability is greater than a preset minimum value (e.g. 0.95).

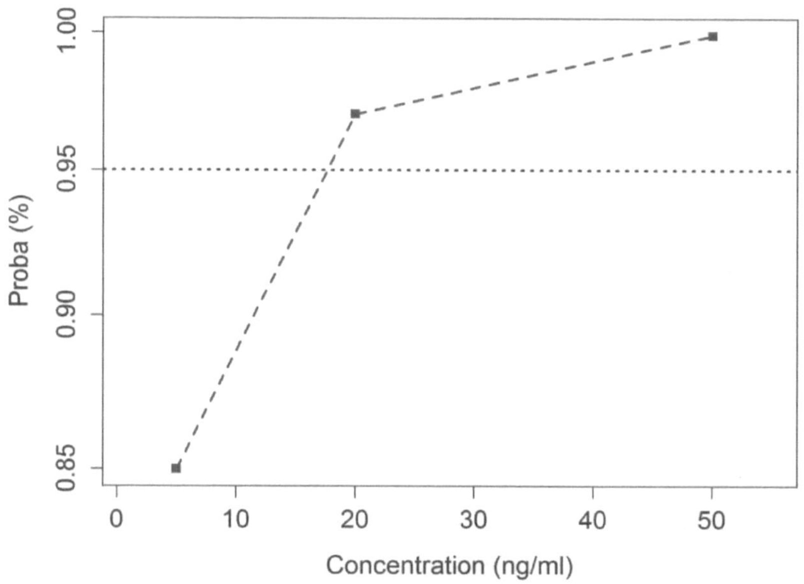

FIGURE 20.9: Probability profile: Illustration of the posterior predictive probability of having measurements falling inside of the acceptance limits at each concentration level. The minimum reliability probability has been set at 0.95 (horizontal dotted line).

The following linear hierarchical model with random slopes, intercepts and residual variance increasing with concentration can be used:

$$X_{ijk} = \beta_0 + \beta_1 \mu_{Ti} + u_{0j} + u_{1j} \mu_{Ti} + \varepsilon_{ijk}, \tag{20.6}$$

where the subscript i stands for the I concentration levels of the validation standards, j for the J number of series or runs and k for the K number of replicates per run. The main difference from the previous model is that the concentration levels are now handled as a continuous factor. μ_{Ti} is the ith concentration level of the validation standard and is considered as a reference or conventional true value. $\boldsymbol{\theta} = (\beta_0, \beta_1)^\top$ are the fixed effects. Additionally, $\boldsymbol{u}_j = (u_{0j}, u_{1j})^\top$ are the random effects of the jth runs and are also assumed to come from a Normal distribution: $\boldsymbol{u}_j \sim \mathrm{N}(\boldsymbol{0}, \Sigma_u)$, with Σ_u a 2×2 covariance matrix. Finally, ε_{ijk} is the residual error assumed to be independent and to come from a Normal distribution of variance σ_i^2. This variance is also given as being dependent on the concentration level i. This phenomenon is frequently observed in real life situations. The general form of this variance function can be defined as a power of the concentration μ_{Ti} (Davidian and Giltinan, 1995):

$$\sigma_i = \sigma \times (\mu_{Ti})^\gamma. \tag{20.7}$$

A probability profile for an analytical procedure using this model and MCMC simulations is shown in Figure 20.10. The probability profile depicts the concentration range over which the analytical procedure is fit for its purpose. This range represents the analytical procedure validation Design Space.

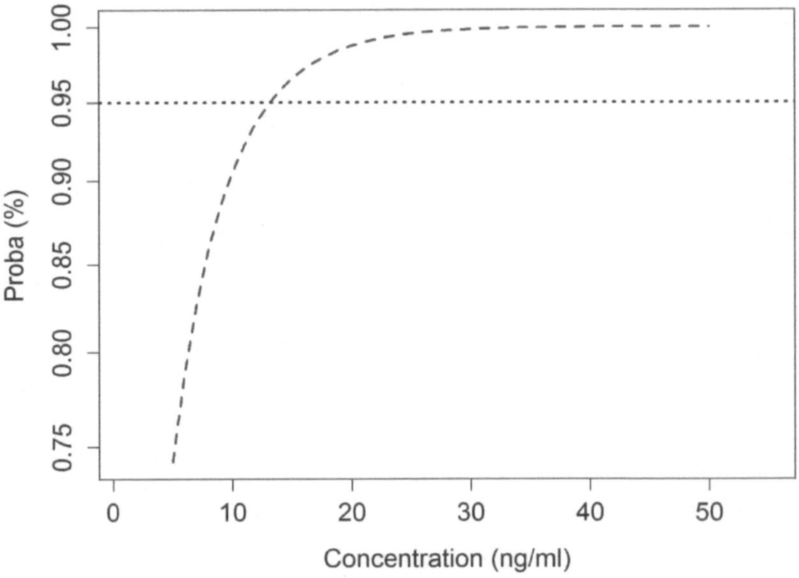

FIGURE 20.10: Bayesian predictive probability profile, modeling over the concentration range studies the probability π_i to have any future analytical result falling within an acceptance value of $\pm$ 15% around the known concentration values of the validation standards. The minimum reliability probability has been set at 0.95. The lower limit of quantification corresponds to the concentration where the predictive probability crosses the minimum probability value of 0.95.

20.4.4 Analytical method transfer

An analytical method transfer is a complete process that consists in transferring a validated analytical method from a "sender" laboratory to a "receiver" laboratory after having experimentally demonstrated that it also masters the method U.S. Pharmacopeia (2019b) and meets the ATP criteria. At the present time, analytical methods transfer is fully integrated into the life cycle of an analytical method in the pharmaceutical industry. Regulatory agencies such as the U.S. Food and Drug Administration (FDA) and European Medicine Agency (EMA) require that a transfer from development to quality control laboratory, or to or from contract or process laboratories, should be performed to certify that the receiver is qualified to execute the methods during their future routine application (EudraLex, 2014; U.S. Food and Drug Administration, 2015). Thus, analytical methods transfer should ensure that the results obtained by the receiver will be reliable and that the receiver laboratory using the transferred method is able to sustain similar decisions as the sender laboratory. This means that the analytical method at the receiver laboratory should be equally fit for purpose. With the exception of the relatively recent USP chapter <1224> (U.S. Pharmacopeia, 2019b), no detailed official guideline exists for transfer methodology in pharmaceutical or bio-pharmaceutical analysis. Note that according to ICH Q9 guideline (ICH Q9, 2005), risk analysis and management should be integrated into a transfer process.

The main aim of analytical method transfers should be to ensure that both laboratories (sender and receiver) will provide similar results with a high degree of confidence. The classical laboratory-to-laboratory comparison used for analytical method transfer (called comparative testing in USP <1224>, (U.S. Pharmacopeia, 2019b)) implies that the sender laboratory has validated the analytical procedure prior to its transfer. Hence, the sender laboratory can be defined as a reference laboratory. In addition, in many applications, the analytical methods used are destructive and do not allow a paired analysis of the samples used in analytical method transfer studies.

The classical design used in analytical method transfer consists of several series of experiments (a minimum of 3) and several replicates per series (usually 3) that the receiver laboratory will perform. The sender laboratory may also perform one or several series if the between series variance has been demonstrated negligible. Based on this common design used in the receiver laboratory, the model that best describes it is also a hierarchical linear model including runs (or series) as factor. For each of the laboratories ($l = 1, 2$), this random ANOVA model with series (or runs) as random factor is the following:

$$X_{ljk} = \mu_l + \alpha_{lj} + \varepsilon_{ljk}, \quad \alpha_{lj} \sim \mathrm{N}(0, \sigma^2_{\alpha,l}), \quad \varepsilon_{ljk} \sim \mathrm{N}(0, \sigma^2_{\varepsilon,l}), \tag{20.8}$$

where μ_l is the overall mean of the lth laboratory, $\mu_l + \alpha_{lj}$ is the mean in run $j = 1, \ldots, J$ of the lth laboratory, ε_{ljk} is the residual error of the kth replicate $(k = 1, \ldots, K)$ of the jth run of the lth laboratory, $\sigma^2_{\alpha,l}$ is the run-to-run variance, and $\sigma^2_{\varepsilon,l}$ is the within-run or repeatability variance, both for the lth laboratory.

Finally, to fully specify the Bayesian model, priors are given to the parameters, as in (20.4).

Let $\pm\lambda$ be the maximum difference allowed for the results of the two laboratories. For the case of the receiver laboratory, using non-informative priors or weakly informative priors is reasonable as there is little knowledge about the behavior of the analytical method at this site. However, for the sender laboratory there is already non-negligible knowledge about the performances of the analytical method in that laboratory. For instance, precision and trueness must be evaluated by the sender laboratory in advance of the evaluation of the results in the receiver laboratory for method transfer performance. At least, there is information about the method precision coming from the analytical method validation that should provide information about the repeatability variance as well as about the intermediate precision variance. If the method has been used for a longer period, historical data may be used, for example coming from the control chart of QC samples.

In order to analyze the success of the assay transfer, the predictive probability of having future differences of results between the two laboratories within the previously chosen acceptance criteria $\pm\lambda$ can be estimated. If this probability is greater than a minimum pre-specified probability level, the analytical method transfer is declared successful.

20.5 Routine

The knowledge gathered during the analytical method's validation and transfer could then be used as informative priors for statistical analyzes of data obtained from subsequent development studies (e.g. processes optimization) or routine applications such as stability studies for drug substances and drug products. The posterior distribution of the intermediate precision variance is indeed available as informative prior for these new studies. As shown in the following sections, the predictive distribution obtained from analytical method's validation can be fine-tuned to find an assay format that can improve the probabilities of success of specific routine applications or even initiate the analytical method control strategy.

20.5.1 Format of the reportable value

A single analytical method or bioassay may be used for different applications such as batch release or shelf-life determination during stability studies. For each of these different applications, the assay format can be optimized based on the information gathered through assay validation, transfer, or even from development studies. The format of the reportable value implies defining how intermediate analytical results will be averaged to define the final result, called reportable value (U.S. Pharmacopeia, 2019a). Generally, only the latter figures on the Certificate of Analysis (CoA). For instance, for release purposes, the reportable value could be defined as the average of two replicates per ELISA plate obtained from two plates. Hence, the reportable value is obtained from four intermediate analytical results. The way to define and justify the format of the reportable value is to assess whether the predictive distribution of the reportable result obtained from a different format is narrow enough, or alternatively, to assess if the probability to fulfill the assay aim is high enough for the different assay format.

From validation studies, the assay variance of an individual result is:

$$\sigma_{IP}^2 = \sigma_{\alpha}^2 + \sigma_{\varepsilon}^2. \tag{20.9}$$

For a different format of n replicates per p runs the reportable result variance is:

$$\sigma_{n\times p}^2 = \frac{\sigma_{\alpha}^2}{p} + \frac{\sigma_{\varepsilon}^2}{np}. \tag{20.10}$$

For each combination of n and p, the predictive distribution of any future result of the defined format can be obtained and the corresponding predictive probability to fulfil the acceptance criteria λ can hence be estimated as shown on Figure 20.11.

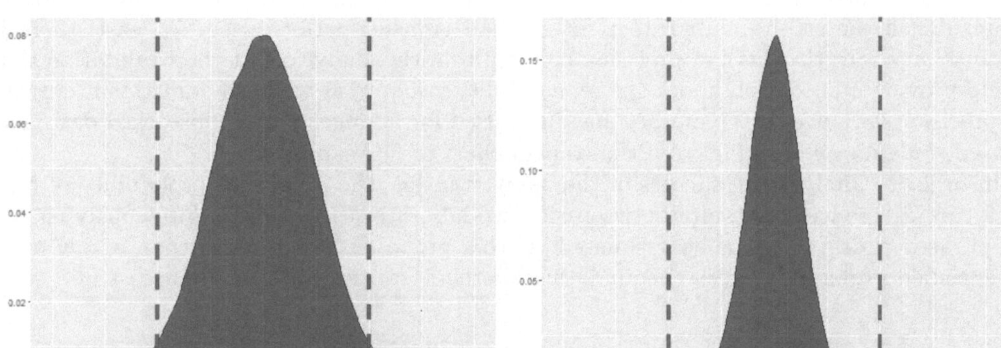

FIGURE 20.11: Predictive distributions of API concentrations of an analytical method for two formats. Left panel: 1×1 ($n \times p$) format for which the predictive probability to have any future result within the acceptance criteria $\lambda = [90\%, 110\%]$ (vertical dashed lines) is 0.79. Right panel: 2×2 format for which the predictive probability to have any future result within the acceptance criteria $\lambda = [90\%, 110\%]$ is 0.98.

The final format of the reportable value will be the $n \times p$ combination that achieves this goal. As expected, this can be extended to more variance components such as operators, equipment, days, plates, etc. These variance components can be easily estimated if the analytical method validation study is designed to explore their impact on the precision of the analytical method.

20.5.2 Control strategy

Quality by Design development of analytical procedure is useless without defining control strategy. This is done to ensure that the procedure remains under control during its routine application and to detect deviations. Again, analytical procedure validation can define a control strategy using quality control samples. For example, the performed experiments can define Bayesian prediction intervals that can be used as initial control limits when building analytical procedure control charts (Rozet et al., 2007). Out-of-control methods can efficiently be detected and corrective actions realized by following daily performances of analytical methods on such charts. Indeed, the use of prediction intervals ensures an adequate balance between consumer and producer risks (Rozet et al., 2007). Finally, when obtaining each new data point of the control chart, the control limits can be updated, providing a more precise estimation of the control limits of the assay.

20.6 Conclusion

The present chapter describes the key role that Analytical Quality by Design plays in the pharmaceutical industry for ensuring adequate analytical method performance and above all high reliability in the analytical results produced. The end result of AQbD is a thorough understanding of the analytical method behavior starting from analytical method development to method transfer and control.

The benefits of implementing pharmaceutical AQbD are to reduce process variability and defects, as a result of enhancing product development, manufacturing efficiencies and post-approval change management. This can be achieved by designing a robust formulation and manufacturing process. The key elements of AQbD include the analytical target profile (ATP) with implemented design of experiments (DoE) and design space (DS). Taken together, these methodologies assess and improve analytical method and assay capability during product lifecycle management.

Bibliography

Borman, P., Roberts, J., Jones, C., Hanna-Brown, M., Szucs, R., and Bale, S. (2010). The development phase of an LC method using QbD principles. *Separation Science*, 2(7):2–8.

Box, G. and Tiao, G. (1973). *Bayesian Inference in Statistical Analysis.* Addison-Wesley, Reading, MA.

Davidian, M. and Giltinan, D. (1995). *Nonlinear Models for Repeated Measurement Data.* Monographs on Statistics and Applied Probability. Chapman and Hall, London.

Deidda, R., Orlandini, S., Hubert, P., and Hubert, C. (2018). Risk-based Approach for Method Development in Pharmaceutical Quality Control Context: A Critical Review. *Journal of Pharmaceutical and Biomedical Analysis*, 161:110–121.

Dewé, W., Marini, R., Chiap, P., Hubert, P., Crommen, J., and Boulanger, B. (2004). Develoment of Response Models for Optimizing HPLC Methods. *Chemometrics and Intelligent Laboratory Systems*, 74:263–268.

Dispas, A., Desfontaine, V., Andri, B., Lebrun, P., Kotoni, D., Clarke, A., Guillarme, D., and Hubert, P. (2017). Quantitative Determination of Salbutamol Sulfate Impurities Using Achiral Supercritical Fluid Chromatography. *Journal of Pharmaceutical and Biomedical Analysis*, 134:170–180.

EudraLex (2014). The Rules Governing Medicinal Products in the European Union, volume 4. *EU Guidelines for Good Manufacturing Practice for Medicinal Products for Human and Vetenary Use - Part 1, Chapter 6: Quality Control.*

Geisser, S. (1965). Bayesian Estimation in Multivariate Analysis. *The Annals of Mathematical Statistics*, 36 (1):150–159.

Hamada, M., Johnson, V., and Moore, L. (2004). Bayesian Prediction Intervals and Their Relationship to Tolerance Intervals. *Technometrics*, 46(4):452–459.

Hanna-Brown, M., Barnett, K., Harrington, B., Graul, T., Morgado, J., Colgan, S., Wrisley, L.AND Szucs, R., Sluggett, G., Steeno, G., and Pellett, J. (2014). Using Quality by Design to Develop Robust Chromatographic Methods. *Pharmaceutical Technology*, 38(9):48–64.

Hubert, C., Houari, S., Rozet, E., Lebrun, P., and Hubert, P. (2015). Towards a Full Integration of Optimization and Validation Phases: An Analytical-Quality-by-Design Approach. *Journal of Chromatography A*, 1395:88–98.

Hubert, P., Nguyen-Huu, J.-J., Boulanger, B., Chapuzet, E., Chiap, P., Cohen, N., Compagnon, P.-A., Dewé, W., Feinberg, M., Lallier, M., Laurentie, M., Mercier, N., Muzard, G., Nivet, C., and Valat, L. (2004). Harmonization of Strategies for the Validation of Quantitative Analytical Procedures, A SFSTP Proposal - Part I. *Journal of Pharmaceutical and Biomedical Analysis*, 36(3):579–586.

Hubert, P., Nguyen-Huu, J.-J., Boulanger, B., Chapuzet, E., Cohen, N., Compagnon, P.-A., Dewé, W., Feinberg, M., Laurentie, M., Mercier, N., Muzard, G., and Valat, L. (2006). Validation des Procédures Analytiques Quantitatives : Harmonisation des Démarches, Partie II - Statistiques. *STP Pharma Pratiques*, 16(1):28–58.

Hubert, P., Nguyen-Huu, J.-J., Boulanger, B., Chapuzet, E., Cohen, N., Compagnon, P.-A., Dewé, W., Feinberg, M., Laurentie, M., Mercier, N., Muzard, G., Valat, L., and Rozet, E. (2007). Harmonization of Strategies for the Validation of Quantitative Analytical Procedures, A SFSTP Proposal-Part III. *Journal of Pharmaceutical and Biomedical Analysis*, 45:82–96.

ICH Q10 (2008). Guidance for Industry, Q10 Pharmaceutical Quality System. *International Conference on Harmonization (ICH) of Technical Requirements for Registration of Pharmaceuticals for Human Use.*

ICH Q2(R1) (2005). Topic Q2 (R1): Validation of Analytical Procedures: Text and Methodology. *International Conference on Harmonization (ICH) of Technical Requirements for Registration of Pharmaceuticals for Human Use.*

ICH Q8 (2009). Guidance for Industry, Q8 Pharmaceutical Development. *International Conference on Harmonization (ICH) of Technical Requirements for Registration of Pharmaceuticals for Human Use.*

ICH Q9 (2005). Guidance for Industry, Q9 Quality Risk Management. *International Conference on Harmonization (ICH) of Technical Requirements for Registration of Pharmaceuticals for Human Use.*

Joint Committee for Guides in Metrology (2018). JCGM 200:2012 - International Vocabulary of Metrology - Basic and General Concepts and Associated Terms.

Lamalle, C., Djang'Eing'A Marini, R., Debrus, B., Lebrun, P., Crommen, J., Hubert, P., Servais, A. C., and Fillet, M. (2012). Development of a Generic Micellar Electrokinetic Chromatography Method for the Separation of 15 Antimalarial Drugs as a Tool to Detect Medicine Counterfeiting. *Electrophoresis*, 33(11):1669–1678.

Lebrun, P., Boulanger, B., Debrus, B., Lambert, P., and Hubert, P. (2012). A Bayesian Design Space for Analytical Methods Based on Multivariate Models and Predictions. *Journal of Biopharmaceutical Statistics.*

Lebrun, P., Sondag, P., Lories, X., Michiels, J., Rozet, E., and Boulanger, B. (2018). Quality by Design Applied in Formulation Development and Robustness. In Coffey, T. and Yang, H., editors, *Statistics for Biotechnology Process Development.* Chapman and Hall/CRC.

Mee, R. (1984). Beta-Expectation and Beta-Content Tolerance Limits for Balanced One-Way ANOVA Random Model. *Technometrics*, 26(3):251–254.

Montgomery, D. (2009). *Design and Analysis of Experiments.* Wiley, New-York.

Nethercote, P., Borman, P., Bennett, T., Martin, G., and McGregor, P. (April 2010). QbD for Better Method Validation and Transfer. *Pharma Manufacturing.com*, pages 37–49.

Nethercote, P. and Ermer, J. (2012). Quality by Design for Analytical Methods: Implications for Method Validation and Transfer. *Pharmaceutical Technology*, 36(10):52.

Peterson, J. (2004). A Posterior Predictive Approach to Multiple Response Surface Optimization. *Journal of Quality Technology*, 36:139–153.

Peterson, J. (2008). A Bayesian Approach to the ICH Q8 Qefinition of Design Space . *Journal of Biopharmaceutical Statistics*, 18:959–975.

Peterson, J. and Lief, K. (2010). The ICH Q8 Definition of Design Space: A Comparison of the Overlapping Means and the Bayesian Predictive Approaches. *Statistics in Biopharmaceutical Research*, 2:249–259.

Peterson, J. and Yahyah, M. (2009). A Bayesian Design Space Approach to Robustness and System Suitability for Pharmaceutical Assays and Other Processes. *Statistics in Biopharmaceutical Research*, 1(4):441–449.

Rausand, M. and Hoyland, A. (2004). *System Reliability Theory: Models, Statistical Methods, and Applications.* John Wiley and Sons, Hoboken, 2nd edition.

Rozet, E., Govaerts, B., Lebrun, P., Michail, K., Ziemons, E., Wintersteiger, R., Rudaz, S., Boulanger, B., , and Hubert, P. (2011). Evaluating the Reliability of Analytical Results Using a Probability Criterion: A Bayesian Perspective. *Analytica Chimica Acta*, 705(1-2): 193–206.

Rozet, E., Hubert, C., Ceccato, A., Dewé, W., Ziemons, E., Moonen, F., Michail, K., Wintersteiger, R., Streel, B., Boulanger, B., and Hubert, P. (2007). Using Tolerance Intervals in Pre-study Validation of Analytical Methods to Predict In-study Results. The Fit-for-Future-Purpose Concept. *Journal of Chromatography A*, 1158(1-2):126–137.

Rozet, E., Lebrun, P., Hubert, P., Debrus, B., and Boualnger, B. (2013). Design Spaces for Analytical Methods. *Trends in Analytical Chemistry*, 42:157–167.

Rozet, E., Lebrun, P., Michiels, J., Sondag, P., Scherder, T., and Boulanger, B. (2015). Analytical Procedure Validation and the Quality by Design Paradigm. *Journal of Biopharmaceutical Statistics*, 25(2):260–268.

Rozet, E., Ziemons, E., Marini, R., Boulanger, B., and Hubert, P. (2012). Quality by Design Compliant Analytical Method Validation. *Analytical Chemistry*, 84((1)):106–112.

Schweitzer, M., Pohl, M., Hanna-Brown, M., Nethercote, P., Borman, P., Hansen, G., Smith, K., and Larew, J. (2010). Implications and Opportunities of Applying QbD Principles to Analytical Measurements. *Pharmaceutical Technology*, 34(2):52–59.

U.S. Food and Drug Administration (2004). PAT, A Framework for Innovative Pharmaceutical Manufacturing and Quality Assurance. *Guidance for Industry.*

U.S. Food and Drug Administration (2009). Pharmaceutical cGMP for the 21st Century – A Risk-Based Approach: Second Progress Report and Implementation Plan. *Department of Health and Human Services, accessed 08/17/2009.*

U.S. Food and Drug Administration (2015). Analytical Procedures and Methods Validation for Drugs and Biologics. *Guidance for Industry.*

U.S. Food and Drug Administration (January 2011). Process Validation: General Principles and Practices. *Guidance for Industry.*

U.S. Pharmacopeia (2019a). Biological Assay Validation. *Chapter <1033>*, Accessed Jan. 2019.

U.S. Pharmacopeia (2019b). Transfer of Analytical Procedures. *Chapter <1224>*, Accessed Jan. 2019.

Verch, T. (2014). Application of Quality by Design and Statistical Quality Control Concepts in Immunoassays. *Bioanalysis*, 6(23):3251–3260.

Wolfinger, R. (1998). Tolerance Intervals for Variance Component Models Using Bayesian Simulation. *Journal of Quality Technology*, 30(1):18–32.

Yarovoi, H., Frey, T., Bouaraphan, S., Retzlaff, M., and Verch, T. (2013). Quality by Design for a Vaccine Release Immunoassay: A Case Study. *Bioanalysis*, 5(20):2531–2545.

Yu, L. (2008). Pharmaceutical Quality by Design: Product and Process Development, Understanding, and Control. *Pharmaceutical Research*, 25:781–791.

21

Bayesian Methods for the Design and Analysis of Stability Studies

Tonakpon Hermane Avohou
University of Liége, Belgium

Pierre Lebrun
Pharmalex, Belgium

Eric Rozet
Pharmalex, Belgium

Bruno Boulanger
Pharmalex, Belgium

Stability testing is required by regulation to obtain marketing approval for any new drug product and ICH Q1 guidance is followed worldwide for that purpose. Based on experimental results, a unique shelf-life and storage instructions applicable to the future batches of the drug product manufactured and packaged under similar conditions should be established. Recently, the entire pharmaceutical regulatory framework has been changing towards a science and risk-based paradigm for process and product development.

As a consequence, stability studies are facing the emergence of new issues related to quality risk management going from the quantification of the risk of Out-of-Specification products in future production, the determination of a shelf-life that guarantees acceptable risks to both patients and manufacturers, the definition of a robust set of storage conditions under which the labelled shelf-life remains valid, to the validation of a process modification and so on. Statistical modelling plays a prominent role in the design and analysis of stability studies. The focus of this chapter is on the benefits of using the Bayesian framework to manage risks and make decisions, in the place of the commonly used traditional frequentist methods to support the evaluation of stability data. Adequate formalization of the stability problem is addressed in this chapter together with proposals of generic designs and models. The pitfalls of the commonly used frequentist approaches are highlighted. Then the Bayesian modelling framework and how it overcomes the limitations of the frequentist methods by enabling a natural, flexible and reliable quality risk management are presented and illustrated by a case study of Bayesian modelling of stability data.

21.1 Introduction

Once a batch of drug is produced, it starts aging, waiting in a warehouse or in pharmacies for its final destination. For the patient, it is however critical that the drug he will take is still fully potent and not toxic at the time of medication, despite degradation(s) that might occur during this aging process. Interestingly, the drug product stability or instability during the time depends upon the ways the manufacturer has designed its process, the drug formulation (excipients, preservatives...). It also depends upon how the manufacturer is able to control appropriate raw materials at reception, and finally how storage conditions are defined and controlled. Hence, for the manufacturer, in turn, the drug stability will be an ultimate control of drug consistency, from release to shelf-life. Degradation might occur naturally, but all (the quality attributes of) commercial batches are expected to degrade the same way during the time a drug is fit for consumption, i.e. during its labelled shelf-life. It should reach and remain a satisfactory level of efficacy and safety. This means a drug substance stored under the recommended conditions is expected to remain within its approved specifications. The role of stability studies is to demonstrate exactly this.

Stability testing is required by regulation to obtain marketing approval for any new drug product. Worldwide, one of the most important guidances that is followed is without contest the ICH Q1 document (ICH, 2003b). The ultimate goal of stability testing is to establish, based on trial data, a unique shelf-life and storage instructions applicable to the future batches of the drug product manufactured and packaged under similar conditions (ICH, 2003b,a; Chow, 2007; Huynh-Ba, 2009).

For a long time, the evaluation of stability data for regulatory approval has almost exclusively focused on estimating the product shelf-life for regulatory compliance, without a real concern for quality assurance (Capen et al., 2012; Quinlan et al., 2013b). In recent years, however, the entire pharmaceutical regulatory framework has been changing towards a science and risk-based paradigm for process and product development. Accordingly, the entire pharmaceutical industry has been moving towards risk-based approaches at any phase of drug development (Capen et al., 2012; Peterson et al., 2009; Stroup and Quinlan, 2016; Yang, 2012, 2017). As a consequence, stability studies are facing the emergence of new issues related to quality risk management. Examples of such issues include: (1) the quantification of the risk of Out-of-Specification (OOS) or compromised products (lots or dosage units) in future production, (2) the quantification of the risk of rejecting conforming products, (3) the choice of a shelf-life that guarantees acceptable risks to both patients and manufacturers, (4) the definition of a robust set of storage conditions under which the labelled shelf-life remains valid, and (5) the guarantees provided on a quality statement on released lots.

Besides setting a valid shelf-life for regulatory approval, stability studies may be exploited for several purposes during post-marketing studies, including for instance: (1) updating the product shelf-life and release limits, (2) providing quality assurance of the robustness of the manufacturing process after a process modification, and other changes such as site, scale, formulation, storage, or shipping conditions (Capen et al., 2012; Quinlan et al., 2013b; Peterson et al., 2009; Stroup and Quinlan, 2016; Yang, 2012, 2017).

Statistical modelling plays a prominent role in the design and analysis of stability studies (ICH, 2003a; Peterson et al., 2009) It is the key decision-making tool to choose a shelf-life and manage risks. Therefore, any statistical method that is meant to support shelf-life establishment should be fully consistent with the quality assurance objectives. In other words, it should enable drug manufacturers to understand, reliably assess, and manage quality risks during the entire product life-cycle (Capen et al., 2012; Stroup and Quinlan, 2016; Yang, 2012, 2017; Quinlan et al., 2013a; Capen et al., 2018).

The focus of this chapter is on the benefits of using the Bayesian framework to manage risks and make decisions, in the place of the commonly used traditional frequentist methods to support the evaluation of stability data. The structure of the chapter is as follows. Section 21.2 summarizes the recent discussions on the objectives and questions to be addressed by stability data modelling. Section 21.3 introduces the generic designs and models generally used in stability studies. Section 21.4 presents an overview of frequentist statistical approaches that are currently used to estimate these models. We underscore their pitfalls as tools to properly make decisions and address the emerging quality risk management issues during stability studies. Section 21.5 presents the Bayesian modeling framework and how it overcomes the limitations of the frequentist methods by enabling a natural, flexible and reliable quality risk management. The chapter ends by an illustrative case study of Bayesian modeling of stability data.

21.2 New perspectives on the objectives and methods of stability data analysis

The ICH Q1 guidance states that stability data evaluation must establish a shelf-life or expiration date applicable to all future batches of the drug product. The implications of this for statistical modeling have been recently revisited in the literature, especially by the Stability Shelf Lives Working Group (SSLWG) of the Product Quality Research Institute (PQRI; see in particular Capen et al., 2012; Quinlan et al., 2013b; Capen et al., 2018). In short, the SSLWG demonstrates that because of natural but uncontrollable variations in the process, a shelf-life computed under ICH Q1E protocol, that would be valid for all future batches, is not practically achievable. The goal of shelf-life estimation should therefore be to determine storage times and conditions providing guarantees that the future production of the batches meets specifications with an acceptably high probability, and without putting manufacturers at risk of prematurely discarding safe and efficacious drug product (Capen et al., 2012; Quinlan et al., 2013b; Yang, 2017; Quinlan et al., 2013a; Capen et al., 2018). Clearly, while not explicitly mentioned by the ICH guidance, the phrase applicable to all future batches of the drug product defines a type of quality (probability) statement. To achieve this goal, one needs to reliably quantify the probability that the future production of the drug substance succeeds or fails to meet specifications (patient risks). One also needs to quantify the probability of rejecting future conforming lots of the product (producer risks).

It must be emphasized that, contrary to the SSLWG, several authors argued that to reliably control patient risks, the labelled shelf-life should be applicable to most future individual dosages or units of any future batch. Hence, shelf-life estimation should focus on minimizing the risk of out-of-specification dosages or units, so as to guarantee that safe drugs are delivered to patients.

From a statistical perspective, properly addressing all these goals involves the need to make predictions and posterior probability statements about the quality of future drug production, given the existing scientific knowledge (e.g. Process Performance Qualification and stability trials) and taking into account as many sources of uncertainty as possible. For such probability statements and risk quantification to be possible, an explicit probability distribution of quality attributes (QA) of interest is required. Clearly, the most appropriate statistical methods to address these needs are the ones able to derive the predictive distribution of the QA of interest, accounting for model parameters' uncertainty and unavoidable process variations (Peterson, 2010; Peterson et al., 2017). Examples of such methods include bootstrap-based methods, fiducial methods and Bayesian methods.

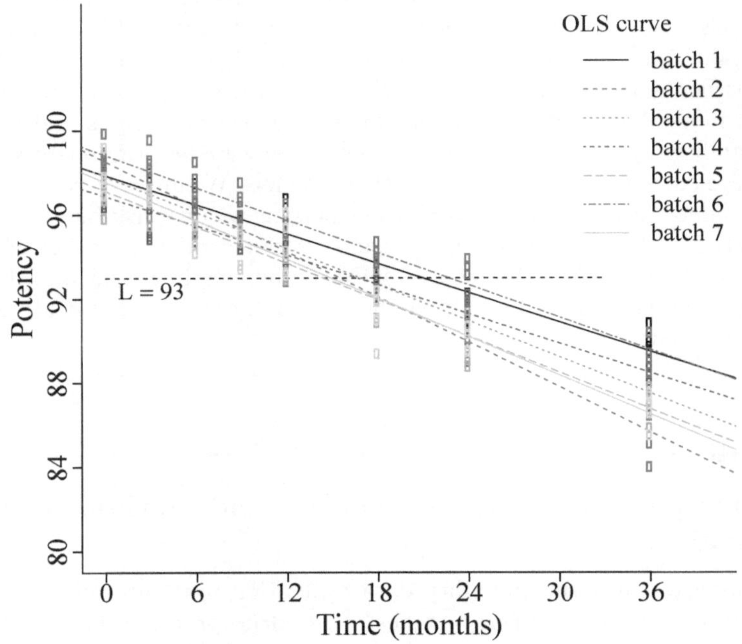

FIGURE 21.1: Illustration of classical ICH Q1 stability data for potency attributes of a drug product.

21.3 Stability designs, models and assumptions

Let Y denote the limiting attribute (QA) of interest in a stability study. We assume that the observed variability of Y at time t, is explained by two sources of variation typical of the manufacturing process, namely the between-batch and the within-batch variabilities. Commonly, the between-batch variability refers to the process variations, while the within-batch variability is related to the measurement of the units used in stability trials. For modeling stability data, the ICH guidance recommends a design including at least three batches. At specified times of release ($t = 0$), and then at $t = 3, 6, 9, 12, 18, 24, 36$ months for a 3-year study, each batch is sampled and Y is measured. This type of design will be used throughout the chapter. As illustration, a representation of such stability data for one attribute (Potency) measured over 7 batches is shown in Figure 21.1.

After generating the data, stability data evaluation starts by postulating a statistical model to describe the relationship between Y and t. Low-order polynomial (linear, quadratic or cubic) or non-linear (exponential or logistic decay) regression models may be chosen depending on the behavior of the stability-limiting attribute (ICH, 2003a; Chow, 2007). In the interest of clarity of the description of various methods throughout the chapter, Y is assumed to be positive and linearly decreasing with the storage time t. The extension to more complex polynomial or non-linear models is straightforward.

In addition to providing a precise approximation of the stability curve, the model should be consistent with the data generation process or design (Quinlan et al., 2013b). Two categories of models differing in the assumptions on the data generation process are in use. The first category, hereto referred as regulatory model, assumes the batch effect is fixed (ICH, 2003a; Chow, 2007). The model is written:

$$\begin{aligned} Y_{ij} &\sim \mathrm{N}(\mu_{ij}, \sigma_\varepsilon^2) \\ \mu_{ij} &= b_{0j} + b_{1j} t_{ij} \quad \text{(separate model for each batch)}, \end{aligned} \tag{21.1}$$

or, more ideally, as

$$\mu_{ij} = b_0 + b_{0j} + b_1 t_{ij} + b_{1j} t_{ij} \quad \text{(common variance model)}.$$

The second category, the random batch-effect (mixed effect) model considers a batch as a random realization of the population of all future batches produced under similar manufacturing conditions. This model, of the form of a mixed model, is written:

$$\begin{aligned} Y_{ij} &\sim \mathrm{N}(\mu_{ij}, \sigma_\varepsilon^2) \\ \mu_{ij} &= \beta_{0j} + \beta_{1j} t_{ij} \\ \boldsymbol{\beta}_j &= (\beta_{0j}, \beta_{1j}) \sim \mathrm{N}(\boldsymbol{b}, \boldsymbol{D}), \end{aligned} \tag{21.2}$$

or in matrix notation

$$\begin{aligned} \boldsymbol{Y} &\sim \mathrm{N}(\boldsymbol{\mu}, \sigma_\varepsilon^2 \boldsymbol{I}_n) \\ \boldsymbol{\mu} &= \boldsymbol{X}\boldsymbol{b} + \boldsymbol{Z}\boldsymbol{\beta} \\ \boldsymbol{\beta} &\sim \mathrm{N}(\boldsymbol{0}, \boldsymbol{G}). \end{aligned}$$

In Equations (21.1) and (21.2), Y_{ij} denotes the measured QA of the i−th unit measured at a particular time t ($i = 1, \ldots, n_j$) drawn from the jth ($j = 1, \ldots, J$) batch; n_j is the total number of tested units from batch j, and J is the total number of batches considered in the stability analysis; $n = \sum_{j=1}^{J} n_j$ is the total number of tested units of the study; t_{ij} is the storage time of the ith unit from the jth batch; In Equation (21.1), b_{0j} and b_{1j} are the variable obtained after the dummy coding for the intercepts and slopes of each batch and b_0 and b_1 are the main intercept and slope (whose interpretation depends upon the aforementioned dummy coding).

In Equation (21.2) $\boldsymbol{\beta}_j$ is a 2×1 vector of latent intercept and slope for batch j ($\boldsymbol{\beta}$ simply stacks all batch latent variables), while $\boldsymbol{b} = (b_0, b_1)^\top$ is a 2×1 vector of global mean intercept and slope for all batches; $\boldsymbol{D} = \begin{bmatrix} \sigma_0^2 & \rho\sigma_0\sigma_1 \\ \rho\sigma_0\sigma_1 & \sigma_1^2 \end{bmatrix}$ is the positive semi-definite covariance matrix of $\boldsymbol{\beta}_j$, where σ_0 and σ_1 are the standard deviations of batch intercepts (β_{0j}) and slopes (β_{1j}) respectively, and ρ the correlation coefficient between β_{0j} and β_{1j}; $\sigma_\varepsilon^2 > 0$ is the variance of the residual; $\boldsymbol{X}$ is the design matrix for fixed effects and $\boldsymbol{Z}$ is the design matrix of random effects; $\boldsymbol{G}$ is a block-diagonal matrix with J identical blocks $\boldsymbol{D}$. Finally, the variance of $\boldsymbol{y}$ is the $n \times n$ matrix $\boldsymbol{V} = \boldsymbol{Z}\boldsymbol{G}\boldsymbol{Z}^\top + \sigma_\varepsilon^2 \boldsymbol{I}_n$.

There have been extensive discussions on which model is most consistent with stability designs. Theoretical and empirical evidences from these discussions showed the random batch-effect model is the most appropriate for the following reasons: first, the degradation model under random batch-effect is more generalizable to future batches of the drug product. Second, it enables shelf-life estimates that are more consistent with the true product shelf-life than the fixed batch-effect, provided a reasonable number of batches is included (Quinlan et al., 2013b; Stroup and Quinlan, 2016). The reader is referred to the relevant literature for more details (Capen et al., 2012; Quinlan et al., 2013b; Stroup and Quinlan, 2016; Kiermeier et al., 2012; Altan et al., 2013).

21.4 Overview of frequentist methods of analysis of stability data and their pitfalls

In this section, we present an overview of the major frequentist methods currently used or proposed to estimate shelf-life. We discuss their limitations for properly addressing the quality risk management issues that are at the heart of the ICH Q1E objective. A comprehensive description of the mathematical development, implementation and performance evaluation of these methods can be found in the relevant literature (Chow, 2007; Quinlan et al., 2013b,a; Stroup and Quinlan, 2016; Yang, 2017). All formulæ below assume a decreasing attribute (e.g. potency) over the time, and hence showcase the computation of a one-sided lower bound for the various intervals. In case of an increasing attribute (e.g. an impurity), the formulae (mainly the quantiles) can be reversed to obtain a one-sided upper boundary. If two-sided estimation is needed, coverage and confidence levels should be adapted accordingly.

21.4.1 Methods for shelf-life estimation

21.4.1.1 Methods based on confidence intervals

Confidence interval methods compute the shelf-life $\widehat{t}_L$ as the time when the 95% one-sided lower confidence interval $L(t)$ of the product mean degradation curve intersects the specification limit L (Chow, 2007). Several strategies are in use to compute the confidence limits of the mean stability curve. The most widespread of these methods is the ICH Q1E method for continuous quality attributes (ICH, 2003a; Chow, 2007; Altan et al., 2013). With this strategy, Equation (21.1) is used to model the data, typically through an analysis of covariance (ANCOVA) scheme. Batch poolability is tested using hypothesis tests of equality of slopes and intercepts and following a specific protocol. In this protocol, as odd as it may seem, the test decision is made with a Type I error rate $\alpha = 0.25$: H_0: $b_{1j} = b_{1k}$ and $b_{0j} = b_{0k}$, $\forall j \neq k$ (Altan et al., 2013). If the intercepts and slopes are judged equal according to the protocol ($P-$value > 0.25), a common slope, or a common slope and intercept regression model for the batches is applied. In case of pooling of batches, the shelf-life is estimated as

$$\widehat{t}_L = \inf\{t \geq 0 : L(t) \leq L\},$$

where $L(t)$ is the 95% lower confidence limit of the mean curve and inf denotes the infimum or smallest lowest bound.

Otherwise, if the batches are not poolable, a regression model is fitted to each batch separately in line with ICH Q1 — or Equation (21.1) might be used to get a common variability — and the shelf-life is estimated as the worst-case shelf-life among the batches::

$$\widehat{t}_L = \min\{\widehat{t}_j\}_{j=1}^{J} \text{ with } \widehat{t}_j = \inf\{t \geq 0 : L_j(t) \leq L\}.$$

where $L_j(t)$ is the lower 95% confidence interval on batch j.

One of the first criticisms of the regulatory method is that it treats batch effect as fixed, hence limiting generalizations to the entire population of batches. Moreover, it may excessively underestimate the true mean shelf-life (Quinlan et al., 2013a). To overcome this limitation, Quinlan et al. (2013b) explored the lower confidence limits of the mean curve using a mixed model framework described in Equation (21.2). The proposed labelled-shelf-life is then computed as:

$$\widehat{t}_L = \inf\left\{t \geq 0 : \widehat{b}_0 + \widehat{b}_1 t - Qt_{\alpha,n-p^*}\sqrt{\boldsymbol{x}'(\boldsymbol{X}'\widehat{\boldsymbol{V}}^{-1}\boldsymbol{X})^{-}\boldsymbol{x}} \leq L\right\}. \tag{21.3}$$

This method is called the *reflection method* by the authors (Quinlan et al., 2013b).

In Equation (21.3), $\widehat{b}_0$ and $\widehat{b}_1$ are the maximum likelihood estimates (ML) of b_0 and b_1; $\widehat{\boldsymbol{V}}$ is the restricted maximum likelihood (REML) of $\boldsymbol{V}$; $\widehat{y}_0$ is the predicted value of Y at the point where the mean curve $\widehat{b}_0 + \widehat{b}_1 t$ intersects L; $(\boldsymbol{X}'\widehat{\boldsymbol{V}}^{-1}\boldsymbol{X})^-$ is the generalized inverse of $\boldsymbol{X}'\widehat{\boldsymbol{V}}^{-1}\boldsymbol{X}$; $Qt_{\alpha,n-p^*}$ is the the quantile of Student distribution with probability $1-\alpha$ and degree of freedom $n-p^*$, n is the sample size and p^* is the rank of $\boldsymbol{X}$.

Whatever the designs used to compute the confidence interval, these methods only provide a quality assurance that the mean of all units of a batch are within the acceptance limits. Therefore, they do not ensure the conformance of most individual dosages to the specifications (Capen et al., 2012; Kiermeier et al., 2012; Quinlan et al., 2013a; Yang, 2017).

21.4.1.2 Methods based on prediction intervals

To address the inconsistency of confidence interval methods with the objective of providing assurance that future individual units meet specifications, some authors use prediction (β−expectation) intervals in the place of confidence intervals, to predict the behaviors of single dosages or units. For a pooled batches scenario for example, the shelf-life is computed as:

$$\widehat{t}_L = \min\left\{ t \geq 0 : \widehat{b}_0 + \widehat{b}_1 t - \widehat{\sigma}_\varepsilon Qt_{\beta,n-2}\sqrt{1 + \left[\frac{1}{n} + \frac{(t-\bar{t})^2}{\sum_{i=1}^n (t-\bar{t})^2}\right]}\right\}.$$

The shelf-life based on the (one sided-lower)$\beta\%$ expected coverage prediction interval has been proven to be more conservative than the one based on confidence intervals. The reader is referred to (Yang, 2017) for further details on theoretical and simulation evidence of the performance of the shelf-life based on frequentist prediction intervals compared to the confidence interval methods. However, in this interval, the coverage is merely expected, and no confidence level can be quantified.

21.4.1.3 Methods based on tolerance intervals

To address the limitations of the frequentist confidence and prediction intervals, some authors proposed the use of a $\beta-\gamma$ tolerance interval of Y (Komka et al., 2010; Capen et al., 2012; Kiermeier et al., 2012; Yang and Zhang, 2012; Quinlan et al., 2013a). The point is to be able to guarantee with $\gamma\%$ confidence that a particular coverage (of dosages or units) will be above the specification. Hence, the shelf-life is estimated as the time when a tolerance interval of Y equals the specification limits. One proposed model to compute the shelf-life is:

$$\widehat{t}_L = \inf\left\{ t \geq 0 : \widehat{b}_0 + \widehat{b}_1 t - Qt_{\beta,df,\delta}\sqrt{\boldsymbol{x}'(\boldsymbol{X}'\widehat{\boldsymbol{V}}^{-1}\boldsymbol{X})^-\boldsymbol{x}} \leq L\right\},$$

where β is the coverage level and γ define a quantile of the distribution of Y, such as $\delta = -\Phi^{-1}(\gamma)\sqrt{J}$ is the $(1-\gamma)$ quantile of a non-central t-distribution with *df* degrees of freedom and non-centrality parameter δ (Quinlan et al., 2013b). Another similar method was proposed by Kiermeier et al. (2012), but these tolerance interval-based methods do not appear to be much used in practice.

21.4.2 Methods for the estimation of probabilities of OOS

As already discussed in Section 21.2, to be able to effectively ascertain the quality of some drug product (e.g. vaccines), drug manufacturers would need to assess the level of risk of

OOS dosage units or batches associated with the chosen product shelf-life during stability studies (Capen et al., 2012; Yang and Zhang, 2012; Quinlan et al., 2013b; Yang, 2017). Given the mixed model (21.2), this probability is defined as the fraction of the marginal distribution of Y that falls within $]0, L]$ at time t. Hence, it is expressed as a function of the model parameters as:

$$
\begin{aligned}
p(\pi(t) \mid \boldsymbol{\theta}) &= \int_0^L p(y \mid \boldsymbol{\theta}; t)\mathrm{d}y \\
&= \Phi\left(\frac{(L - \boldsymbol{x}(t)^\top \boldsymbol{\beta})}{\sqrt{\sigma_\varepsilon^2 + \boldsymbol{x}(t)^\top \boldsymbol{D}\boldsymbol{x}(t)}}\right),
\end{aligned}
\tag{21.4}
$$

where $\pi(t) \in [0, 1]$ denotes the probability OOS of the entire production at time t; $\Phi(\cdot)$ denotes the cumulative standard Normal distribution function; $\boldsymbol{\theta} = \{\boldsymbol{b}, \boldsymbol{D}, \sigma_\varepsilon^2\} \in \boldsymbol{\Theta}$ denotes a set of the parameters $\boldsymbol{b}$, $\boldsymbol{D}$, and σ_ε^2.

As for previous equations, computing Equation (21.4) in the frequentist framework is mathematically challenging. A naïve approach would consist of plugging in the crude point estimates of the mixed model parameters. The resulting point estimate would be highly sensitive to the uncertainty of the estimates of $\boldsymbol{\theta}$. A possible method to overcome this flaw is to use the concepts of fiducial statistics and generalized pivotal quantity. However, these methods are also mathematically engaged and non-trivial (Weerahandi, 1993).

21.4.3 Pitfalls of risk management with frequentist methods

As already discussed in Section 21.2, the confidence interval methods perform poorly in providing quality assurance that the product meets specifications at the shelf-life. This can be slightly improved by computing a confidence interval accounting for the batch random effect, but this would still fail at providing guarantee that the (individual) drug a patient would take is still of sufficient quality. The prediction interval and tolerance interval methods perform better as they enable control of patient risks. However, they inherit drawbacks common to all frequentist methods: they can only use the information provided by the data from the stability trial (no prior knowledge) and quickly become difficult to compute. The mathematical issue of plug-in point estimates might also give concern when the parameter uncertainty is high (high variability, low degrees of freedom).

21.5 Bayesian methods of analysis of stability data

In this section, we present the Bayesian approach for modeling stability data. We show that it offers a unified and coherent modeling and decision-making framework that can reliably and flexibly address most quality risk management issues of interest in a stability study. Particularly, it enables one to easily and reliably derive the predictive distribution of the quality attribute. Using the Monte-Carlo framework of Bayesian simulation allows making use of such distribution to derive any other quantity of interest such as shelf-life or risk of OOS. Moreover, it enables a natural and principled way of combining prior knowledge of the drug with the stability data, possibly making inference more precise.

21.5.1 Bayesian estimation of the drug stability models

In the Bayesian framework, model (21.2) is estimated as follows. First, any existing information on the drug is summarized and translated into prior probability density of the model parameters that represents the belief about these parameters before the current stability data are examined. Prior belief is generally and preferably based on existing data. If no substantial prior information is available, then non-informative or weakly informative prior densities may be used. Let $p(\boldsymbol{b})$, $p(\sigma_\varepsilon)$ and $p(\boldsymbol{D})$ denote our prior densities of $\boldsymbol{b}$, σ_ε and $\boldsymbol{D}$ respectively. The most common form of $p(\boldsymbol{b})$ is a bivariate Normal. $p(\sigma_\varepsilon)$ is generally assumed to be an Inverse-Gamma or a Half-Cauchy density. Possible forms for $p(\boldsymbol{D})$ are either product of independent uniform priors on the standard deviations and the correlation coefficient of the batch intercepts and slopes, or product of Half-Cauchy densities on the standard deviations and an LKJ density on the correlation matrix of of the batch intercepts and slopes (Gelman, 2006).

Second, the likelihood of the parameter given the data is written:

$$\begin{aligned}\mathcal{L}(\boldsymbol{\beta}, \boldsymbol{D}, \sigma_\varepsilon^2 \mid \mathcal{D}) &= p(\boldsymbol{Y} \mid \boldsymbol{\beta}, \sigma_\varepsilon^2, D) p(\boldsymbol{\beta} \mid \boldsymbol{b}, \boldsymbol{D}) \\ &= \prod_{j=1}^{J} \prod_{i=1}^{n_j} N(Y_{ij} \mid \boldsymbol{x}'_{ij}\boldsymbol{\beta}_j, \sigma_\varepsilon^2) \times \prod_{j=1}^{J} N(\boldsymbol{\beta}_j \mid \boldsymbol{b}, \boldsymbol{D})\end{aligned}$$

where $\mathcal{L}(\cdot)$ is the likelihood function and $\mathcal{D}$ denotes the observed stability data.

Third, the joint posterior distribution of the model parameters is derived using the Bayes theorem as the product of the likelihood and the prior densities as follows,

$$p(\boldsymbol{b}, \boldsymbol{D}, \tau_e \mid \mathcal{D}) \propto \mathcal{L}(\boldsymbol{b}, \boldsymbol{D}, \sigma_\varepsilon \mid \mathcal{D}) \times p(\boldsymbol{b}) \times p(\boldsymbol{D}) \times p(\sigma_\varepsilon).$$

Often, the analytic form of this joint posterior distribution is not tractable, and it can be approximated using one of the several Markov Chain Monte Carlo techniques. This posterior distribution is the key output to Bayesian stability data modelling. It summarizes our uncertainty about model parameters after the data have been observed and all subsequent inferences follow from it. Particularly, the predictive distribution of any quantity — e.g. predictive distribution of Y, predictive distribution of batch shelf-life, probability of OOS — which is a function of the model parameters can be derived by propagating uncertainty from a Monte Carlo sample of the posterior distribution of the parameters to the quantity or function of interest. Of specific interest, the predictive distribution of Y at any time t, denoted $p(\tilde{y} \mid t; \mathcal{D})$, can be computed by propagating uncertainty from the posterior distribution of the parameters to Y as follows :

$$p(\tilde{y} \mid t; \mathcal{D}) = \int_{\boldsymbol{\Theta}} p(\tilde{y} \mid \boldsymbol{\theta})\, p(\boldsymbol{\theta} \mid t; \mathcal{D})\, \mathrm{d}\boldsymbol{\theta}, \tag{21.5}$$

where $\tilde{y}$ denotes a future value of Y, $\boldsymbol{\theta} = \{\boldsymbol{b}, \boldsymbol{D}, \sigma_\varepsilon^2\} \in \boldsymbol{\Theta}$ denotes a set of the parameters $\boldsymbol{b}$, $\boldsymbol{D}$, and σ_ε^2, and $\boldsymbol{\Theta}$ represent the parameters space. It is noted that to obtain the predictive distribution of any future value of Y, it is first mandatory to get the distribution of the random effects $\tilde{\boldsymbol{\theta}}$ for the future batches:

$$p(\tilde{y} \mid t; \mathcal{D}) = \int_{\Theta} p(\tilde{y} \mid t, \tilde{\boldsymbol{\theta}}) p(\tilde{\boldsymbol{\theta}} \mid \boldsymbol{\theta}) p(\boldsymbol{\theta} \mid \mathcal{D}) d\boldsymbol{\theta}. \tag{21.6}$$

21.5.2 Methods for shelf-life estimation

21.5.2.1 Method based on tolerance interval

In the Bayesian framework, a one-sided β-expectation tolerance interval is derived as the $(1-\beta)$-quantile of the predictive distribution of Y (Guttman, 1988). A shelf-life based on the β-expectation tolerance interval can then be estimated as timepoint when the $(1-\beta)$-quantile of the predictive distribution of Y (Equations 21.5 and 21.6), intersects the specification limit L. Formally,

$$\widehat{t}_L = \inf\{t \geq 0 : Q_{1-\beta}(\tilde{y} \mid t) \leq L\}, \tag{21.7}$$

where $Q_{1-\beta}(\tilde{y} \mid t)$ is the $(1-\beta)$-quantile of the predictive distribution of Y at time t.

21.5.2.2 Method based on the predictive distribution of batch shelf-life

Similar to what has been proposed by Quinlan et al. (2013a), the predictive distribution of the batch shelf-life can be derived by propagating the uncertainty from the posterior distribution of the model parameters to the batch shelf-life, as follows:

$$p(\tilde{T}_m \mid \mathcal{D}) = \int_{\boldsymbol{\Theta}} p(\tilde{T}_m \mid b_{0m}, b_{1m}) \times p\,(b_{0m}, b_{1m} \mid \boldsymbol{\theta}) \times p\,(\boldsymbol{\theta} \mid \mathcal{D})\,\mathrm{d}\boldsymbol{\theta}. \tag{21.8}$$

In practice, one can simply back-predict the predictive distribution through the model and proceed using Monte Carlo simulations as $T^{(m)} = \left(L^{(m)} - b_{0m}\right)/b_{1m}$, with $L^{(m)}$ being the mth sample generated from a Normal distribution centered on L with variance equal to the posterior variance $\sigma_\varepsilon^2 \mid \mathcal{D}$; and b_{0m} and b_{1m} being the mth samples of the (predictive) posterior distribution of the random effects.

21.5.3 Methods for estimation of probabilities of OOS

The predictive distribution of $\pi(t)$, denoted $p\big(\pi(t) \mid \mathcal{D}\big)$, can be derived by propagating uncertainties from the joint posterior distribution of the model parameters to the expression for $\pi(t)$ as follows:

$$p\big(\pi(t) \mid \mathcal{D}\big) = \int_{\boldsymbol{\Theta}} p\big(\pi(t) \mid \boldsymbol{\theta}\big) p(\boldsymbol{\theta} \mid \mathcal{D}) \mathrm{d}\boldsymbol{\theta}, \tag{21.9}$$

where $p(\pi(t) \mid \boldsymbol{\theta})$ is defined as in (21.4). Then this distribution can be summarized by its mean, median or mode.

Alternatively, the expected value of $\pi(t)$, denoted $\mathrm{E}\big[\pi(t) \mid \mathcal{D}\big]$, can be computed by taking the expectation of (21.9) with respect to the joint posterior distribution of the model parameters. This is equivalent to integrating the posterior predictive density of Y in Equations 21.5 and 21.6 over the OOS domain, $[0, L]$, that is,

$$\mathrm{E}\big[\pi(t) \mid \mathcal{D}\big] = \int_0^L p\big(\tilde{y} \mid t; \mathcal{D}\big) \mathrm{d}\tilde{y}. \tag{21.10}$$

The integral in Equation (21.10) is not tractable and is evaluated numerically using a Monte Carlo integration as follows:

$$\int_0^L p\big(\tilde{y} \mid t; \mathcal{D}\big) \mathrm{d}\tilde{y} \quad \approx M^{-1} \sum_{m=1}^{M} \mathbb{I}\big(\tilde{y}(t)^{(m)} \leq L\big), \tag{21.11}$$

where $\mathbb{I}(\cdot)$ represents the indicator function and M the number of iterations.

21.5.4 Examples

In this subsection, we illustrate through a case study how Bayesian modeling can flexibly enable efficient risk understanding and management during stability studies by computing any of the above discussed quantities of interest for decision-making.

The drug product considered is a vaccine whose potency degradation model is $y = 98.00 - 0.30t$; the covariance matrix of batch intercepts and slopes was $\boldsymbol{D}_r = \begin{bmatrix} 0.400 & -0.0078 \\ -0.007 & 0.002 \end{bmatrix}$ the within-batch variance was $\sigma_r^2 = 0.5625$; the lower specification limit was $L = 93.0$ and the corresponding mean shelf-life was $t_r = 16$ months. Using this model as a reference, stability data are simulated, including 7 batches and 5 measurements per batch at each timepoint (0, 3, 6, 9, 12, 18, 24 and 36 months) — see Figure 21.1 for illustration. The Bayesian mixed model of Equation (21.2) was applied to the data, as described in Section 21.5.1 using weakly informative priors on model parameters.

For model estimation, `rstan` 2.18.2 has been used from within the `R` environment 3.5.1 (R Core Development Team, 2011; Stan Development Team, 2014). After a warmup of 1000 iterations on 4 parallel chains, 5,000 samples from the posterior distribution of the parameters are obtained on each chain, leading to 20,000 posterior samples. The code ran during 15 seconds on `Mac OS Mojave` on a 2.7 GHz quad-core laptop architecture from year 2013. The set of posterior samples of $\boldsymbol{\theta} = \boldsymbol{b}, \boldsymbol{D}, \sigma_\varepsilon^2$ is presented in Figure 21.2 and summarized in Table 21.1.

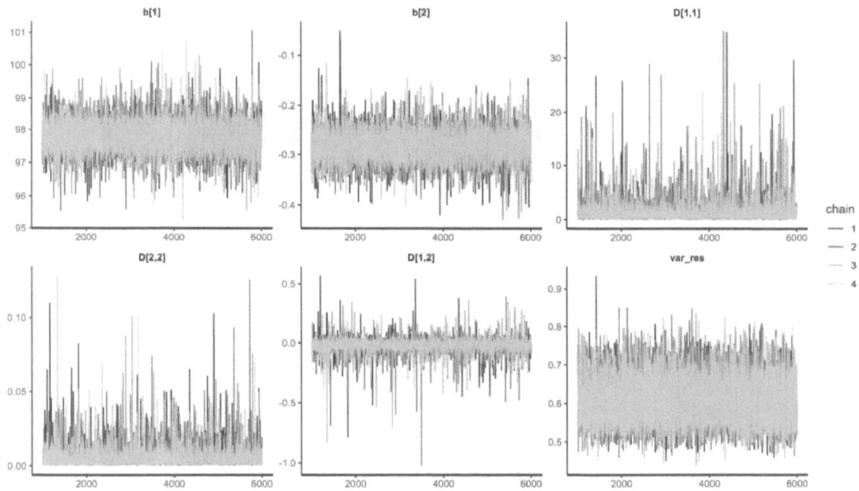

FIGURE 21.2: Traceplots of the sampled posterior parameters $\boldsymbol{\theta} = \boldsymbol{b}, \boldsymbol{D}, \sigma_\varepsilon^2$ using 4 chains (`rstan`).

TABLE 21.1: Posterior summaries. `n_eff` represents the effective sample size of the posterior samples, and `Rhat` illustrate the successful convergence to the same stationary distribution

Parameter	Mean	Mode	SD	5%	95%	`n_eff`	`Rhat`
b_1	97.81	97.81	0.4	97.18	98.43	13606	1
b_2	-0.28	-0.28	0.03	-0.32	-0.24	9778	1
$D[1,1]$	1.06	0.34	1.26	0.25	2.92	10967	1
$D[2,2]$	0	0.0014	0.01	0	0.01	7214	1
$D[1,2]$	-0.01	-0.0050	0.04	-0.07	0.03	10933	1
σ_ε^2	0.61	0.58	0.05	0.53	0.7	26883	1

Figure 21.3 illustrates the (mean) predicted degradation curves (using $y^{(m)} = b_0^{(m)} + b_1^{(m)}t$). With 7 batches available, degrees of freedom for the batch random effects are quite low, and it is likely that the stability behaviors that may be expected from future batches would dramatically increase the uncertainty and lead to difficult visualization, when predicting from Equation (21.6). However, insights on the characteristics of interest (shelf-life and risk of OOS) can be obtained easily. Figure 21.4 shows Bayesian estimation of labelled shelf-life using various methods, namely the lower 95% confidence interval and the lower 95% coverage $\beta-$expectation tolerance interval (left) and the batch shelf-life distribution method (right).

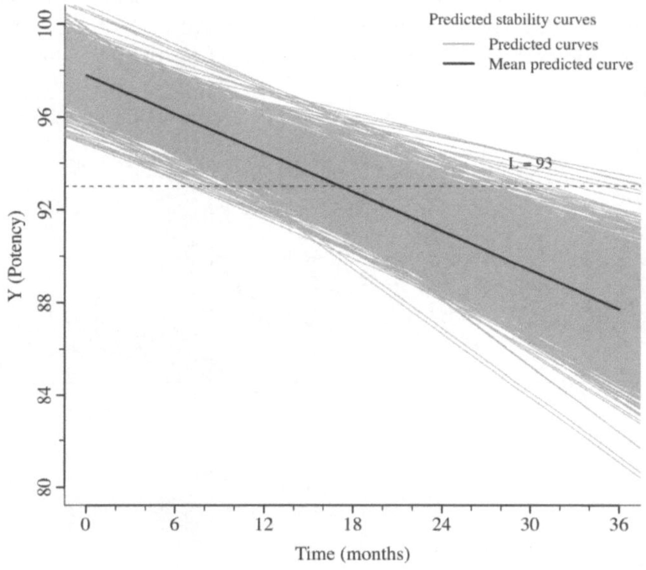

FIGURE 21.3: Predicted mean stability curves.

Altogether, this information may enable the manufacturer to understand and manage risks and appropriately choose a shelf-life. For example, the shelf life based on the $\beta-$expectation tolerance interval is $\widehat{t}_2 = 9$ months, with a probability of OOS dosages of 0.05, approximately (Figures 21.2 and 21.3). Using a 5%-quantile for the batch shelf-life predictive distribution, a shelf-life of $\widehat{t}_3 = 9$ months is obtained, logically similar to the one obtained using a $\beta-$expectation tolerance interval.

Finally, Figure 21.5 shows the expected risk of out-of-specification as function of storage time, that is similar to the risk that a patient is injected a vaccine dosage with low potency (Equations 21.10—21.11). At a time of 9 months, the probability (risk) of OOS is about 5% as expected from previous results.

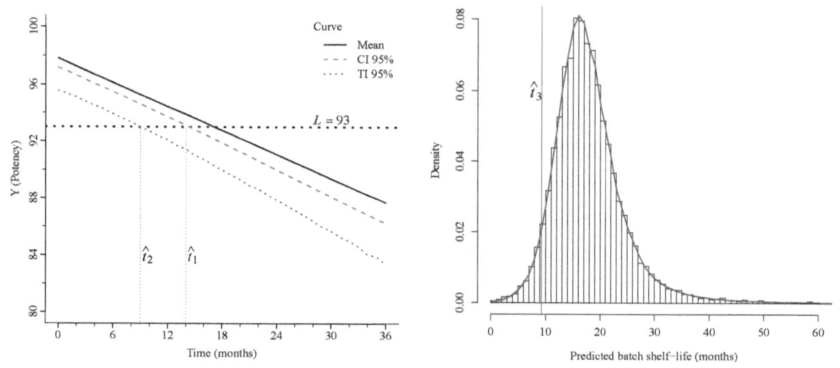

FIGURE 21.4: Various methods of shelf-life estimation. Left: Classical confidence interval (Equation 21.3) and (Bayesian) β−expectation tolerance intervals methods (Equation 21.7). Right: Shelf-life distribution methods (Equation 21.8). The grey vertical line is the 5% quantile of the distribution.

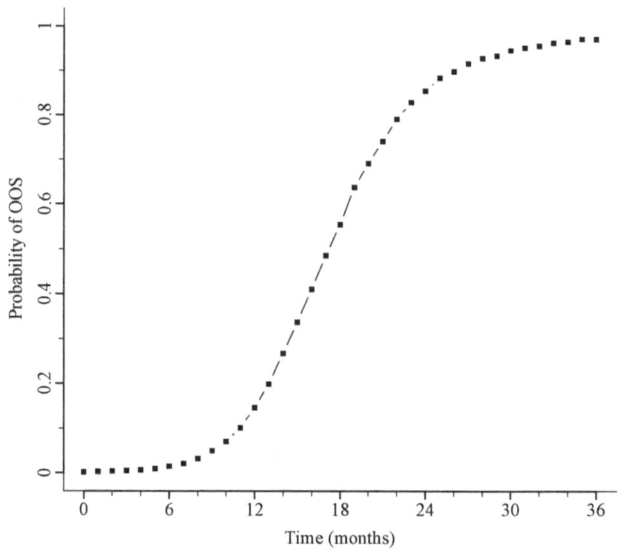

FIGURE 21.5: Expected probability of Out-of-Specifications as function of storage time.

21.6 Conclusions

Regulations are changing towards a quality-by-design and risk-oriented approach to development, approval and post-marketing monitoring of drug substances. As a consequence, stability data evaluation has seen the emergence of new quality management issues. To fully address these issues, a change of statistical modeling paradigm from non-probabilistic to probabilistic or predictive statistical methodologies is required. Bayesian methods are more flexible, and their results are more clinically interpretable, but require more careful development and specialized software.

Bibliography

Altan, S., Manola, A., Shoung, J.-M., and Shen, Y. (2013). Perspectives on Pooling as Described in the ICH Q1E Guidance. In *Joint Statistical Meetings (JSM) Proceedings, Statistical Computing Section, Alexandria, VA*, pages 1121–1131, Alexandria, VA. American Statistical Association.

Capen, R., Christopher, D., Forenzo, P., Huynh-Ba, K., LeBlond, D., Liu, O., O'Neill, J., Patterson, N., Quinlan, M., Rajagopalan, R., Schwenke, J., and Stroup, W. (2018). Evaluating current practices in shelf life estimation. *American Association of Pharmaceutical Scientists PharmSciTech*, 19(2):668–680.

Capen, R., Christopher, D., Forenzo, P., Ireland, C., Liu, O., Lyapustina, S., O'Neill, J., Patterson, N., Quinlan, M., Sandell, D., Schwenke, J., Stroup, W., and Tougas, T. (2012). On the shelf life of pharmaceutical products. *American Association of Pharmaceutical Scientists PharmSciTech*, 13(3):911–918.

Chow, S.-C. (2007). *Statistical Design and Analysis of Stability Studies.* Chapman & Hall/CRC, Boca Raton, FL.

Gelman, A. (2006). Prior distributions for variance parameters in hierarchical models. *Bayesian Analysis*, 1(3):515–534.

Guttman, I. (1988). Tolerance regions, statistical. In Kotz, S. and Johnson, N., editors, *Encyclopedia of Statistical Sciences*, volume 9, pages 272–287. John Wiley, New York, NY.

Huynh-Ba, K. (2009). *Handbook of Stability Testing in Pharmaceutical Development: Regulations, Methodologies, and Best Practices.* Springer Science+Business Media,, New-York, USA.

ICH (2003a). *ICH Harmonised Tripartite Guidelines. Evaluation for Stability Data, Q1E.* ICH.

ICH (2003b). *ICH Harmonised Tripartite Guidelines. Stability Testing of New Drug Substances and Products Q1A(R2).* ICH.

Kiermeier, A., Verbyla, A., and Jarrett, R. (2012). Estimating a single shelf-life for multiple batches. *Australian and New Zealand Journal of Statistics*, 54(3):343–358.

Komka, K., Kemény, S., and Bánfai, B. (2010). Novel tolerance interval model for the estimation of the shelf life of pharmaceutical products. *Journal of Chemometrics*, 24(3-4):131–139.

Peterson, J. (2010). What your ICH Q8 design space needs: a multivariate predictive distribution. *Pharma Manufacturing.com*, 8(10):23–28.

Peterson, J. J., Snee, R. D., McAllister, P. R., Schofield, T. L., and Carella, A. J. (2009). Statistics in pharmaceutical development and manufacturing. *Journal of Quality Technology*, 41(2):111–134.

Peterson, J. J., Yahyah, M., Lief, K., and Hodnett, N. (2017). Predictive Distributions for Constructing the ICH Q8 Design Space. In Reklaitis, G. V., Seymour, C., and García-Munoz, S., editors, *Comprehensive Quality by Design for Pharmaceutical Product Development and Manufacture*, chapter 4, pages 55–70. John Wiley & Sons, Ltd.

Quinlan, M., Stroup, W., Chistopher, D., and Schwenke, J. (2013a). On the distribution of batch shelf lives. *Journal of Biopharmaceutical Statistics*, 23(4):897–920.

Quinlan, M., Stroup, W., Schwenke, J., and Christopher, D. (2013b). Evaluating the performance of the ICH guidelines for shelf life estimation. *Journal of Biopharmaceutical Statistics*, 23(4):881–896.

R Core Development Team (2011). *R: A Language and Environment for Statistical Computing*. R Foundation for Statistical Computing, Vienna, Austria.

Stan Development Team (2014). *Stan Modeling Language: User's Guide and Reference Manual, Version 2.2.0.* Stan Development Team.

Stroup, W. and Quinlan, M. (2016). Statistical Considerations for Stability and the Estimation of Shelf Life. In Zhang, L., editor, *Nonclinical Statistics for Pharmaceutical and Biotechnology Industries*, pages 575–604. Springer International Publishing, Cham, Switzerland.

Weerahandi, S. (1993). Generalized confidence intervals. *Journal of the American Statistical Association*, 88(283):899–905.

Yang, H. (2012). Ensure product quality and regulatory compliance through novel stability design and analysis. *Journal of GXP Compliance*, 16(3):43.

Yang, H. (2017). *Emerging Non-clinical Biostatistics in Biopharmaceutical Development and Manufacturing.* Chapman & Hall/CRC, Boca Raton, FL.

Yang, H. and Zhang, L. (2012). Evaluation of statistical methods for estimating shelf-life of drug products: A unified and risks-based approach. *Journal of Validation Technology*, Spring 2012:67–74.

22

Content Uniformity Testing

Steven Novick

AstraZeneca, US

Buffy Hudson-Curtis

GlaxoSmithKline Pharmaceuticals, US

Content uniformity is a measure of the amount of active pharmaceutical ingredient in the units of a batch of drug product. Before a batch of newly manufactured drug product is released to consumers, content uniformity testing is used to establish that the dosage units of a drug product consistently contain the specified amount of drug (active pharmaceutical ingredient). Content uniformity testing establishes whether a sample of units from a batch of drug product meets specified criteria on the amount of drug present. The foundation for most content uniformity testing stems from USP guidelines, namely USP<905> for solid dosage units, USP<3> for topical and transdermal products, and USP<601> for inhaled products. Two drawbacks of the USP guidelines are that they do not expressly provide a level of statistical confidence nor do they directly characterize the population of units in the batch. These deficiencies may be remedied through the ASTM E2810 and PTI-TOST testing methods. Although none of these approaches were crafted as Bayesian in nature, several authors in recent times have placed a Bayesian spin on E2810 and PTI-TOST methods. In this chapter, a thorough review of the USP guidelines, ASTM E2810 and PTI-TOST are provided along with their Bayesian counterparts and extensions. The methods are illustrated by looking at operating characteristics and example data.

22.1 Introduction

Before a batch of a newly manufactured drug product is released to consumers, *content uniformity testing* is used to establish that the dosage units of a drug product consistently contain the specified amount of drug (active pharmaceutical ingredient). For dosage units from a batch to be of uniform content the amount of active pharmaceutical ingredient in the dosage units of a batch must be reasonably close to the intended (target) dose, thus avoiding the patient risk of under/over dosing. Tests of content uniformity assess the assayed results of a sample of units from a batch against a predetermined set of criteria.

To illustrate the concept, consider the amount (i.e. content) of acetylsalicylic acid in tablets from a newly manufactured batch of 500 mg aspirin. As stated on the tablet container label intended for consumers, the individual dosage units should all (i.e. uniformly) contain doses reasonably close to 500 mg. A comprehensive testing of all tablets from the batch would provide 100% certainty of content uniformity; however, resource constraints may be prohibitory or the test may be destructive. Thus, a representative sample of tablets from the batch is examined. Upon assaying the contents of a random sample of ten aspirin tablets from the batch, perhaps eight values fall within 90-110% of the label claim of 500 mg and two fall within 80-120%. How can we tell if the batch is acceptable for public consumption?

The United States Pharmacopeia (USP) chapters provide testing standards for content uniformity that are used by more than 140 countries. The specifics of most modern USP content uniformity tests may be found in USP<905> for solid dosage units, USP<3> for topical and transdermal drug products, and USP<601> for aerosols, nasal sprays, metered-dose inhalers, and dry-powder inhalers. A listing and discussion of the USP and other guidelines for content uniformity may be found in Chapter 23 "Assessing Content Uniformity" of Nonclinical Statistics for Pharmaceutical and Biotechnology Industries (Hudson-Curtis and Novick, 2016). In addition, the approach discussed in ASTM E2810 (a.k.a., the CuDAL approach), see E2810-11 (2011), and the PTI-TOST have been suggested as techniques for batch release.

Content uniformity measurements are typically given as percent of label claim (%LC). USP Standards for Content Uniformity <905> and <601> are two-tiered procedures for testing content uniformity using a sample of units from a batch of drug product (U.S. Pharmacopeia, 2014, 2006, 2011b,a). They are implemented by selecting a set $n_1 + n_2$ dosage units for evaluation. For Tier 1, the n_1 dosage units are evaluated against the Tier 1 acceptance criteria. If the criteria are not met, the second set of n_2 dosage units may be evaluated. The second tier testing combines the results of the n_2 dosage units with those from Tier 1 and then evaluates the n_1+n_2 total dose units against a second set of acceptance criteria. It is worth noting that these tests are revised and updated over time; the latest USP chapter should be referenced to ensure the most up to date standard is utilized. The USP methods are not necessarily harmonized with the European Pharmacopoeia and the Japanese Pharmacopoeia, and so those resources should be consulted when applicable. USP and other regulatory guidance documents may specify the method used to obtain content uniformity results (e.g. content uniformity, weight variation), and is beyond the scope of this chapter.

Though currently accepted, content uniformity tests by regulatory agencies are not Bayesian in nature. Bayesian approaches can be extremely useful in assessing batch and process performance against these tests as well as in addressing more complex data structures when applying these tests. Some proposed Bayesian approaches to content uniformity testing from the current literature and Bayesian procedures used to assess the risk of meeting content uniformity testing requirements will be given in this chapter. USP<905> is discussed in detail and is used as an illustrative example throughout this chapter.

22.2 Classical procedures for testing content uniformity

USP chapters provide binary tests so that, by measuring content uniformity on a sample of units from a batch, the batch either meets or does not meet the USP requirements. The criteria for solid dosage units, given by USP<905>, are shown in Table 22.1.

A common question that arises in practice is whether or not a particular batch or process is likely to meet the requirements of content uniformity testing. Operational characteristic (OC) curves are often used to address this concern. The OC represents the probability that a batch meets criteria (e.g. pass the USP criteria) under an assumption about the batch population characteristics. Thus, operating characteristics are conditional probabilities $\Pr(Success \mid \boldsymbol{\theta})$, where $\boldsymbol{\theta}$ denotes the set of model parameters (e.g. the mean for a particular batch and within-batch standard deviation), and *Success* indicates that the

TABLE 22.1: Criteria for meeting USP<905> for content uniformity testing of solid dosages

1. Calculate the mean ($\overline{Y}$) and standard deviation (s) of the assay results (in %) where $n = 10$ for Tier 1, and $n = 30$ for Tier 2, $\overline{Y} = \frac{1}{n}\sum_{i=1}^{n} Y_i$, and $s = \sqrt{\frac{1}{n-1}\sum_{i=1}^{n}(Y_i - \overline{Y})^2}$.
2. Establish the Reference Value (M). This value depends on the target content (T) per dosage unit at the time of manufacture and the observed mean of the sample ($\overline{Y}$). The value T is expressed as a percent of the label claim, and is typically 100%.
   a. Case 1: $T \leq 101.5$
      i. If $98.5 \leq \overline{Y} \leq 101.5$, then $M = \overline{Y}$
      ii. Otherwise, $M = 98.5$ if $\overline{Y} < 98.5$ and $M = 101.5$ if $\overline{Y} > 101.5$
   b. Case 2: $T > 101.5$
      i. If $98.5 \leq \overline{Y} \leq T$, then $M = \overline{Y}$
      ii. Otherwise, $M = 98.5$ if $\overline{Y} < 98.5$ and $M = T$ if $\overline{Y} > T$
3. Calculate the Acceptance Value ($\text{AV} = \mid M - \overline{Y} \mid + ks$) using the acceptability constant k, where $k = 2.4$ for Tier 1 ($n = 10$), and $k = 2.0$ for Tier 2 ($n = 30$).
4. The requirements for dosage uniformity are met if:
   a. Tier 1: the AV of the first ten dosage units is less than $L_1 = 15.0\%$
   b. Tier 2: if the AV for the first ten dosage units is greater than $L_1 = 15.0\%$, the criteria are met if the final acceptance value of the 30 dosage units is less than $L_1 = 15.0\%$ and if all individual dosage units ($Y_i, i = 1, \ldots, 30$) meet the requirement $[1 - (0.01)L_2]M \leq Y_i \leq [1 + (0.01)L_2]M$, where $L_2 = 25.0\%$.

criteria of the test are met. Monte Carlo computer simulation is a helpful tool for evaluating risks through the OC of a test, particularly when the tests (such as given by USP<905>) are complex in nature and do not lend themselves to closed-form solutions to evaluate the relevant properties. Using USP<905>, and assuming that content uniformity assay values for a batch follow a Normal distribution with mean μ and standard deviation σ, the OC of USP<905> may be calculated by the outline given in Table 22.2.

Operating characteristic curves were generated to illustrate the probability to pass USP<905> when $T = 96$, 98, 100, 102 and 104, the true batch mean is μ, and the true batch standard deviation is σ. These curves, shown in Figure 22.1, were created by the algorithm in Table 22.2 with B=10,000 and are very useful in evaluating whether or not a particular batch of known mean and standard deviation will meet the USP<905> test criteria.

A common critique of the complex acceptance criteria given in Table 22.1 is that USP<905> is not associated with a set of hypotheses for testing nor is there an assumption about the distribution of the data (Bergum and Li, 2007; Novick and Hudson-Curtis, 2018a). Thus, there is no concept of statistical power or test size associated with USP<905>. Two other test methods for establishing the content uniformity of solid dosage units that, to differing degrees, ameliorate the issues with USP<905> are now discussed.

TABLE 22.2: Monte Carlo algorithm to evaluate the operating characteristics of a batch against USP<905>

1. Generate 30 observations from a Normal distribution with mean μ and standard deviation σ.
2. Using the criteria given in Table 22.1, evaluate the first 10 observations via the Tier 1 test and, if needed, evaluate all 30 observations via the Tier 2 test.
3. Repeat steps 1 and 2 a large number of times (e.g. B=10,000 times). The operating characteristic is the proportion of times (out of B) that a simulated data set meets the USP<905> criteria.

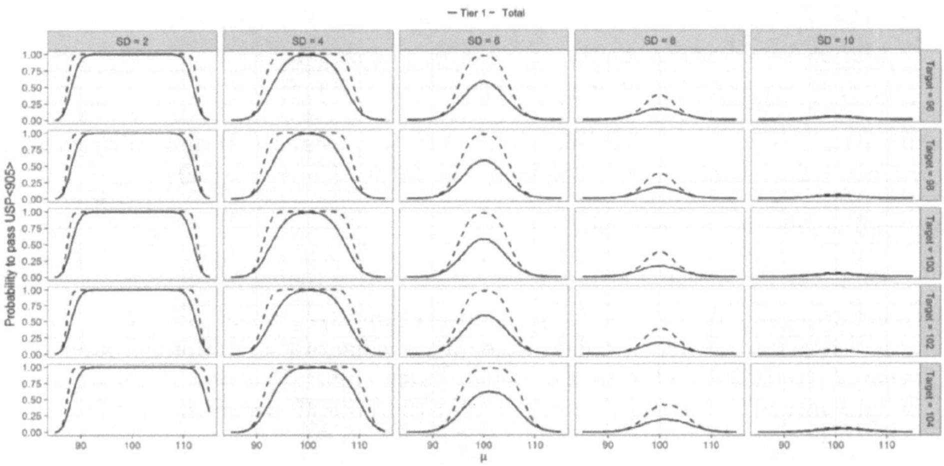

FIGURE 22.1: OC curves for USP<905>: Rows display T (Target) values between 96-104. Solid and dashed lines show the probability to meet USP<905> in Tier 1 and after Tier 2 (total), if needed.

Bergum and Li (2007) published a novel method called *content uniformity and dissolution acceptance limits* (CuDAL) to estimate a lower bound for the probability that a random sample from a batch would pass the USP<905> standard for content uniformity with statistical confidence. Based on a random sample of size n of solid dosage units from a batch and a given confidence level, the CuDaL calculation involves the creation of a simultaneous $100(1-\alpha)\%$ frequentist confidence region for (μ, σ). If the operating characteristic probabilities (see Figure 22.1) are all larger than p_0 for the set of every (μ, σ) in the confidence region, then with $100(1-\alpha)\%$ confidence, the acceptance probability for a random sample from the tested manufactured batch is at least p_0. The CuDaL method was incorporated into ASTM E2709 and E2810. As an example, consider a sample from a batch with n=30 units, sample mean $\overline{y} = 96$, and sample standard deviation SD $= 3.41$. For this scenario, ASTM E2810 provides (p_0 % =) 90% confidence that at least 95% of samples from the same batch would meet the USP<905> criteria.

While providing confidence that any random sample (of size 30 dosage units) from the batch at hand would meet with the USP<905> criteria, ASTM E2810 does not overcome a shortcoming of USP<905>, namely its lack of meaningful batch characterization. Lostrito (2005) proposed an alternative to USP<905> testing content uniformity with a two one-sided parametric tolerance interval test (PTI-TOST). Unlike USP<905> and ASTM E2810, the PTI-TOST is associated with hypotheses of the batch parameters. Letting L% and U% denote lower and upper testing bounds, the hypotheses are

H_0: fewer than $100(1+p)/2\%$ of units lie at or above L% or fewer than $100(1+p)/2\%$ of units lie at or below U%.
H_a: at least $100(1+p)/2\%$ of units lie at or above L% and at least $100(1+p)/2\%$ of units lie at or below U%. (22.1)

To examine the hypotheses in (22.1) for a test size α and given a sample of units from a batch, one calculates test statistics T_L and T_U, where T_L is the $100(1-\alpha)\%$ lower confidence limit for the $100(1-p)/2\%$ quantile of the batch population of %LC values and T_U is the $100(1-\alpha)\%$ upper confidence limit for the $100(1-p)/2\%$ quantile of the batch population of %LC values. The alternative hypothesis in (22.1) is accepted if $T_L > L\%$ and $T_U < U\%$. For two-tier testing, Novick et al. (2009) suggest using the Lan-DeMets alpha-spending approach (Lan and DeMets, 1983) (with Pocock boundary) to maintain the correct overall significance testing level. The values T_L and T_U are respectively called the lower $100(1-\alpha)\%/100(1-p)/2\%$ and upper $100(1-\alpha)\%/100(1+p)/2\%$ tolerance limits. For the PTI-TOST tolerance limits are calculated assuming that the data stem from a univariate Normal distribution and are given as $T_L = \overline{y} - Ks$ and $T_U = \overline{y} + Ks$, where K is a function of the sample size, confidence $100(1-\alpha)\%$, and desired coverage $100p\%$. Though there is no set guidance for the PTI-TOST parameters, Lostrito (2005) proposed the test with $\alpha = 0.05, p = 0.875, L = 80\%$ and $U = 120\%$. As an example calculation, consider a single-tier test with $L\%$=80 and $U\%$=120 for a sample of $n = 30$ dosage units with $\overline{y} = 96$, and sample standard deviation SD $= 3.41$. With 95% confidence to cover 87.5% of all dosage units in the batch, $K = 2.08, T_L = 88.9$ and $T_U = 103.1$. Since $88.9 > 80$ and $103.1 < 120$, the dosage units in the batch are declared to exhibit content uniformity.

The PTI-TOST is also given as an alternative to USP<601>, which was developed to establish criteria for batches of oral, inhaled, and nasal drug products (OINDPs). Sampling content from an OINDP batch is more complicated than tablet sampling because OINDPs require a device (e.g. a nasal inhaler) to deliver the dose. Doses are not delivered at random from an OINDP, but are imparted sequentially. As suggested in USP<601>, inhaled devices are selected at random from the batch (or possibly through stratified sampling of the batch) and at least two doses (usually the first and the last) are sampled from each inhaler.

Like USP<905>, the USP<601> is not associated with parametric hypotheses, nor does meeting/not meeting the USP criteria characterize the units in a batch. Novick et al. (2009) detail a PTI-TOST alternative to USP<601> that compares the hypotheses (22.1) via a test of the tolerance limits T_L and T_U, originally proposed by the FDA at the October 2005 Advisory Committee meeting (Lostrito, 2005).

22.3 Bayesian procedures for testing content uniformity and risk

Regulated content uniformity testing is not commonly performed with Bayesian procedures. This may be due to the difficulty in implementing Bayesian methods without a statistician or pre-canned software. Still, there are some notable Bayesian or Bayesian-like procedures in the literature for testing content uniformity. Some of the authors use generalized pivotal quantity (GPQ) methods (Weerahandi, 2004), a frequentist method that may be used to calculate confidence intervals. Hannig (2009) demonstrated that GPQ analysis is a special case of fiducial inference, a frequentist framework that resembles Bayesian methods. This section gives a brief overview of some of the available resources for implementing Bayesian approaches. Though all of the Bayesian methods in this section use vague or non-informative priors, the authors of each work note that real information could be incorporated into the prior distribution. In the first part of this section, we will discuss Bayesian techniques that can be used to improve upon or augment frequentist approaches, particularly relevant to ASTM E2810, which assesses a batch relative to USP<905>, and the PTI-TOST approach. In the second part of this section we will discuss statistical assurance, a Bayesian technique that can be used to assess risk by examining the expected performance of a batch against a particular test. Statistical assurance may be seen as an extension of the operational characteristic curves used in the frequentist framework.

The ASTM E2810 procedure introduced in Section 22.2 is based on a frequentist confidence region for (μ, σ) with which one determines the minimum probability that any random sample from the same batch would meet with USP<905> and may be used to demonstrate content uniformity of a batch. Lewis and Fan (2016) show that the classical statistical approach to ASTM E2810 is conservative at each step of construction, leading to overly restrictive acceptance limits. Using Bayesian methods, Lewis and Fan (2016) create a $100(1-\alpha)\%$ credible limit for the USP<905> OC (Figure 22.1), vastly improving upon the testing acceptance limits. Recall the example from Section 22.2 for which a sample from a batch with $n = 30$ units and sample mean $\overline{y} = 96$ provides 90% confidence that at least 95% of samples from the same batch would meet the USP<905> criteria, so long as the sample standard deviation is no larger than SD = 3.41. By exploiting a straight-forward Bayesian mechanism and without making any additional assumptions, Lewis and Fan (2016) show that the sample standard deviation can be as large as SD = 4.07 while still maintaining the 90% probability (90% confidence in ASTM E2810) that at least 95% of samples would meet USP<905>.

In Section 22.2, the discussed tolerance limits for the PTI-TOST are built under classical statistical methods for a sample from a univariate Normal population. For independent, univariate Normal data, one arrives at the same tolerance limits via GPQ or via Bayesian methods with a Jeffreys' prior (Krishnamoorthy and Mathew, 2009), meaning that the current PTI-TOST can already be judged a Bayesian test method. Two notable publications propose a PTI-TOST method for use with bivariate Normal data. In both cases, the authors constructed GPQ tolerance limits. Novick and Hudson-Curtis (2018a,b) extend the PTI-TOST as an alternative to USP<905> for the situation in which samples are drawn from a batch, stratified by time or batch location. The authors note that with independent vague priors on model parameters, the GPQ-based T_L and T_U could be equivalently provided as Bayesian tolerance limits. Lewis and Novick (2012) consider the PTI-TOST alternative to USP<601>, noting the potential for correlation between beginning and end doses from the same OINDP device. The authors construct GPQ tolerance limits from a bivariate Normal distribution and point out that their method is equivalent to a Bayesian procedure with a Jeffreys' prior.

A Bayesian PTI-TOST is also equivalent to a Bayesian posterior probability calculation in which the alternative hypothesis in (22.1) is declared based on the posterior probability that at least $100(1+p)/2\%$ of units lie at or above $L\%$ and at least $100(1+p)/2\%$ of units lie at or below $U\%$. Recall the example in Section 22.2 with $n = 30$ dosage units, $\overline{y} = 96$, SD=3.41 and testing limits $L\%$=80 and $U\%$=120. With $p = 0.9$, the 95%/90% tolerance limits are 88.4 and 103.6, which fall inside 80 – 120%. Using a Jeffreys' prior, the posterior probability in favor of the alternative hypothesis is given by $\Pr(\mu - 1.645\sigma >$

$80, \mu + 1.645\sigma < 120 \mid \text{Data}) \geq 0.999$, where μ and σ are the batch mean and standard deviation parameters and 1.645 is the 95th percentile of the standard Normal distribution. As such, the posterior probability and PTI-TOST approaches agree.

A very natural question follows: "Will our manufacturing process lend itself to a high probability to pass the test?" While the OC curves in Figure 22.1 reflect the mean and standard deviation from dosage units within a particular batch, to evaluate the process capability, at a minimum, one must consider the mean and two components of variation: batch-to-batch standard deviation and within-batch standard deviation. Of course, it is possible that other sources of variability might also be of interest (and hence should be measured and estimated), such as variability introduced by manufacturing site, analyst, or machine line. While one can estimate these probabilities using more complex Monte Carlo simulations, there is a Bayesian approach that utilizes a modern statistical method called *assurance*, see also Chapter 1.

O'Hagan et al. (2005) detail a modern statistical method called *assurance* that calculates the unconditional probability of success of a process of a clinical trial, but may also be used for process capability. Assurance is the expected value of the operating characteristic, integrated over the posterior distribution; i.e. assurance $= \int \Pr(Success \mid \boldsymbol{\theta}) p(\boldsymbol{\theta} \mid \text{Data})\, d\boldsymbol{\theta}$ where $p(\boldsymbol{\theta} \mid \text{Data})$ is the posterior distribution for the model parameters. Assurance may also be stated as the mean posterior predictive probability of the success of the process. Following the outline given by LeBlond and Mockus (2014), one may use Monte Carlo methods to estimate the integral. Let $\boldsymbol{\theta}$ denote the model parameters that describe the content uniformity population; e.g. $\boldsymbol{\theta} = (\mu, \sigma_{\boldsymbol{\beta}}, \sigma_e)^\top$, where μ denotes the overall process mean, $\sigma_{\boldsymbol{\beta}}$ is the batch-to-batch standard deviation, and σ_e is the within-batch standard deviation. The LeBlond and Mockus (2014) algorithm for calculating assurance is outlined in Table 22.3, which is in fact an MCMC algorithm.

TABLE 22.3: Algorithm for Monte Carlo estimation of assurance

1. With an appropriate prior on $\boldsymbol{\theta}$ and an appropriate data likelihood, fit the model to a data set that allows estimation of the posterior distribution $\boldsymbol{\theta} \mid \text{Data}$;
2. Draw one posterior sample for the set of parameters $\boldsymbol{\theta}$ in step 1;
3. Generate a posterior predictive data set for a single batch with sample size suitable for testing content uniformity. Data are generated from the likelihood model assumed in step 1 and from the parameters $\boldsymbol{\theta}$ drawn in step 2;
4. Determine the content uniformity test success or failure of the data set created in step 3. A success results in the estimate $\Pr(Success \mid \boldsymbol{\theta}) = 1$ and a failure results in the estimate $\Pr(Success \mid \boldsymbol{\theta}) = 0$;
5. Repeat steps 2 – 4 many times, say 10,000 times;
6. Assurance (the process capability) is the average value of the zeros and ones from step 4.

In this manner, the posterior predictive distribution of content uniformity may be sampled to estimate the probability that a future batch will meet the USP<905> criteria. The process capability is calculated by replacing Step 1 of Table 22.3 with 30 draws from a random batch taken from the posterior predictive distribution.

To illustrate the concept of assurance, suppose a manufacturing process must be evaluated against USP<905> and target T = 100 with the data shown in Table 22.4 and Figure 22.2. Process capability against USP<905> will be estimated via statistical assurance, incorporating our knowledge and uncertainty about the data distribution under three different realistic scenarios. Though this section focuses on USP<905>, similar procedures may be followed to evaluate the risk that a process will/will not meet the content uniformity requirements for other USP guidelines, ASTM E2810, a PTI-TOST, or an appropriate Bayesian hypothesis testing method.

TABLE 22.4: Example development and production data: Content uniformity from six batches with 10 units per batch.

	Batch					
	Development			Production		
Unit	1	2	3	1	2	3
1	109.3	109.8	102.5	93.3	98.0	97.1
2	104.8	108.1	103.7	93.5	99.3	94.7
3	106.3	110.2	100.9	94.8	104.4	95.6
4	108.0	109.8	103.1	94.0	100.7	97.7
5	107.7	111.0	102.9	96.7	98.1	94.5
6	106.1	108.5	104.9	96.6	98.1	97.2
7	108.4	107.8	103.2	92.8	99.5	98.9
8	106.3	113.8	101.3	91.5	99.6	97.3
9	109.2	107.9	96.9	94.1	100.7	97.6
10	110.2	107.7	101.7	91.6	101.3	99.6

22.3.1 Example: Production data only

After collecting development content data, one may try to estimate the probability that future production data will meet with USP<905>. As a starting point, using Table 22.1, all three development batches met with the USP<905> criteria in Tier 1 testing. By placing a Bernoulli (pass/fail) distribution on the three development batches, the estimated frequentist point estimate for the probability to meet with USP<905> is 3/3 = 1. Pairing the Bernoulli data with the conjugate Jeffreys' Beta(0.5, 0.5) prior distribution, the posterior mean probability is about 0.88. While these comprise valid point estimates, the richness of the data may be better exploited by fitting a distribution to the content uniformity measurements.

We will assume that a linear hierarchical model may be fitted to the development data with the model given by

$$Y_{ij} \mid \boldsymbol{\beta}_i, \sigma_e \sim \mathrm{N}(\boldsymbol{\beta}_i, \sigma_e^2)$$
$$\boldsymbol{\beta}_i \mid \mu_{\mathrm{Dev}}, \sigma_{\boldsymbol{\beta}} \sim \mathrm{N}(\mu_{\mathrm{Dev}}, \sigma_{\boldsymbol{\beta}}^2),$$

whereby Y_{ij} is the content of the jth tablet ($j = 1, 2, \ldots, 10$) of the ith batch ($i = 1, 2, 3$). Using frequentist REML modeling, point estimates with 95% confidence intervals are given by $\widehat{\mu}_{\mathrm{Dev}} = 106.4(101.8, 110.9)$, $\widehat{\sigma}_{\boldsymbol{\beta}} = 3.8(1.4, 10.3)$, and $\widehat{\sigma}_e = 1.9(1.5, 2.5)$; but, where does this place the process on the OC curve in Figure 22.1? A Monte Carlo simulation was run

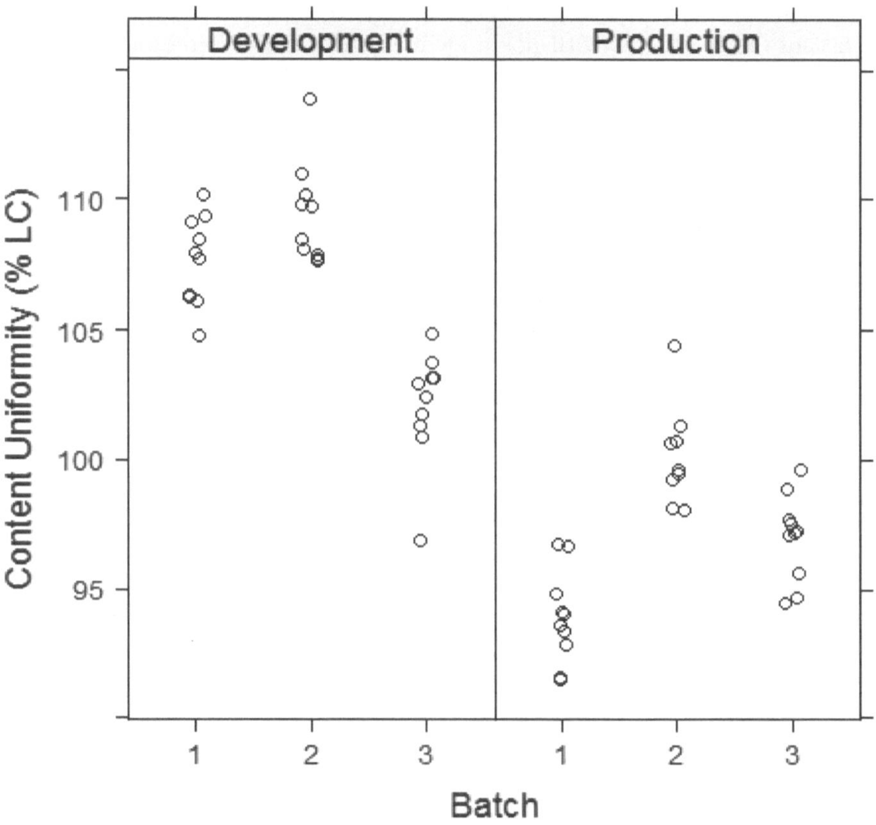

FIGURE 22.2: Example development data and production data: Six total batches with 10 units per batch.

to estimate the probability to meet the USP<905> criteria by setting the parameters equal to the REML point estimates, generating the mean of a batch as $\boldsymbol{\beta}^* \sim \mathrm{N}(\widehat{\mu}_{\mathrm{Dev}}, \widehat{\sigma}^2_{\boldsymbol{\beta}})$, and then finding the probability on the OC curve in Figure 22.1 using $(\mu = \boldsymbol{\beta}^*, \sigma_e = \widehat{\sigma}_e)$. After repeating this procedure 10,000 times, the average OC curve value was calculated as a 0.95 probability to meet the USP<905> criteria. This value, however, is likely to be overly optimistic as it does not account for the uncertainty in the model parameter estimates $(\widehat{\mu}_{\mathrm{Dev}}, \widehat{\sigma}_{\boldsymbol{\beta}}, \widehat{\sigma}_e)$.

By using the technique to calculate statistical assurance, practitioners have a direct method to calculate the probability to meet USP<905> while incorporating model parameter uncertainty. Independent vague prior distributions were assigned to each of the parameters $(\mu, \sigma_{\boldsymbol{\beta}}, \sigma_e)$, where the term *vague* may be taken to mean that the prior distributions are more diffuse when compared to the uncertainty in the likelihood. Three independent MCMC chains were run using `JAGS` software (Plummer, 2003) with burn-in = 20,000, thinning = 10, and sampling (after thinning) = 20,000 for a total of 60,000 posterior draws. MCMC convergence was checked by inspecting the trace plots. Further, we have run enough iterations until the effective sample size is greater than 10,000 for each parameter and the ratio of MC error to the posterior SD (MC error/SD) is less than 5%. Effective sample sizes for each of the three parameters was larger than 21,000 and MCerrSD < 1% for all parameters. Unsurprisingly, because vague priors were used, posterior results closely match those from REML with posterior medians and 95% credible intervals given as $\widehat{\mu}_{\text{Dev}} = 106.4(100.5, 112.0)$, $\widehat{\sigma}_{\boldsymbol{\beta}} = 3.5(1.7, 11.5)$ and $\widehat{\sigma}_e = 2.0(1.5, 2.6)$.

The REML point estimate for the USP<905> process capability probability may be written as the value of

$$\int \Pr(\text{OC} \mid \boldsymbol{\beta} = b, \widehat{\sigma}_{\boldsymbol{\beta}}, \widehat{\sigma}_e) \left(\frac{1}{\widehat{\sigma}_{\boldsymbol{\beta}}}\right) \phi\left(\frac{b - \widehat{\mu}_{\text{Dev}}}{\widehat{\sigma}_{\boldsymbol{\beta}}}\right) db,$$

which integrates only over the hierarchical data distribution conditioned on parameter estimates $(\widehat{\mu}_{\text{Dev}}, \widehat{\sigma}_{\boldsymbol{\beta}}, \widehat{\sigma}_e)$, where $\phi(\cdot)$ is the standard Normal probability density function. Statistical assurance, however, given as

$$\int \Pr(\text{OC} \mid \boldsymbol{\beta} = b, \sigma_{\boldsymbol{\beta}}, \sigma_e) \left(\frac{1}{\sigma_{\boldsymbol{\beta}}}\right) \phi\left(\frac{b - \mu_{\text{Dev}}}{\sigma_{\boldsymbol{\beta}}}\right) p(\mu_{\text{Dev}}, \sigma_{\boldsymbol{\beta}}, \sigma_e \mid \text{Data})\, d(b, \mu_{\text{Dev}}, \sigma_{\boldsymbol{\beta}}, \sigma_e),$$

integrates over both the hierarchical data distribution and the posterior distribution of the parameters. The integration required to calculate assurance may be approximated via the steps in Table 22.3. After drawing 10,000 posterior samples, the average OC curve value (i.e. the Monte Carlo approximation for the integral) was calculated as 0.90 assurance to meet the USP<905> criteria with the current process. Because assurance utilizes all elements of uncertainty, this probability value should be considered more reflective of our knowledge of the process compared to the REML estimate.

22.3.2 Example: Full data with vague priors

After collecting production data, we assume that the production data and development data may be combined to estimate the capability of the process to meet USP<905>. Using a Bayesian approach, we illustrate the assurance calculation on the combined development and production data sets. It is assumed that a linear hierarchical model is appropriate for the data distributions as $Y_{ijk} \mid \boldsymbol{\beta}_i, \sigma_e \sim \text{N}(\boldsymbol{\beta}_i, \sigma_e^2)$ and $\boldsymbol{\beta}_i \mid \mu_k, \sigma_{\boldsymbol{\beta}} \sim \text{N}(\mu_k, \sigma_{\boldsymbol{\beta}}^2)$, $(i = 1, 2, \ldots, 6)$ representing the batches, $j = 1, 2, \ldots, 10$ the tablets per batch and k the Development (Dev) or Production (Prod). By specifying separate means for the development and product data, we are allowing for potential differences in the two processes while assuming that the magnitude in the components of variability are equal. An example of this situation may occur after noting the development mean of 106.4, which is higher than the target 100%. The content may be purposely reduced in the production batches to avoid the appearance of overfill.

As before, independent vague prior distributions were assumed for $(\mu_{\text{Dev}}, \mu_{\text{Prod}}, \sigma_{\boldsymbol{\beta}}, \sigma_e)$. Posterior medians and 95% credible intervals are given as $\widehat{\mu}_{\text{Dev}} = 106.4(101.8, 110.9)$, $\widehat{\mu}_{\text{Prod}} = 97.0(92.4, 101.6)$, $\widehat{\sigma}_{\boldsymbol{\beta}} = 3.3(1.8, 7.6)$, and $\widehat{\sigma}_e = 1.9(1.6, 2.3)$. Graphs of the marginal posterior distributions for each parameter are shown in Figure 22.4. The assurance that a future batch will meet USP<905> was estimated following the steps in Table 22.3 and given as 0.94.

22.3.3 Example: Production data with informative priors

In Section 22.3.1 the development data were modeled in order to predict the behavior of production batches and ultimately to estimate the probability that a future production batch would meet with the USP<905> criteria. In Section 22.3.2 we assumed that the development and production process were compatible in terms of components of variability, while allowing for a mean shift. In this subsection we assume that, though the development data analysis is relevant and informative when considering the production data, the development and production data cannot be directly combined for analysis. For example, we may have only point estimates and confidence intervals for the variance components from the development data. This information may become the basis for an informative prior distribution for use in an analysis of the production data.

Suppose that the only information given from the development data is the point estimate for $\sigma_\beta = 3.8$ with upper 95% confidence limit 8.8 and the point estimate for $\sigma_e = 1.9$ with upper 95% confidence limit 2.4. Two popular prior distributions for variance components are the Half-t distribution for standard deviations (the vague Half-Cauchy is a Half-t distribution with 1 degree of freedom) and the Gamma distribution for the inverse variance. We show one of each for illustrative purposes. A Half-t prior for σ_β was constructed with scale parameter 3.8 (set somewhat arbitrarily to the point estimate for σ_β) and 8 degrees of freedom. The degrees of freedom were determined so that the Half-t 95% quantile was approximately equal to 8.8. A Gamma prior for σ_e^{-2} was constructed by finding parameters (a, b) such that $E(\sigma_e^{-2}) = (a/b) = 1/1.9^2$ and the 5% quantile of the Gamma distribution is equal to $1/2.4^2$). Rounding to the nearest integer, the prior is given by $\sigma^{-2} \sim \text{Gamma}(15, 55)$. Graphs of the priors for σ_β and σ_e are shown in Figure 22.3.

The content uniformity data of the production batches were analyzed, assuming the linear hierarchical model $Y_{ij} \mid \boldsymbol{\beta}_i, \sigma_e \sim \text{N}(\boldsymbol{\beta}_i, \sigma_e^2)$ and $\boldsymbol{\beta}_i \mid \mu_{\text{Prod}}, \sigma_\beta \sim \text{N}(\mu_{\text{Prod}}, \sigma_\beta^2)$ and $(i = 1, 2, 3)$ representing the batches, $j = 1, 2, \ldots, 10$ the tablets per batch. We set a vague prior for the mean μ_{Prod} and informative priors $\sigma_\beta \sim \text{half} - t(3.8, 8)$ and $\sigma_e^{-2} \sim \text{Gamma}(15, 55)$ for the variance components.

Posterior medians and 95% credible intervals are for $\mu_{\text{Prod}} = 97.0(92.0, 101.9)$, for $\sigma_\beta = 3.3(1.5, 8.2)$, and for $\sigma_e = 1.9(1.6, 2.3)$. Graphs of the marginal posterior distributions for each parameter are shown in Figure 22.4. The assurance that a future batch will meet USP<905> was estimated following the steps in Table 22.3, yielding the value 0.97. As expected, these results match closely with those from Section 22.3.2 as they utilized approximately the same amount of information, though in very different ways. As seen in Figure 22.4, the marginal posterior distributions are nearly indistinguishable.

22.4 Challenges for the Bayesian procedures

By now, the reader has been introduced to the various regulatory guidelines for testing content uniformity and to some of its alternatives. To the authors' knowledge, none of the published Bayesian methods for content uniformity testing is officially sanctioned by a regulatory body. Regulatory agencies appear hesitant to implement test methods that cannot be performed by a lay person with simple spreadsheet functions or through a table look-up. Such a policy limits test methods to simple data assumptions. In addition, agencies appear reluctant to allow prior information when assessing the results of a newly manufactured batch. The thought process relates the belief that the quality of the last $(K - 1)$ batches cannot be used to infer the quality of the Kth batch.

Given the uptake in ASTM E2810 use, we offer two arguments in favor of using the (Lewis and Fan, 2016) improvement based on Bayesian posterior probability. First, given a prior distribution for the univariate Normal parameters, the acceptance limits from the Lewis and Fan method can be made into a table. For example, with a prior, acceptance

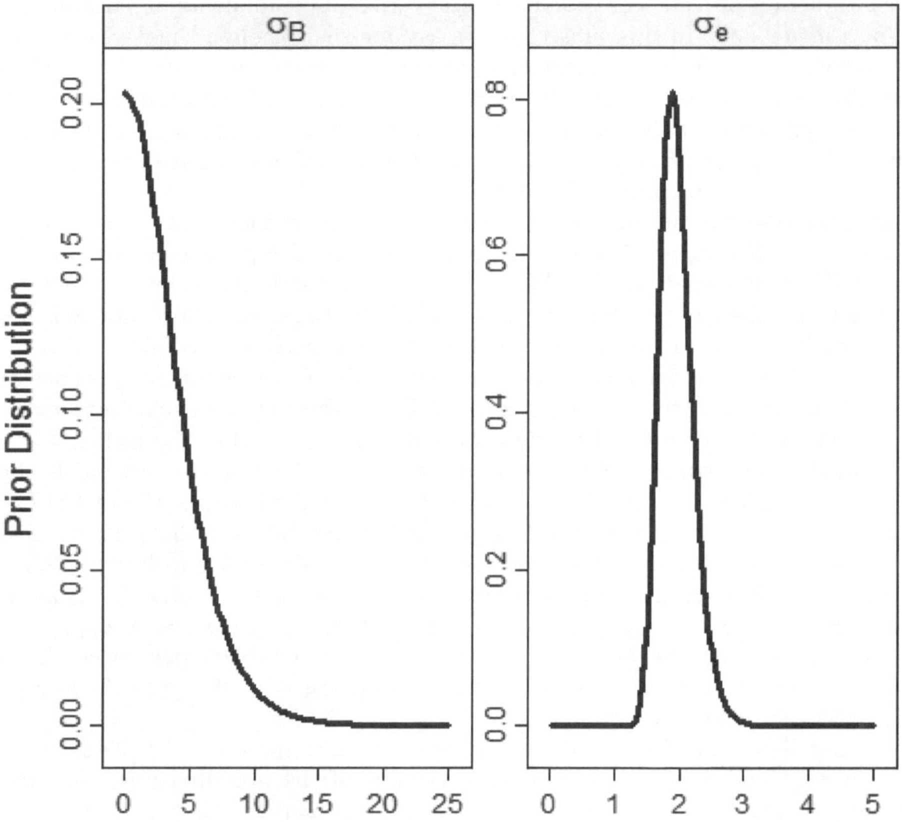

FIGURE 22.3: Prior distributions for $(\sigma_{\beta}, \sigma_e)$ based on point estimates and upper confidence limits from development data

limits can be created for all conceivable outcomes. Second, the Lewis and Fan method can easily accommodate a non-standard data distribution, such as, for example, when the data follow a Log-Normal distribution or should the data be provided with interval-censoring.

For those who prefer the PTI-TOST, one can argue that the test method is already Bayesian. Like the Lewis and Fan method, and as shown by Lewis and Novick (2012) and Novick and Hudson-Curtis (2018a), the PTI-TOST is easily altered for non-standard data distributions. Further, as noted in Section 22.3, the content uniformity assessments may equivalently be made via a posterior probability calculation.

As for issues with informative priors, we agree that one must take care not to overwhelm the assayed results from sampled units of a new batch with historical information. On the other hand, there should also be room to debate the level of historical data that may be incorporated when declaring whether or not a batch exhibits content uniformity.

Finally, we are pleased to see the rise in the number of risk analyses performed with Bayesian posterior predictive probabilities to assess process performance. As illustrated in the scenarios in Section 22.3, this Bayesian method of computing statistical assurance is a direct way of assessing how a product may perform against a particular test while accounting

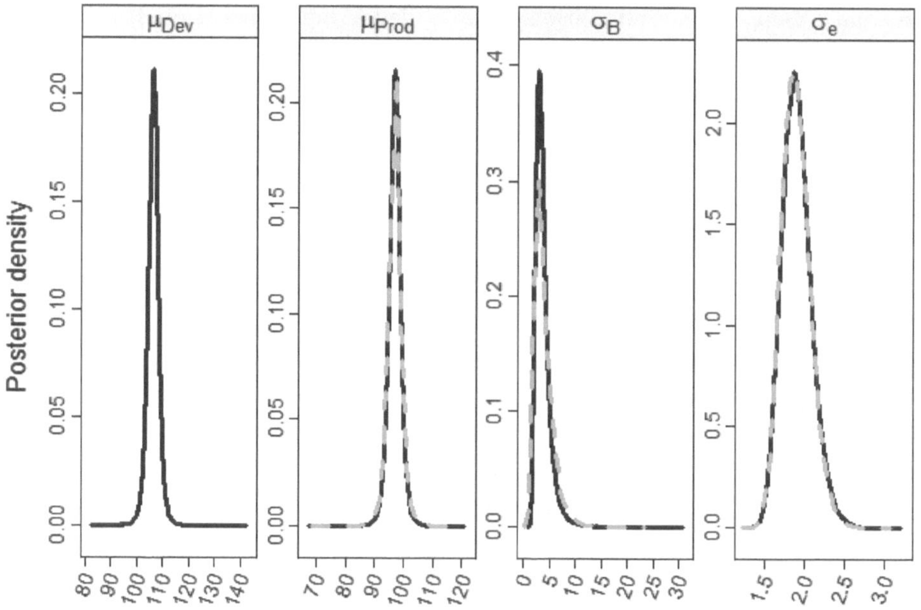

FIGURE 22.4: Analysis of full data with vague priors versus analysis of production data with informative priors: Posterior marginal distributions for $(\mu_{\text{Dev}}, \mu_{\text{Prod}}, \sigma_{\boldsymbol{\beta}}, \sigma_e)$ from analysis of full data with vague priors (black lines). Posterior marginal distributions for $(\mu_{\text{Prod}}, \sigma_{\boldsymbol{\beta}}, \sigma_e)$ from analysis of production data with informative priors (grey lines).

for the different sources of variability within the data, as well as the uncertainty in the estimates of process performance. As for the future, we think that as Bayesian methods continue to gain traction in the pharmaceutical industry, it is only a matter of time before a posterior probability or posterior quantile becomes a commonly applied test statistic for content uniformity testing of a batch of drug product.

Bibliography

Bergum, J. and Li, H. (2007). Acceptance limits for the new ICH USP 29 content uniformity test. *Pharmaceutical Technology*, 30(10):90–100.

E2810-11, A. (2011). Standard Practice for Demonstrating Capability to Comply with the Test for Uniformity of Dosage Units, ASTM E2810-11.

Hannig, J. (2009). On generalized fiducial inference. *Statistica Sinica*, 19:491–544.

Hudson-Curtis, B. and Novick, S. (2016). Assessing Content Uniformity (Chapter 23). In L. Zhang, editor, *Nonclinical Statistics for Pharmaceutical and Biotechnology Industries*, pages 631–652. Springer, New York, NY.

Krishnamoorthy, K. and Mathew, T. (2009). *Statistical Tolerance Regions. Theory, Applications, and Computation.* 2nd edition. John Wiley & Sons, Inc., Hoboken, New Jersey, USA.

Lan, K. K. G. and DeMets, D. L. (1983). Discrete sequential boundaries for clinical trials. *Biometrika*, 70:659–663.

LeBlond, D. and Mockus, L. (2014). The posterior probability of passing a compendial standard, part 1: Uniformity of dosage units. *Statistics in Biopharmaceutical Research*, 6(3):270–286.

Lewis, R. and Fan, A. (2016). Improved acceptance limits for ASTM standard E2810. *Statistics in Biopharmaceutical Research*, 8(1):40–48.

Lewis, R. and Novick, S. (2012). A generalized pivotal quantity approach to the parametric tolerance interval test for dose content uniformity batch testing. *Statistics in Biopharmaceutical Research*, 4(1):28–36.

Lostrito, R. (2005). Advisory Committee for Pharmaceutical Science Meeting (in transcripts). `"http://www.fda.gov/ohrms/dockets/ac/05/transcripts/2005-4187T1.pdf"` (accessed 4 Dec 2017).

Novick, S., Christopher, D., Dey, M., Lyapustina, S., Golden, M., Leiner, S., Wyka, B., Delzeit, H., Novak, C., and Larner, G. (2009). A two one-sided parametric tolerance interval test for control of delivered dose uniformity. Part 1 — characterization of FDA proposed test. *American Association of Pharmaceutical Scientists PharmSciTech*, 10(3):820–828.

Novick, S. and Hudson-Curtis, B. (2018a). Content uniformity testing via two variance components parametric tolerance interval test. *Journal of Biopharmaceutical Statistics*, 28(3):463–474.

Novick, S. and Hudson-Curtis, B. (2018b). Efficient computing for one and two variance components parametric tolerance interval testing. *Statistics in Biopharmaceutical Research*, 11(2):146–151.

O'Hagan, A., Stevens, J., and Campbell, M. (2005). Assurance in clinical trial design. *Pharmaceutical Statistics*, 4(3):187–201.

Plummer, M. (2003). JAGS: A Program for Analysis of Bayesian Graphical Models Using Gibbs Sampling. In *Proceedings of the 3rd International Workshop on Distributed Statistical Computing (DSC 2003), Vienna, Austria, March 20–22.* ISSN 1609-395X.

U.S. Pharmacopeia (2006). Uniformity of dosage units. The sixth interim revision announcement (1st supplement to USP 30–NF 25). *Pharmacopeial Forum*, 32(6):1649—-1659.

U.S. Pharmacopeia (2011a). Explanatory note "USP-NF harmonized chapter <905> uniformity of dosage units". `"http://www.usp.org/USPNF/notices/generalChapter905.html"`, Accessed 11 September 2018.

U.S. Pharmacopeia (2011b). Uniformity of Dosage Units. `"https://tinyurl.com/lc8exx5"`, Accessed 02 March 2016.

U.S. Pharmacopeia (2014). Inhalation and nasal drug products: Aerosols, sprays, and powders – Performance quality tests, first supplement to USP 37-NF32, August 2014.

Weerahandi, S. (2004). *Generalized Inference in Repeated Measures: Exact Methods in MANOVA and Mixed Models.* John Wiley & Sons, New Jersey.

23

Bayesian Methods for In Vitro Dissolution Drug Testing and Similarity Comparisons

Linas Mockus

Purdue University, US

Dave LeBlond

CMC Statistical Studies, US

The rationale for, and current practice of, in vitro dissolution testing is reviewed. The non-linear Weibull dissolution profile equation is described and employed in hierarchical Bayesian modeling. Use of this modeling is illustrated with actual multi-batch dissolution studies to predict the posterior predictive probability that a) a single manufacturing process will produce tablets that meet the requirements of the compendial standard, and b) two manufacturing processes produce tablets with "similar" dissolution profiles. The fundamental importance of having a parametric quality standard, in the first case, and a parametric definition of similarity, in the second case, are emphasized.

23.1 Introduction

In order for an oral dosage form (tablet, capsule or other unit) to provide the desired benefit, the active pharmaceutical ingredient (API) must first dissolve in the patient's gastrointestinal tract. Drug molecules must be in a dissolved form to diffuse to their sites of biological transport, circulation, activity, storage, metabolism, and elimination. When the dissolution is rate limiting due to inherent low API solubility or intentional dosage form design (i.e. modified, controlled, or extended release), it can directly impact bioavailability, and thus the efficacy and/or safety of the medication. Consequently, the understanding and control of the dissolution rate of a pharmaceutical product is a key goal of both pharmaceutical sponsors and regulators.

Because it is difficult to determine dissolution rates in vivo, in vitro (IV) dissolution methodologies have evolved as surrogate measures, which, ideally, are predictive of in vivo performance, bioavailability, blood levels, pharmacokinetic behavior, and ultimately, safety and efficacy of the drug product.

In this chapter, we give a brief review of current practice in IV dissolution. More comprehensive recent reviews of the field are available in Burdick et al. (2017); LeBlond et al. (2015); Long and Chen (2009) and Tsong et al. (2009). We provide some motivation for Bayesian approaches in this field and give two examples that rely on Bayesian paradigms and methodology. Data and computer code used in these examples are available from the book's web site `http://www.statistica.it/gianluca/book/bmpr/`.

23.2 Current statistical practices in IV dissolution and their limitations

23.2.1 Role of compendial standards in lot disposition decisions

Regulatory authorities require most solid oral dosage forms to meet compendial standards for lot release (e.g. World Health Association, 2006; U.S. Food and Drug Administration, 1997b,a; European Medicine Agency, 2008). Compendial standards such as USP<711> for immediate release or USP<724> for modified release dosage forms specify multistage tests performed in a well-defined commercial apparatus (see U.S. Pharmacopeia, 2008).

In harmony with the European and Japanese Pharmacopoeia, USP<711> describes the multi-stage testing that serves as a market standard for the expected quality of dissolution performance for many immediate or extended release drug products. USP<711> specifies the conditions for IV dissolution determination, such as dissolution medium and apparatus, gives the number of units to be tested, and places limits on the expected measurement results. IV dissolution measurements consist of the estimated amount of drug dissolved (usually expressed as a percent of the unit active ingredient label claim, %LC) as a function of time during agitation within a commercial dissolution apparatus. Rapidly dissolving or immediate release (IR) product units must generally exhibit a minimum % dissolution (referred to as Q) at some specified early time (e.g. 30 or 45 minutes) to assure adequate bioavailability. Extended release (ER) products generally have minimum and/or maximum % dissolution limits at an early, intermediate, and later time to assure the integrity of the release mechanism.

The Q and other % dissolution limits and times for a given product are originally set by negotiation between sponsors and regulators and may be codified in respective compendial monographs (see discussion in Hofer and Gray, 2003). For example, the USP monograph on Metformin Hydrochoride Tablets (an IR product) specifies a Q of $\geq$ 70%LC at 60 minutes. The USP monograph on the 500mg Metformin Hydrochoride ER Tablets specifies that the % dissolved at 1, 3, and 10 hours be within the ranges 20 to 40%LC, 45 to 60%LC, and $\geq$ 85%LC, respectively.

The USP<711> three stage sampling and acceptance table for IR products is summarized in Table 23.1.

TABLE 23.1: USP<711> Sampling and acceptance table for IR dosage forms.

Stage	Number of units sampled and tested	Acceptance criteria for observed % dissolution and decision
1	6	If the 6 individual results are all $\geq Q + 5\%$, pass. Otherwise continue to stage 2
2	6 more	If the average of the 12 results is $\geq Q$, and all 12 results are $\geq Q - 15\%$, pass. Otherwise continue to stage 3
3	12 more	If the average of the 24 results is $\geq Q$, and not more than 2 of the 24 results are $< Q - 15\%$, and all 24 results are $\geq Q - 25\%$, pass. Otherwise, fail.

A lot of drug product that passes the USP<711> standard test at Stage 1, 2, or 3 is considered to have met the compendial standard. However, the USP General Notices implies that compendial standards such as USP<711> and the associated monographs serve as benchmarks of performance and are not intended to be used per se for lot release decisions. Manufacturers are presumably expected to implement their own demonstration tests to assure that the compendial market standard can be met with high probability.

23.2.1.1 Parametric vs. empirical market standards

USP<711> is an empirical standard in that expected quality is stated in terms of measurements (i.e. the acceptance region is defined in the space of observed data). From the perspective of inference, it would have been preferable to specify an acceptance region based on limits for key population parameters such as true means and standard deviations. Such a parametric standard would motivate understanding of underlying sampling distributions and facilitate development of coherent risk based statistical tests for lot disposition decisions for a given product. Parametric standards are desirable because they are independent of the measurement or estimation methods used and provide a basis for statistical tests of hypothesis or equivalence.

In order to construct a proper parametric standard for risk-based decision making, a manufacturer must "reverse engineer" the intent of empirical standards such as USP<711>. A notable procedure for doing so is described in ASTM E2709 (Practice for demonstrating capability to comply with an acceptance procedure). This methodology, originally proposed by Bergum (1990) and encoded into a SAS program commonly referred to as "CuDAL" (see Chapter 22), uses computer simulation and/or conservative approximations to generate the probability of passing USP<711> as a function of the true lot mean and standard deviation (assuming Normality). Cholayudth (2011) gives a nice summary and a spreadsheet implementation.

In the ASTM E2709 approach, a bivariate $C\%$ confidence region on the sample average and standard deviation is estimated from observed testing on some specified number of units from the lot. The extremes of this confidence region are compared to a lower bound perimeter defined by a minimum, P, of the probability of passing USP <711>. If the confidence region is within the perimeter, then the lot has a probability P of meeting the market standard with at least $C\%$ confidence in a repeated sampling sense. While the ASTM E2709 methodology is statistically valid, it is inherently conservative in that many truly acceptable lots will fail the test with traditional sample sizes. De los Santos et al. (2015) have proposed less conservative methodologies involving alternative confidence region shapes or tolerance interval approaches. These authors suggested Bayesian approaches as a subject for future research, which we consider in this chapter.

23.2.2 Statistical modeling of IR dissolution profiles

Key product development and pivotal clinical lots of IR products are usually tested at 3 to 6 time points (e.g. 15, 20, 25, 30, 45, and 60 minutes). However, Kielt et al. (2016) illustrate technology permitting continuous dissolution monitoring. Dissolution testing over time provides a dissolution profile (plot of observed % dissolution over time) for each unit tested. A wide variety of linear and nonlinear mathematical models have been fitted to dissolution profiles. Zhang et al. (2010) provide a comprehensive description of such models. An empirical model we have found useful in our work, and which we illustrate here, is the Weibull drug dissolution model. The 3-parameter Weibull drug dissolution model is obtained by adding a scale parameter M (described below) to the cumulative 2-parameter Weibull distribution function (the complement of which is the Weibull survival function which is useful in reliability analysis). This model expresses % dissolution, w, as a function of dissolution time, t, conditional on parameters M, T and b. Namely,

$$w = M\left[1 - \exp\left(-\left(\frac{t}{T}\right)^b\right)\right]. \tag{23.1}$$

Its inverse function is also of interest given by

$$t = T\left[\log\left(\frac{M}{M-w}\right)^{1/b}\right].$$

Unless otherwise noted, all log transformations used in this chapter will be natural log, denoted $\log(\cdot)$.

Figure 23.1 provides insight into the effect of changes in Weibull parameter values on profile shape.

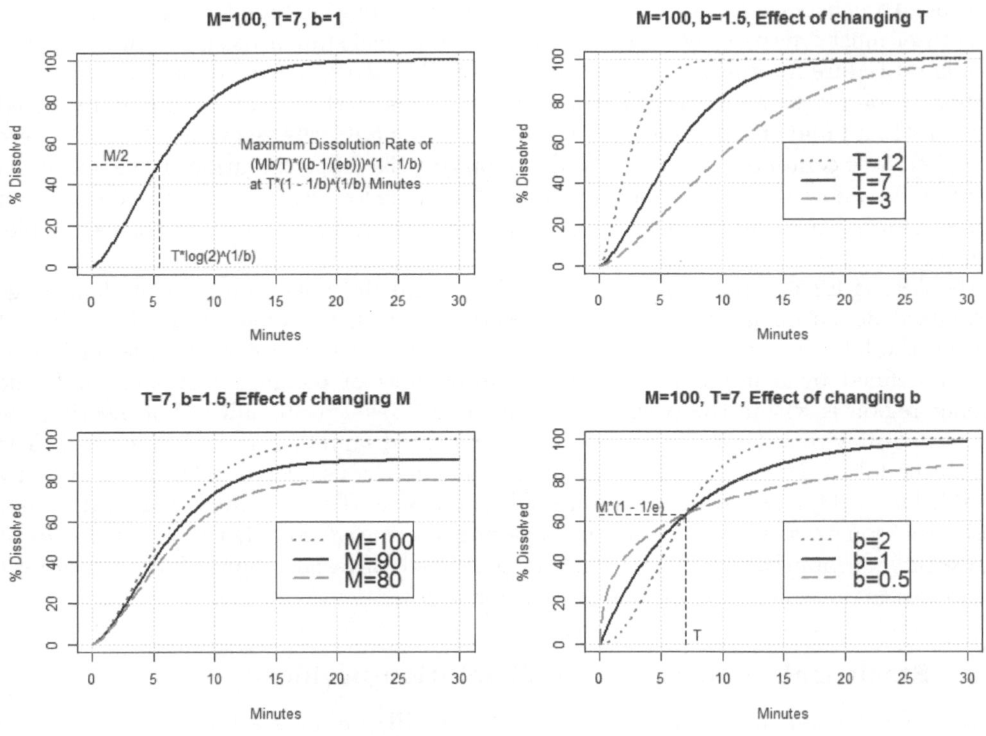

FIGURE 23.1: Illustration of a typical dissolution profile (upper left) and the impact of changes in parameters T (upper right), M (lower left) and b (lower right) on profile shape based on Equation (1). See accompanying text for details.

The upper left graph represents a typical IR dissolution profile. The predicted time at which half of the drug is dissolved is $T\left[\log(2)\right]^{1/b}$. The maximum dissolution rate is $\left[Mb/T\right)\left((b-1)/(eb)\right]^{1-1/b}$, which occurs at time $T\left[1-1/b\right)\right]^{1/b}$. The effect of changing M (lower left) or T (upper right) is a proportional change in the vertical or horizontal direction, respectively. While variation in any of the three parameters may result in between- and/or within-lot unit dosage non-uniformity, variation in M would have a proportional impact. Increasing b (lower right) accentuates sigmoidicity producing an initial delay, commonly seen in IV dissolution profiles. Regardless of the value of b, the profile always predicts a % dissolution of $M(1 - 1/e)$ at time T. If dissolution profiles from multiple tablets from multiple lots of a process are available, proper modeling can provide insight into the relative amount of each type of variation from within and between lot sources.

23.2.3 Extending inferences to the process that makes lots

Deming (1975) distinguished two kinds of statistical studies:

- Enumerative study: action is taken only on the material studied.
- Analytic study: action is taken on the process that produced the material studied.

Any "one-lot-at-a-time" release test, including the approach recommended in ASTM E2709 methodology, is enumerative and provides no actionable inferences regarding the process that makes lots. Analytic inferences, on the other hand, are essential to risk-based process validation as advocated by U.S. Food and Drug Administration (2011). Bayesian hierarchical process modeling provides a flexible paradigm for such analytic inferences. Bayesian approaches were introduced by LeBlond and Mockus (2014) for analytic process inference regarding unit dose uniformity based on the USP<905> market standard. In this chapter, we apply similar Bayesian models to process inference based on USP<711>. In the first example below, we illustrate how dissolution profiles from multiple lots from a process can be used to estimate the probability that future lots made by the process will pass the USP<711> compendial standard.

23.2.4 Comparison of IR dissolution profiles

Because IV dissolution often reflects drug bioavailability, European Medicine Agency (2010); U.S. Food and Drug Administration (1995, 1997b,a,c, 2000, 2001, 2003) EMA (2010) and FDA (1995, 1997a-c, 2000, 2001, 2003) require a demonstration of dissolution similarity for process / method change or manufacturing site change or to obtain a bio-waiver that avoids the need for a costly clinical study. For dissolution method validation, there is sometimes also a need to demonstrate IV dissolution "non-equivalence" to prove that the in-vitro method can detect formulation / process differences. Zhang et al. (2010) provide a comprehensive description of statistical metrics and criteria often used for such comparison studies.

A coherent similarity test requires an unambiguous and actionable definition of what is meant by "similar". Ideally, the requirements for similarity would be based on those aspects of the dissolution profile critical for safety and efficacy. U.S. Food and Drug Administration (1997b) indicates that this can be achieved if the relationship between IV and in vivo performance is understood (referred to as an in vitro in vivo correlation or IVIVC). In the absence of such a correlation, a number of arbitrary standards of similarity have been advanced in the interest of regulatory due diligence. A comprehensive review of these is found in Zhang et al. (2010).

European Medicine Agency (2010) and U.S. Food and Drug Administration (1995, 1997a,c, 2017) recommend the use of the f_2 statistic, first proposed by Moore and Flanner (1996), as a metric for IV dissolution similarity. The f_2 metric is a "plug in statistic" in which the observed % dissolution (averaged across lots and units within lots) for each product version ($\bar{y}_{1,n}$ and $\bar{y}_{2,n}$ e.g. manufacturer 1 and 2, respectively) obtained at a number of time points ($n = 1, \ldots, N_{times}$) are substituted into Equation (23.2).

$$f_2 = 50 \log_{10} \left(\frac{100}{\sqrt{1 + \frac{1}{N_{times}} \sum_{n=1}^{N_{times}} (\bar{y}_{2,n} - \bar{y}_{1,n})^2}} \right). \tag{23.2}$$

The f_2 statistic is 100 when both profiles are identical and approaches zero as dissimilarity increases. An f_2 of 50 corresponds to profiles vertically displaced by about 10%. Regulatory guidance recommends that an observed $f_2 \geq 50$ implies that the 2 mean dissolution profiles are considered similar. The f_2 test outcome is known to be sensitive to the number and choice of time points. Traditionally, f_2 is obtained using only a few data points (e.g. $N_{times} = 3$ or 4). U.S. Food and Drug Administration (1995, 1997a) recommends no more than one time point with over 85% dissolution. As with the compendial market standards noted above, f_2 is an empirical standard for dissolution profile similarity because there is no underlying parametric definition of similarity. An alternative parametric metric, F_2, was defined by Novick et al. (2015) as

$$F_2 = F_2(\boldsymbol{w}_1, \boldsymbol{w}_2) = 50 \log_{10} \left(\frac{100}{\sqrt{1 + \frac{1}{N_{times}} \sum_{n=1}^{N_{times}} (w_{2,n} - w_{1,n})^2}} \right), \tag{23.3}$$

with

$$\boldsymbol{w}_i = \begin{bmatrix} w_{i,1} \\ w_{i,2} \\ \vdots \\ w_{i,N_{times}} \end{bmatrix}, \qquad \text{for } i = 1, 2.$$

F_2 is not an observed sampling statistic, but is a fixed function of $w_{2,n} - w_{1,n}$, where $w_{1,n}$ and $w_{2,n}$ are the true mean levels of the nth time point, (e.g. for process 1 and 2, respectively), replacing their sample estimates $\bar{y}_{1,n}$ and $\bar{y}_{2,n}$, respectively, from Equation (23.2).

It is convenient to introduce a reparameterization of Equation (23.1):

$$w \sim \text{Weibull}(t; M, \alpha, \beta) = M \left[1 - \exp\left(- \left(\frac{t}{\exp(\alpha)} \right) \exp(\beta) \right) \right].$$

where $\alpha = \log(T)$ and $\beta = \log(b)$.

If justified, the mean parameters may in turn be expressed in terms of a Weibull dissolution profile model where for process i,

$$w_{i,n} \sim \text{Weibull}(t_n; \mu_{1,i}, \mu_{2,i}, \mu_{3,i}), \qquad \text{for } i = 1, 2. \tag{23.4}$$

This reparameterization of Equation (23.1) is helpful in avoiding convergence and numerical challenges during MCMC computation (to be described below) because $\mu_2 \equiv \log(T)$

and $\mu_3 \equiv \log(b)$ need not be strictly positive as T and b must be. The upper asymptote parameter $\mu_1 = M$, can take on any real value. We illustrate the F_2 approach to similarity testing in the second example below.

To allow use of mean data, i.e. $\bar{y}_{1,n}$ and $\bar{y}_{2,n}$ in Equation (23.2) above, the U.S. Food and Drug Administration (1997a) recommends that the percent coefficient of variation at the earlier time points (e.g. 15 minutes) should not be more than 20%, and at other time points should not be more than 10%. In instances where within batch variation is more than 15% CV, a multivariate statistical distance (MSD) procedure is more suitable for dissolution profile comparison (U.S. Food and Drug Administration, 1997a). In the MSD approach, individual tablet % dissolution results at multiple time points are treated as vectors. Tsong et al. (2009) illustrate the calculations and suggest that similarity be accepted if the multi-dimensional confidence ellipse for the mean dissolution difference vector lies within a perimeter about zero based on the observed within formulation variability at each time point. The MSD approach would seem to require a greater burden of proof of similarity in those cases where variability is high.

The f_2 and multivariate metrics can only be used when both profiles being compared have the same time points. This limitation can be removed if the dissolution profile is modeled (e.g. using a Weibull model). As suggested by U.S. Food and Drug Administration (1997a), profile similarity can be based on the MSD between the estimates of the underlying model parameters for the two profiles being compared. Sathe et al. (1996) illustrate a model-based MSD approach by pre-defining a similarity acceptance region and constructing a confidence region in a manner analogous to the methods used in the model independent MSD approach of Tsong et al. (2009). We illustrate a model dependent MSD approach using a Bayesian approach in the second example below.

23.2.5 Importance of a clear definition of the similarity inference space

The aforementioned regulatory guidance discusses the conditions when each similarity approach (f_2, model independent / dependent MSD) may be applicable. However, these guidance rules are silent regarding the intended inference space for the similarity determination. Are conclusions limited to the units and lots studied (empirical study) or is there an intent to make inferences to a larger process or processes (analytic study)? In some studies, it may be important to determine similarity between two lots made by a single manufacturing process. In other studies, the comparison may be between two groups of lots made by a single process. More generally, it may be necessary to compare groups of lots from two or more manufacturers or sites. The apparent objectives of most regulated studies include inferences about the safety and efficacy of future lots made by a process. In such a case, an analytic perspective is appropriate in order to have a coherent statistical approach that assures drug product quality. Eaton et al. (2003) have outlined normative requirements for a sound statistical approach to similarity testing.

In order to treat the similarity decision from a risk-based perspective, probabilities must be estimated. A probabilistic approach to such determinations encourages consideration of inference space issues because the focus of such an approach is on the specific events to which the estimated probabilities refer. Probabilistic modeling is the hallmark of the Bayesian approach. In this chapter, we illustrate how Bayesian approaches can be used to model dissolution profiles and further how these models can facilitate risk-based dissolution similarity decisions.

23.3 The value of adopting Bayesian paradigms

In this section, we provide some motivation for Bayesian approaches in the context of dissolution similarity testing based on the F_2 metric. While this illustration is limited, the same concepts and arguments apply generally to any pharmaceutical setting in which risk-based decisions are conditional on observed data. Consider the three approaches to similarity testing illustrated in Figure 23.2.

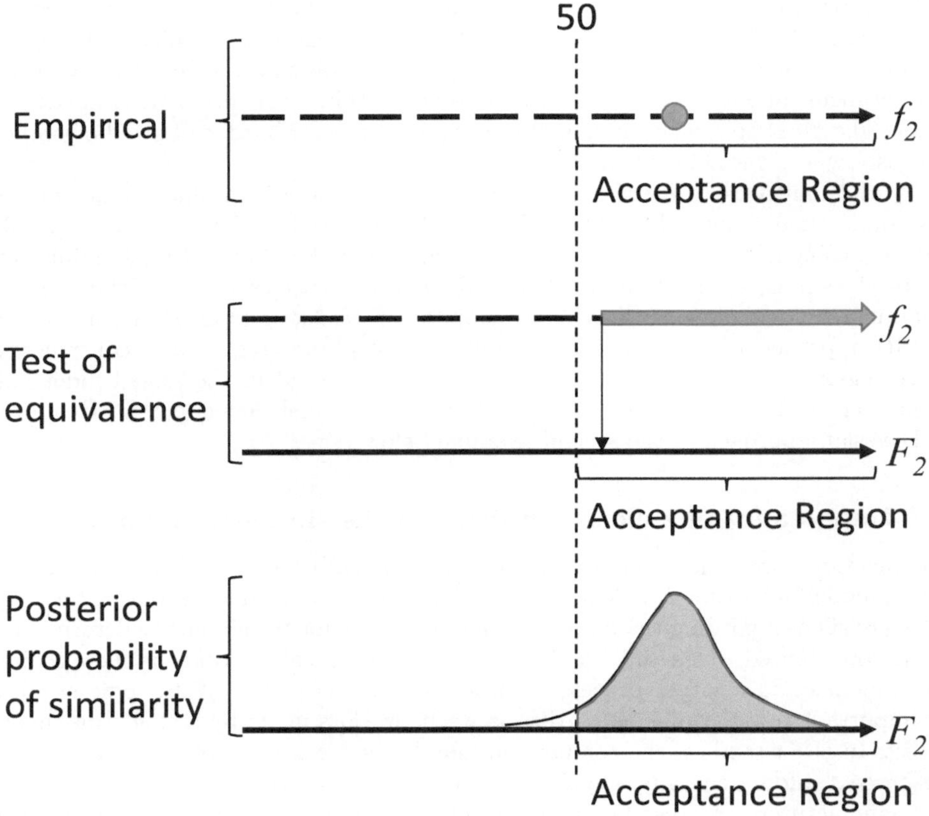

FIGURE 23.2: Illustration of conceptual differences between the current non-parametric f_2 approach (Empirical), a parametric model-based approach that uses a one-sided lower 95% confidence interval of F_2 (Test of equivalence), and a Bayesian F_2 approach (Posterior probability of similarity). The space (f_2 or F_2) on which the acceptance region is defined is indicated based on the currently accepted regulatory decision limit of 50.

Current practice is illustrated by the top approach ("Empirical") in Figure 23.2. The f_2 statistic is simply calculated from the data and if the resulting statistic (circle) is at or above 50, a conclusion of similarity is accepted. The empirical approach does not require any underlying parametric statistical model that describes how dissolution profile data are generated. There is no standard practice detailing how data from multiple lots from multiple processes/sites (if available) are to be summarized. There is no statistical test of similarity because f_2 is not conceived as an estimator of any model parameter. There is no basis for predicting the frequentist behavior of this approach.

The middle approach ("Test of equivalence") in Figure 23.2 is related to the methodology recommended by the U.S. Food and Drug Administration (2000, 2001, 2003, 2017) for a test of bioequivalence. A test of dissolution equivalence based on the F_2 metric requires a proper statistical model that takes into account the experimental and treatment designs and all sources of variance and error distributions impacting the observed dissolution profile data. A region of similarity must also be defined in the inference parameter space of F_2 (arguably ≥ 50). Based on a statistical estimator f_2 of F_2, a one-sided lower 95% confidence interval on F_2 is derived. If the lower bound of that interval is ≥ 50, a conclusion of similarity is accepted with at least 95% confidence. The confidence interval is a random statistic based on repeated sampling, which is the basis for the 95% confidence claim. Thus, the interval is shown as being associated with the sample (estimator) space of f_2 although the repeated sampling inference is mapped to the parametric (estimand) space of F_2. The confidence claim (95%) is fixed in advance and is associated with the statistical methodology, not with any particular pair of formulations being compared. The repeated sampling decision error rates and operating characteristics associated with this approach can be anticipated from theory or computer simulation. This inference procedure is clearly superior to the empirical approach. A test of equivalence treats f_2 as a statistical estimator of F_2. Unfortunately, Shah et al. (1998) concluded that the sampling distribution of f_2 is analytically intractable making it challenging to model its frequentist properties, although bootstrapping has been considered by Paixão et al. (2017).

The bottom approach ("Posterior probability of similarity") in Figure 23.2 requires a proper Bayesian model as well as prior distributions for model parameters. As with the "Test of equivalence" approach, the region of similarity is defined in the F_2 parameter space. However, unlike the "Test of equivalence" approach, the inference is also based on the F_2 parameter space. Modern Bayesian procedures provide (a sample from) the posterior distribution of F_2. As discussed in the previous section, F_2 is a fixed function of model parameters. Therefore, F_2 is obtained from each draw of a parameter joint posterior sample and thus a sample from the posterior distribution of F_2, conditional on observed data, is easily obtained by Bayesian methodology. The posterior probability of similarity can then be estimated by integrating, by a simple counting exercise, the area of the F_2 posterior distribution over the acceptance region. Unlike the fixed confidence coefficient associated with the test of equivalence confidence interval, this posterior probability is not fixed in advance, but is estimated and refers directly to the hypothesis of interest. This probability of similarity can serve as a direct, quantitative, risk-based metric of the degree of similarity without any analytical approximations. If the estimated posterior probability of similarity is high (arguably $\geq 95\%$), a conclusion of similarity can be accepted. While the repeated sampling behavior of this approach is often not known from theory, it can be determined by computer simulation. Such simulations by Novick et al. (2015) have shown that Bayesian approaches incorporating F_2 have performance that is comparable to or in many cases superior to the f_2 statistic as a decision rule.

Traditional non-linear mixed modeling based on restricted maximum likelihood estimation often depends on analytical and/or distributional approximations that can impact the estimation and inference in unexpected ways and sometimes lead to embarrassing outcomes (e.g. negative variance component estimates). We have found that Bayesian hierarchical non-linear models, such as those illustrated in this chapter, can be implemented without such approximations, translate naturally into the intuitive syntax of Bayesian software such as `BUGS` (see Lunn, 2013), `JAGS` (see Plummer, 2017), `Stan` (see Stan Development Team, 2018), or `SAS Proc MCMC` (see SAS Institute, Inc, 2018) contribute to a deeper understanding of the process being modeled, and to greater insight into its future performance. Long before modern Bayesian tools were widely available, Aitchison and Dunsmore (1975) and Geisser (1993) provided arguments in favor of the Bayesian approach to predictive inference and decision making. In the modern era, we can employ these tools to make better health care decisions.

23.4 Applying Bayesian approaches: Two examples

In this section, we model actual dissolution profiles measured on tablets from two different solid oral dosage forms that we refer to as SODF1 and SODF2. Multiple tablets from each of multiple lots were tested from both dosage forms. Dissolution profiles for SODF1 were obtained from tablets made at a single manufacturing site, but SODF2 data include tablets made at two different manufacturing sites. We thus have the recipe for a hierarchical model: tablets within lots within a process (and for SODF2, within a manufacturing site). For both products we use a three parameter Weibull dissolution model to describe each tablet dissolution profile and estimate random effects of lot and tablet-within-lot on the three Weibull parameters to determine between-lot and within-lot variability. In Section 23.4.1 below, the data and models are presented in a form which most closely matches the variable and iteration structure used when coding in software such as `BUGS`, `JAGS`, or `Stan`. We find this coding structure intuitive and directly relevant to the model assumptions regarding data generation.

23.4.1 SODF1: Estimating the probability of meeting the USP<711> standard

The USP<711> result (Pass or Fail) is a quality metric for individual lots. However, due to sampling and analytical variability errors in lot dispositioning (pass truly substandard lots or fail truly acceptable lots) are possible. The probabilities of such disposition errors serve as quality metrics for the process that makes lots. From a regulatory perspective, it would be desirable to know the posterior probabilities, conditional on dissolution data $\boldsymbol{y}$, Pr(Pass at Stage $X \mid \boldsymbol{y}$), where $X = 1, 2, 3$, and Pr(Fail $\mid \boldsymbol{y}$) for future lots made by the process. The objective of this SODF1 example is to estimate these probabilities. Such estimates would also be of value to a manufacturer because additional stages incur added analytical costs and failures incur investigation and replacement costs. Costs need to be anticipated to support proper life-cycle budgeting. In order to estimate these probabilities for a given process, we require dissolution testing results on multiple units from multiple lots made by the process.

23.4.1.1 Data description

The SODF1 monograph specifies a minimum % dissolution of $Q = 80\%$ at 30 minutes. The data consist of $N_{lots} = 6$ SODF1 lots made by a single manufacturer. Twelve units (tablets) from each lot were tested (total number of units $N_{units} = 72$). Repeated measures of % dissolution were taken from each unit at 1, 2, 5, 10, 15, 20, and 30 minutes of dissolution time. Thus there were $N = 6 \times 12 \times 7 = 504$ total observations. The variables l_n, u_n, t_n, and y_n identify the unique lot (1 to 6), unique unit (1 to 72), dissolution time , and observed % dissolution, respectively, for each observation $n = 1, \ldots, N$.

23.4.1.2 Sampling model description

The observed % dissolution is assumed here to have Normally distributed errors of measurement,

$$y_m \overset{iid}{\sim} \mathrm{N}(w_m, \sigma^2), \tag{23.5}$$

with a common standard deviation, σ. While error diagnostics (not presented here) verify that this is a reasonable approximation for the examples in this chapter, there are at least two issues with this naïve approximation worth pointing out. First, the standard deviation of dissolution measurements is often greater near 50% dissolution and smaller near the limits of 0 and 100% dissolution where the analytical error distributions may also be skewed toward 50%. Second, the range of % dissolution is limited to 0 to 100% whereas the Normal distribution is unbounded. To model variance heterogeneity, a Normal error distribution with σ being a quadratic function of dissolution time might suffice. If both spread and skewness are excessive, a family of Skew-Normal error distributions might be appropriate. Alternatively, a logit transformation or a Beta error distribution (which is similarly bounded) for y might be considered. For the sake of simplicity, we continue with the naïve assumption of Equation (23.5), while recognizing that, in general, more elaborate assumptions may be appropriate.

The unobserved true dissolution, w_n, of observation n is modelled using the Weibull dissolution model as

$$w_n \sim \mathrm{Weibull}(t_n; M_n, T_n, b_n),$$

where the three Weibull parameters of the dissolution model are each modelled hierarchically (units within lots within process) as vectors composed of a process mean, $\boldsymbol{\mu}$, a lot specific effect, $\boldsymbol{\varepsilon}_{l_n}$, and a unit specific effect, $\boldsymbol{\delta}_{u_n}$:

$$\begin{aligned} \begin{bmatrix} M_n \\ T_n \\ b_n \end{bmatrix} &= \boldsymbol{\mu} + \boldsymbol{\varepsilon}_{l_n} + \boldsymbol{\delta}_{u_n} \\ &= \begin{bmatrix} \mu_1 \\ \mu_2 \\ \mu_3 \end{bmatrix} + \begin{bmatrix} \varepsilon_{1,l_n} \\ \varepsilon_{2,l_n} \\ \varepsilon_{3,l_n} \end{bmatrix} + \begin{bmatrix} \delta_{1,u_n} \\ \delta_{2,u_n} \\ \delta_{3,u_n} \end{bmatrix}. \end{aligned} \tag{23.6}$$

The subscripts l_n and u_n identify the unique lot and unit associated with the nth observation.

Analyses of dissolution data generally include too few lots (e.g. 6 to 13) to allow reasonable estimation of inter-parameter error correlations. Therefore, the lot level effects are assumed to be mutually uncorrelated random samples from Normal populations with zero mean and standard deviation vector $\boldsymbol{\sigma}_l = (\sigma_1^l, \sigma_2^l, \sigma_3^l)^\top$ as follows:

$$\boldsymbol{\varepsilon}_{l_n} \overset{iid}{\sim} \mathrm{N}(\mathbf{0}, \boldsymbol{\Lambda}), \tag{23.7}$$

where $\boldsymbol{\Lambda} = \boldsymbol{\sigma}_l^\top \boldsymbol{I} \boldsymbol{\sigma}_l$, $\boldsymbol{I}$ is a 3×3 identity matrix and $i = 1, \ldots, N_{lots}$.

Because of the large number of unique units available in the data set, modeling covariance among the unit level effects is feasible. Consequently, unit level effects are assumed drawn from a multivariate Normal population having zero mean and a non-diagonal symmetric covariance matrix, $\boldsymbol{\Upsilon}$.

$$\boldsymbol{\delta}_{u_n} \overset{iid}{\sim} \mathrm{N}(\mathbf{0}, \boldsymbol{\Upsilon}), \tag{23.8}$$

where $\boldsymbol{\Upsilon} = \boldsymbol{\sigma}_u^\top \boldsymbol{\Omega} \boldsymbol{\sigma}_u$, $\boldsymbol{\Omega}$ is a correlation matrix and $i = 1, \ldots, N_{units}$.

This decomposition facilitates prior specification as discussed in the next sub-section. Had there been a larger number of lots in the data set it would be preferable to model correlations in $\boldsymbol{\Lambda}$ as well as in $\boldsymbol{\Upsilon}$.

23.4.1.3 Prior distributional assumptions

The full Bayesian model requires specification of proper prior distributions for the 11 underlying model parameters, $\boldsymbol{\mu}, \boldsymbol{\sigma_u}, \boldsymbol{\sigma_l}, \sigma$ and $\boldsymbol{\Omega}$. We employed weakly informative priors here, but — if scientifically justified — informative priors might have been used to advantage. Our approach to identifying priors was iterative. Starting with informative priors, we monitored the impact on the estimated posteriors while successively reducing the prior information content (widening the spread of the prior distributions) until prior choice was not impacting the posterior estimate. For instance, we initially employed Normal prior distributions for location parameters, μ_1, μ_2 and μ_3 centered near parameter point estimates obtained from nonlinear regression fits of the mean profile to the Weibull dissolution model. For the scale parameters $\sigma_1^l, \sigma_2^l, \sigma_3^l, \sigma_1^u, \sigma_2^u, \sigma_3^u$ and σ, we initially employed folded Normal prior distributions left truncated at zero. Ultimately, final posterior distributions were obtained using uniform prior distributions for both location and scale parameters. Of course, if justifiable and convincing prior knowledge were available, it would be preferable to leverage that prior knowledge for better-informed and more efficient decision making.

For the correlation matrix $\boldsymbol{\Omega}$, we used the prior distribution $\boldsymbol{\Omega} \sim$ LKJ Corr(1). The LKJ distribution (Lewandowski et al., 2009) is a distribution over correlation matrices and has the density $f(\boldsymbol{\Omega} \mid \eta) \propto \mid \boldsymbol{\Omega} \mid^{\eta-1}$, so $\eta = 1$ leads to a uniform distribution on correlation matrices, while the magnitude of correlations between components decreases as $\eta \to \infty$. LKJ prior is recommended for the Hamiltonian Monte Carlo based software (`Stan`) we were using — see Gelman et al. (2013), Stan Development Team (2018) and Chapter 21. An alternative choice is a Wishart prior which might be more effective for Gibbs-sampler based software such as `BUGS`.

23.4.1.4 Computational methods

The statistical model, given by Equations (23.5) through (23.8), was fit to the data using the `R` package `rstan` (Stan Development Team, 2018) under `R` version 3.3.2 and `RStudio` version 1.0.136 (with `Rtools`) under `Windows 7` using a 4-core, 2GHz 64bit processor. Four chains, 20,000 iterations each, were collected after a 20,000 warmup and random initialization. This produced an 80,000 draw sample from the joint posterior distribution.

The following `R` packages were required and are freely available from `https://cran.r-project.org/` : `rstan`, `lattice`, `latticeExtra`, `MASS`, `coda`. We found the MCMC diagnostic utilities `mcmcCoda`, `diagMCMC`, and `plotPost` from the `DBDA2-utilities.R` file (available from `https://sites.google.com/site/doingbayesiandataanalysis/software-installation`) described in Kruschke (2015) useful for monitoring convergence and mixing.

23.4.1.5 Marginal summary of model parameter joint posterior distribution

The utilities from Kruschke (2015) were used to visually assure convergence and mixing.

TABLE 23.2: Marginal summary of model parameter joint posterior distribution for SODF1.

Parameter	Mean	SD	2.5%	50%	97.5%	ESS	$\widehat{R}$	Standard Error of Mean as a % of SD
μ_1	95.47	1	93.54	95.46	97.46	4893	1.002	1.4
μ_2	2.32	0.05	2.22	2.33	2.43	18203	1.001	0.7
μ_3	0.276	0.027	0.226	0.276	0.327	1124	1.003	3
σ	1.56	0.06	1.45	1.56	1.68	80000	1.002	0.4
σ_1^l	2.09	1.16	0.88	1.81	4.99	2844	1.002	1.9
σ_2^l	0.106	0.064	0.033	0.092	0.266	1302	1.003	2.8
σ_3^l	0.053	0.031	0.019	0.046	0.128	17292	1	0.8
σ_1^u	0.325	0.247	0.026	0.27	0.925	508	1.012	4.4
σ_2^u	0.145	0.014	0.122	0.144	0.175	80000	1.002	0.4
σ_2^u	0.046	0.007	0.032	0.045	0.061	1378	1.003	2.7

The standard deviations of the marginal posterior distributions in Table 23.2 are reasonably low compared to the respective means. The estimated medians are reasonably close to the respective means and based on the 2.5% and 97.5% percentile estimates, the marginal distributions are reasonably symmetrical. The $\widehat{R}$ values are all below 1.02, suggesting good mixing among the four chains. The effective sample size (ESS — see Chapter 1) values are all near or above 1000, except for σ_1^u, which is associated with the between unit covariance matrix. The standard error of the posterior mean is below 5% of the standard deviation of the posterior for all parameters. The relatively low ESS of some parameters suggests that a larger MCMC sample should have been taken. Nevertheless, we continue with the example for illustration.

23.4.1.6 Fitted dissolution profiles

In Figure 23.3, the dissolution profiles of each tablet in the data set are plotted with lot identified using different plot symbols and line types. Each line corresponding to a given lot connect the posterior means corresponding colored lines connect the posterior mean of predicted % dissolved. The posterior mean of the nth observation was calculated as:

$$\bar{w}_n = \frac{1}{N_{draws}} \sum_{i=1}^{N_{draws}} \text{Weibull}\left(t_n; \mu_1^{[i]}, \mu_2^{[i]}, \mu_3^{[i]}\right),$$

with $N_{draws} = 80,000$ and where the superscripts in brackets denote the ith MCMC posterior draw. The posterior mean of predicted % dissolved appears to correspond well with the observed data and the fitted Weibull model matches the observed dissolution profile shapes adequately. The Bayesian hierarchical Weibull profile model thus appears to be a useful representation of the mechanism of the underlying IV dissolution process for SODF1.

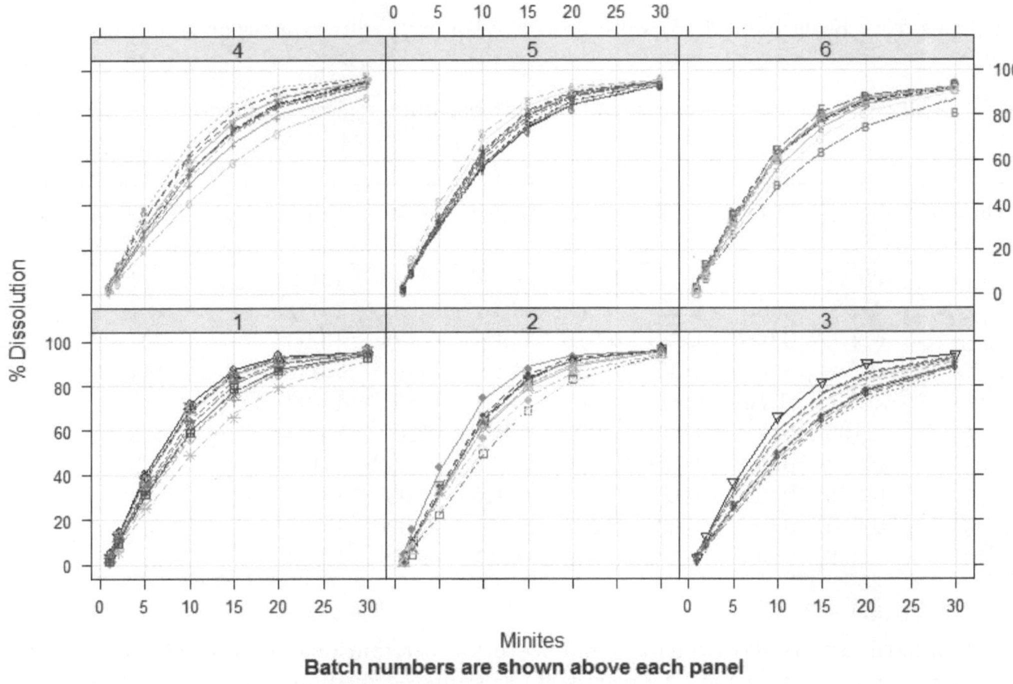

FIGURE 23.3: Comparison of model predictions (joined with colored lines) with observed data (correspondingly colored circles).

23.4.1.7 Estimating the posterior predictive probability of future USP<711> outcomes

Four possible mutually exclusive and exhaustive outcome events result from an execution of the USP<711>: Pass at Stage 1, Pass at Stage 2, Pass at Stage 3, or Fail. We estimated the USP<711> outcome probabilities of each of these events for future lots made by the SODF1 process and tested using USP<711> using the MCMC posterior sample summarized in Table 23.2 . From the 80,000 draw posterior sample, 16,000 draws of future observations were randomly sampled. For each of these 16,000 posterior draws (indexed by the superscript $[i]$), predicted effects of 4,000 future lots (indexed by l) were simulated based on Equation (23.7), i.e.

$$\boldsymbol{\varepsilon}_l^{[i]} \overset{iid}{\sim} \mathrm{N}(\mathbf{0}, \boldsymbol{\Lambda}^{[i]}),$$

for $l = 1, \ldots, 4,000$ and $i = 1, \ldots, 16,000$.

For each posterior draw, $[i]$, and predicted future lot l, unit level effects from 24 future units (indexed by $u(l)$) were simulated based on Equation (23.8)

$$\boldsymbol{\delta}_{u(l)}^{[i]} \overset{iid}{\sim} \mathrm{N}(\mathbf{0}, \boldsymbol{\Upsilon}^{[i]}),$$

for $u(l) = 1, \ldots, 24$.

For each posterior draw $[i]$, and unit level effect within lot level effect, $u(l)$, Weibull parameters were simulated based on Equation (23.6), i.e.

$$\begin{bmatrix} M_{u(l)}^{[i]} \\ T_{u(l)}^{[i]} \\ b_{u(l)}^{[i]} \end{bmatrix} = \boldsymbol{\mu}^{[i]} + \boldsymbol{\varepsilon}_l^{[i]} + \boldsymbol{\delta}_{u(l)}^{[i]}.$$

For each posterior draw $[i]$, and unit level effect within lot level effect, $u(l)$, a future true % dissolved at 30 minutes,

$$w_{u(l)}^{[i]} \sim \text{Weibull}(t_n; M_{u(l)}^{[i]}, T_{u(l)}^{[i]}, b_{u(l)}^{[i]}),$$

and future observed % dissolved,

$$\widehat{y}_{u(l)}^{[i]} \overset{iid}{\sim} \text{N}\left(w_{u(l)}^{[i]}, \left(\sigma^{[i]}\right)^2\right),$$

were simulated. The 24 simulated results for each lot were applied to the USP<711> algorithm in Table 23.1 using the monograph Q value of 80 and the four mutually exclusive USP<711> outcomes were tallied for each set of 4,000 lots. Thus 16,000 samples from the posterior predictive distributions of the marginal probabilities Pr(Pass at Stage $X \mid \boldsymbol{y}$) (with $X = 1, 2, 3$) and Pr(Fail $\mid \boldsymbol{y}$) were obtained for this process. Note that these four marginal probabilities sum to one for each of the 16,000 draws. Kernel density estimates of these marginal USP <711> outcome probabilities are presented in Figure 23.4.

Figure 23.4 clearly shows that these probabilities exhibit skewed distributions and would be poorly represented by a single value. It is clear, however, that, based on the model and data used, at least 99% of future SODF1 lots should pass at stage 1 or 2 USP<711>. Stage 3 testing (required either when a lot passes at stage 3 or when a lot fails) should occur with a posterior predictive probability below 1%. Of those lots that do require Stage 3 testing, most will ultimately fail. However, the overall failure rate will be below 1%. Very rarely should a lot require stage 3 testing and it is very unlikely that a future lot will fail. However, we can express risk more quantitatively. For example, in Table 23.3 are the percentiles of the distributions illustrated in Figure 23.4, obtained by a simple counting exercise from the simulation output.

TABLE 23.3: Cumulative posterior predictive probabilities of USP<711> outcome events when testing SODF1.

Percentile:	1%	5%	50%	95%	99%
USP<711> outcome event					
Pass at stage 1	0.625	0.767	0.9518	0.9848	0.9928
Pass at stage 2	0.0073	0.0153	0.0483	0.2198	0.3185
Pass at stage 3	0	0	0	0.0015	0.0053
Fail	0	0	0	0.0068	0.0605

Summaries such as in Table 23.3 allow us to place credible bounds on the true values of the event probabilities and make "worst-case" risk statements such as "A 95% one-sided lower credible bound on the probability of a future SODF1 lot passing USP<711> at stage 1 is 0.767" or "A 95% one-sided upper credible bound on the probability of a future SODF1 lot failing the USP<711> test is 0.0068". More informative risk assessments are available from a perspective of power (see Kruschke, 2015, Section 13.1.2).

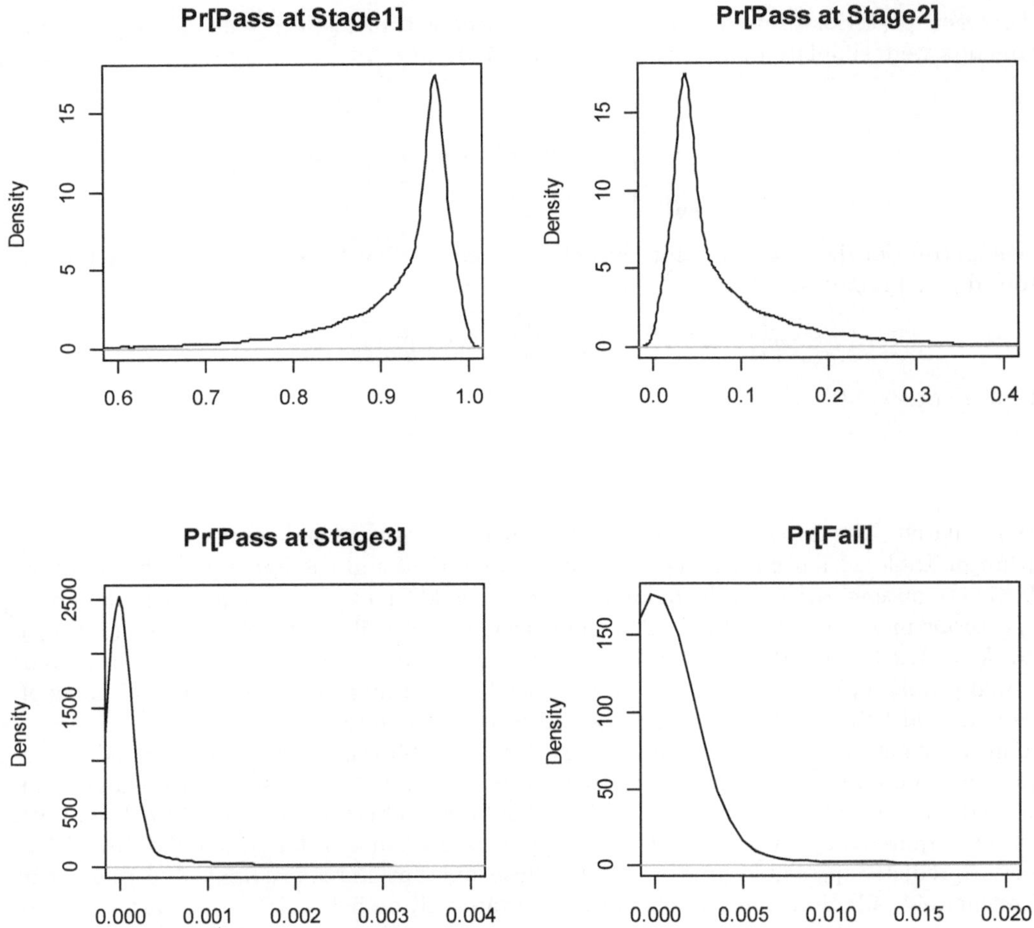

FIGURE 23.4: Kernel density estimates of posterior predictive probabilities of USP<711> outcome probabilities based on dissolution profiles obtained from 6 lots of Product1. Each estimate is based on 16,000 posterior draws.

While such statements provide intuition into the quality level of the SODF1 process, it may be of more practical interest to estimate the expected cost of providing the SODF1 product over its life-cycle (at least related to risk of dissolution testing and failure). Such costs could be of interest to both manufacturers and regulators. USP<711> testing costs double (quadruple) when stage 2 (3) testing is required. A USP<711> failure entails both an investigation cost and an additional manufacturing cost to replace the failed lot. LeBlond and Mockus (2014) provide approximate lot manufacturing, testing, and failure investigation costs. We can use these estimates to illustrate expected cost determination for the SODF1 product. The approximate costs associated with each USP<711> outcome are given in Table 23.4.

We can average these costs, weighted by the posterior predictive distributions illustrated in Figure 23.4. Let $P_e^{[i]}$ be the ith draw from the posterior predictive distribution of the

TABLE 23.4: Approximate cost per lot for various USP<711> test outcome events for testing of SODF1.

USP<711> outcome event	e	Manufacturing	USP<711> Testing	Failure investigation	Total Cost (C_e)
Pass at stage 1	1	200	3	0	203
Pass at stage 2	2	200	6	0	206
Pass at stage 3	3	200	12	0	212
Fail	4	400	12	2	414

probability of event e, then

$$\text{Expected Cost per lot} \cong \frac{1}{N_{draws}} \sum_{i=1}^{N_{draws}} \sum_{e=1}^{4} P_e^{[i]} C_e,$$

for $N_{draws} = 80,000$.

The expected cost per lot for SODF1, based on the assumed costs and the posterior predictive distributions illustrated in Figure 23.4 is $203,715. Thus, a manufacturer should factor an additional $715 cost per lot, above the initial manufacturing cost of $200,000, into the product budget to account for additional testing and expected lot failures. In this example, the additional cost is a small fraction of the overall manufacturing cost, but when unfortunate events occur, the impact can be problematic if not anticipated, particularly to affected stakeholders in an organization (e.g. an analytical laboratory).

If actual costs are available for testing, investigations, and lot replacement, then these can be integrated with respect to these predictive posterior distribution samples to estimate mean or worst-case costs for life-cycle resource management. This kind of knowledge should be of utility to regulators and sponsors alike in assessing the impact of product quality on the cost of health care interventions.

23.4.2 IV dissolution similarity of SODF2 made at two manufacturing sites

In this second example, we compare the dissolution profiles of a tablet product (SODF2) made at two different manufacturing sites, referred to as sites 1 and 2. We treat site 1 as the approved (or reference) site and site 2 as an unapproved (or test) site. We illustrate Bayesian model dependent tests of similarity based on both F_2 and multi-parameter space similarity regions.

23.4.2.1 Data description

We index the SODF2 manufacturing site with $m = 1, 2$. $N_{1,lots} = 8$ lots were obtained from manufacturer 1 and $N_{2,lots} = 5$ lots from manufacturer 2. Twelve units (tablets) from each lot were tested ($N_{1,lots} = 96$ and $N_{2,lots} = 60$). Percent dissolution measurements were obtained from each unit at 1, 2, 4, 8, 16, 32, and 45 minutes. Thus, there were $N_{1,obs} = 8 \times 12 \times 7 = 672$ and $N_{2,obs} = 5 \times 12 \times 7 = 420$ total observations from these sites. The vectors $l_{m,n}, u_{m,n}, t_{m,n}$ and $y_{m,n}$ identify the unique lot, unique unit, dissolution time (0 to 45), and observed % dissolution, respectively, for observation n from site m. The dissolution profiles for each lot (AKA batch) and unit are shown in Figure 23.5 below. Each of the 13 panels includes dissolution profiles for 12 tablets with circle symbols indicating individual observed dissolution values.

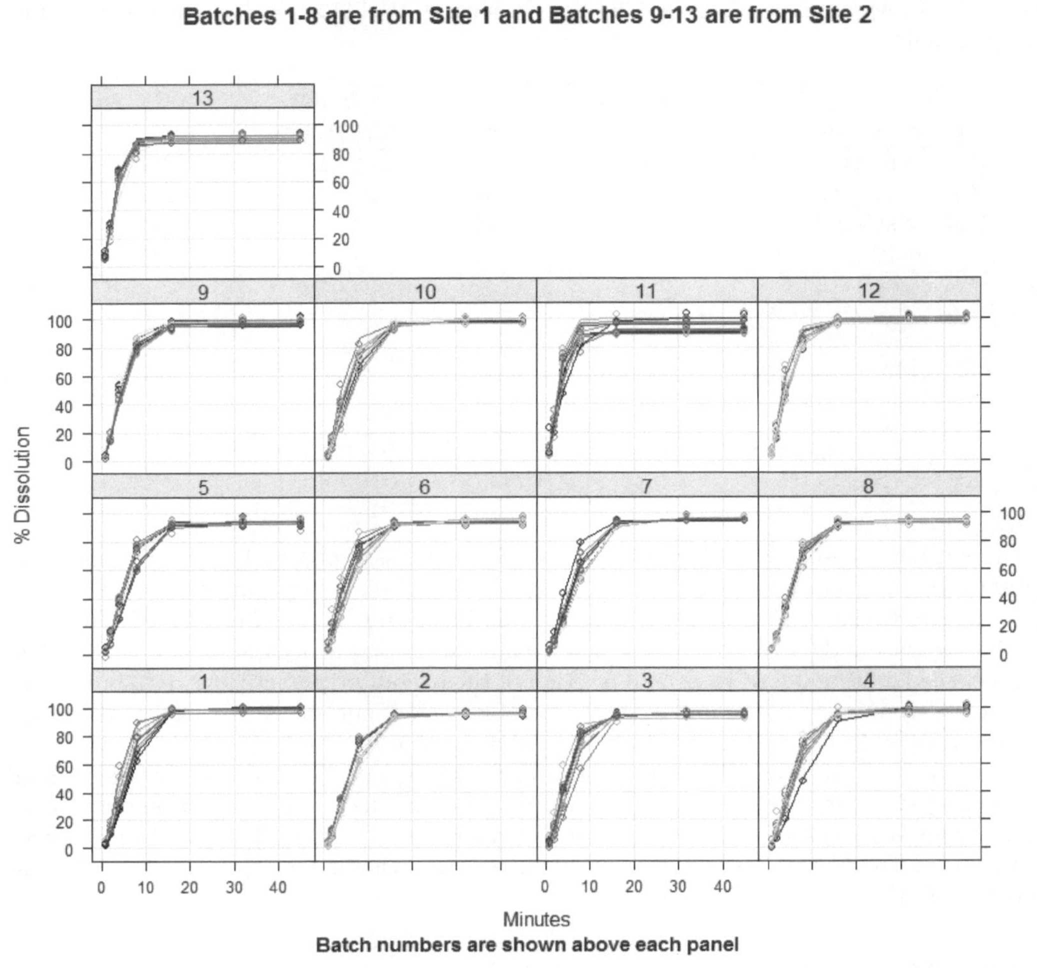

FIGURE 23.5: SODF2 data: Dissolution profiles for each batch.

23.4.2.2 Model description

The model used for SODF2 was identical to that used for SODF1 described above. Data from both SODF2 manufacturing sites were analyzed together in the same computational run with all model parameters (except for σ) duplicated for each site. Analytical variance, σ^2, was assumed common between manufacturers because all the analytical work was completed in the same analytical laboratory using the same equipment.

23.4.2.3 Computational methods

The computational methods used for SODF2 were identical to those described for SODF1 above, with the following exceptions. Four independent chains of 4,000 draws each (after a 4,000 draw warmup) were obtained to provide a 16,000 draw sample from the joint posterior distribution of all model parameters. The smaller MCMC sample size was based on the ESS and relative standard error of the mean estimate. We felt the sample size was adequate for the required inference.

23.4.2.4 Comparison of observed and predicted dissolution profiles

The dissolution profiles of each tablet for both sites were plotted as done previously for SODF1 (results not shown here). Again, the posterior predicted % dissolution results appeared to correspond well with the observed data and the fitted Weibull model matched the observed dissolution profile shapes adequately. The Bayesian hierarchical Weibull profile model thus appears to be a useful representation of the mechanism of the underlying IV dissolution process for SODF2.

23.4.2.5 Comparison of grand mean dissolution profiles for sites 1 and 2

The grand mean dissolution profiles for sites 1 and 2 are compared in Figure 23.6. The maximum dissolution for SODF2 tablets appears nearly the same at both sites. However, test site (site 2) clearly exhibits a more rapid dissolution than the reference site (site 1). The dissolution profile for site 2 is 10-20% higher than for site 1 at dissolution times between 2 and 8 minutes.

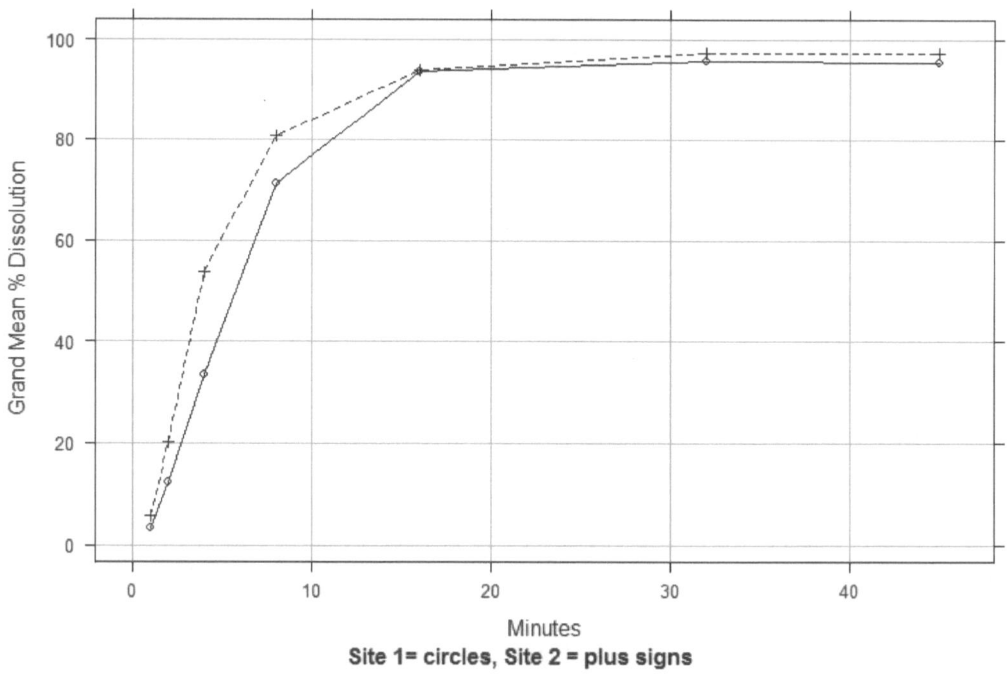

FIGURE 23.6: Comparison of the mean dissolution profiles of manufacturing sites 1 and 2. Each symbol plots the grand mean % dissolution over all batches and units for each site and time point.

23.4.2.6 Similarity of SODF2 process level mean Weibull parameters

Table 23.5 presents a statistical summary of the marginal posterior distributions of model parameters. The maximum asymptote, μ_1, and sigmoidicity, μ_3, are similar for both sites.

However the scale parameter, μ_2, is greater for site 1 and this appears to be driving the slower dissolution rate for site 1.

TABLE 23.5: Posterior distribution summary for process level mean parameters for two manufacturers of SODF2.

Parameter	Mfg. Site	Mean	SD	2.5%	50%	97.5%	ESS	$\widehat{R}$	Standard Error of Mean as a % of SD
μ_1	1	95.57	0.95	93.7	95.56	97.46	3330	1	1.7
	2	95.73	3.09	90.02	95.76	101.42	1875	1.001	2.3
μ_2	1	1.88	0.04	1.81	1.88	1.96	4571	1.001	1.5
	2	1.56	0.18	1.2	1.56	1.94	4108	1.002	1.6
μ_3	1	0.544	0.021	0.503	0.544	0.587	4596	1.001	1.5
	2	0.504	0.037	0.433	0.504	0.58	3691	1.001	1.6

The question is whether the difference in the dissolution profiles between site 1 and 2 is large enough to be considered dissimilar. To address this question, we need a clear definition of similarity. Below we illustrate two of many possible similarity definitions. In both cases considered here similarity is defined parametrically, that is — we define similarity as a region in the space of true model parameter values, or more accurately, in the space of the values of function(s) of the true model parameters.

23.4.2.7 Posterior probability of manufacturing site similarity based on F_2

F_2 is defined by Equation (23.3) as a univariate function of model parameters. By analogy with the f_2 statistic, we define the region of similarity as $F_2 > 50$. The behavior of the f_2 statistic is known to be sensitive to the number and choice of dissolution time points. Regulatory guidance recommends including no more than one time point having mean % dissolution of 85% or greater in the f_2 calculation. Therefore, for illustration of the F_2 approach here, we use only the time points 1, 2, 4, 8, and 16 minutes. From the 16,000 draw posterior sample, Equation (23.4) was used to obtain the predicted mean % dissolution at t_n minutes for site m:

$$w_{m,n}^{[i]} \sim \text{Weibull}\left(t_n; \mu_{1,m}^{[i]}, \mu_{2,m}^{[i]}, \mu_{3,m}^{[i]}\right),$$

for $m = 1, 2$ and $i = 1, \ldots, N_{draws} = 16,000$.

Equation (23.3) was then used to obtain a sample from the posterior distribution of F_2, i.e.

$$F_2^{[i]} = F_2\left(\boldsymbol{w}_1^{[i]}, \boldsymbol{w}_2^{[i]}\right).$$

Here, the vectors $\boldsymbol{w}_m^{[i]} = \left(w_{m,1}^{[i]}, w_{m,2}^{[i]}, w_{m,3}^{[i]}, w_{m,4}^{[i]}, w_{m,5}^{[i]}\right)^\top$ correspond to time points 1, 2, 4, 8 and 16 minutes.

Figure 23.7 provides a kernel density estimate of the posterior distribution of F_2 for the comparison of IV dissolution similarity of the products from manufacturing sites 1 and 2.

We take the probability of similarity for these two products to be equal to the posterior probability that $F_2 > 50$. For a conclusion of similarity to be credible, we would expect the posterior probability that $F_2 > 50$ to be high (e.g. 90%). We can estimate this posterior probability from our posterior sample by a simple counting and averaging process.

$$\Pr\left(F_2 > 50 \mid \boldsymbol{y}\right) \cong \frac{1}{N_{draws}} \sum_{i=1}^{N_{draws}} \mathbb{I}\left(F_2^{[i]} > 50\right).$$

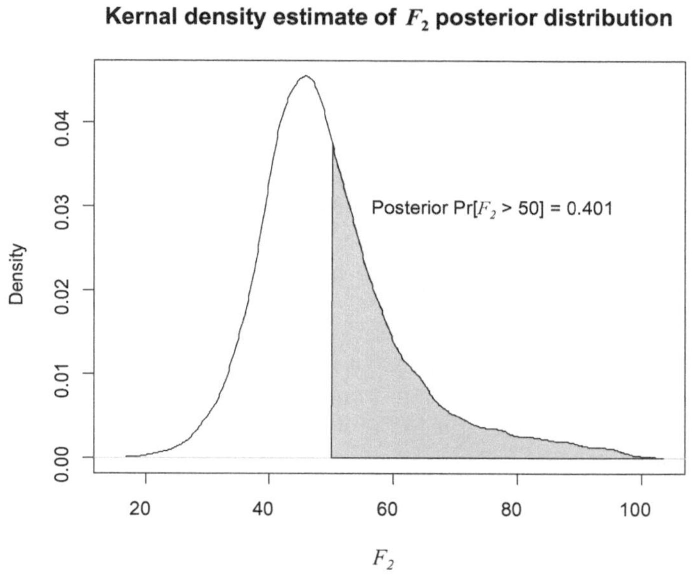

FIGURE 23.7: IV dissolution similarity of SODF2 made by two manufacturers: Kernel density estimate of the posterior distribution of F_2.

As indicated in Figure 23.7, this probability is 0.401, which is not compelling for a conclusion of similarity. This outcome is not unexpected as the observed mean % dissolution differs by 10-20% between 2 and 8 minutes as shown in Figure 23.5.

23.4.2.8 Multivariate similarity based on Weibull model parameter differences

Below we apply a Bayesian approach to an analytic study that includes multiple lots from each process being compared. The approach is based on the work of Sathe et al. (1996) who employed a frequentist procedure. The Bayesian approach permits inferences about the processes and properly accounts for both sampling variation and estimation uncertainty. It employs a sample from the joint posterior distribution of the three Weibull parameter differences obtained by simple subtraction at each MCMC draw, i.

$$\begin{aligned}\Delta\mu_1^{[i]} &= \mu_{1,1}^{[i]} - \mu_{1,2}^{[i]}\\ \Delta\mu_2^{[i]} &= \mu_{2,1}^{[i]} - \mu_{2,2}^{[i]}\\ \Delta\mu_3^{[i]} &= \mu_{3,1}^{[i]} - \mu_{3,2}^{[i]}.\end{aligned}$$

We define a similarity region in parameter space, as

$$\begin{aligned}\text{SR1} &= \left(-3\widehat{S}_1 \le \Delta\mu_1 \le 3\widehat{S}_1\right) \cap \left(-3\widehat{S}_2 \le \Delta\mu_2 \le 3\widehat{S}_2\right) \cap\\ &\quad \left(-3\widehat{S}_3 \le \Delta\mu_3 \le 3\widehat{S}_3\right),\end{aligned}$$

where $\widehat{S}_p$ are univariate standard deviations that include both between and within lot variation estimated for the pth parameter from reference site 1 and is obtained as follows:

$$\widehat{S}_p = \frac{1}{N_{draws}} \sum_{i=1}^{N_{draws}} \sqrt{\left(\sigma_{p,1}^{l[i]}\right)^2 + \left(\sigma_{p,1}^{u[i]}\right)^2}, \tag{23.9}$$

for $p = 1, 2, 3$.

In Equation (23.9), the superscripts $l[i]$ and $u[i]$ indicate the ith posterior draw of the between-lot or within-lot variances respectively. The subscript indicates the pth parameter from reference site 1.

SR1 is based on quantities estimated from the data set, which means this standard of similarity will vary from experiment to experiment. Ideally, the quantities $\widehat{S}_p$ should be fixed constants for all such comparisons for a given product. Their value should be based on the characteristics of the dissolution profile critical for safety, efficacy, manufacturability, and/or quality assurance.

The 16,000 draw MCMC sample is plotted in three scatter plots in the lower left of Figure 23.8. The grey boxes are projections of the 3-dimensional SR1 similarity region onto each of the three bivariate marginal posterior sample scatter plots. The black ellipses identify quantiles containing 90% of the mass of a bivariate Normal distributions fitted to the posterior sample separately in each of the three bivariate projections. The probabilities in the respective panels of the upper right in Figure 23.8 are estimated from the percentages of the posterior draws within the grey bivariate projections of the SR1 similarity region in the corresponding lower left panels.

It is clear from Figure 23.8 that both $\Delta\mu_1$ and $\Delta\mu_3$ are well within their respective limits. However, $\Delta\mu_2$ shows considerable probability mass outside its limits. However, Figure 23.8 is presented largely for visual and diagnostic purposes. The desired posterior probability that the true vector of Weibull parameter true values is contained within SR1 can be estimated by a simple counting exercise as follows

$$\Pr\left(\boldsymbol{\mu} \in \text{SR1(Bayes)} \mid \boldsymbol{y}\right) \cong \frac{1}{N_{draws}} \sum_{i=1}^{N_{draws}} \prod_{p=1}^{3} \mathbb{I}\left(-3\widehat{S}_p \leq \Delta\mu_p \leq 3\widehat{S}_p\right) = 0.895.$$

This result can be compared to the $\Pr(F_2 > 50)$, which was only 0.401. The difference should not be surprising. While F_2 is based only on the Weibull parameter mean differences, SR1 makes allowances for intra- and between lot variability. Both definitions of similarity are arbitrary. There is no reason to think they should result in the same conclusion because they are based on fundamentally different definitions of what similar means.

23.5 Conclusions

Bayesian applications in the in vitro dissolution field are not new. Examples have been described by Novick et al. (2015); LeBlond et al. (2015). These include inferences on lot release, process quality, and dissolution similarity as considered in this chapter. In this section, we focus on the value of Bayesian statistics in supporting in vitro dissolution decisions and highlight some aspects not covered in this chapter.

Our own experiences with Bayesian approaches and tools in the field of in vitro dissolution have been very positive. We want to highlight the following advantages:

- As illustrated in this chapter, posterior inference permits statements such as "The probability that future lots will pass USP<711> is X" or "The probability that dissolution profiles at site 1 and 2 are similar is Z". Such statements are not permitted using frequentist methods.

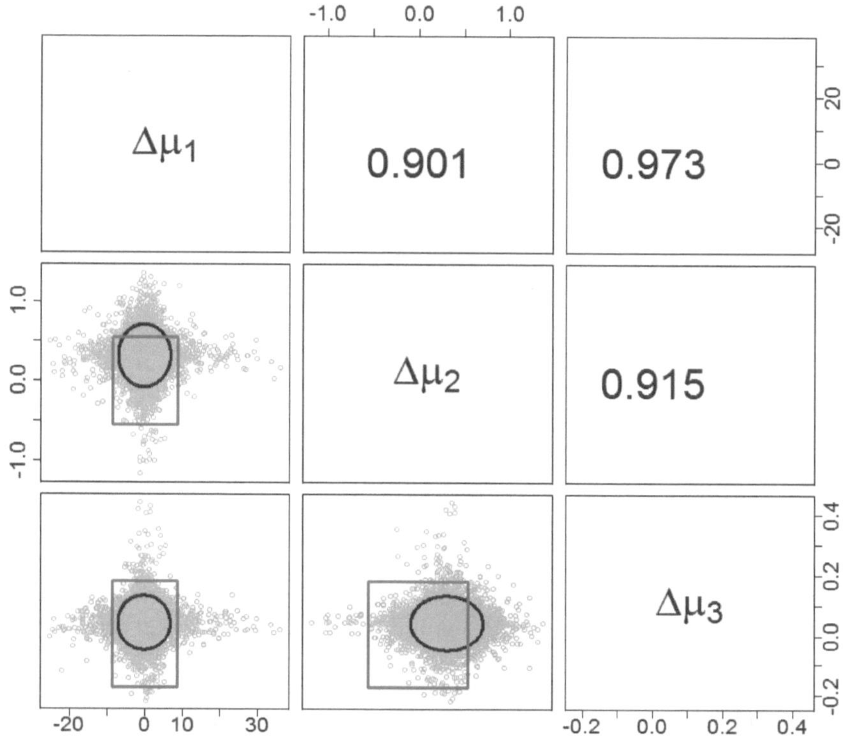

FIGURE 23.8: Scatter plot matrix of a 16,000 draw sample from joint posterior distribution of process level Weibull parameter differences. The grey circles are individual posterior draws. The black contour lines are ellipses that include approximately 90% of the posterior mass of the 2 parameters plotted in each panel. The variable names along the diagonal indicate the parameter whose difference is plotted on the adjoining axes. The grey rectangles are $\pm 3 \times \mathrm{SD}_p$ similarity limits as defined in the text. The probabilities in the upper right panels are estimated from the percentages of the posterior draws within the grey bivariate projections of the SR1 similarity region in the corresponding lower left panels.

- The posterior distributions of complex functions of model parameters such as F_2, whose estimator f_2 exhibits an intractable sampling distributions, are easily explored using MCMC samples. Estimation of posterior probabilities is reduced to a simple counting and averaging exercise. Nonlinear models such as the Weibull function and hierarchical models (required for analytic study inference and essential features of IV dissolution analysis) are easily accommodated. We feel that compendial and other standards such as USP<711> and similarity standards are best expressed as functions of model parameters and modern Bayesian software makes it easy to get the posterior distribution of such functions.
- While not illustrated in this chapter, the Bayesian paradigm provides a rigorous and quantitative basis for leveraging scientifically justified prior information, for continuous

knowledge building, an essential component of better (and more efficient) scientific decision making.

At the same time, we must acknowledge some challenges. Verifying MCMC chain convergence, mixing, prior impact, and calibrating the repeated sampling properties (if required) can be time consuming and requires persistence. Some aspects we have not considered in this chapter that may deserve future attention include the following.

- Application of Bayesian methodology to develop IV dissolution lot disposition rules and similarity regions based on predicted pharmacokinetic outcomes more directly to clinical safety and efficacy along the lines presented by Qiu et al. (2016).
- More realistic profile models (e.g. modeling variance heterogeneity across the % dissolution range).
- Bayesian modeling of in vitro dissolution stability data for shelf life estimation.
- Regulatory approvals that depend on analytic (rather than solely enumerative) studies and inference.

In this chapter, similarity has only been addressed from a process average point of view by comparing the population means either via F_2 or parameters of the Weibull model. But is average performance really the question of interest? From a patient's risk perspective, one may be interested in knowing the probability that a process will produce individual lots (or tablets) not having an adequate IV dissolution profile. An alternative perspective might be to treat similarity through the lens of predicting process capability. The ability of Bayesian methodology to provide the posterior predictive distribution of characteristics of future lots (or tablets) can be used to advantage to address this question and connect the ICH guidance concepts of quality by design and design space to the patient's risk and assessment of similarity (see for example Lebrun et al., 2015).

Bibliography

Aitchison, J. and Dunsmore, I. R. (1975). *Statistical Prediction Analysis.* Cambridge University Press, Cambridge, UK.

Bergum, J. S. (1990). Constructing acceptance limits for multiple stage tests. *Drug Development and Industrial Pharmacy,* 16(14):2153–2166.

Burdick, R. K., LeBlond, D. J., Pfahler, L. B., Quiroz, J., Sidor, L., Vukovinsky, K., and Zhang, L. (2017). *Statistical Applications for Chemistry, Manufacturing and Controls (CMC) in the Pharmaceutical Industry.* Springer, Cham, Switzerland.

Cholayudth, P. (2011). Using the bergum method and `MS Excel` to determine the probability of passing the USP dissolution test. *Pharmaceutical Technology,* 30(1).

De los Santos, P., Phahler, L., Vukovinsky, E., Liu, J., and Harrington, B. (2015). Performance characteristics and alternative approaches for the ASTM E2709/2810 (CUDAL) method for ensuring that a product meets USP <905> uniformity of dosage units. *Pharmaceutical Engineering,* 35(5):44–57.

Deming, W. E. (1975). On probability as a basis for action. *The American Statistician,* 29(4):146.

Eaton, M., Muirhead, R., and Steeno, G. (2003). Aspects of the dissolution profile testing problem. *Biopharmaceutical Report*, 11(2):2–7.

European Medicine Agency (2008). Guideline on the Investigation of Bioequivalence. Committee for Medicinal Products for Human Use. `https://www.ema.europa.eu/en/investigation-bioequivalence`; accessed March 31, 2020.

European Medicine Agency (2010). Guideline on the Investigation of Bioequivalence. Committee for Medicinal Products for Human Use. `http://www.ema.europa.eu/docs/en_GB/document_library/Scientific_guideline/2009/09/WC500003011.pdf`; accessed March 31, 2020.

Geisser, S. (1993). *Predictive Inference: an Introduction.* Number 55 in Monographs on statistics and applied probability. Chapman & Hall, New York, NY.

Gelman, A., Carlin, J., Stern, H., Dunson, D., Vehtari, A., and Rubin, D. (2013). *Bayesian Data Analysis.* Chapman Hall/CRC, New York, NY, 3rd edition.

Hofer, J. D. and Gray, V. A. (2003). Examination of selection of immediate release dissolution acceptance criteria. *Dissolution Technologies*, 10:16–20.

Kielt, A., Nir, I., Seely, J., and Inman, G. (2016). Analysis of two active pharmaceutical ingredients (API) products using UV spectrophotometry with multi-component analysis and a fiber optic dissolution analyzer. *American Pharmaceutical Review.* Posted online September 30, 2016, `http://tiny.cc/r52q6y`.

Kruschke, J. K. (2015). *Doing Bayesian Data Analysis: A Tutorial with R, JAGS, and Stan.* Academic Press, Boston, edition 2 edition.

LeBlond, D., Altan, S., Novick, S., Peterson, J., Shen, Y., and Yang, H. (2015). In vitro dissolution curve comparisons: A critique of current practice. *Dissolution Technologies*, 23(01):14–23.

LeBlond, D. and Mockus, L. (2014). The posterior probability of passing a compendial standard, Part 1: Uniformity of dosage units. *Statistics in Biopharmaceutical Research*, 6(3):270–286.

Lebrun, P., Giacoletti, K., Scherder, T., Rozet, E., and Boulanger, B. (2015). A quality by design approach for longitudinal quality attributes. *Journal of Biopharmaceutical Statistics*, 25(2):247–259.

Lewandowski, D., Kurowicka, D., and Joe, H. (2009). Generating random correlation matrices based on vines and extended onion method. *Journal of Multivariate Analysis*, 100(9):1989–2001.

Long, M. and Chen, Y. (2009). Dissolution testing of solid products. In Qiu, Y., Chen, Y., Zhang, G. G. Z., Liu, L., and Porter, W., editors, *Developing Solid Oral Dosage Forms: Pharmaceutical Theory & Practice.* Elsevier Science.

Lunn, D. (2013). *The BUGS Book: A Practical Introduction to Bayesian Analysis.* Texts in Statistical Science. CRC Press, Taylor & Francis Group, Boca Raton, FL.

Moore, J. and Flanner, H. (1996). Mathematical comparison of curves with an emphasis on in vitro dissolution profiles. *Pharmaceutical Technology*, 20(6):64–74.

Novick, S., Shen, Y., Yang, H., Peterson, J., LeBlond, D., and Altan, S. (2015). Dissolution curve comparisons through the F_2 parameter, a Bayesian extension of the f_2 statistic. *Journal of Biopharmaceutical Statistics*, 25(2):351–371.

Paixão, P., Gouveia, L. F., Silva, N., and Morais, J. A. (2017). Evaluation of dissolution profile similarity – Comparison between the f2, the multivariate statistical distance and the f2 bootstrapping methods. *European Journal of Pharmaceutics and Biopharmaceutics*, 112:67–74.

Plummer, M. (2017). JAGS: Just another gibbs sampler. http://mcmc-jags.sourceforge.net; accessed March 31, 2020.

Qiu, J., Martinez, M., and Tiwari, R. (2016). Evaluating in vivo-in vitro correlation using a Bayesian approach. *The American Association of Pharmaceutical Scientists Journal*, 18(3):619–634.

SAS Institute, Inc. (2018). SAS/STAT©15.1 User's Guide: The MCMC Procedure.

Sathe, P. M., Tsong, Y., and Shah, V. P. (1996). In-vitro dissolution profile comparison: statistics and analysis, model dependent approach. *Pharmaceutical Research*, 13(12):1799–1803.

Shah, V. P., Tsong, Y., Sathe, P., and Liu, J. P. (1998). In vitro dissolution profile comparison–statistics and analysis of the similarity factor, f2. *Pharmaceutical Research*, 15(6):889–896.

Stan Development Team (2018). RStan: the R interface to Stan. R package version 2.17.3. http://mc-stan.org; accessed March 31, 2020.

Tsong, Y., Sathe, P., and Shah, V. (2009). In vitro dissolution profile comparison. In Dekker, M., editor, *Encyclopedia of Biopharmaceutical Statistics*. Taylor & Francis.

U.S. Food and Drug Administration (1995). Guidance for Industry: Immediate Release Solid Oral Dosage Forms. Scale-Up and Postapproval Changes: Chemistry, Manufacturing and Controls, In Vitro Dissolution Testing and In Vivo Bioequivalence Documentation. U.S. Department of Health and Human Services, FDA. Center of Drug Evaluation and Research (CDER): Rockville, Maryland. http://www.fda.gov/downloads/drugs/guidancecomplianceregulatoryinformation/guidances/ucm070636.pdf; accessed March 31, 2020.

U.S. Food and Drug Administration (1997a). Guidance for Industry: Dissolution Testing of Immediate Release Solid Oral Dosage Forms. U.S. Department of Health and Human Services, FDA. Center of Drug Evaluation and Research (CDER): Rockville, Maryland. http://www.fda.gov/downloads/drugs/guidancecomplianceregulatoryinformation/guidances/ucm070237.pdf; accessed March 31, 2020.

U.S. Food and Drug Administration (1997b). Guidance for Industry: Extended Release Oral Dosage Forms: Development, Evaluation, and Application of In Vitro/In Vivo Correlations. U.S. Department of Health and Human Services, FDA. Center of Drug Evaluation and Research (CDER): Rockville, Maryland. http://www.fda.gov/downloads/drugs/guidancecomplianceregulatoryinformation/guidances/ucm070239.pdf; accessed March 31, 2020.

U.S. Food and Drug Administration (1997c). Guidance for Industry: SUPAC-MR: Modified Release Solid Oral Dosage Forms. Scale-Up and Post Approval Changes: Chemistry, Manufacturing and Controls; In Vitro Dissolution Testing and In Vivo Bioequivalence Documentation. U.S. Department of Health and Human Services, FDA. Center of Drug Evaluation and Research (CDER): Rockville, Maryland. `http://www.fda.gov/downloads/drugs/guidancecomplianceregulatoryinformation/guidances/ucm070640.pdf`; accessed March 31, 2020.

U.S. Food and Drug Administration (2000). Guidance for Industry: Waiver of In Vivo Bioavailability and Bioequivalence Studies for Immediate-Release Solid Oral Dosage Forms Based on Biopharmaceutics Classification System; U.S. Department of Health and Human Services, FDA. Center of Drug Evaluation and Research (CDER): Rockville, Maryland. `http://www.fda.gov/downloads/drugs/guidancecomplianceregulatoryinformation/guidances/ucm070246.pdf`; accessed March 31, 2020.

U.S. Food and Drug Administration (2001). Guidance for Industry: Statistical Approaches to Bioequivalence; U.S. Department of Health and Human Services, FDA. Center of Drug Evaluation and Research (CDER): Rockville, Maryland.

U.S. Food and Drug Administration (2003). Guidance for Industry: Bioavailability and Bioequivalence Studies for Orally Administered Drug Products – General Considerations. U.S. Department of Health and Human Services, FDA. Center of Drug Evaluation and Research (CDER): Rockville, Maryland. `http://www.fda.gov/downloads/drugs/guidancecomplianceregulatoryinformation/guidances/ucm070124.pdf`; accessed March 31, 2020.

U.S. Food and Drug Administration (2011). Guidance for Industry Process Validation: General Principles and Practices. U.S. Department of Health and Human Services, FDA. Center of Drug Evaluation and Research (CDER): Rockville, Maryland. `https://www.fda.gov/downloads/drugs/guidances/ucm070336.pdf`; accessed March 31, 2020.

U.S. Food and Drug Administration (2017). Guidance for Industry: Waiver of In Vivo Bioavailability and Bioequivalence Studies for Immediate-Release Solid Oral Dosage Forms Based on a Biopharmaceutics Classification System. U.S. Department of Health and Human Services, FDA. Center of Drug Evaluation and Research (CDER): Rockville, Maryland. `https://www.fda.gov/downloads/Drugs/Guidances/ucm070246.pdf`; accessed March 31, 2020.

U.S. Pharmacopeia (2008). General chapters: Dissolution <711>, Drug release <724>, Intrinsic dissolution <1087>, In vitro and in vivo evaluation <1088>, Assessment of product performance <1090>, The dissolution procedure <1092>, Unit dose uniformity <905>, Washington D.C. `https://www.usp.org/`; accessed March 31, 2020.

World Health Association (2006). WHO Expert Committee on Specifications for Pharmaceutical Preparations. WHO Technical Report Series Fortieth Report. Dissolution Profile Comparison. `http://whqlibdoc.who.int/trs/WHO_TRS_937_eng.pdf`; accessed March 31, 2020.

Zhang, Y., Huo, M., Zhou, J., Zou, A., Li, W., Yao, C., and Xie, S. (2010). DDSolver: an add-in program for modeling and comparison of drug dissolution profiles. *The American Association of Pharmaceutical Scientists Journal*, 12(3):263–271.

24

Bayesian Statistics for Manufacturing

Tara Scherder
SynoloStats LLC, US

Katherine Giacoletti
SynoloStats LLC, US

Biopharmaceutical manufacturing processes are considered in three stages: Process Development and Design, Process Qualification, and Continued Process Verification. The use of statistical modelling in pharmaceutical process design and validation has only relatively recently become prevalent. The use of frequentist methods (e.g. tolerance intervals) is common, but a Bayesian approach is increasingly more popular, particularly as Bayesian probability statements can be derived for complex testing schemes, for which frequentist tolerance intervals can not provide a quantification of the risk. These concepts will be described in detail in this chapter using three illustrative examples.

24.1 Introduction

Under the paradigm of the lifecycle approach to Process Validation (PV) as described in the 2011 U.S. Food and Drug Administration Guidance for Industry Process Validation (U.S. Food and Drug Administration, 2011), biopharmaceutical manufacturing processes are considered in three stages: Process Development and Design (Stage 1), Process Qualification (PQ, Stage 2), and Continued Process Verification (CPV, Stage 3). The first commercial batches are made during Process Performance Qualification (PPQ), the second element of PQ. The lifecycle approach is also cited in EU guidance documents (2016 EMA PV Guideline, 2015 EU GMP Annex 15) using slightly different terminology: Stage 2 is termed Process Validation (PV) rather than Process Qualification, and Stage 3 is termed Ongoing Process Verification (OPV) rather than Continued Process Verification. Prior to these guidance documents, the use of statistics in pharmaceutical process design and validation was rather limited. Although some increase in the use of experimental design occurred following publication of Quality by Design principles in ICH Q8, the adoption was not widespread. Process design continued to rely heavily on previous experience and first principles to determine a formulation and process. Process parameters were varied within a limited range of key parameter settings, typically one factor at a time (OFAT), to determine allowable operating ranges. A successful process validation required the manufacture of three consecutive commercial batches, with sampling and analysis limited to the amount specified in the regulatory filing for release to the patient market (batch release testing). Statistical design of experiments and analyses to understand the multivariate relationships between inputs and outputs, or to estimate process variability to evaluate risk, were neither routinely expected nor widely utilized. In routine manufacturing, performance testing was limited to batch release requirements, and results were typically trended only once per year. The lifecycle approach, and the greater regulatory emphasis on process understanding and assessment of the population of units of product through more rigorous design, validation, and process monitoring represent a major shift in the pharmaceutical industry. The goals of the lifecycle approach necessitate increased application of statistics throughout the lifecycle, with obvious benefit to both patients and businesses.

The focus of this chapter is the commercial manufacturing process, Stages 2 and 3 of the product lifecycle. Stage 2 (PPQ/PV) batches must demonstrate with "a high degree of assurance" (U.S. Food and Drug Administration, 2011) that the process is capable of reproducibly manufacturing a product which meets its quality requirements. The objectives of Stage 3 (CPV/OPV) are to understand routine manufacturing (batch to batch) variability, detect unusual variability or changes in process performance, and enable process improvement. In many cases, simple statistical tools available in off-the-shelf statistical software such as `Minitab` or `JMP`, such as statistical intervals (for instance, Normal tolerance intervals) in Stage 2, and control charts and capability indices in Stage 3, are used to meet these objectives. In many cases, these simple tools are adequate; however, there are limitations to their use and interpretation. The application of Bayesian methods to address these limitations is the subject of this chapter.

Process capability (or inversely, the risk of future results outside of product (quality) specifications), is a critical measurement of the commercial manufacturing process, and is assessed periodically starting in Stage 2. The use of frequentist tolerance intervals to assess process capability is common, particularly at the conclusion of Stage 2. These intervals cover at least a specified proportion of the population with a stated confidence. They are simple to compute (for a single population with one source of variability) and can enable the goal of demonstrating process capability with a high degree of assurance. The typical analysis compares the tolerance interval for each product quality attribute computed from samples of each batch to the attribute specification range (typically the product release specification). The interpretation is limited, however. If each tolerance interval falls entirely within the respective range, the process is deemed capable. But if the tolerance interval for one or more batches is not entirely within specifications, the conclusion may be ambiguous. The process capability may still be quite high, but a decision about whether a sufficiently "high degree of assurance" has been demonstrated is difficult in this situation. And importantly, in either case, this approach does not provide an estimate of the key value of interest — the probability that future product (batches or units) will be outside the product specification range.

In contrast, a direct answer to the fundamental question of "What is the probability that future product will meet specification?" is indeed achievable using Bayesian methods. This clear statement of process capability incorporates all current knowledge (data and, if applicable, prior information) regarding the process and the uncertainty of that knowledge (represented by the width of the posterior predictive distribution). Unlike with frequentist intervals, this is possible regardless of the data structure — it is just as simple with multiple variance components as with a single one. The Bayesian probability statement can also be derived for complex testing schemes, for which frequentist tolerance intervals could not provide a quantification of the risk. These concepts will be described in detail in this chapter using illustrative examples, namely:

1. Optimizing sampling without compromising patient risk for revalidation/transfer of an existing process;
2. Characterizing process capability with a direct, simple statement of patient risk; and,
3. Estimating the risk of future out-of-specification results in the presence of multiple sources of variability and staged testing.

24.2 Manufacturing situation 1: Revalidation/transfer

During the commercial supply stage of a pharmaceutical product (Stage 3), process changes (e.g. equipment changes, site transfers, etc.) can trigger revalidation. By this time, substantial process understanding should exist. This is particularly true for processes developed using the lifecycle approach, with greater process understanding developed during Stage 1 and Stage 2 than under the traditional development and validation paradigm, and a large body of data collected regarding within and between batch variability of the process during Stage 2 and Stage 3.

A frequent challenge, especially for older processes, is that the (sometimes lengthy) process history may consist of a relatively small amount of data if developed, validated, and commercially manufactured using traditional approaches — e.g. limited or no data from designed experiments and sampling limited to product release testing levels during validation and commercial supply stages. Yet, even though the sample size per batch may be limited, the process knowledge gained from years of production is relevant and applicable when considering revalidation or transfer of such a process. Manufacturers and patients benefit when this prior information is leveraged to reduce sampling and testing during revalidation, thereby minimizing costs without compromising quality and safety.

For these "legacy" (existing) products, it is often logical and justifiable to use the body of previous manufacturing data as the basis for the prior for an informative Bayesian analysis. Doing so can reduce the sample size (number of batches and/or number of samples per batch) required to precisely characterize performance in the revalidation, by "borrowing strength" from prior manufacturing experience in the analysis of the revalidation/transfer results. "Informative" in this context refers to the explicit incorporation into the statistical analysis of previously existing knowledge about the parameters to be analyzed by way of the "prior" or "prior distribution" for each parameter for which such knowledge exists. When an informative prior is used, this prior knowledge about the parameters becomes part of the analysis and affects any estimates or predictions. Bayesian analyses can be, and often are, performed using vague or weak priors (sometimes referred to as "non-informative" priors), in which case little or no prior information is used in the analysis and all information comes from the data (i.e. through the likelihood).

24.2.1 Example 1: Use of prior information to reduce sample size without increasing patient risk

The analysis of PPQ batches, including batches for a revalidation or transfer during Stage 3, must include an assessment of product quality throughout the batch. It is a classical inference problem, whereby a statement about population performance (all product units, such as vials within a batch) derived from a sample of product units is sought. Manufacturers must design sampling plans for the PPQ batches, which will provide the data required to provide a high degree of assurance that the untested dosage units in the batch will be within finished drug product or substance specification. As previously noted, a commonly employed method in the pharmaceutical industry to obtain such a statement is the computation of a tolerance interval (TI), typically a Normal (frequentist) TI.

The general formula for a $100(1-\alpha)\%/\beta\%$ tolerance interval is:

$$\text{Average} \pm k[\text{Standard deviation Estimate}],$$

where k depends upon the confidence level, $(1-\alpha)$, the proportion covered, β, and the number of samples, n. Note the industry naming convention orders the TI parameters as confidence/coverage, while statistical references order the parameters coverage/confidence.

The number of samples per PPQ batch is determined before manufacture of the PPQ batches and is estimated such that, if performance is as expected based on representative development batches, the tolerance intervals computed for the product quality attributes from the PPQ batches will fall within product release specifications. A Bayesian approach to this sample size determination will be illustrated using the example of revalidation of a legacy product following a manufacturing process change.

The quality attribute of interest in this example is product potency, a common measurement of the strength of drug activity. Assume that the process change was not expected to change the mean or variability of the drug potency. The historical batch data, representing one potency measurement per batch, are summarized in Table 24.1 below. Table 24.1 also includes an estimate of the potency measurement variability, derived from test method validation studies.

TABLE 24.1: Summary statistics from historical data for legacy revalidation case study.

Number of Batches	Mean Potency (%) (SE)	Standard Deviation (%)
25	100.3 (0.59)	2.94
Estimated measurement variability (SD)		1.5

Before applying any statistical models, the historical data are evaluated for trends or other non-random behavior using a run chart such as the one displayed in Figure 24.1. The historical batch measurements are displayed in chronological order with the overall mean indicated by the dashed horizontal line. Control charts, which include lower and upper control limits (LCL and UCL, respectively) to bracket the range of results expected if the process is subject only to random, inherent variability are also often used, but are beyond the scope of this discussion (Montgomery, 2012).

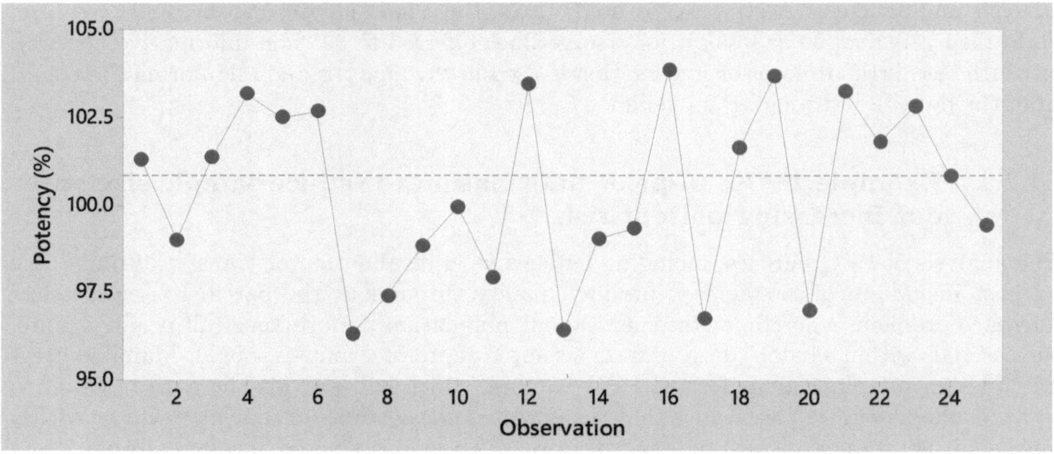

FIGURE 24.1: Legacy revalidation case study: run chart of historical potency results.

Figure 24.1 shows a well-behaved process that randomly varies around a common mean. While there are individual points close to the specification limits (95.0% - 105.0%), which is not uncommon for such products, the process history observed in Figure 24.1 along with a well-established manufacturing control strategy would reasonably support the conclusion that there is little risk of producing a batch of drug product with potency outside of the specification range. However, despite this evidence, a 95% confidence/95% coverage TI derived from the historical mean and SD extends beyond the specification range even with a within-batch sample size as large as 30. While this sample size may not seem unreasonable in many fields or industries, it can be untenable in many pharmaceutical manufacturing situations due to the high cost of testing methods and the product lost to testing. The sample size seems particularly excessive considering the historical performance, which indicates a low risk of out of specification results.

The reasons for a conservative sample size required for this application of a frequentist TI are twofold: (1) for high confidence and coverage (95%/95% in this case), the multiplier k for a frequentist TI is quite large with smaller sample sizes, and (2) regardless of how large the sample size, the frequentist TI makes no use of prior knowledge regarding process performance. In other words, a frequentist TI ensures the stated confidence and coverage by increasing the width for smaller n, reflecting uncertainty due to not having much information (only the information in the sample). For example, for sample sizes ranging from 3 to 8, the k multiplier of the standard deviation for the frequentist 95% confidence/95% coverage TI ranges from 9.99 ($n = 3$) to 3.74, for $n = 8$ (Howe, 1969). As the sample size increases, the TI gets narrower, but still incorporates only the information in the current sample. Additionally, in this example, the variability estimate from the data set (based on a single result per batch), does not provide a good estimate of the within-batch variability.

In contrast, a Bayesian approach can leverage other information, such as the historical evidence of robust process performance, while also exploring the range of plausible sample means and standard deviations in predictions of future performance. An informative Bayesian analysis expresses available knowledge — in this case the historical manufacturing data — as probability distributions for one or more parameters of interest. For example, the historical potency data in this case study have an overall mean of 100.3 and standard error of 0.59, which can be expressed by saying that mean potency follows a $\mathrm{N}(100.3, 0.592)$ distribution. Since the simple standard deviation of the historical data (2.94%) includes batch-to-batch variability, and the batch is expected to be homogeneous, the measurement variability estimate for the test method could be leveraged to determine a more appropriate prior for the within-batch variability. The choice of information for the priors should incorporate all relevant knowledge representative of the process to be analyzed.

To implement an informative Bayesian approach, one could use the summary statistics from Table 24.1 to formulate priors for the mean and variability both within and between batches. Sample sizes are explored for the Bayesian analysis using simulation, as follows:

(i). The historical data are used to formulate a prior for the batch means, i.e. $\mu_p \sim \mathrm{N}(100.3, 0.592)$. The measurement variability estimate is used to formulate a prior for the within-batch variance, i.e. $\sigma_p^2 \sim \mathrm{IG}(24.4, 53.5)$.

(ii). In each simulation run, a new batch mean μ_p and new within-batch variance σ_p^2 are drawn from the priors described in (i). For a given within-batch sample size n, n future PPQ results are drawn as a random sample from a $\mathrm{N}(\mu_p, \sigma_p^2)$ distribution (referred to as the prior predictive distribution).

(iii). An informative Bayesian analysis is performed using the simulated PPQ sample drawn as described in (ii), with prior distributions for the mean and variance being the same as were used in step (i). This results in a joint posterior distribution for μ and σ^2, the (simulated) PPQ batch mean and variance.

(iv). A Bayesian 95% confidence/95% coverage TI is estimated based on the posterior distributions of the 2.5th and 97.5th quantiles, generated in the analysis in (iii) of all $\mathrm{N}(\mu, \sigma^2)$ distributions over the joint posterior distribution of μ and σ^2.

Other intervals may be computed as well (prediction intervals, frequentist and/or Bayesian, for example), if desired.

(v). This process is repeated a large number of times for a range of candidate PPQ sample sizes. For each sample size, the proportion of 95% confidence/95% coverage TIs within specifications is the probability of meeting the criterion for that PPQ sample size (referred to as assurance, as opposed to the concept of frequentist power). The Bayesian TI is often referred to as a β/γ tolerance interval ("BGTI"; Wolfinger, 1998); which describes the range within which a stated proportion (β) of future individual results is predicted to fall with stated confidence (γ).

Note that the use of the historical data to generate both the prior and the simulated PPQ data for the likelihood is appropriate for the PPQ sample size simulations, before the PPQ data have been observed. However, at the completion of PPQ, the analysis will consist of steps (ii) through (iv), replacing the simulated PPQ data with the actual observed PPQ data. The benefit of using informative Bayesian analyses is that the prior information (here, the estimated measurement variability as information about within-batch variability, as well as a plausible distribution of batch means) is combined with the PPQ data, essentially basing interval estimates (and widths) on a larger, combined data set. Consequently, the use of an informative Bayesian analysis can permit substantial reduction in the number of samples within a PPQ batch needed to make acceptable claims of capability, while ensuring quality for the patient.

Depending on the desired risk statement and interpretation, other intervals, such as a frequentist prediction interval or a Bayesian β-expectation tolerance interval may be

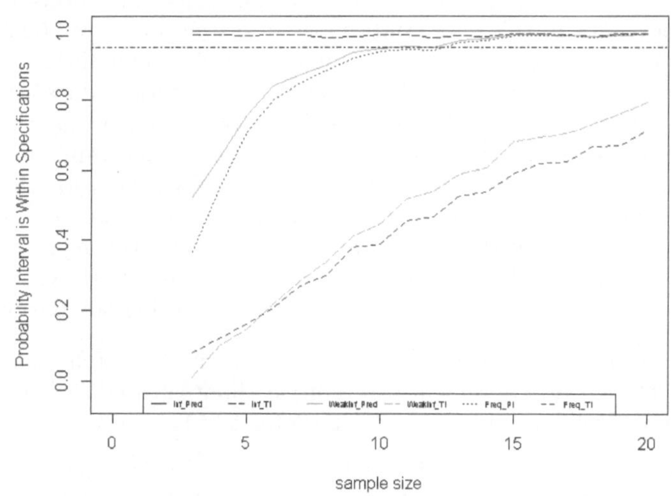

FIGURE 24.2: Simulated probability of various frequentist and Bayesian statistical intervals (95% confidence and 95% coverage, as applicable for each interval) being within specifications for range of sample sizes ("Inf_Pred" = Bayesian informative prediction interval (black solid line), "Inf_TI" = Bayesian informative tolerance interval (dashed black line), "WeakInf_Pred" = Bayesian informative prediction interval with weaker prior (solid light grey line), "WeakInf_TI" = Bayesian informative tolerance interval with weaker prior (dashed light grey line), "Freq_PI" = frequentist prediction interval (solid dotted dark grey line), "Freq_TI" = frequentist tolerance interval (dashed dark grey line).

applicable. A Bayesian β-expectation tolerance interval ("BETI") is also referred to as Bayesian prediction interval and describes the range within which an expected proportion (β) of individual results is predicted to fall (Hamada et al., 2004). Figure 24.2 shows the probability of the interval being within specifications for a range of PPQ batch sample sizes for various methods, using the example data and the prior described above. The figure also shows the results for a Bayesian analysis using a weaker prior, which increases the uncertainty in the prior distributions, thereby reducing the influence of the prior on the results. The sample size reduction from a Bayesian informative analysis is clear from these results; and, as expected, the non-informative Bayesian method performs nearly identically to the frequentist analysis in this equal-tailed scenario.

The prior for the informative sample size determination in an example such as this is most appropriately based on historical data. Sensitivity analyses may be requested by regulatory reviewers to explore the influence of alternative priors for the specific modelling circumstances. This is really no different than the recommendation to use a range of plausible means and standard deviations as assumptions for frequentist power and sample size calculations. However, in the Bayesian setting the use of distributions for both the prior and the posterior, rather than single point estimates, inherently incorporates the exploration of a range of possible means and standard deviations. This is another advantage of the Bayesian approach, whether or not an informative analysis is used.

24.3 Manufacturing situation 2: Evaluating process capability

The FDA Guidance for Process Validation describes the use of heightened (sometimes referred to as "enhanced") sampling, i.e. taking more samples per batch than is required for batch release to market, in order to better understand intra-batch variability. This level of sampling during Stage 2, especially when combined with greater process understanding obtained by more rigorous development (employing designed experiments, etc.), provides statistical confidence regarding the quality of the entire batch, allowing risk-based quality decisions before proceeding to commercial manufacturing, including ongoing sampling needs.

Although frequentist Normal TIs are often used to make risk statements based on enhanced sampling in Stage 2, and are popular because of the simplicity of calculation, they can lead to ambiguous results, and can be cumbersome or impossible with complex data structures. On the other hand, a Bayesian model leads to a clear and direct statement of patient risk, and has the added advantage of elegantly accommodating complex data structures with multiple sources of variability.

24.3.1 Example 2: Use Bayesian methods to make clear predictions of patient risk

Consider the example of a product for which Assay (measured amount of the active pharmaceutical ingredient; API) must be within 95.0 — 105.0% (% of the label-claim amount of API). Five PPQ batches were manufactured for Stage 2, with additional samples taken beyond routine batch release testing in order to statistically evaluate capability prior to commercial manufacturing. The results are displayed in Figure 24.3. Before proceeding to Stage 3, the data are analyzed to confirm confidence in the capability of the process to meet specifications.

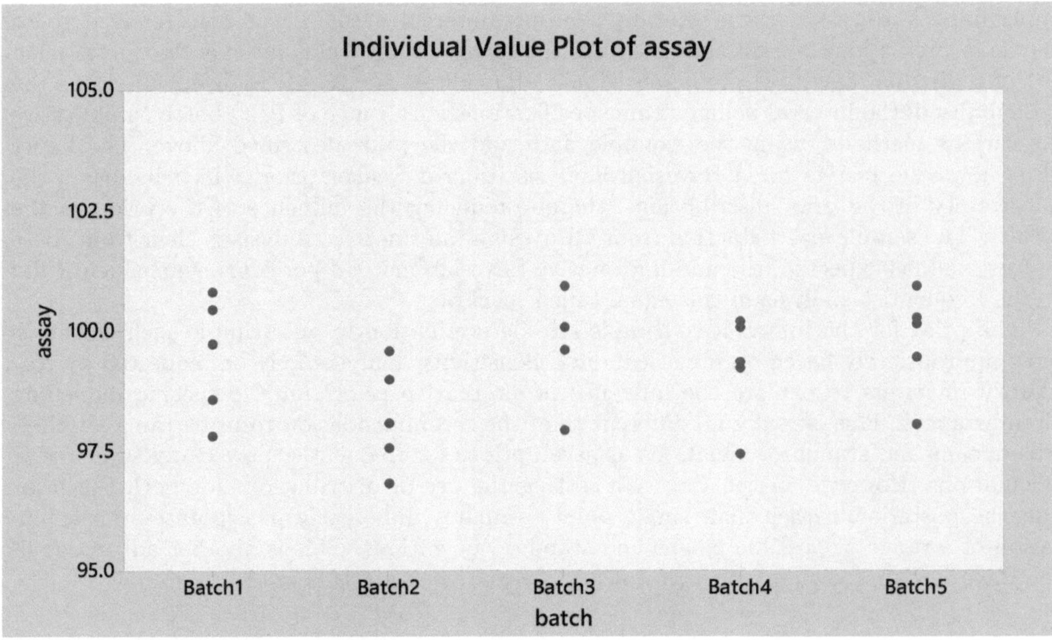

FIGURE 24.3: Individual value plot of Assay (%) from five PPQ batches (n = 5/batch). The graph is scaled to the specification limits of 95.0 – 105.0%.

The results in Figure 24.3 indicate a reproducible process, with consistent performance from batch to batch; most of the variability appears to be due to within-batch sources – most likely primarily if not entirely analytical measurement variability. The individual results from each batch are well within the specification limits and the spread of assay results within a batch is consistent among batches, indicating that this within-batch variability is predictable. The means, standard deviations, and frequentist 95/95 TIs for these batches are shown in Table 24.2 below.

TABLE 24.2: Batch means, SDs, and frequentist 95/95 TIs for Assay (%).

Batch	Mean Assay (%) (SD) (n = 5/batch)	Frequentist 95/95 TI
1	99.5 (1.27)	93.0 – 105.9
2	98.2 (1.10)	92.6 – 103.8
3	99.6 (1.10)	94.0 – 105.2
4	99.2 (1.11)	93.6 – 104.9
5	99.8 (1.10)	94.2 – 105.3

Note all intervals extend beyond the specification range of 95-105%, even though the batch means and within-batch SDs are quite consistent, and visual examination of the data indicate a predictable process with little risk of failing specifications. Yet the manufacturer is left without a strong statistical statement of this assurance. Further analysis might include a TI which includes both between and within batch components. However, the interpretation will still be limited to simply whether or not the TI falls within the specification range. A more elegant approach — and one that more directly addresses the question of interest to patients and regulators — is to use a Bayesian model to directly calculate the predicted probability of a future individual value being out of specification.

Using a Bayesian approach, the first step is to fit a hierarchical model to the process data, such as:

$$\text{Assay}_{ij} \sim \text{N}(\mu + \beta_i, \sigma^2_{\varepsilon ij}),$$

where μ is the overall process mean and β_i are the individual batch differences from the overall mean $\beta_i \sim \text{N}(0, \sigma^2_\beta)$.

Using any Bayesian modeling software, one can obtain the posterior distribution of the parameters μ, σ^2_β, and σ^2_ε. Using non-informative priors such as $\mu \sim \text{N}(0, 1e+52)$, $\sigma^2_\beta \sim \text{Inv-Gamma}(0.5, 0.5)$ and $\sigma^2_\varepsilon \sim \text{Inv-Gamma}(0.5, 0.5)$, the posterior distributions in this example are summarized in Table 24.3.

TABLE 24.3: Posterior parameter estimates (and 95% credible intervals) from Bayesian hierarchical model of Assay (%) data from five batches.

Parameter	Posterior Mean (95% Credible Interval)
Mean	99.2 (98.7, 99.8)
Inter-batch SD	0.19 (0.00, 0.38)
Intra-batch SD	1.23 (0.85, 1.57)

The advantage of the Bayesian analysis is that it generates distributions of the model parameters, allowing calculation of any intervals or probabilities of interest. Further, if available and appropriate, prior information can be incorporated regarding some or all of the model parameters. Thus, these distributions reflect the full knowledge and uncertainty regarding the process performance. Additionally, a posterior predictive distribution can be computed and used to calculate intervals and probabilities related to future individual results, which is of primary interest, as it is individual results that are directly related to patient risk.

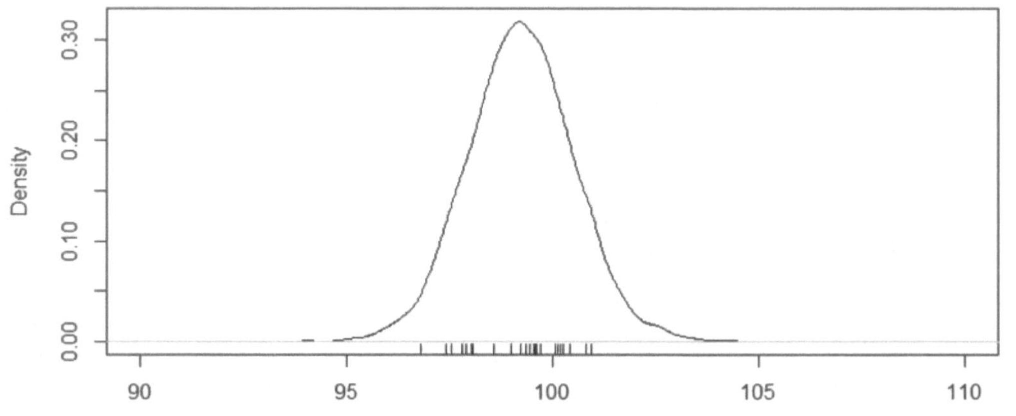

FIGURE 24.4: Posterior predictive distribution of Assay (%). The batch data are indicated by markers on the x-axis.

The results of these computations are displayed in Figure 24.4, the posterior predictive distribution of assay measurements based on the joint posterior distribution from the Bayesian model. The posterior predictive distribution is obtained by taking a random draw from a Normal distribution with mean μ_i and variance $\sigma^2_{\beta i} + \sigma^2_{\varepsilon i}$, where i refers to the i–th member of the joint posterior distribution of the parameters. Based on this distribution, the predicted probability of a future individual result to be within the specification range is directly estimated to be 99.9%. This conclusion regarding expected process performance is a far more informative assessment of capability than the simple affirmation that a TI falls within the specification range.

24.4 Manufacturing situation 3: Use Bayesian modeling of complex testing schemes as justification for reducing sampling

It is not uncommon to continue the heightened sampling described in the previous section into Stage 3 to further understand process variability and gain confidence of quality, for at least some product attributes, In-Process-Controls, and/or process parameters. When this confidence is provided for multiple batches, assurance is obtained regarding the process (not just individual batches), thus establishing a statistical justification for reducing the level of sampling for future batches. The desire to optimize sampling and monitoring is not restricted to the manufacturer; unnecessary sampling and testing do not ultimately benefit the patient. Quite often, the decision to reduce the level of sampling in manufacturing does not require statistical inference. However, there are situations where statistical modelling is quite useful, and Bayesian statistics are particularly appropriate to inform this decision, as illustrated in the next case study.

In this example, the risk of future out-of-specification results is sought to confidently reduce the level of sampling within each batch, in the presence of multiple sources of variability and staged testing criteria. The product quality attribute is evaluated according to staged acceptance criteria as specified by the U.S. Pharmacopoeia (USP), with units tested and criteria specified at each stage, conditional on results from the previous stage. Using a Bayesian approach, risk statements regarding the probability of passing each stage of the testing scheme can be made, taking into account the conditional nature of the staged testing and the structure of the data (multiple sources of variability). This example is clearly applicable to other staged testing, such as dissolution or content uniformity, and for attributes which have specification profiles rather than a single value, such as modified-release products (see, for example, Lebrun et al., 2015).

24.4.1 Example 3: Evaluate risk by predicting probability of meeting batch release criteria

Consider a transdermal product with a routine batch release test for in-vitro release (IVR) based on a single sample of six units per batch. IVR is a measure of the rate at which the active pharmaceutical ingredient (API) is released from the product matrix. It is typical to use a staged testing scheme to assess product quality, such as USP <724> Transdermal Delivery Systems – General Drug Release Standards (U.S. Pharmacopeia, 2018) in this case. Such testing schemes increase sampling over multiple testing stages or levels, beginning with the smallest sample size and strictest criteria. Progression to the next stage is only required if product fails the current stage, thereby optimizing sampling without compromising quality. The specific stages and criteria for this example are listed in Table 24.4.

TABLE 24.4: USP <724> in-vitro release acceptance criteria

Level	Number Tested	Criteria per USP <724>	Criteria for this Example
L1	6	No individual value outside stated range	Each unit $\geq$80%
L2	6	The average of the 12 units (L1 + L2) lies within the stated range. No individual value is outside the stated range by more than 10% of the average of the stated range.	Average of 12 $\geq$ 80% AND Each unit $\geq$71%
L3	12	The average of the 24 units (L1 + L2 + L3) lies within the stated range. Not more than 2 of the 24 units are outside the stated range by more than 10% of the average of the stated range; and none of the units is outside the stated range by more than 20% of the average of the stated range.	Average of 24 $\geq$ 80% AND No more than 2 units $<$ 71% AND Each unit $\geq$ 62%

Such testing schemes can substantially reduce routine testing costs to manufacturers, though modeling such data to make predictions about future performance is a complex task. In this example, heightened sampling above routine batch release level was performed for the three PPQ and first three CPV/OPV batches, in order to better understand the within-batch variability of IVR. Sampling would be reduced to the routine batch release level once the manufacturer has confidence that the process performance justifies the reduction. Any performance assessment must not only consider the multiple sources of variability (within and between samples within a batch, and also between batches); it must also account for the staged testing criteria for IVR, with the evaluation of the criteria at levels 2 and 3 conditional on a sample failing to meet the criteria at the previous level(s). A Bayesian analysis is appropriate to quantify this risk, because one can model the hierarchical variability structure and directly compute the probability of success at each successive IVR testing level, conditional on the previous level(s).

Suppose that the IVR results from the PPQ and first three commercial batches are as shown in Figure 24.5 below.

All results are above 80%, the minimum IVR in Level 1 testing. Although the within batch variability differs slightly from batch to batch, the results in Figure 24.5 indicate relatively consistent variability both between and within batches. (Evidence of systematic trends would require closer examination before proceeding with statistical modeling).

A Bayesian hierarchical model was fit to these data to estimate the overall mean and the variability between batches, between locations within a batch and within a sample:

$$\mathrm{IVR}_{ijk} \sim \mathrm{N}(\mu + \beta_i + \delta_{ij}, \sigma^2_{\varepsilon ijk}),$$

where μ is the overall process mean, β_i are the individual batch deviations from the overall mean $\beta_i \sim \mathrm{N}(0, \sigma^2_\beta)$ and δ_{ij} are the sample-to-sample deviations $\delta_{ij} \sim \mathrm{N}(0, \sigma^2_\delta)$.

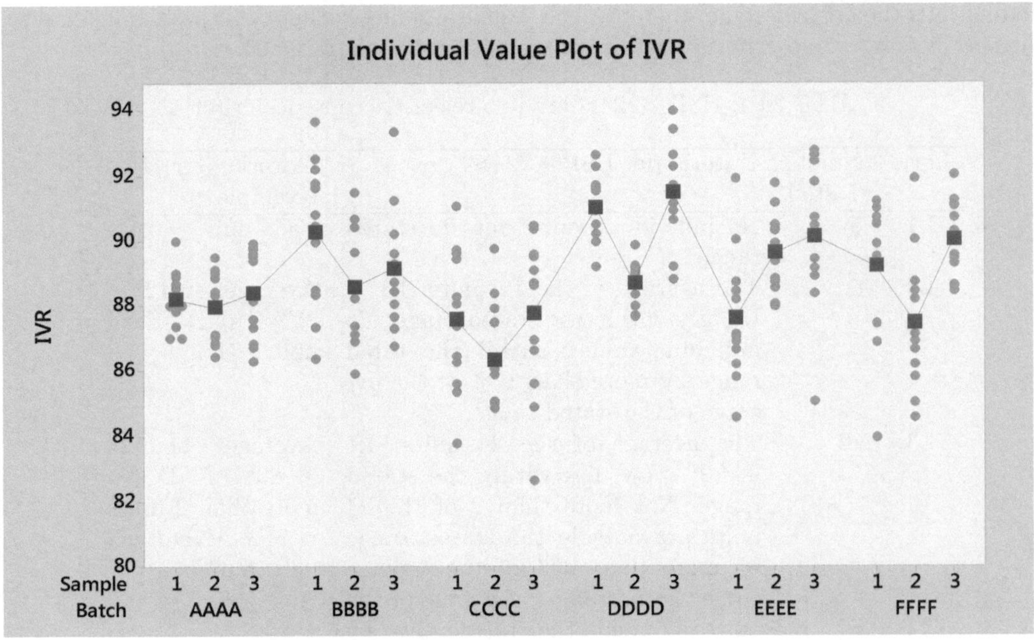

FIGURE 24.5: Individual value chart of IVR (%) from six batches, with the mean of each sample indicated by squares and connected from sample to sample.

Using non-informative priors on $\mu, \sigma_\beta^2, \sigma_\delta^2$ and σ_ε^2, e.g. $\mu \sim$ N$(0, 1e+52)$, $\sigma_\beta^2 \sim$ Inv-Gamma$(0.5, 0.5)$, $\sigma_\delta^2 \sim$ Inv-Gamma$(0.5, 0.5)$, and $\sigma_\varepsilon^2 \sim$ Inv-Gamma$(0.5, 0.5)$, the posterior distribution of the model parameters is summarized in Table 24.5 below.

TABLE 24.5: Posterior parameter estimates (and 95% credible intervals) from Bayesian hierarchical model of IVR

Model Parameter	Median Estimate (95% Credible Interval)
Overall Mean	88.9 (87.6, 90.1)
Between Batch SD	1.09 (0.58, 2.54)
Between Sample SD	0.62 (0.00, 1.57)
Within Sample SD	1.81 (1.64, 2.01)

The predicted probability of a future individual IVR result outside of specification can be derived from the posterior predictive distribution of IVR results. In this case, the probability of a single IVR result less than 80% is estimated to be 0.5%. As in the previous example, this estimate represents a direct risk statement (probability of a result below an acceptable limit), which incorporates all sources of variability and the uncertainty in the estimates of the mean and variability. However, in this case, the probability of a single future IVR result being less than 80% is not a complete and accurate estimate of the process risk. Instead, the probability associated with each testing stage as listed in Table 24.4 is more useful, beginning with the probability that all 6 samples of Level 1 are greater than or equal to 80%, followed by the probability that a sample of 12 (comprising the original 6 plus 6 more) fails Level 2 *if the original sample of 6 failed Level 1*, and finally if required, the probability that a sample of 24 (comprising the 6 from Level 1, the 6 from Level 2, plus 12 more) fails to meet Level 3 criteria *if the Level 1 and 2 samples from the same batch failed both of those previous stages.* These probabilities simply cannot be evaluated directly using frequentist techniques, but are quite simple to calculate using simulation based on the Bayesian model.

To estimate the relevant conditional probabilities, random samples of 24 units from a random batch were selected over the joint posterior distribution of model parameters, rather than the single draw from each point in the joint posterior as used in the probability calculation above. From each sample of 24 the first 6 are evaluated against the Level 1 criterion and, if the criterion is not met, the original 6 and the next 6 are evaluated against the Level 2 criteria, and if those criteria are not met the entire sample of 24 is evaluated against the Level 3 criteria. The probabilities of passing each level of the USP <724> testing criteria for this example are presented in Table 24.6.

TABLE 24.6: Conditional probabilities of meeting USP <724> staged testing criteria using Bayesian posterior distributions.

USP <724> Test Level	Probability of Meeting Criterion(a) Conditional on Progressing from Previous Level
L1	98.80%
L2	63.60%
L3	4.50%

The probabilities in Table 24.6 clearly indicate that the risk of failing the Level 1 USP <724> criterion (1.2%) is greater than the 0.5% probability of a single unit less than 80% IVR, which is not unexpected since the Level 1 criterion requires that all 6 units have IVR greater than or equal to 80%. The prediction of overall probability failing a batch, that is, the probability of failing Level 3, given failure at Levels 1 and 2, is a very useful metric for decision making, easily computed from the results in Table 24.6.

Using Bayesian modeling, it is possible to simulate the USP <724> staged testing scheme using samples which reflect the expected process performance based on all knowledge accumulated at this point in the lifecycle, including multiple variance components, and the uncertainty in the estimates of the process performance parameters (mean and variability parameters). Because the probability estimates in Table 24.6 have clear and relevant interpretation, the Bayesian approach enables risk-based decisions regarding the continuation of heightened sampling for this process. This kind of staged testing occurs for many dosage forms, and the use of Bayesian modeling to provide an easily interpretable estimate of risk at each testing stage is extremely valuable for process understanding, resource planning, and risk-management.

24.5 Discussion

Evaluation of manufacturing performance and risk, whether to plan or analyze PPQ batches or monitor commercial manufacture, is often performed using traditional statistical techniques such as TIs, control charts, and capability indices. While these statistical workhorses of manufacturing may not always be exact, they are often sufficient to meet the objectives of detecting changes in performance or prioritizing process improvement efforts by identifying sub-par performance. However, a Bayesian approach offers two distinct advantages not possible with traditional approaches: 1) incorporation of all relevant knowledge (past and current) in assessment of risk and 2) a direct statement of quality, for instance, the probability that a batch or individual result (such as the dosage unit) will meet product specifications. Quality statements related to individual dosage units are of obvious importance to the patient, regulators, and manufacturers. While frequentist TIs have an interpretation that is related to individual units, comparing a TI to specifications can lead to ambiguous results. A Bayesian probability statement, on the other hand, is quite clear and provides an explicit answer to the question of risk, thereby enabling decision making. In addition to these two advantages, applicable to any manufacturing situation, there are common manufacturing situations for which solutions are either far simpler or only possible using Bayesian methodology.

The first example in this chapter, leveraging prior information to reduce sample size for a PPQ, demonstrates how the use of historical manufacturing data can dramatically reduce the sampling and testing required in re-validation or technology transfer situations, without sacrificing statistical rigor or confidence about the process. In other words, the patient risk is protected, but the manufacturers' cost (which ultimately is passed on to payors) is reduced. This philosophy is consistent with the lifecycle approach to process validation, in which information is meant to accumulate throughout the lifecycle and, at each stage in the lifecycle, inform decision making over time, thereby ensuring quality and patient benefit. Neither re-validation nor tech transfer should be treated as an isolated snapshot of the process with no prior knowledge of performance, or expectation of future monitoring. The use of prior information is reasonable and even preferred, because only by using all information gained throughout the lifecycle can the quality of the product be accurately characterized — with the added benefit of optimizing sample size.

It should be noted, however, that the term "prior" does not mean that the information used in an informative analysis must come from previous manufacturing history. Prior knowledge can also refer to plausible ranges of a parameter, such as limits on biologically/chemically/physically possible results or on the potential variability of a test method or process. Thus, the benefits of using prior information in a Bayesian approach described for the legacy product of Example 1 also applies to new products. Frequentist techniques assume no such boundaries on the range of plausible results, resulting in very wide TIs for small sample sizes. The use of prior information of this type (i.e. not based on historical manufacturing data) — e.g. purity bounded in [0, 100], or assay variability $\leq$20% – adds "strength" to the analysis compared to a frequentist analysis, and is quite justifiable based on scientific fundamentals. The term "borrowing strength" in Bayesian analysis is recognized in numerous regulatory guidance documents related to clinical trials for medical devices and small populations (U.S. Food and Drug Administration, 2010, 2016; European Medicines Agency, 2006).

While only the first example presented in this chapter makes use of prior information, the other two examples are easily extended to an informative analysis if appropriate and desired. The use of prior information should be justified based on: 1) the relevance of the information to the process to be modeled (termed "exchangeability" in Bayesian methodology literature), and 2) the benefits of an informative analysis weighed against the complexity of justifying and explaining the model. This note is not meant to discourage the use of prior information when appropriate — in fact it may seem strange to ignore the substantial information that exists by the time a product reaches Stage 2 or 3 of the lifecycle (if not earlier) — but rather to acknowledge that the choice of statistical methodology in the regulated environment of biopharmaceutical development and manufacturing is not a purely mathematical one. Further, the non-informative analyses presented as examples in this chapter demonstrate that important benefits and advantages of Bayesian methodology are found in the ease of computation (given available software) and interpretation, regardless of whether prior information is used.

In addition to the computation of the probability that an individual dosage unit will meet quality specifications, a value only quantifiable using Bayesian methods, the 2nd and 3rd examples highlight the advantages of Bayesian modeling for commonly encountered complex data structures and staged testing scenarios.

Additional examples where Bayesian methods provide the only statistical solution to the risk associated with product performance include:

- Control limits for orphan drugs or other expedited approval products for which extremely limited data are available at the time of commercialization: Bayesian modeling of hierarchical data structures and potential use of platform information for informative analysis.
- Capability of complex data structures and unique distributions such as in-process-control measurements: Bayesian modeling of hierarchical data structures with the constraint of truncated distribution at alert/action limits.
- Control limits for product attributes exhibiting auto-correlation due to long-term expected sources of variability such as raw material lots — use of short-term variability may result in limits that are too narrow; long-term variability may in some cases result in limits which are too wide: Bayesian modeling of hierarchical data structures.

Bibliography

European Commission (2015). EU GMP Annex 15: Qualification and Validation. "https://ec.europa.eu/health/sites/health/files/files/eudralex/vol-4/2015-10_annex15.pdf".

European Medicines Agency (2006). Guideline on Clinical Trials in Small Populations. "http://www.ema.europa.eu/docs/en_GB/document_library/Scientific_guideline/2009/09/WC500003615.pdf".

European Medicines Agency (2016). Guideline on Process Validation for Finished Products. "https://www.ema.europa.eu/en/documents/scientific-guideline/guideline-process-validation-finished-products-information-data-be-provided-regulatory-submissions_en.pdf".

Hamada, M., Johnson, V., Moore, L. M., and Wendelberger, J. (2004). Bayesian prediction intervals and their relationship to tolerance intervals. *Technometrics*, 46(4):452–459.

Howe, W. G. (1969). Two-sided tolerance limits for normal populations—some improvements. *Journal of the American Statistical Association*, 64(326):610–620.

International Council for Harmonisation (2005). Q8 (core) - Pharmaceutical Development. "https://database.ich.org/sites/default/files/Q8_R2_Guideline.pdf".

Lebrun, P., Giacoletti, K., Scherder, T., Rozet, E., and Boulanger, B. (2015). A quality by design approach for longitudinal quality attributes. *Journal of Biopharmaceutical Statistics*, 25(2):247–259. PMID: 25360720.

Montgomery, D. (2012). *Introduction to Statistical Quality Control, 7th Ed.* John Wiley & Sons.

U.S. Food and Drug Administration (2011). Guidance for Industry: Statistical Approaches to Bioequivalence; U.S. Department of Health and Human Services, FDA. Center of Drug Evaluation and Research (CDER): Rockville, Maryland.

U.S. Food and Drug Administration (2010). Guidance for Industry and FDA Staff. Guidance for the Use of Bayesian Statistics in Medical Device Clinical Trials. U.S. Department of Health and Human Services, FDA. Center of Drug Evaluation and Research (CDER): Rockville, Maryland.

U.S. Food and Drug Administration (2011). Guidance for Industry. Process Validation: General Principles and Practices. U.S. Department of Health and Human Services, FDA. Center of Drug Evaluation and Research (CDER), Center for Biologics Evaluation and Research (CBER), Center for Veterinary Medicine (CVM): Rockville, Maryland.

U.S. Food and Drug Administration (2016). Guidance for Industry and FDA Staff. Leveraging Existing Clinical Data for Extrapolation to Pediatric Uses of Medical Devices. U.S. Department of Health and Human Services, FDA. Center of Drug Evaluation and Research (CDER): Rockville, Maryland.

U.S. Pharmacopeia (2018). U.S. Pharmacopeia and National Formulary. USP 41-NF36. Rockville, MD.

Wolfinger, R. D. (1998). Tolerance intervals for variance component models using bayesian simulation. *Journal of Quality Technology*, 30(1):18–32.

Part V

Additional topics

25

Bayesian Statistical Methodology in the Medical Device Industry

Tarek Haddad

Medtronic, US

In the medical device industry, Bayesian methods are generally being used in two areas. The first is in the creation of stochastic engineering models (SEM) to analyze the performance of the device during its design stage prior to release to market. A SEM attempts to simulate the performance of a medical device in the intended patient population. These SEMs typically combine many sources of information, such as in vitro testing and numerical modeling, then use Bayesian modeling to combine and incorporate sampling error/bias into the simulations. In this chapter we will be discussing the elements used to construct a SEM.

The second area in which Bayesian methods are used is in modeling and analysis of clinical trials to demonstrate the safety and efficacy of the device. These methods include adaptive Bayesian device trials, and augmenting trials with historical data using dynamic borrowing informative prior methods. These methods reduce uncertainty in trial outcomes, can reduce total enrollment size, and trial time. Finally, we discuss new opportunities and activities around augmenting clinical trials with stochastic engineering models as a prior data source. Discussion and examples in this chapter will be structured primarily around the model of a class III cardiac lead medical device and will include a summary of a mock submission, conducted in a collaboration by the FDA and industry, detailing the use of both SEMs and adaptive Bayesian trials.

25.1 Introduction

A medical device is broadly defined as a device designed through mechanical and electrical engineering intended to affect the structure or any function of the human body and which does not achieve its primary purpose through use of a pharmacological substance. The medical devices industry is a highly-regulated industry. In the United States, like pharmaceuticals, medical devices are regulated by the Food and Drug Administration (FDA) Center for Devices and Radiological Health (CDRH).

Regulatory authorities around the world recognize different classes of medical devices based on their design complexity, their use characteristics, and their potential for harm if misused. In this chapter, when we use the term "medical device" or "device," we refer primarily to Class III devices, as defined by the FDA, devices that sustain or support life or are implanted (U.S. Food and Drug Administration, 2017). Examples of Class III medical devices are electrical stimulators (pacemakers, defibrillators, leads, etc.), structural products (stents and heart valves, etc.), and procedural devices (ablation catheters, etc.).

The industry relies on Bayesian statistical models in two stages of testing a medical device prior to release to market. The first is in the use of Bayesian methods, coupled with *stochastic engineering models (SEM)* to analyze the performance of the device during its design stage. This will be discussed in Section 25.2. The second area, discussed in Section 25.3, is the use of Bayesian methods in the modeling and analysis of clinical trial evidence to demonstrate the safety and effectiveness of the device.

Discussion and examples in this chapter will be structured primarily around the model of a Class III cardiac lead medical device. Leads are a critical element for electrical stimulators. Because they are exposed to many high stress environments in both the shoulders and the heart, leads may fracture, resulting in the need for additional surgery, possible injury, and, in some cases, death. Consequently, the medical device industry has invested much time and resources to safely and efficiently bring a lead to market. Section 25.3 will end with a summary of an initiative undertaken by industry and FDA to use stochastic engineering models as a prior in a clinical trial of cardiac leads (MDIC, 2017).

25.2 Use of stochastic engineering models in the medical device design stage

In the past, the industry evaluated the safety of a medical device prior to market release by conducting a set of bench tests; this would entail subjecting the medical device to the specific bench tests for a length of time under certain external conditions. For example, under a fatigue bench test, the device would have to withstand a specified minimal number of cycles at a particular stress. In the past, if all samples passed these bench tests, the device was considered acceptable for clinical use. Because these are attribute tests, simple binomial assumptions can be made. This allows for construction of confidence and reliability estimates based on simple equations.

Unfortunately, in many cases these tests did not accurately simulate the true underlying stresses due to patient and environmental variability. As a result, these engineering tests were not capable of differentiating the safety of a good device from a defective one. An example is the Medtronic Fidelis lead, which successfully passed all bench testing, but still had substantially poor performance in the field. It was removed from the market. As a result, new methodologies, called stochastic engineering models, were developed to assess and predict the performance of the devices. These methods were more statistical in nature and utilized advanced engineering as well as advanced statistical methods.

A SEM creates a clinically relevant simulation of the performance of a medical device in the intended patient population, i.e. a simulation that will predict the results of a patient clinical trial or the assessment of the performance of the product once it is released to the market. Common SEMs include mechanical models to predict rates of fractures in cardiac leads, stents, valves and tines; electrical models that simulate the interaction of a device and the body in the presence of external forces, such as electrical forces during an Magnetic Resonance Imaging (MRI) scan; and biological models, such as those controlling blood glucose through delivery of insulin (Wilkoff et al., 2013; Kovatchev et al., 2009; Viceconti et al., 2017).

SEMs vary in complexity, typically incorporating one or more of the following elements:

i. **Use Conditions**. Use conditions are potential stresses to which the device may be exposed during the implant procedure or once it is in the body. Often these use conditions can be quantified and represented by a distribution that accounts for patient-to-patient variability. Use condition data may come from imaging studies representing the underlying population, such as an MRI imaging study demonstrating the amount of stress a device is exposed to in the body;

ii. **Bench testing/In vitro testing**. Testing is performed on device specimens in a laboratory to assess the reliability of the product. In the medical device industry, the majority of these tests attempt to replicate the environment of the device in its intended use. However, much of the testing is done under use conditions in excess of the device's normal service parameters in order to reduce the time it takes to assess the performance. These excess conditions include increasing the stress, the strain, temperatures, voltage, etc.;

iii. **Numerical modeling/Finite element analysis**. In many cases, bench testing cannot accurately impose the same use conditions on a device as those that occur in the real world. In this case, numerical modeling creates a linkage method between the complex real-world conditions and the simplified use conditions implemented in a bench test;

iv. **Sampling error/bias**. In each element, i. through iii. above, parameters and distributions are being constructed. Limited sample size and uncertainties associated with those parameter estimations should be accounted for in the final calculation. Normally, sampling error does not exist in numerical modeling. However, bias must be addressed. If Bayesian methods are used for constructing estimates of all parameters and distributions, then the predictive distribution is a convenient and appropriate method for accounting for uncertainty in the final calculation. As detailed below, we must construct these predictive distributions to appropriately account for these uncertainties.

In situations where the primary mechanisms contributing to device safety or effectiveness are well understood and modeled it is possible to simulate the clinical outcomes for a new iteration of the device in its intended population (Haddad et al., 2017). We refer to these simulations as "virtual patient" data representing a continuum of information that can be exchangeable for real patient outcomes in a clinical study. Examples of virtual patient data include blood glucose level control in diabetes therapy (Kovatchev et al., 2009) or (Haddad et al., 2014).

25.2.1 Notation

Let the virtual patient cohort $\boldsymbol{y}_0 = \{y_{01}, \ldots, y_{0,N_0}\}$ represent N_0 individual virtual patient outcomes. Each $\boldsymbol{y}_0$ can be thought of as a vector from a multivariate distribution, where $\boldsymbol{\eta}$ are parameters that index the distribution $f_0(\boldsymbol{y}_0 \mid \boldsymbol{\eta})$. Note that $f_0(\boldsymbol{y}_0 \mid \boldsymbol{\eta})$ may not be based on closed form known distributions, but may instead be a complex set of stochastic statistical simulations or numerical physics-based engineering models.

25.2.2 Example of a stochastic engineering model to create virtual patients for cardiac leads

As an example of a SEM that creates virtual patients, we consider the case of cardiac lead fracture rate inside the heart (Haddad et al., 2014). See Figure 25.1 for three different lead models. The heart contracts with every heartbeat, causing the lead to bend. Lead fracture occurs when the accumulated cycles of bending stress exceed the fatigue strength of the lead. In this example, the model assumes that the number of cycles to fracture, C, depends on the applied bending stress, S, measured as geometric curvature. We first collect samples of bending stress $D_{0S} = \{s_1, \ldots, s_n\}$ by imaging leads in real patients throughout a full cardiac cycle (Baxter and McCullouch, 2001). Meanwhile, a bench top fatigue strength test can be used to obtain samples of the number of cycles to fracture $D_{0C} = \{c_1, \ldots, c_n\}$, given an applied bending stress S.

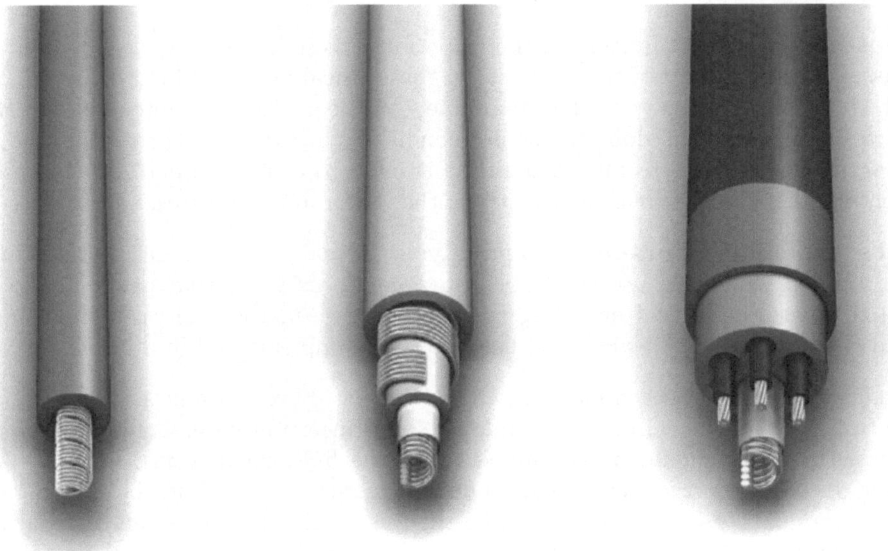

FIGURE 25.1: Medtronic Lead Models 4193 (left), 5076 (center), and 6947 (right). From left to right, the leads are intended for pacing in the left and right ventricles, and for defibrillation in the right ventricle.

The statistical model assumes that S follows a distribution, $f_0(S \mid \boldsymbol{\eta}_S)$ parameterized by $\boldsymbol{\eta}_S$. $f_0(S \mid \boldsymbol{\eta}_S)$ reflects the variability from patient anatomy and physician implantation technique. Given S, we assume that C follows the distribution $f_0(C \mid S, \boldsymbol{\eta}_C)$ with parameters $\boldsymbol{\eta}_C$ leading to a joint distribution $f_0(C, S \mid \boldsymbol{\eta})$ with $\boldsymbol{\eta} = \{\boldsymbol{\eta}_S, \boldsymbol{\eta}_C\}$. The variability of C given a particular S can be due to manufacturing tolerances or material properties. The uncertainty about $\boldsymbol{\eta}$ is described by prior distribution $p_0(\boldsymbol{\eta})$. The data collected in $D_0 = \{D_{0S}, D_{0C}\}$ are used to derive posteriors for $\boldsymbol{\eta}$, denoted as $p_0(\boldsymbol{\eta} \mid D_0)$, where $p_0(\boldsymbol{\eta} \mid D_0)$ represents the joint posterior distribution of the engineering parameters. From the joint posterior of $\boldsymbol{\eta}$, we can then derive the marginal posteriors $p_0(\boldsymbol{\eta}_S \mid D_0)$ and $p_0(\boldsymbol{\eta}_C \mid D_0)$.

Finally, to generate relevant clinical outcome information from engineering data, $\boldsymbol{y}_0$, we assume that we have identified a suitable transfer function, t, relating each bending stress S_k and number of cycles C_k to a clinically relevant time-to-lead fracture, $y_{0k} = t(C_k, S_k)$ $(k = 1, \ldots)$ for survival analysis and $\boldsymbol{y}_0 = \{y_{01}, \ldots, y_{0,N_0}\}$.

Using the joint distribution of S and C above, we can represent the distribution of y_0 given $\boldsymbol{\eta}$ as $f_0(y_0 \mid \boldsymbol{\eta})$. To draw samples of y_0 we must construct the multivariate predictive distribution of y_0 where $\boldsymbol{\eta}$ has been integrated out, as follows:

$$p_0(\boldsymbol{y}_0 \mid D_0) = \int f_0(\boldsymbol{y}_0 \mid \boldsymbol{\eta}) p_0(\boldsymbol{\eta} \mid D_0) d\boldsymbol{\eta}. \tag{25.1}$$

The elements of each $\boldsymbol{y}_0$ vector, capture patient-to-patient variability for each realization of $\boldsymbol{\eta}$. The multiple $\boldsymbol{y}_0$ vectors (one for each $\boldsymbol{\eta} = \{\boldsymbol{\eta}_C, \boldsymbol{\eta}_S\}$ combination) also capture the uncertainty in $\boldsymbol{\eta}$. Since Equation (25.1) has no closed form solution we implement Algorithm 1 in order to draw samples of $\boldsymbol{y}_0$, see Table 25.1.

There are two nested loops in Algorithm 1. The outer loop draws posterior values of $\boldsymbol{\eta}$ from $p_0(\boldsymbol{\eta} \mid D_0)$, and the inner loop draws a vector of N_0 patients with outcomes $\boldsymbol{y}_0$ from

TABLE 25.1: Algorithm 1: Example stochastic engineering model.

```
for i = 1...m_0 {    # draw posterior parameters
Draw η_{C_i} from p_0(η_C | D_0)
Draw η_{S_i} from p_0(η_S | D_0)
...
    for j = 1...N_0 {    # construct N_0 virtual patients
    Draw S_{ij} from f_0(S | η_{S_i})
    Draw C_{ij} from f_0(C | S, η_{C_i})
    y_{0,ij} = t(C_{ij}, S_{ij})    # convert C and S to y_0 (years to failure)
    }
y_{0i} = {y_{0,i1}, ..., y_{0,iN_0}}
}
```

$f_0(\boldsymbol{y}_0 \mid \boldsymbol{\eta})$. In our example, the clinical outcome of interest is years to lead failure. Combining the two loops together is equivalent to Equation (25.1). The nested loops in Algorithm 1 separate the natural variation between patients from the parameter uncertainties due to sampling error. This separation accurately accounts for the two types of variability, and is why Equation (25.1) is a multivariate distribution as opposed to univariate (unless you only want to simulate one virtual patient).

For this example, the transfer function t is to divide C by the number of heartbeats per year to obtain time to failure in years. In Figure 25.2, we use Algorithm 1 to generate a survival curve of years to lead failure for each of the m_0 vectors of $\boldsymbol{\eta}$.

25.2.3 Updating and calibration

As noted above, each virtual patient cohort represents a simulated set of virtual patients conditioned on a single set of posterior parameters from the engineering models. Thousands of cohorts of virtual patients are created, each with a unique set of posterior parameters (each corresponding to a generated $\boldsymbol{\eta}$ in Algorithm 1). When real clinical data becomes available it is possible to compare the simulated cohorts to the real data. Intuitively, the virtual cohorts that more closely match the clinical data are more likely to be accurate representations of the real population. This similarity implies that the corresponding posterior parameters for the virtual patient cohorts are likely to be the actual parameter values, and we can update the posterior distributions accordingly. With the new posterior distributions, we can draw new virtual cohorts that will have distributions aligning more closely with the clinical performance.

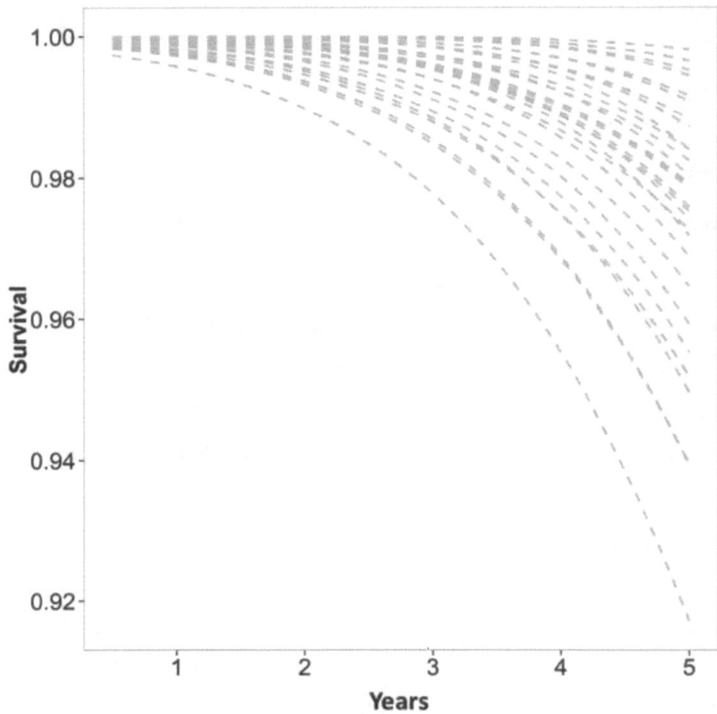

FIGURE 25.2: Lead survival curves generated using virtual patients from Algorithm 1. The curves represent Kaplan-Meir estimates from $\boldsymbol{y}_{0i}$ where i runs from 1 to m_0.

25.3 Use of Bayesian statistics in the design and analysis of medical device clinical trials

25.3.1 Uniqueness of medical device trials

Because of the unique characteristics of medical devices, adapting traditional drug clinical trial designs, which rely primarily on blinding and large participant populations, to a medical device clinical trial design presents formidable practical challenges.

Most medical devices must be implanted through an in-hospital procedure. As a result, it is very difficult to incorporate blinding as part of the trial; and it is nearly impossible to implement double blinding. For example, when an artificial valve is implanted, neither the patient nor the physician can be blinded. Creating a sham group is also extremely challenging. The patients would have to undergo a surgical procedure where no device, or a fake device, is implanted; and this presents significant medical risks and ethical concerns, and would be highly expensive (Campbell and Yue, 2016). Additionally, a doctor's expertise in the implant procedure can play a critical role in the success of the device. Therefore, careful consideration of physician training and physician randomization is important.

Each hospital procedure for a device can cost thousands of dollars. That cost makes large clinical trials prohibitive. As a result, medical device trials are usually in the hundreds of participants, while drug trials are in the thousands (Pibouleaua and Chevret, 2011).

There are also positive advantages in the design of device clinical trials, as opposed to drug clinical trials. In nearly all cases, medical devices are targeted treatments and have few interactions with other parts of the body. A non-localized drug can have ancillary effects, known and unknown, on the entire body. Furthermore, in a drug trial there almost always exist uncertainties related to patient adherence to the required drug regimen; in a device trial, the device will perform its function without patient action. Unlike drug trials, early phase dosing studies are generally not needed in device clinical trials. And, finally, many device trials assess iterative improvements on previous generation devices leading to readily available historical data (Pibouleaua and Chevret, 2011).

Because of these differing considerations and requirements in the design of the two types of clinical trials, and especially the difference related to trial size, device trials require more flexible designs and sophisticated statistical analysis. Here again, Bayesian techniques can be highly useful in designing medical device clinical trials, particularly in the use of adaptive Bayesian trials and informative priors to model and analyze clinical evidence (Bonangelino et al., 2011).

25.3.2 Adaptive Bayesian trials

The considerable expense and the surgery risks associated with each patient in a medical device trial necessitate a clinical trial design that minimizes the number of participants to the smallest number demonstrating the safety and efficacy of a device. Determining this appropriate sample size is a challenge. An adaptive Bayesian trial with sample size re-estimation procedures can help by adaptively determining the appropriate sample size needed.

A typical adaptive trial would sequentially enroll a set number of patients; and then use a predictive distribution to impute the results for patients that have not reached follow up to determine the probability that the trial will be effective under current enrollment. This is called an *expected success determination* which was also called assurance by O'Hagan et al. (2005) and introduced in Chapter 1, but described in greater detail in Chapters 4, 5, 3 and 22. We can also use the predictive distribution to impute the probability of success at the maximum enrollment that the trial design has planned to determine whether the trial has a low probability of ultimately achieving its goal. If so, then we can declare futility and end the trial early. This minimizes costs and avoids exposing patients to unnecessary, ineffective treatments. This is especially critical for device trials, because the implant procedure can involve a higher risk than simply taking a pill.

An adaptive Bayesian trial may need to account for three kinds of patients at each interim analysis (Berry et al., 2010):

i. Patients with complete data;

ii. Patients with partially complete data. These patients have been enrolled in the study and have some follow up time, but have not reached final follow up;

iii. Patients with a total absence of data because they have not yet been enrolled in the study.

Many trials have time to event, or survival as endpoint. In cases where the endpoint is hospitalization or death, we will have partial data at interim analysis. For these cases, one option is to use the piecewise exponential distributions to impute patients' final outcomes using the posterior predictive distribution (PPD). While the PPD is a general concept that has been introduced in Chapter 1, and used in many other chapters in this book, it is illustrative to apply it in the context of medical device studies. First note that generating data from the PPD can be considered as imputing fictive data.

The method of imputation proceeds as follows: at interim analysis, construct posterior distributions for piecewise hazard rates using the data from the existing enrolled patients in the trial. Draw a set of posterior values; use the conditional predictive distribution to impute a complete data set for patients that have been enrolled at the interim analysis (we use the conditional distribution in order to incorporate the partial information we have on these patients. Closed form solutions to the conditional distribution are available for piecewise exponential). Impute a second data set of all patients including patients that may be enrolled based on the maximum allowable enrollment. Construct final test statistics for both data sets. Repeat this process M times. Determine the number of times you pass the trial for both data sets. If this number is greater than expected success probability for the current enrollment data set, stop enrollment for expected success. If the rate of failed trials is greater than the futility probability for the second data set, stop the trial for futility.

As an example, an adaptive Bayesian study design was used in the BLOCK HF study (Curtis et al., 2013), which compared bi-ventricular cardiac pacing to single chamber pacing in heart failure patients. The design allowed for up to 1200 patients to undergo randomization and featured sample size re-estimation and two interim analyzes with pre-specified trial-stopping rules. Finally, consult Chapter 8 for an extensive treatment of Bayesian adaptive designs.

25.3.3 Informative priors and dynamic borrowing

As stated above, medical devices are usually targeted therapies with few ancillary reactions, and the device industry tends to have many iterative products with similar functions, thereby making historical data from past trials accessible and relevant (Campbell and Yue, 2016). Additionally, sources of prior data for devices could come from early phase trials when very little has changed between the early phase trial and the pivotal study thus making this kind of data an optimal prior. All of these characteristics would support the use of an informative prior for statistical purposes in designing and analyzing the subsequent trial. Even so, the use of the informative prior has been fraught with misunderstanding and controversy. Details on eliciting prior information from experts can be found in Chapter 5.

The greatest concerns with use of the informative prior are the possible inflation of traditional frequentist Type I error rate and the potential point estimate bias in the treatment effect or complication rate in cases where the prior was based on data substantially different from the current data (Mandrola et al., 2018).

Concerns related to a prior differing from current data can be addressed using dynamic borrowing methods (Viele et al., 2014) where the weight of the prior is determined through a statistical comparison between the prior and the current data, which will then give the prior a weight relative to its similarity to the current data. Extensive details of this approach can also be found in Chapter 6.

However, the use of dynamic borrowing may increase uncertainty in trial outcome due to variability in study power. Because of this greater uncertainty, dynamic borrowing is best performed in conjunction with an adaptive Bayesian trial (see Chapter 8) where there is the ability to reassess sample size requirements at interim analyses. Pairing dynamic borrowing with an adaptive trial gives the trial the flexibility to leverage the prior data when there are similarities between the prior and current data, but also allows the flexibility of converting the trial to a traditional non-informative Bayesian trial if discrepancies are observed between the prior and current data.

However, adaptive Bayesian trials require an enormous number of simulations to assess operating characteristics. For example, a statistician may need to construct the posterior hundreds of millions of times to assess operating characteristics, such as Type I error rate, power, etc. Also, if construction of the posterior entails MCMC procedures using standard software such as `Stan`, `JAGS` or `SAS PROC MCMC`, which generally require many seconds to run a single calculation, the time required for the process would be prohibitive. The medical device industry is unlikely to tolerate such long delays and may choose less complex non-Bayesian designs.

There are several dynamic borrowing methods proposed in literature, such as hierarchical, power prior, commensurate prior, and test & pool methods, see Viele et al. (2014) as well as Chapter 8. The *discount prior method* (Haddad et al., 2017) is a more recent method that provides both computational efficiency (avoiding MCMC procedures) and a mechanism to reduce the weight of the prior to zero when there is a high level of discordance between the prior and the current data. The discount prior method uses similar notation as the power prior where the level of borrowing is described in terms of a single parameter α_0 that ranges from 0 to 1; a value of 0 indicates no historical borrowing while a value of 1 indicates full historical borrowing. The discount prior provides a robust approach to adaptively determining the weight α_0. Note that the notation $\widetilde{\alpha}_0$ is used below to distinguish the discount prior approach from other power prior methods.

Briefly, the discount prior method consists of three steps:

1. Comparison between historical data and current data to get an agreement measure $a(\cdot)$ where $0 \leq a(\cdot) \leq 1$;
2. A discount function $W(\cdot)$ to compute the weight given to the historical data via $\widetilde{\alpha}_0 = W(a)$;
3. Implementation of the power prior to construct the appropriate prior distribution.

The agreement measure $a(\cdot)$ is constructed using a Z-score. The function $W(\cdot)$ should be such that $W(a)$ ranges between 0 and 1 and is close to 0 when a is close to 0, indicating a high level of disagreement between the historical and current data. The discount function $W(a)$ should be pre-specified. Additionally, the discount function should be tailored specifically to the needs of the clinical trial in terms of a clinician's comfort level with the historical data. The choice of discount function will affect trial characteristics such as power, Type I error rate, bias, etc.. The use of a Weibull cdf, multiplied by a fixed scalar value α_{max}, as the discount function has been suggested (Haddad et al., 2017). The scalar α_{max} represents the maximum amount of historical borrowing when the Weibull cdf is 1. The Weibull cdf is written

$$W(a \mid \lambda, \gamma) = \alpha_{max}\left[1 - \exp\{-(a/\lambda)^{\gamma}\}\right], \tag{25.2}$$

where γ and λ are the shape and scale parameters, respectively. The Weibull cdf works well as a discount function when $\lambda < 1$ since $1 - \exp\{-(a/\lambda)^{\gamma}\} \leq 1$ for $a \leq 1$. The shape parameter γ controls the rate at which changes in a cause changes in $\widetilde{\alpha}_0$. Increasing λ results in conservative borrowing of historical data. The identity function $a = W(\cdot)$ has also been proposed as a good choice for the discount function due to its simplicity and understandability. The identity function can be interpreted as having prior weight equal to the probability that the prior data and current data come from the same underlying population. In many cases with the discount prior approach, analytical closed forms exist for the posterior distributions.

25.3.3.1 Discount prior example

As an example of the use of the discount prior, we turn our attention to a previous analysis that incorporated historical data using a non-dynamic approach (Holmes et al., 2014). We use the results of the PREVAIL (Watchman Left Atrial Appendage Closure Device in Patients with Atrial Fibrillation Versus Long Term Warfarin Therapy) trial. The goal of the PREVAIL study was to assess the safety and efficacy of left atrial appendage (LAA) occlusion for stroke prevention in patients with non-valvular atrial fibrillation compared with long-term warfarin therapy. Atrial fibrillation affects your heart's ability to pump blood normally. This can cause blood to pool in an area of the heart called the LAA. There, blood cells can stick together and form a clot. When a blood clot escapes from the LAA, and travels to another part of the body, it can cut off the blood supply to the brain, causing a stroke. The Watchman Device (Figure 25.3) is designed to prevent the clotting of blood in the LAA. This device is an alternative to the lifelong use of warfarin for people with atrial fibrillation.

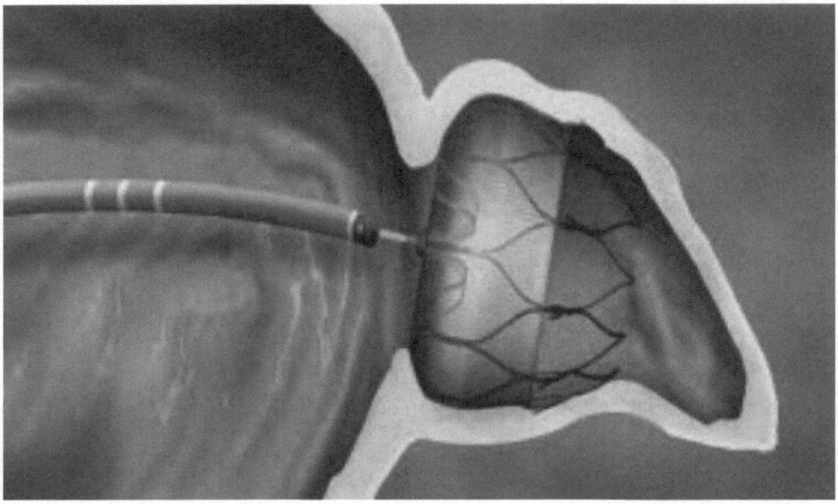

FIGURE 25.3: Watchman Left Atrial Appendage Closure Device: Designed to prevent clotting of blood in the left atrial appendage.

The analysis of the PREVAIL study data incorporated previous data from the earlier PROTECT study. During the PROTECT study, 463 patients were randomized to the Watchman treatment arm while 244 patients were randomized to the control arm. In total, there were $y_{0t} = 39$ events in $N_{0t} = 1,720$ patient-years of follow-up in the treatment arm and $y_{0c} = 34$ events in $N_{0c} = 901$ patient-years of follow-up in the control arm. The PREVAIL study randomized 269 patients to the Watchman treatment arm (Holmes et al., 2014) while 138 patients were randomized to the control arm. At the 18 month analysis time, there were $y_t = 14$ events in $N_t = 259$ patient-years of follow-up in the treatment arm and $y_c = 4$ events in $N_c = 141$ patient-years of follow-up in the control arm. The historical PROTECT trial data was previously given a fixed weight of 50% and combined with the PREVAIL trial data to carry-out a survival analysis using a piecewise exponential model. In the present case study, the composite primary endpoint of stroke, systemic embolism, or cardiovascular/unexplained was used during the follow-up period. Previously, the Watchman treatment was found to be non-inferior to warfarin based on the 95% credible interval (CI) of the rate ratio being below the non-inferiority margin of 1.75. In the present analysis, we use the Poisson count model as described below to approximate the results of the previous analysis as well as to estimate the historical data weight dynamically using the discount prior.

In this example, we derive the discount prior for Poisson count data. We start with the definition of the power prior as:

$$p(\theta \mid y_0, \widetilde{\alpha}_0) \propto L(\theta \mid y_0)^{\widetilde{\alpha}_0} p_0(\theta), \tag{25.3}$$

where $L(\theta \mid y_0)$ is the likelihood function for the historical data, $p_0(\theta)$ denotes the initial non-informative prior distribution for θ, and $\widetilde{\alpha}_0$ is a "discount" parameter that controls the influence of historical data y_0 on the final power prior $p(\theta \mid y_0, \widetilde{\alpha}_0)$. Note that when we are using the discount prior method, as opposed to the traditional power prior, we substitute $\widetilde{\alpha}_0$ for α_0.

$\widetilde{\alpha}_0$ varies between 0 and 1. Suppose we have data collected on N subject-years, and we observe y events. Further, suppose that we have N_0 historical subject-years and we observe y_0 events. We are interested in estimating an event rate θ and we assume $Y \sim \text{Poisson}(N\theta)$ and $Y_0 \sim \text{Poisson}(N_0\theta_0)$. Further, suppose for notation purposes that $Y \sim \text{Poisson}(N\widetilde{\theta})$. The difference between $\widetilde{\theta}$ and θ is how it is being estimated. θ is the parameter of interest and is estimated using the current study data as well as the prior data weighted appropriately using the discount prior method, whereas $\widetilde{\theta}$ is estimated from the current data only with no historical data influence and is considered a nuisance parameter. $\widetilde{\theta}$ is used for estimating the appropriate weighting of the prior based on the pre-specified discount function $W(\cdot)$. If it is determined by the discount function that the historical weight equals 0 (i.e. $\widetilde{\alpha}_0 = 0$) then $\widetilde{\theta} = \theta$.

We assume that the sampling distribution of the historical data, conditional on θ and the weight $\widetilde{\alpha}_0$ is

$$L(y_0 \mid \theta)^{\widetilde{\alpha}_0} \propto \left[\theta^{y_0} \exp(-N_0\theta)\right]^{\widetilde{\alpha}_0}. \tag{25.4}$$

Assuming for simplicity a conjugate Gamma prior distribution on the success rate, the discount prior is obtained by combining this prior with the Expression in (25.4) and is written as:

$$p(\theta \mid y_0, \widetilde{\alpha}_0) \propto \text{Gamma}(\theta \mid \widetilde{\alpha}_0 y_0 + c, \widetilde{\alpha}_0 N_0 + d),$$

with discount parameter $\widetilde{\alpha}_0 = W\left(a(\widetilde{\theta}, \theta)\right)$ determined from $p(\widetilde{\theta} \mid y) = \text{Gamma}(\widetilde{\theta} \mid y + \widetilde{c}, N + \widetilde{d})$ and $p(\theta_0 \mid y) = \text{Gamma}(\theta_0 \mid y_0 + c_0, N_0 + d_0)$, where each of $c, c_0, \widetilde{c}, d, d_0$, and $\widetilde{d}$ are prior hyperparameters of the respective Gamma distributions. The agreement measure $a(\cdot)$ has the form:

$$\begin{aligned} a &= 2\left(1 - \Phi(Z)\right), \\ Z &= \mid \widetilde{\theta} - \theta_0 \mid (\widetilde{\tau}^2 + \tau_0^2)^{-1/2}, \end{aligned}$$

where Φ is the standard Normal cdf, and each of $\widetilde{\tau}^2$ and τ_0^2 are posterior variance estimates of $\widetilde{\theta}$ and θ_0, respectively. The value of a is input into the discount function $W(\cdot)$, with here the Weibull function as discount function, to compute $\widetilde{\alpha}_0$. Given the discount prior of θ, the posterior distribution that weights the historical data via $\widetilde{\alpha}_0$ has the form:

$$p(\theta \mid y, y_0, \widetilde{\alpha}_0) \propto \text{Gamma}(\theta \mid y + \widetilde{\alpha}_0 y_0 + c, N + \widetilde{\alpha}_0 N_0 + d).$$

In the calculation of Z, $\widetilde{\tau}^2 = \widetilde{\theta}/N$ and $\tau_0^2 = \theta_0/N_0$ the variance estimates derived via the Fisher Information under the Poisson likelihood.

Formally, we are interested in augmenting the PREVAIL trial data, i.e. the current data, with the PROTECT trial, i.e. historical data, to estimate the rate ratio, $\theta = \theta_t/\theta_c$, where θ_t and θ_c are the event rates for the control and test arm, respectively. We assume $Y_t \sim \text{Poisson}(N_t\theta_t)$, $Y_c \sim \text{Poisson}(N_c\theta_c)$, $Y_{0t} \sim \text{Poisson}(N_{0t}\theta_{0t})$ and $Y_{0c} \sim \text{Poisson}(N_{0c}\theta_{0c})$. We use the current data of each arm to facilitate calculation of the agreement measure. To construct the historical data weight, we estimate $\widetilde{\alpha}_{0t}$ and $\widetilde{\alpha}_{0c}$ separately for the treatment and control arms, respectively. We use a Weibull cdf discount function with shape 1.5 and scale 0.4. (These values were chosen because of their intuitive properties; for example, if the measure of agreement $a(\cdot)$ equals 0.1 or 0.05, then the historical data will be given a weight of about 0.1 and 0.05 respectively). We fit two model types to the data: (1) fix the historical data weight at 0.5 as in the PREVAIL analysis and carry out posterior estimation of the event rate, denoted $\theta_{0.5}$; and (2) estimate the historical data discount weight dynamically with a maximum weight of 0.5 and carry out posterior estimation of the event rate, denoted as θ. Model fit was performed using the `bayesDP` package in `R`, which implements the Bayesian Discount Prior methods (Musgrove, 2018). Results are displayed in Figure 25.4. We see the densities of the current data only, the historical data only, and two curves of the posterior of the current data augmented by the historical data. The Poisson rate ratio mean posterior estimate and credible interval of the historical PROTECT data alone was $\theta_0 = \theta_{0t}/\theta_{0c} = 0.58$ (95% CI:0.37,0.91) while the estimate of the current PREVAIL data alone was $\widetilde{\theta} = \widetilde{\theta}_t/\widetilde{\theta}_c = 1.68$ (95% CI:0.62,5.29). The posterior estimate when fixed $\widetilde{\alpha}_0 = 0.5$ is $\theta_{0.5} = 0.83$ (95% CI:0.49,1.46) while the posterior estimate when estimating $\widetilde{\alpha}_0$ dynamically is $\theta = 1.41$ (95% CI: 0.63,3.36).

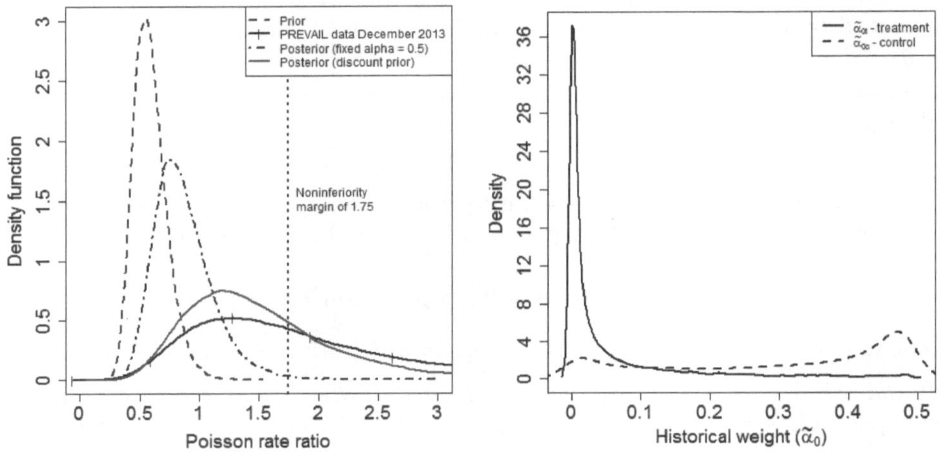

FIGURE 25.4: Poisson data application to PREVAIL Watchman data. (a) Dashed line: Prior density of historical PROTECT data; solid line with vertical dash: Likelihood of the current PREVAIL data; black-dotted-dashed line: Posterior density with historical data weight fixed at 0.5; solid line: Posterior density with historical data weight estimated dynamically with max weight of 0.5. (b) Distributions of the discount weights for the treatment arm (solid) and control arm (dashed).

The 95% credible interval of $\theta_{0.5}$ supports non-inferiority since 1.75 is above the upper limit. Meanwhile, our discount prior approach results in a 95% CI that does not support non-inferiority. As can be seen in Figure 25.4, when $\widetilde{\alpha}_0$ is fixed at 0.5, augmentation with the historical data causes much of the mass of the current data to shift below 1. On the other hand, when $\widetilde{\alpha}_0$ is estimated dynamically, the posterior density appears similar to the current data density. For the discount prior model, the median estimate of the historical control data weight was $\widetilde{\alpha}_{0c} = 0.35$ (95% CI: 0.00,0.49) and the historical treatment data weight was $\widetilde{\alpha}_{0t} = 0.01$ (95% CI: 0.00,0.38). Thus, we see that very little weight is given to the historical treatment data while a marginal amount of weight is given to the control data. This analysis indicates that dynamic borrowing may be prudent in pivotal clinical trials where historical borrowing is being used.

25.3.3.2 Stochastic Engineering Models as priors

SEMs are being used in pre-clinical evaluations to predict the safety and efficacy of medical devices. For example, a SEM was used in demonstrating the safety of cardiac rhythm devices during Magnetic Resonance Imaging (Gold et al., 2015). In the case of the MRI example for cardiac rhythm devices, some computational models are sufficiently mature that future pre-market human clinical evaluation may not be necessary (Shiren and Jeffrey, 2017). However, the modeling framework for MRI safety took more than a decade of development. During that time, the SEMs were only used as a supplemental source of evidence and were not used to reduce the size or duration of the clinical trials. Therefore, the industry did not gain the maximum amount of efficiency because the engineering model was not explicitly incorporated into the design of the clinical trial to reduce the cost of the trial. Large investments were made in both clinical trials and engineering models creating redundant information.

An alternative to using SEMs only for supplemental sources of evidence is possible. One alternative is to incorporate a SEM as an informative prior in a Bayesian trial. This would have the effect of efficiently utilizing the engineering model while also reducing the cost and size of the trial. This would also allow for the validation of the model if the results of the prior were consistent with the real trial results. Thus, a synergistic relationship would be created.

Analogous to the framework described above for incorporation of historical data with a discount function, the prior weight could be proportional to the maturity of the model. For example, in the MRI case the SEM in the first trial might have been given a relatively small amount of weight relative to real patients because the MRI model was in its infancy. In subsequent trials the SEM might have been given a larger weight, but still rely on real patients; and in the final stages the trial would be completely dominated by virtual patients. This tiered approach is highly efficient when information is utilized commensurate with the maturity levels of the SEMs.

The medical device industry and regulatory agencies have had much recent discussion about the possibility of augmenting a clinical trial using SEMs or "virtual patients" as discussed in Section 25.1 (Shiren and Jeffrey, 2017; Mullin et al., 2018). A mock FDA submission was conducted to test the approach of using a SEM as a prior, see Section 25.3.3.4.

25.3.3.3 Implementation

In a clinical trial, the primary focus is on clinical outcomes, such as the failure rate in patients, θ. That is, for real patient outcomes y, we assume a standard distribution $f(y \mid \theta)$ indexed by the parameter of interest θ. If the SEM accurately predicts clinical outcomes, then the outcomes of virtual and clinical patients will be similar. Therefore, the virtual patients should provide relevant information about θ. Using this assumption, we interpret y_0 as having been generated from a distribution governed by the clinical parameter θ (i.e. $Y_0 \sim f(y_0 \mid \theta)$ instead of generated from $p_0(y_0 \mid D_0)$ — Equation (25.1), which, as mentioned above, may be complex with no closed form. This interpretation is done for notational and mathematical convenience, as the power prior approach discussed in detail in the beginning of Section 25.3.3 requires the selection of a closed form likelihood function governed by the clinical parameter θ. This assumption is similar to standard statistical practice, where a standard distribution (e.g. Normal) is selected because it fits the data reasonably well. Data from a well-developed SEM will frequently be highly similar to clinical data.

Unlike historical data, data created by a SEM have virtually unlimited sample size. Therefore, an appropriate weighting approach is required. Additionally, we would like a method for discounting the virtual patients in cases where there is heterogeneity between current and virtual patient studies. One approach is to use the power prior framework introduced by Ibrahim and Chen (2000) and discussed in Chapter 6 to discount the prior generated by virtual patients.

Let $\boldsymbol{y}$ be a response vector of length n from the current study and $L(\theta \mid \boldsymbol{y}) = \prod_{j=1}^{n} f(y_j \mid \theta)$ its likelihood function. Similarly, we can construct the likelihood function for a single cohort of virtual patients, $L(\theta \mid \boldsymbol{y}_0) = \prod_{j=1}^{N_0} f(y_{0j} \mid \theta)$. The cohort likelihood is then used to form a prior as shown next.

Let $p_0(\theta)$ denote the initial non-informative prior distribution for θ. We define the power prior distribution of θ for the current study given one virtual patient cohort y_0 as: $p(\theta \mid y_0, \alpha_0) \propto L(\theta \mid y_0)^{\alpha_0} p_0(\theta)$, where the parameter α_0 is a "discount" parameter that controls the influence of virtual patient data $\boldsymbol{y}_0$ on $p(\theta \mid \boldsymbol{y}_0, \alpha_0)$, with α_0 varying between 0 and 1, and as α_0 approaches 1, more weight is given to the virtual patient data $\boldsymbol{y}_0$.

When historical data is used, α_0 represents the weight placed on its prior. For virtual simulations it is convenient to write $\alpha_0 = n_0/N_0$, where n_0 is the effective sample size of the prior and then the power prior can be rewritten as follows:

$$p(\theta \mid \boldsymbol{y}_0, n_0) \propto L(\theta \mid \boldsymbol{y}_0)^{(n_0/N_0)} p_0(\theta). \tag{25.5}$$

Up until this point we have dealt with only one virtual cohort $\boldsymbol{y}_0$. As noted above, we need to account for the uncertainty in the parameters governing the SEM, $\boldsymbol{\eta}$. To incorporate the entire distribution of $p_0(\boldsymbol{y}_0 \mid D_0)$ we integrate (25.5) over $\boldsymbol{y}_0$ given D_0, the engineering data, to obtain the prior in (25.5):

$$p(\theta \mid n_0, D_0) = \int p(\theta \mid \boldsymbol{y}_0, n_0) p_0(\boldsymbol{y}_0 \mid D_0) d\boldsymbol{y}_0. \tag{25.6}$$

The integral in (25.6) has no closed form solution but one can generate data from $p(\theta \mid n_0, D_0)$ with draws of $\boldsymbol{y}_0$ from $p_0(\boldsymbol{y}_0 \mid D_0)$, then drawing θ from each instance of the power prior $p(\theta \mid \boldsymbol{y}_0, n_0)$ (25.5). We repeat this process m_0 times using ordinary Monte Carlo methods, setting m_0 large enough to appropriately construct the posterior distribution for parameters $\boldsymbol{\eta}$. This generates values of θ that incorporate the uncertainty in the virtual patient data $\boldsymbol{y}_0$ while weighting virtual patient data to the effective prior sample size of n_0. Note there are two sources of Monte Carlo error, i.e. the number of virtual patients in a cohort, N_0 and the number of cohorts, m_0.

25.3.3.4 Mock submission

In order to demonstrate the usefulness of augmenting virtual patients into a clinical trial, an initiative was undertaken by the Medical Device Innovation Consortium (MDIC) made up of industry and FDA to create a *mock submission* with regard to a new mock lead model, called 2015v (MDIC, 2017). This lead model was similar to a predicate lead, but had moderate design changes which might have had an effect on its reliability in terms of lead fracture in the heart. However, SEMs were created to be able to predict lead fracture performance and virtual patients were created to simulate the clinical performance of the new product. An adaptive Bayesian clinical trial was designed where the virtual patient results were used as the prior (Haddad et al., 2017).

The mock submission involved both a sponsor team and a review team. The sponsor team was composed of several individuals familiar with ICD lead technology, other members of the medical device industry, and several FDA representatives. The review team was formed with FDA representation from several divisions within the Center for Devices and Radiological Health (CDRH), led by the Office of Device Evaluation / Division of Cardiovascular Devices.

The mock submission team constructed virtual patients using a method identical to the example shown in Section 25.2.3. The trial was designed as a single arm, with an objective performance goal (OPG) of less than 3% fracture rate at 18 months for the trial endpoint. The adaptive design had a minimum of $N = 200$ real subjects enrolled. Interim analyses were conducted in increments of 30 subjects to a max sample size of $N = 410$. If expected success at any of the interim analyses was greater than 90% enrollment would stop. Additionally, if the probability of success for the trial was less than 1%, futility would be called. Success of the trial was defined by a posterior probability of greater than 95%. In addition, to incorporate these virtual patients as a prior, the mock submission team used the discount prior approach discussed in Section 25.3.3 above for down weighting the virtual patients. A Weibull cdf was used as the discount function with varying parameters to achieve certain clinical operating characteristics, such as Type I error rate less than 10%, and power greater than 80%. Two types of sample size re-estimation methods were utilized in the trial design. The first was a traditional adaptive re-estimation based on the clinical endpoint response variable. The second was adapting the prior based on input data used in the SEM, collected from the (real) enrolled patients (Berry et al., 2010). Both cases were used for sample size re-estimation or stopping the trial early for success or futility. In addition, two mock pre-submission meetings were conducted. The mock submission process created a template for industry and the FDA to follow when developing a real clinical study where SEMs are being utilized as a prior.

Table 25.2 below shows the results of the simulation. The table consists of four scenarios that were simulated. One used a fixed power prior where the virtual patients received a weight of $n = 160$; two used Weibull discount priors, and the last used a non-informative prior. Additionally, the table shows the power, Type I error rate, average number of virtual patients enrolled, and average number of real patients enrolled. As can be seen, the fixed power prior had excellent power, but unacceptable Type I error rate. The non-informative prior had good Type I error rate but insufficient power. Only the Weibull(0.1,1.5) discount priors were able to meet required power and Type I error rate requirements.

TABLE 25.2: VP Mock submission simulation results.

Prior	Power $\theta = 1\%$	Type I error $\theta = 3\%$	Average #VP(n_0) $\theta = 1\%$	Average enrolled $\theta = 1\%$
Fixed prior ($n_0 = 160$)	0.96	0.29	160	209
Weibull(0.05, 1.5)	0.78	0.05	89	244
Weibull(0.1, 1.5)	0.85	0.10	121	240
Weak prior Beta(1,1)	0.64	0.03	0	248

25.4 Challenges

Use of informative priors in pivotal trials is still rare, even with the enhancement of dynamic borrowing. This is due to a lack of understanding as to how these methods work and how they affect operating characteristics of clinical trial results. To mitigate these issues, more retrospective studies should be performed, as well as mock submissions similar to the ones described above, which will allow clinicians and statisticians to understand how these borrowing methods affect a clinical trial.

Additionally, there are opportunities to expand on the dynamic borrowing methodologies currently being used. For example, in the discount prior methodology described in Section 25.3.3, a Z-score is used to measure the similarities between historical and current data. Other measures of similarity might have the potential for improving operating characteristics using a discount prior approach.

Only a limited number of SEMs have been created to generate clinical evidence for safety and efficacy. There exists tremendous potential for the development of new SEMs in other applications in the medical device field, pharmaceuticals and elsewhere. Additionally, new SEMs could be based on machine learning algorithms and artificial intelligence as opposed to physics and chemistry based SEMs. However, development of successful new SEMs will require a closer collaboration among engineers, chemists and statisticians.

Bibliography

Baxter, W. and McCullouch, A. (2001). In vivo finite element model-based image analysis of pacemaker lead mechanics. *Medical Image Analysis*, 5(4):255–270.

Berry, S., Carlin, B., Lee, J., and Müller, P. (2010). *Bayesian Adaptive Methods for Clinical Trials.* CRC Press, Boca Raton, FL.

Bonangelino, P., Irony, T., Liang, S., Li, X., Mukhi, V., Ruan, S., Xu, Y., Yang, X., and Wang, C. (2011). Bayesian approaches in medical device clinical trials: a discussion with examples in the regulatory setting. *Journal of Biopharmaceutical Statistics*, 21(5):938–953.

Campbell, G. and Yue, L. (2016). Statistical innovations in the medical device world sparked by the fda. *Journal of Biopharmaceutical Statistics*, 26(1):3–16.

Curtis, A., Worley, S., Adamson, P., Chung, E., Niazi, I., Sherfesee, L., Shinn, T., and Sutton, M. (2013). Biventricular pacing for atrioventricular block and systolic dysfunction. *New England Journal of Medicine*, 368:1585–1593.

Gold, M., Kanal, E., Schwitter, J., Sommer, T., Yoon, H., Ellingson, M., Landborg, L., and Bratten, T. (2015). Preclinical evaluation of implantable cardioverter-defibrillator developed for magnetic resonance imaging use. *Heart Rhythm*, 12(3):631–638.

Haddad, T., Himes, A., and Campbell, M. (2014). Fracture prediction of cardiac lead medical devices using Bayesian networks. *Reliability Engineering & System Safety*, 123:145–157.

Haddad, T., Himes, A., Thompson, L., Irony, T., Nair, R., and MDIC Computer Modeling and Simulation Working Group Participants (2017). Incorporation of stochastic engineering models as prior information in Bayesian medical device trials. *Journal of Biopharmaceutical Statistics*, 10:1–15.

Holmes, D., Kar, S., Price, M., Whisenant, B., Sievert, H., Doshi, S., Huber, K., and Reddy, V. (2014). Prospective randomized evaluation of the Watchman Left Atrial Appendage Closure device in patients with atrial fibrillation versus long-term warfarin therapy: the PREVAIL trial. *Journal of the American College of Cardiology*, 64(1):1–12.

Ibrahim, J. and Chen, M. (2000). Power prior distributions for regression models. *Statistical Science*, 15(1):46–60.

Kovatchev, B., Breton, M., Man, C., and Cobelli, C. (2009). In vivo finite element model-based image analysis of pacemaker lead mechanics. *Journal of Diabetes Science and Technology*, 3(1):44–55.

Mandrola, J., Foy, A., and Naccarelli, G. (2018). Percutaneous left atrial appendage closure is not ready for routine clinical use. *Heart Rhythm*, 15(2):298–301.

MDIC (2017). Medical device innovation consortium. `"http://mdic.org/computer-modeling/virtual-patients/"`.

Mullin, C., Vincent, L., Haddad, T., White, R., Carlson, M., Cetnarowski, W., Duncan, B. et al. (2018). The clinician role in trial innovation using bayesian methods and a novel engineering model (in review). *Journal of the American College of Cardiology.*

Musgrove, D. (2018). bayesDP R Package: Tools for the Bayesian discount prior function. `"https://cran.r-project.org/web/packages/bayesDP/vignettes/bdpbinomial-vignette.html"`.

O'Hagan, A., Stevens, J., and Campbell, M. (2005). Assurance in clinical trial design. *Pharmaceutical Statistics*, 4(3):187–201.

Pibouleaua, L. and Chevret, S. (2011). Bayesian statistical method was underused despite its advantages in the assessment of implantable medical devices. *Journal of Clinical Epidemiology*, 64(3):270–279.

Shiren, O. and Jeffrey, J. (2017). An FDA viewpoint on unique considerations for medical-device clinical trials. *New England Journal of Medicine*, 376:1350–1357.

U.S. Food and Drug Administration (2017). Medical Devices. `"https://www.fda.gov/MedicalDevices/DeviceRegulationandGuidance/Overview/GeneralandSpecialControls/default.htm"`.

Viceconti, M., Cobelli, C., Haddad, T., Himes, A., Kovatchev, B., and Palmer, M. (2017). In silico assessment of biomedical products: The conundrum of rare but not so rare events in two case studies. *Journal of Engineering in Medicine*, 231(5):455–466.

Viele, K., Berry, S., Neuenschwander, B., Amzal, B., Chen, F., Enas, N., Hobbs, B., Ibrahim, J., Kinnersley, N., Lindborg, S., Micallef, S., Roychoudhury, S., and Thompson, L. (2014). Use of historical control data for assessing treatment effects in clinical trials. *Pharmaceutical Statistics*, 13(1):41–54.

Wilkoff, B., Albert, T., Lazebnik, M., Park, S., Edmonson, J., Herberg, B., Golnitz, J., Wixon, S., Peltier, J., Yoon, H., Willey, S., and Safriel, Y. (2013). Safe magnetic resonance imaging scanning of patients with cardiac rhythm devices: a role for computer modeling. *Heart Rhythm*, 10(12):1815–1821.

26

Program and Portfolio Decision-Making

Nitin Patel
Cytel Inc, US

Charles Liu
Cytel Inc, US

Masanori Ito
Astellas Pharma Inc., Japan

Yannis Jemiai
Cytel Inc, US

Suresh Ankolekar
Cytel Inc, US and Maastricht School of Management, Netherlands

Yusuke Yamaguchi
Astellas Pharma Inc., Japan

Recent analysis by the Tufts Center for the Study of Drug Development estimates an average cost of $2.6 billion to develop and gain marketing approval for a new drug. Despite this massive investment, the probability of clinical success was estimated to be a dismal 11.8%. Clearly drug development expenses need to be managed more efficiently and effectively. The key is to integrate cross-functional information in a structured manner that permits comparison of different development strategies. Layered onto that is the understanding of uncertainty and the balancing of risk and reward. Decisions at the program and portfolio levels should be supported by optimal choice theory and a quantitative modeling of risk and uncertainty. Statisticians, being essentially trained in the science of uncertainty, are perfectly placed to influence the decision-making process, supporting it with tools like decision analysis, optimization, modeling and simulation. Furthermore, the Bayesian approach to statistical inference is incredibly well-suited to the task, since it naturally supports decision theory by way of intuitive probability statements on meaningful events, formal incorporation of prior or external information, quantification of trade-offs with loss functions, and regular updates of the picture as data accrue. In this chapter we provide clinical trial statisticians and decision analysts with an overview of the area of quantitative modeling to support drug development decisions at program and portfolio levels. We give an overview of classical statistical approaches currently used to manage programs and portfolios, and discuss their pitfalls. We describe how Bayesian inference can inform and improve decisions made to promote or abort programs or products in development. We focus on approaches that explicitly model the relationship between trial designs and performance criteria. We include detailed case studies on program and portfolio level decision support models and conclude with an outlook for future developments, open problems, and emerging opportunities.

26.1 Introduction

The development of medicines and devices to improve human health is a noble, yet onerous and risky endeavor. The most recent analysis by the Tufts Center for the Study of Drug Development estimated a cost (averaged across a range of therapeutic areas) of $2.6 billion to develop and gain marketing approval for a new drug (DiMasi et al., 2016). Despite this massive investment, the probability of clinical success (i.e. the likelihood that a drug that enters clinical testing will eventually be approved) was estimated to be a dismal 11.8%. Meanwhile, capturing the promised return on investment remains elusive in the post-blockbuster drug (multi-billion dollar product targeting large disease population) era. This is especially true given the rising regulatory and societal scrutiny faced by the pharmaceutical industry when it comes to safety and cost. Newer regulatory requirements for ever more intense monitoring of safety and benefit-risk, coupled with pressure from payers to demonstrate cost-effectiveness, though both justified, have increased the burden on drug developers. This has created an environment full of constraints, in which smart and judicious decisions need to be made to maximize return and minimize risk for the drug developers, in view of the modern portfolio theory (Brealey, 1983; Sharpe, 1981). Antonijevic (2015) highlights the need for optimization in the drug development process to improve cost-effectiveness, productivity, and quality in drug development at program and portfolio levels. He notes that the pharma industry is far behind other major industries in deployment of quantitative methods.

Smart and judicious decisions, whether made at the trial, program or portfolio level, should be supported by quantitative modeling of risk and uncertainty. Statisticians, essentially trained in the science of uncertainty, are perfectly placed to quantitatively inform the decision-making process, supporting it with tools like decision analysis, optimization, modeling and simulation. Furthermore, the Bayesian approach to statistical inference is well-suited to the task, since it naturally supports decision theory by way of intuitive probability statements on meaningful events, formal incorporation of prior or external information, quantification of trade-offs with loss functions, and regular updates of the picture as data accrue.

The key is to integrate information from multiple stakeholders in a structured manner that permits comparison of different development strategies. The value of a pharmaceutical product comes down to a delicate balance between cost of development, expected revenues, and *Probability of Success (PoS)*, otherwise expressed as risk. One way to capture this value and all three of its key components is via the *Expected Net Present Value (ENPV)*, the difference between the present value of future returns from an investment and the amount of investment itself, weighted by its PoS. Other measures such as *Return on Investment (ROI)*, or *Benefit-Cost Ratio (BCR)*, where benefits and/or costs may be expressed in non-financial terms, can also be optimized in the Bayesian framework.

These measures can be optimized at the program level to weigh different clinical development strategies against each other and select the most promising one. At the portfolio level, ENPV is also a good measure by which to promote promising products and stop work on others. Of course, portfolio management also comprises strategic goals that may not be directly captured by ENPV, such as reaching multiple market segments or taking advantage of economies of scale in advertising, sales, manufacturing and logistics. Ultimately, however, insights gained from modeling and simulation of different portfolio strategies are meant to be supportive to decision-making, and do not eliminate the need for judgment and experience.

In this chapter we address the Phase IIa (Ph2a) or Proof-of-Concept (POC), Phase IIb (Ph2b) and Phase III (Ph3) stages of clinical development. The reason for this focus is that these stages account for the majority of drug development costs in clinical research and are the area in which most of our own research efforts have been concentrated. All the models we discuss use trial designs to optimize PoS employing what Spiegelhalter et al. (2004) call the *hybrid classical Bayesian* approach. Here, a prior is used at the design stage to determine design variables, while assuming that the data resulting from the trial will be analyzed using classical hypothesis testing and estimation methods. This approach is appropriate for decision analysis since a sponsor decides on the trial design based on available information, with the objective of deriving economic or social benefit, whereas regulatory review for drug approval is typically conducted using classical frequentist theory. Also, our focus is on models that highlight the relationship between trial designs and criteria like PoS, clinical utility, ENPV, ROI and BCR. Bayesian priors are necessary to compute overall PoS for a program since classical methods provide conditional estimates given specific parameter values.

The chapter is organized as follows. In each section, we first discuss decision-making approaches at the program level before continuing to the portfolio optimization challenge. In Section 26.2 we give an overview of classical statistical approaches currently used to manage programs and portfolios, and discuss their pitfalls. We then describe (Section 26.3) how Bayesian inference can inform and improve decisions made to promote or abort programs or products in development. Case studies follow (Section 26.4) to illustrate the proposed approaches. Finally, we conclude (Section 26.5) with an outlook on future developments, open problems, and emerging opportunities.

26.2 Classical approaches

26.2.1 Classical approaches to program design

Quantitative program level models link model components for individual trials by developing models for Go/No-Go decisions between trials. The traditional approach to program design uses the frequentist paradigm. In most situations, the focus is designing to detect a clinically meaningful effect of the drug under development. Let us consider the important case of the Go/No-Go decision to launch a Ph3 trial based on Ph2 results. For simplicity, we assume that a single Ph2 trial will be followed by a single Ph3 trial with both efficacy endpoints having Normal distributions differing in Ph2 and Ph3 effect sizes due to differences between populations, sites and other factors. The PoS is the power at the "true", but unknown Ph3 effect size (δ_t). Generally, the targeted power $(1-\beta)100\%$ is 80% or more for Ph3 trials, where β is the Type II error rate. In practice, however, only around 50% of the drugs going into the Ph3 trials are successful. One of the reasons for this phenomenon is the 'regression to the mean' effect due to the Go choice being triggered by higher values of efficacy observed in Ph2 while the No-Go alternative is triggered by lower observed values. Other reasons are greater heterogeneity of the Ph3 population and substantially different populations in Ph2 and Ph3 trials. Wang et al. (2006) use a simulation model to explore three choices for the assumed effect size for Ph3 (δ_a): (i) the Ph2 point estimate (δ_p), and two conservative estimates: (ii) one standard deviation below the point estimate (L_1); and (iii) two standard deviations below the point estimate (L_2). A launching threshold for the effect size based on the minimum clinically and economically meaningful effect size is specified as a criterion to launch Ph3. The Ph2 trial, and the related Ph3 trial when the launch criterion is met, are simulated over various scenarios. The authors report a wide range of variations in the average PoS for the three choices for δ_a. It should be noted that a higher average PoS in Ph3 for a conservative choice of effect size is also associated with a lower probability of launching the Ph3 trial. In addition to simulation and discounting δ_p to obtain conservative values for δ_a, Chuang-Stein and Kirby (2014) recommend reducing the bias due to regression to the mean through replication by conducting dose finding trials after POC trials, reducing Ph2 estimates using meta-analysis and PK/PD modeling. Kirby et al. (2012) investigate multiplicative methods for discounting where $\delta_a = f \times \delta_p$. They studied the same scenarios as Wang et al. Based on simulations and empirical analysis of data of completed Ph2 and Ph3 studies between 1998 and 2009 at Pfizer, their broad recommendation is to use a multiplicative discount factor of 0.9 and a Ph3 launch criterion equal to about half of the target effect size for the drug.

De Martini (2013) combines the Ph2 and Ph3 success probabilities in an expression for the overall PoS at the program level. This expression includes a parameter, γ, a measure of conservativeness in the effect size estimate for powering the Ph3 trial. γ is the confidence level for a one-sided confidence limit of the estimate of the effect size from the Ph2 trial. The lower limit of Ph2 effect size is used for powering the Ph3 trial. Higher γ would lead to lower probability of launching the Ph3 trial but a higher expected PoS on average, while lower values of γ have the opposite effect. De Martini finds an optimal value of γ using Ph2 data to devise a calibrated optimal sample size strategy and reports that it is the best Ph3 sample size estimator among several competing strategies when the ratio of true effect sizes of Ph3 and Ph2 is in the range 0.8 to 1.0.

While it is important to optimize Ph3 sample sizes to ensure that the trials are not underpowered, the sample size and the PoS play a critical role in determining the value of drug development at the program and portfolio levels. De Martini (2014) extends the above approach to allocate resources to Ph2 and Ph3 sample sizes to maximize overall PoS for the Ph2/Ph3 program. Antonijevic (2015) highlights key components for assessing the value as costs, expected revenues, and risks that are influenced by the trial design and its implementation. For example, the Ph2 and Ph3 sample sizes determine the program duration, which affects time to market if the program is successful, thus impacting revenue. This adds another dimension to the optimization of the Ph3 sample size. Typically, ENPV is a concave function of the sample size, with a maximum ENPV at an optimum sample size that could be different from conventional sample sizes.

26.2.2 Classical approaches to portfolio optimization

One simple, but effective, approach to portfolio decision making is to set consistent Go/No-Go criteria. One large pharmaceutical company that has adopted a uniquely consistent approach to decision making is AstraZeneca (Frewer et al., 2016). Specifically, all trials planned in early clinical development undergo a standardized procedure for deriving pre-specified Go/No-Go criteria. The criteria are calculated using two target values for the primary endpoint, and two threshold probabilities relating to these targets (1) the false stop risk (similar to a Type II error rate) is set to 10%, and (2) the false go risk (similar to the Type I error rate) is set to 20%. Deviations from these fixed probability thresholds are exceptional, and must be justified. However, this approach does not provide quantitative measures of portfolio performance.

Drug development portfolio management is fundamentally a multi-faceted problem in terms of scope, uncertainties, tools, techniques and process. The scope includes choice of the program designs, scheduling of the drug development projects, in-licensing/out-licensing/partnering of the projects, resource allocations to ongoing and planned projects and reallocation of resources of terminated projects. Uncertainties related to the PoS in multiple phases determine the probability of launching the next phase, the trial duration, and the market risk impacts the value and downside risk of the portfolio.

Persinger (2015) highlights two key challenges in prioritizing and choosing drug development investments at a portfolio level in a resource constrained environment. Firstly, allocating resources between different programs at a given point of time is difficult as they are at various stages of development. Secondly, the periodic nature of the portfolio review leads to delay in reallocating resources of a terminated project. A project-driven approach that optimizes programs individually may lead to undesirable portfolio from a strategic perspective, in addition to being sub-optimal. Persinger proposes a "hybrid" approach, where the project-level decisions are made in the context of regular or real-time portfolio reviews and availability of updated information.

Sharpe and Keelin (1998) describe a three-phase decision-making process developed at SmithKline Beecham involving management and project teams. The first phase primarily focuses on the alternatives where the project teams iteratively generate options to modify the current plan adding, deleting, and changing the scope of programs under the "What-Ifs" guidance of management teams. The second phase focuses on valuing the alternatives with the project teams performing the detailed evaluations that are calibrated by management teams to ensure consistency across the alternatives and clarity among teams. The third phase completes the resource-allocation process with project teams involved in further refinements and evaluations of the final set of alternatives and decision-making by the management teams. The projects are ranked on the basis of the return on investment (ROI=ENPV/Budget) and selected in decreasing order of ROI until the total available budget is allocated. The emphasis here is on the iterative and refined process that promotes shared understanding among the decision-makers and development teams and addresses soft issues around resource allocation including information quality, credibility, and trust.

Various tools and techniques have been proposed and deployed to support the decision-making at the project and portfolio level. Bode-Greuel and Nickisch (2008) proposed value-driven project management tools to align the projects with the portfolio decisions. Kloeber and Kim (2012) outlined various portfolio management methods for different stages of drug development based on key project characteristics including cost, timing, risk, and value. Nie et al. (2012) presented a stochastic combinatorial optimization decision-support tool to address several interacting decisions involved in portfolio management at program and portfolio level. The tool uses a genetic algorithm to search for the optimal solutions in the decision space, linked to an evaluation model of the drug development pathway that captures the interdependencies, value and risks of critical events for a portfolio of drugs. The tool evaluates combinations of strategic decisions by simulating the event flow of parallel projects using simulations to generate probability distributions of the NPV. These and other papers in the engineering literature do not model the impact of trial designs on portfolio value. As mentioned earlier, our focus in this chapter is on portfolio models that explicitly model the relationship between trial designs and performance criteria like PoS, ENPV and BCR.

26.3 Current Bayesian approaches to program design

26.3.1 Conceptual overview

The primary focus of drug development has for a long time been on the cost and the timeline of development. The most important parameter, PoS, has largely been overlooked, and drugs were developed as if the success was imminent (Bonabeau et al., 2008). However, failing drugs yield only the cost of development, and the later they fail, the greater the cost. When pharmaceutical companies evaluate PoS, it is typically evaluated by a committee of experts, with limited use of data. Another way is to estimate the PoS as the industrial average from benchmarking. This is a more objective approach, but often there is no reference data for compounds in a new disease area. In this case, a range of possible values can be estimated from subjective estimates by experts. This approach is commonly applied in practice, but is done without a Bayesian model for deriving the PoS from trial design parameters. Julious and Swank (2005) describe a Bayesian decision tree model that goes beyond individual trials to apply Bayesian analysis to the clinical development plan of a compound.

Following a study, we can update the PoS of Ph2 and Ph3 as posterior probabilities sequentially in a Bayesian framework. The later the development stage, the smaller the uncertainty about PoS. Figure 26.1 shows a decision tree with the distribution of PoS at various stages of a clinical development plan.

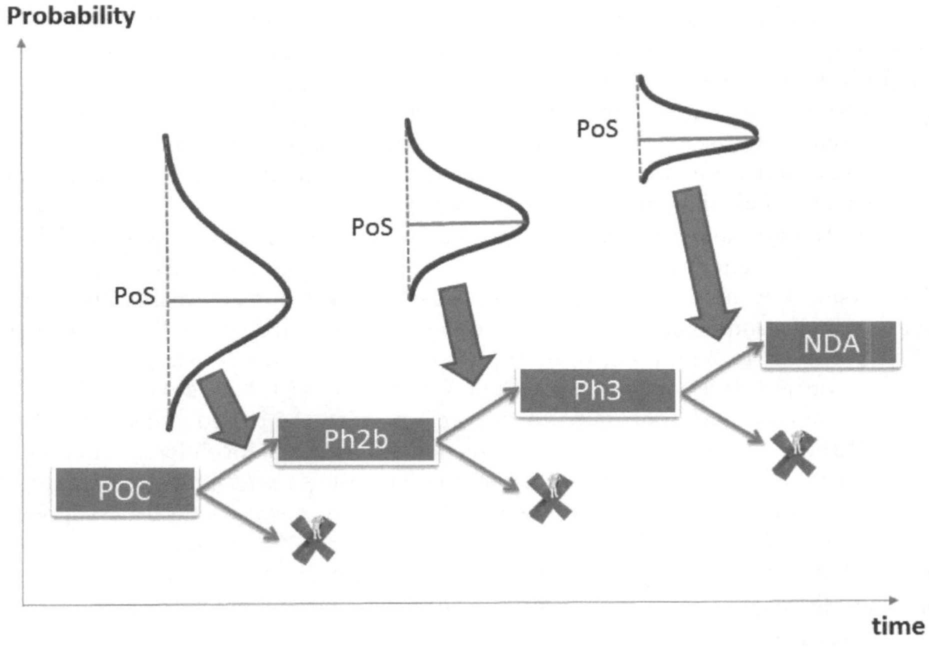

FIGURE 26.1: Schematic representation of the sequential nature of clinical development. Go/No-Go decisions are made following results of POC (Ph2a), Ph2b, and Ph3 trials. The uncertainty in PoS estimates is depicted as reducing after results of each phase become available in the case of Go decisions.

POC study results are used to determine if the project will go to the next phase or not. This decision is usually made using efficacy criteria, while checking that there are no serious safety concerns. However, the best decision may change dynamically, depending on various internal or external factors. For example, the minimum requirement of the treatment difference against comparator for the compound may increase following the launch of a new competitor. The ENPV may decrease due to news of safety concerns for a similar compound developed elsewhere. Factors which should be considered in the Go/No-Go decision include: timeline, cost, and value of the compound (commercial value, strategic fit for the company, unmet medical needs). One way to tackle this complex problem is to conduct program level analysis under various scenarios. Once the POC study is conducted, we can model design elements of subsequent stages such as sample sizes, trial costs, and timelines. Finally, we can calculate the predictive probability to meet the target product profile (PoS), ENPV and other metrics, to support decisions regarding this project.

The typical cash flow over time for a drug that is launched is shown in Figure 26.2. It has two components: the pre-launch drug development cost profile and the post-launch net revenue profile.

The drug development costs include all expenditures directly related to preparation for the *New Drug Application (NDA) submission.* It includes costs of POC, Ph2b and Ph3 trials and other costs incurred related to developing the drug. For simplicity we assume two confirmatory Ph3 trials are required, and that they are conducted in parallel. If the Ph3 trials are successful and regulatory approval is obtained, and the decision is made to launch, there are major additional set-up costs for manufacturing, training and recruiting sales staff, and marketing expenses. This leads to the trough at the time of launch prior to generation of revenue from sales of the drug.

The net revenue profile is the cash flow from sales revenue less the cost of goods sold, marketing and sales costs. Net revenue rises after launch as market penetration increases. Over time (generally around 5 years from launch) it flattens out at a peak level due to market saturation. When the patent life of the drug expires net revenue begins to decline because competing and generic drugs enter the market resulting in decrease in market share and large reductions in the drug price.

After the POC study is conducted, we can plan the study design of later phases (Ph2b and Ph3) and estimate launch timing. The planned sample size of Ph2b and Ph3 may be changed according to the results from the POC study. Of course the changes of planned sample sizes affect the total cost and timeline. ENPV is calculated by time discounting the revenue and cost profiles, with consideration of remaining patent life. Other measures of value can also be updated. The revenue profile generally drops rapidly for small molecule drugs after patent expiry due to generic versions marketed by competitors and so is not likely to contribute significantly to overall ENPV. However, biosimilar drugs often come to market at prices that are not inexpensive and it would be important to model comparative cost effectiveness of competing products after patent expiry for such drugs.

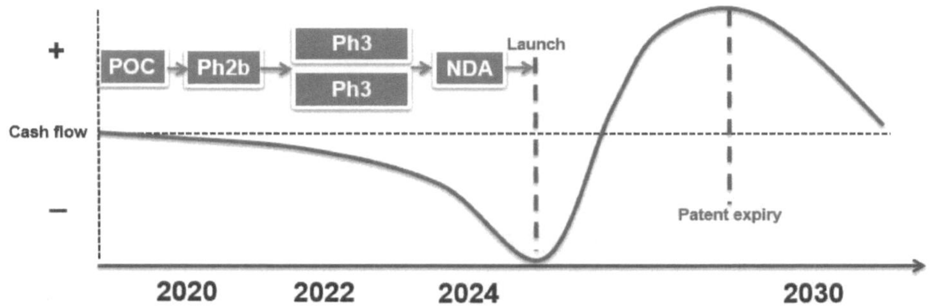

FIGURE 26.2: Typical cash flow profile for drug development program.

The Go/No-Go decision can be made on the basis of ENPV from updated parameters. For example, if the efficacy result from the POC trial is weaker than expected, the sample sizes of Ph2b and Ph3 will increase, delaying the launch, and shortening the remaining patent life, which ultimately decreases the ENPV. Thus, a value-driven approach can lead to a No-Go decision after POC, even if the treatment difference against the comparator satisfies the efficacy criteria.

Go/No-Go decision criteria should be set at the planning stage of the POC. A natural and intuitive approach is to decide to Go if the Bayesian posterior probability, Pr(treatment difference $> \delta \mid D) > \theta$, where θ is a threshold value. The critical treatment difference, δ, is a clinically meaningful difference or defined values in the target product profile.

26.3.2 Simulation methods

Program-level simulation can be used to optimize the threshold posterior probability, θ, in the value-driven approach. For example, we can calculate the ENPV for several thresholds (e.g. 0.7, 0.8, 0.9, etc.) and examine their operating characteristics. Figure 26.3 shows an example of the simulation cycle for a simple illustrative program.

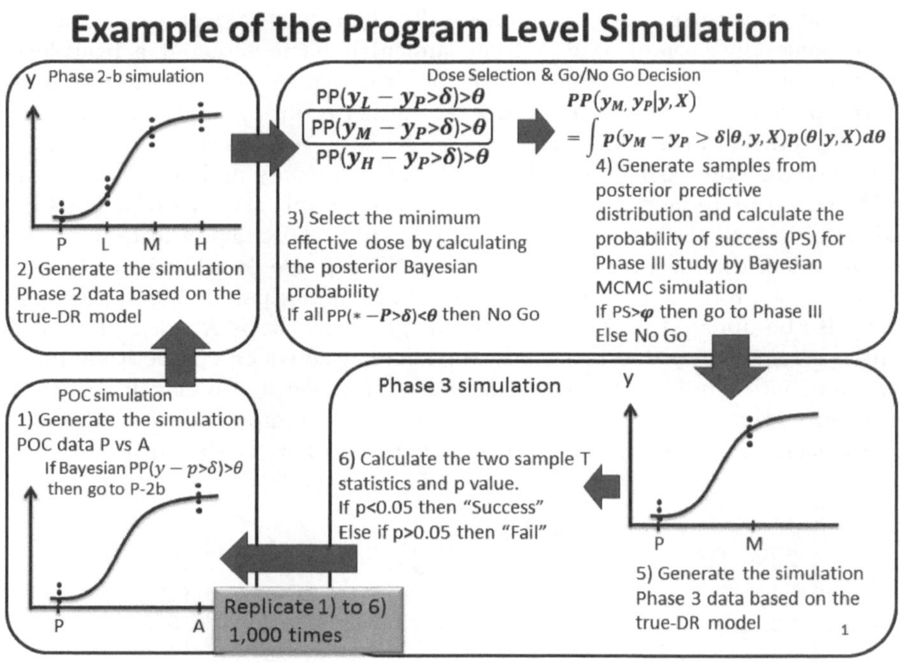

FIGURE 26.3: High level overview of the flow of simulations for an example program depicted as consisting of 6 steps that are iterated 1000 times.

The program consists of the following 6 steps:

- Draw a Monte Carlo (MC) sample of patient responses in a 2-arm POC trial of the study drug (A) vs. Placebo (P) that follow a stipulated dose response curve and compute the Bayesian posterior probability (PP) that the difference between the A and P arms exceeds a hurdle difference δ. If the PP is greater than a threshold value θ, proceed to the next step;
- Draw a MC sample of responses for a 4-arm Ph2b trial with Low (L), Medium (M) and High (H) doses versus placebo;

- Select the smallest dose that clears the hurdle value with a PP that exceeds θ to carry to Ph3. If no dose is available stop; otherwise go to the next step. In Figure 26.3, the Medium dose is chosen for this sample;

- Compute the PoS for the selected dose. If it exceeds a cut-off value ϕ, go to the next step; otherwise stop the program after Ph2b.

- Draw a Monte Carlo (MC) sample of patient responses for a 2-arm Ph3 trial;

- Conduct a 2-sample t test on the Ph3 sample at a 2-sided significance level of 0.05. If the null hypothesis is rejected, the simulated program is considered a success. Otherwise, record a program failure.

From the results of 1000 simulated trials calculate performance metrics such as PoS, ENPV, downside risk of NPV falling short of a target value, and probability of meeting the Minimum Effective Dose at Ph2b for various values of θ and ϕ can be calculated for a sufficient number of simulations. The entire process can be repeated for different true dose response curves to explore robustness to dose response specification errors.

Over the last few decades, several authors have proposed Bayesian approaches to program design. For example, Whitehead (1985) represents an early Bayesian reference on program design, although he relied on analytic calculations, rather than simulations. Inoue et al. (2002) proposed a fully Bayesian sequential approach for expanding a randomized Ph2 trial to Ph3. The decisions to stop early, continue, or proceed to Ph3 were made repeatedly during a time interval. Their simulations showed clear advantages for this Bayesian sequential design (smaller sample sizes, and shorter trial durations) over conventional group sequential designs.

Chuang-Stein et al. (2011) observe that often sponsors make Go/No-go decisions based on various probabilities under different assumptions of treatment effect. They do not assess how likely the assumed treatment effect is to be true in a rigorous fashion. Chuang-Stein et al. argue that successive milestones such as end of Ph1, Ph2a or Ph2b provide natural decision points to evaluate accumulating data. In modeling terms, this leads to the hybrid classical-Bayesian approach of Spiegelhalter et al. (2004) that we have referred to earlier in Section 26.1. Chuang-Stein et al. (2011) advocate the use of assurance (O'Hagan et al., 2005) to make the sample size decision for confirmatory trials, see also Chapters 4, 5, 3 and 17. They illustrate the value of using assurance in making Go/No-Go and sample size decisions through two case studies. The first is related to development of SC-75416, a COX-2 inhibitor for acute and chronic pain, and the second to Axitinib, a treatment of pancreatic cancer.

More recent work explicitly uses ENPV as a key metric to compare fixed versus adaptive trial designs within a program. As discussed earlier, one of the advantages of this metric is that it naturally incorporates an explicit tradeoff between PoS and time delays or trial costs. We summarize below examples of this approach reported by the Adaptive Program subteam of the Adaptive Design Scientific Working Group (ADSWG) of the Drug Information Association (DIA) and include a more detailed case study on neuropathic pain (Patel et al., 2012) in a later section.

Marchenko et al. (2013) compared five hypothetical programs for treatments in advanced pancreatic cancer, and the goal was to select the better dose in Ph2 to take to Ph3. Three prior settings (optimistic, uniform, and pessimistic) were represented by discrete prior distributions over possible values of the hazard ratio. Out of the five programs, the best ENPV was found for the most complex program, which included features such as adaptive randomization and early stopping for futility and efficacy. In an extension of the paper, Parke et al. (2017) considered eight different Ph2/Ph3 development programs. For each program, a positive result in Ph2 led to the selected treatment to be studied in a single two-arm Ph3 clinical trial, which was assumed to be sufficient for regulatory approval in this case study. A Bayesian approach was utilized in the adaptive trial designs. For example, in designs with an option to drop an arm, this decision was based on the posterior probability that the hazard ratio was less than one: $\Pr(HR < 1)$. A distribution of treatment effects was assumed, for which they assigned prior weights to discrete values of HR (1, 0.9, 0.8, 0.7, and 0.6). An additional constraint was that the expected PoS in Ph3 should be at least 50%: designs that did not meet this criterion were selectively penalized, so that programs that included those Ph3 designs were rarely optimal. Their principal conclusions were that the addition of a group sequential design in Ph3 increased the ENPV by around 35%, while the use of adaptive elements in Ph2 design increased ENPV by about 15%. Overall, similar to previous findings, the optimal program (highest ENPV) here was the most complex one: a three-arm response adaptive randomization design in Ph2, plus a group sequential design with five analyses in Ph3.

In a similar study, Antonijevic et al. (2013) presented an example of optimizing design aspects of Ph2b and Ph3 in a treatment for type 2 diabetes. Like Marchenko and Parke, they created different dose efficacy and safety profiles, with random variation in patient responses. Fixed versus adaptive design, as well as Ph2b and Ph3 sample sizes were compared on ENPV. The authors found that the adaptive design was superior to the fixed design at identifying the best dose at Ph2b, and that larger sample sizes in Ph3 (ranging from 200 to 600 patients) led to improvements in ENPV.

De Martini (2016) builds on the ADSWG work to optimize a measure of profit that adjusts the ENPV for volatility. He uses the Bayesian concept of assurance to incorporate ideas from his approach (described in Section 26.2.1) to determine Ph2 sample size. The measure of profit that he uses is the classical mean-variance criterion of Levy and Markowitz (1979).

26.3.3 Analytic methods

26.3.3.1 Chen-Beckman approach

In a series of publications, Chen and Beckman have investigated how to maximize the efficiency or cost-effectiveness of trial, program, or portfolio decisions, in terms of optimal Type I and Type II error rates or sample sizes, e.g. Beckman et al. (2011); Chen and Beckman (2009a,b). Their approach can be considered a Bayesian one, in which they place a two-point prior on the treatment effect: a prior probability p that the alternative hypothesis is true, and prior probability $1-p$ that null hypothesis is true. In this approach, optimum power for a POC trial is the one that maximizes a Benefit Cost Ratio (BCR). The numerator (benefit) is proportional to the expected number of truly active drugs correctly identified for Phase III, while the denominator (cost) is the expected sample size required. Alternative measures of benefits or costs, e.g. in terms of NPV, or quality adjusted life years (QALY) can also be used to define this ratio.

For a fixed, finite budget, the Chen-Beckman approach can be used to determine how large (and how many) POC trials should be conducted. In several analyses, they have found that the optimal power, and equivalently optimal sample size, tend to be lower than the desired power and sample sizes of traditional designs. At the program level, it is more cost-effective to conduct more (and smaller) POC trials, and to set the corresponding Go/No-Go criteria high. This is because for a fixed budget, one needs to account for the opportunity cost of failing to fund additional POC trials that could have detected a successful treatment. For example, Chen et al. (2015) showed a typical example where two POC studies at 60% power were up to 30% more efficient than a single POC study at 80% power.

26.3.3.2 Holmgren approach

Holmgren (2013) advocates the use of a measure for sponsor companies to optimize Ph2/Ph3 programs and portfolios. This measure, which he calls efficiency, is the same as the BCR measure as defined by Chen and Beckman.

To illustrate his approach consider a setting where there is a single Ph2 trial followed by a Ph3 trial if the Ph2 trial, that has the same Normally distributed endpoint as the Ph3 trial, is significant at a one-sided level of α_2. Both the Ph2 and Ph3 trials are balanced 2-arm trials of drug vs. control. The mean treatment effect size is δ, where $\delta < 0$ if the drug is effective and $\delta = 0$ if it is not. Ph3 is successful if the null hypothesis $\delta = 0$ is rejected at α_3, the one-sided significance level, and p is the prior probability that the drug is effective. In this case, he shows:

$$\text{Efficiency} = \frac{p \times \Phi\left(Z_{\alpha_2} - [Z_{\alpha_3} - Z_\beta] f_\delta \sqrt{f_N}\right) \times \Phi\left(Z_{\alpha_3} - [Z_{\alpha_3} - Z_\beta] f_\delta\right)}{N\left[f_N + p \times \Phi\left(Z_{\alpha_2} - [Z_{\alpha_3} - Z_\beta] f_\delta \sqrt{f_N}\right) + (1-p)\alpha_2\right]},$$

where $\Phi(\cdot)$ denotes the cumulative standard Normal distribution, and $\Phi(Z_x) = x$, N is the Ph3 sample size for power $= (1 - \beta)$, f_N is the Ph2 sample size expressed as a fraction of N, f_δ is the actual value of δ expressed as a multiple of the value of δ used to compute N.

For an intuitive understanding of this formula note that:

- The numerator is the PoS for the program. It is the product of three terms. The first term is the prior probability that the drug is effective, the second term is the probability of Ph2 trial success, and the third term is the probability of Ph3 success;
- The denominator is the expected number of subjects enrolled in the program. The first term in the square bracket is the Ph2 sample size expressed as a fraction of N, the Ph3 sample size; the second term and third terms are the expected sample sizes for Ph3 if the drug is effective and not effective respectively expressed as fractions of N;
- If we visualize a situation where many similar programs are undertaken, efficiency is the rate per expected number of subjects enrolled in the Ph2+Ph3 program at which the clinical development strategy identifies effective drugs through successful programs.

Holmgren argues that efficiency is a better measure than ENPV to support decision making at both program and portfolio levels. His main reason for advocating efficiency as opposed to ENPV is that it does not require estimates of market revenues for drugs under development. However, despite the difficulty in estimating revenues for new drugs, ENPV along with ROI (and other measures based on cash flow) are key financial yardsticks for late stage trials, and are widely used in pharmaceutical companies.

Holmgren develops several models that use the efficiency measure to provide insight into different aspects of drug development.

At the portfolio level, he shows that maximizing efficiency is equivalent to maximizing the expected number of effective drugs that have success at Ph3 subject to a constraint limiting the size of the overall Ph2/Ph3 budget. However, he makes the strong assumptions that Ph3 cost as well as prior probability of success are the same for all the drugs, and ignores potential market value differences among the drugs.

26.3.4 Current Bayesian approaches to portfolio design

Chen and Beckman have extended their approach to optimizing program level to portfolio level decisions (Chen et al., 2015). Their model was developed for application to oncology trials to optimally allocate resources when there are more POC trials of interest than the budget available for them. Mallinckrodt et al. (2012) and Lindborg et al. (2014) describe an approach that is similar to that of Chen et al. (2015) in that they use 2-point priors for drug effectiveness to optimize α and β of POC trials for a portfolio of candidate drugs for clinical development from POC trials to be carried forward to Ph3. However, they do not explicitly consider budget allocation to candidate drugs but use methodology similar to classical discriminant analysis to construct classification rules that incorporate the total expected cost of development. Mallinckrodt et al. (2012) point out that a limitation of their own work is that they have assumed that all drugs in the portfolio are at the same stage of development. They recognize that: "In practice, research enterprises typically have drugs at all stages of development with decisions made one at a time" In Case study 3, we examine the paper by Patel and Ankolekar (2015), which models this sequential aspect of portfolio decision making. A key advantage of their model is that it integrates knowledge from experts in diverse areas of expertise such as clinical research, trial management, clinical operations, statistics, financial analysis, and marketing. Their formulation is rich in scope and provides the basic framework for quantitative analysis to support a variety of practical decisions arising in the portfolio optimization context.

26.4 Case studies of program and portfolio-level Bayesian decision analysis models

In this section we provide details of applications that illustrate use of a Bayesian decision theoretic approach to support program and portfolio decision making.

26.4.1 Case study 1

The examples of Ph2/Ph3 programs we have discussed so far all involve a Ph2 trial followed by one or two confirmatory Ph3 trials. There are situations when a Ph2/Ph3 program has to be designed where the rate of availability of patients for trials is slow relative to that of new treatments. This case study (Hee and Stallard, 2012) illustrates a model for a Ph2/Ph3 program of such a situation that arises in the context of developing a treatment for severe asthma using mediator antagonists that target the inflammatory mediator receptors. The total patient population size of 300 is small. There are three promising treatments.

The primary endpoint is binary and is the same for both Ph2 and Ph3. For each patient, absence of moderate or severe asthma exacerbation during the treatment period of 4 weeks is considered to be a success. The program design consists of a series of decision-theoretic single-arm Ph2 trials followed by a randomized balanced two arm Ph3 trial. For the Ph3 trial a classical frequentist analysis is used to test significance at a two-sided level of 0.05. There is a gain of 1 unit if the Ph3 trial is successful. There is a fixed cost associated with setting up a trial. For each Ph2 trial the fixed cost is 0.002 units while for the Ph3 trial the fixed cost is 0.02. There is a variable cost per patient of 0.0001 units. There is a common beta prior for the Pr(success) parameter for a patient for each of the Ph2 trials which are conducted sequentially. Also, there is sequential decision-making within each Ph2 trial based on the posterior after observing each subject. After each update one of four decisions is made: (i) recruit one more patient to the current Ph2 trial; (ii) stop the trial and proceed to Ph3; (iii) stop the current Ph2 trial and start another trial with a new candidate treatment; or (iv) stop the trial and abandon the development plan. At every decision point the action that gives the maximum expected utility is chosen. Expected utility for an action is the maximum achievable expected value of the difference between gain and future trial costs. These values are computed for each action by using a dynamic programming algorithm that employs backward recursion. This corresponds to working back from the end nodes of a decision tree in steps until the root node of the tree is reached.

The optimum strategy that maximizes expected utility is to have a minimum of 19 patients in the first Ph2 trial and continue recruitment up to a maximum of 84 patients. If 78 successes are observed in the 84 patients, then proceed to Ph3; otherwise initiate the second Ph2 trial for which the corresponding optimum values are minimum = 11, maximum = 44, proceed to Ph3 if 41 successes are observed; otherwise stop the second Ph2 trial and proceed to Ph3. The third Ph2 trial is not worth undertaking because at this stage there are only 172 patients in the population that have not already been enrolled in Ph2 trials and it is better to go directly into Ph3.

26.4.2 Case study 2

Patel et al. (2012) presented a case study for Ph2 trial design based on program-level considerations. The various design elements included the number of doses, the sample sizes for Ph2 and Ph3, and the dose selection rule. Simulations within a Bayesian framework allowed for a number of program-level metrics (such as the PoS, ENPV, and probability of exceeding a threshold NPV value) to be used for optimizing trial design.

In this case study, the simulations followed a five-step procedure:

1. The primary measure of efficacy was a 0 to 10 numeric rating scale (NRS). The mean change from baseline between the investigational product and placebo is 1 NRS unit, so this represented the target efficacy response. Results were generated for a single Ph2 study, which would determine whether Ph3 (two identical pivotal trials) should be launched. Ph2 data were simulated under various assumptions for number of doses (4 vs. 8), sample size, and dose-response relationships for both efficacy and safety. Seven dose-response profiles were for efficacy (Figure 26.4). Six of these profiles (all except the NULL response) were multiplied by 3 levels of maximum response, creating 19 (18 + NULL) dose response relationships. These 19 dose response relationships were crossed with three possible profiles for safety (Table 26.1), making a total of 57 scenarios. The safety profile is expressed as the probability of a patient experiencing nuisance adverse events (AEs) commonly associated with products for neuropathic pain (e.g. weight gain and decrease in sexual function). These AEs will not cause stoppage of development or prevent drug approval, but will lower the benefit/risk profile and negatively impact sales.

TABLE 26.1: Probability profiles for adverse events (AE) at each dose.

Pr(AE)	Dose levels						
AE Profile	0	1,2,3	4	5	6	7	8
Low	0.1	0.10	0.10	0.10	0.13	0.15	0.18
Moderate	0.1	0.10	0.15	0.20	0.25	0.30	0.35
High	0.1	0.15	0.23	0.30	0.38	0.45	0.53

The standard deviation of subject response was 2 units. These values were assumed to be the same for Ph2 and Ph3 within each program simulation for both Ph2 and Ph3. Recall that the target efficacy response was 1 NRS unit (difference from placebo). The three levels of maximum efficacy response for each profile

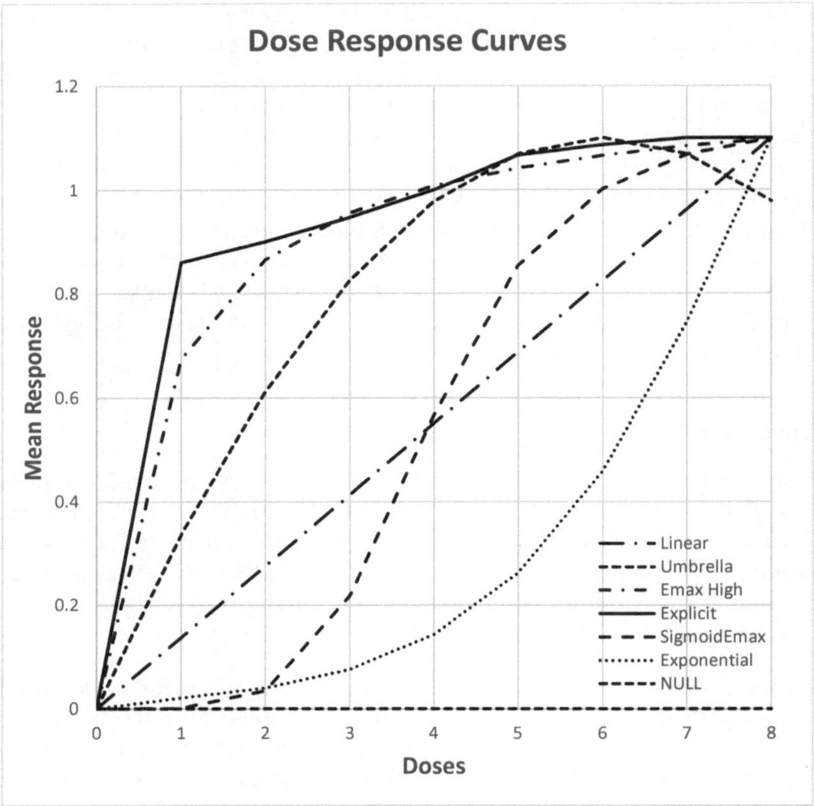

FIGURE 26.4: Dose-response profiles considered in simulations.

were: 1.1 as the base level, and 50% higher and lower levels. The Ph2 efficacy data were fitted using a 4-parameter logistic (4PL) model, with "almost flat" priors to the model parameters and the variance. Note that the prior is on 4 model parameters, rather than the treatment effect size. Samples from the posterior distributions were drawn using a Gibbs block sampling algorithm that was found to be much better than a Metropolis within Gibbs procedure. The Ph2 safety data are analyzed using a frequentist isotonic regression model to estimate the mean safety response at each dose. The responses are generated for each patient as independent Bernoulli trials. The simulations were performed using a custom software tool known as CytelSim, written in C++.

2. Following each simulated Ph2 trial, one dose was selected for Ph3, using one of two criteria: (a) the target dose selection method, i.e. the dose whose estimated efficacy was closest and above the target (of 1 NRS unit), or (b) the maximum utility method, i.e. select the dose that would yield the maximum utility that was based on a combination of efficacy and tolerability as described in item 4 below. If no dose satisfied either criterion, the development program was terminated. Before either method is applied, a linear trend test is conducted on the efficacy endpoint. Because doses are equally-spaced on the log scale, the trend test is equivalent to fitting a linear regression model on the log dose. The two methods

for selecting a dose for Ph3 trials are applied only if the trend test is significant at the one-sided 5% level.

3. If the simulated program proceeds to Ph3, two Ph3 trials are simulated by generating responses that follow the same true underlying distributions used in Ph2. A program was considered as successful only if both Ph3 trials demonstrated a statistically significant treatment effect.
4. The expected net present value (ENPV) was calculated, reflecting factors such as: time to patent expiry, trial costs, and efficacy and safety at the recommended dose. The safety and efficacy values are combined into a clinical utility function of the marketed dose as shown in Figure 26.5. This clinical utility function was estimated by two experienced clinicians who were co-authors of the case study. The net revenue over time after market release was constructed to ramp up in 5 years to a peak that was proportional to the clinical utility and to decline sharply after expiry of the patent. This approach aligns societal and sponsor objectives.
5. Steps 1-4 were repeated many times to calculate a number of key metrics such as: probability of entering Ph3, probability of success, the average total development time, and the probability of achieving certain thresholds for ENPV.

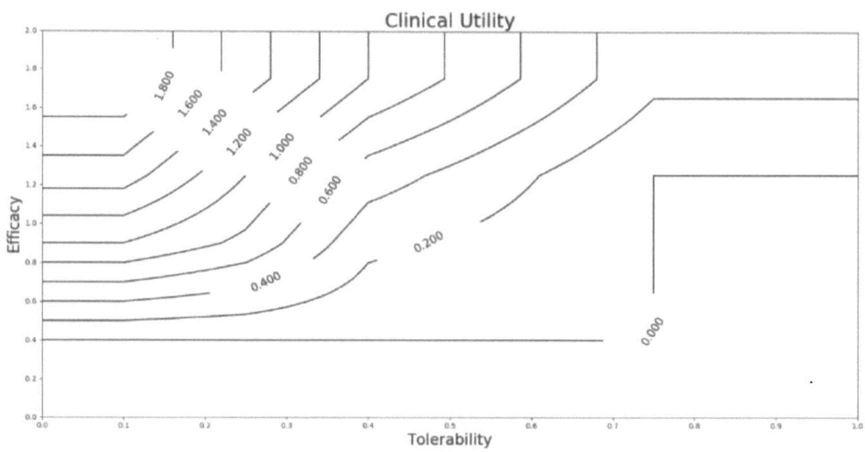

FIGURE 26.5: Clinical Utility function reflecting trade-off between efficacy and tolerability ($\Pr(AE)$).

The principal findings from simulations are described below.

i. **Probability of Success**. PoS for the Ph2+Ph3 program maximum utility dose selection method dominated the target dose selection method across all scenarios and all sample sizes. In Table 26.2 we show detailed results for all the dose profiles (except the NULL profile) and where the maximum response was 1.1 and the tolerability profile was moderate. The improvement in PoS for a sample size of 270 ranges from 4 to 64%;

ii. **Expected Net Present Value**. In the case study, maximizing ENPV was the criterion used to determine the optimal sample size for the Ph2 trial. Table 26.3 gives ENPV values for different sample sizes for all dose profiles (except the NULL profile) where the maximum response was 1.1 and the tolerability profile was moderate.

TABLE 26.2: Probability of Success for the Program: comparison of target and maximum utility dose selection methods for all dose profiles (except NULL) with maximum response = 1.1 and moderate AE profile.

	SigmoidEmax		EmaxHigh		Explicit		Exponential		Linear		Umbrella	
Ph2 Sample Size	Target Dose	Max Utility Dose	Target Dose	Max Utility Dose	Target Dose	Max Utility Dose	Target Dose	Max Utility Dose	Target Dose	Max Utility Dose	Target Dose	Max Utility Dose
135	0.54	**0.80**	0.28	**0.43**	0.25	**0.38**	0.43	**0.55**	0.63	**0.63**	0.49	**0.55**
225	0.55	**0.95**	0.38	**0.61**	0.37	**0.55**	0.56	**0.77**	0.85	**0.85**	0.54	**0.76**
270	0.60	**0.98**	0.43	**0.70**	0.42	**0.64**	0.59	**0.83**	0.85	**0.89**	0.58	**0.82**
405	0.53	**0.99**	0.44	**0.84**	0.47	**0.78**	0.61	**0.93**	0.85	**0.97**	0.55	**0.93**
540	0.57	**1.00**	0.54	**0.93**	0.53	**0.87**	0.61	**0.98**	0.83	**0.99**	0.61	**0.98**
675	0.57	**1.00**	0.53	**0.96**	0.55	**0.94**	0.68	**0.99**	0.84	**1.00**	0.61	**1.00**
810	0.55	**1.00**	0.50	**0.99**	0.49	**0.95**	0.62	**0.99**	0.80	**1.00**	0.58	**1.00**

The ENPV for the optimal sample sizes for each dose response profile are shown in the shaded cells for both target and maximum utility dose selection methods. For every profile, the latter method is superior. The utility maximization method dominated even when the target was reduced from 1.0 NRS to 0.2 NRS with a step size of 0.1 NRS. Reducing the target increases the probability of going to Ph3. However, this does not improve the performance of the target method in selecting the right dose or improving the ENPV;

iii. **Effect of different AE profiles**. The maximum utility dose selection method continues to be the preferred method for low and high tolerability scenarios. For example, for the Sigmoid Emax dose response profile with maximum response 1.1 NRS and a moderate tolerability scenario the optimal ENPV under the maximum utility selection method is greater than that under the target efficacy selection method for the low, medium and high AE profiles by 113%, 89% and 66%, respectively. A similar preference is shown when the maximum response dose response profiles are 50% higher or lower than the base value of 1.1 NRS;

iv. **Sample size decision for Ph2 trial**. To determine the optimal sample in Ph2 assuming that we did not know the maximum level or the shape of the true efficacy dose response profile, two methods were considered: (a) yielding the highest expectation of ENPV with respect to prior probabilities across the full range of 54 non-NULL scenarios or (b) a minimax approach, i.e. minimizing the maximum loss, defined as the difference of the ENPV for that sample size from the best ENPV across all sample sizes for that scenario. For method (a), if we assume that all the non-NULL scenarios are equiprobable, the optimum sample size is 270 for both 4 dose and 8 dose designs. Under this method, another assumption could be that the dose response profiles and tolerability profiles are equiprobable and independent, and that the maximum efficacy is independent of these, with the base level being twice that of the lower and higher levels. In this case the optimal sample size depends on the number of doses tested: 270 patients for 4-dose designs and 405 for 8-dose designs, whereas in (b), the optimum sample size was 270 for the 4-dose design as well as for the 8-dose design;

TABLE 26.3: ENPV comparison of target and maximum utility dose selection methods for all dose profiles (except NULL) with maximum response = 1.1 and moderate AE profile.

	SigmoidEmax		EmaxHigh		Explicit		Exponential		Linear		Umbrella	
Ph2 Sample Size	Target Dose	Max Utility Dose	Target Dose	Max Utility Dose	Target Dose	Max Utility Dose	Target Dose	Max Utility Dose	Target Dose	Max Utility Dose	Target Dose	Max Utility Dose
135	1.23	**2.02**	0.85	**1.51**	0.85	**1.42**	0.4	**0.91**	**1.42**	1.35	1.35	**1.85**
225	1.16	**2.29**	1.18	**2.04**	1.18	**1.95**	0.61	**1.26**	**1.78**	1.77	1.48	**2.43**
270	1.22	**2.32**	1.31	**2.32**	1.32	**2.23**	0.69	**1.39**	1.75	**1.79**	1.65	**2.61**
405	1.03	**2.23**	1.28	**2.61**	1.35	**2.53**	0.76	**1.42**	1.6	**1.83**	1.46	**2.77**
540	1.04	**2.13**	1.47	**2.68**	1.42	**2.61**	0.71	**1.36**	1.46	**1.74**	1.54	**2.71**
675	0.97	**2.01**	1.33	**2.61**	1.37	**2.62**	0.76	**1.3**	1.36	**1.63**	1.42	**2.56**
810	0.88	**1.86**	1.16	**2.46**	1.14	**2.45**	0.68	**1.19**	1.19	**1.49**	1.27	**2.36**

v. **Sample size decision for Ph3 trials.** When a dose has been identified for the Ph3 trials, two Ph3 trials were designed with the same sample size. Usually, a Ph3 trial is designed to have a pre-specified power (e.g. 90%) to detect a clinically meaningful difference (e.g. 1 NRS unit) at the two-sided 5% significance level. The standard deviation for the Ph3 trials is assumed to be at two NRS units. In the case study, the usual sample size consideration is overridden by the need to satisfy an ICH E1 safety data requirement. ICH E1 states the extent of pre-marketing product exposure needed to support marketing authorization of drugs intended for long-term treatment of non-life threatening conditions. In general, it is anticipated that the total number of individuals treated with the investigational drug at the dosage levels intended for clinical use should be about 1500. Due to the safety database requirement, Ph3 sample sizes are driven by the need to satisfy the safety database requirement in the base case. This safety database requirement results in Ph3 being over-powered for efficacy in every scenario, i.e. the sample size for the Ph3 trials has greater than 95% power to detect an effect size of 0.5 at the two-sided 5% significance level;

vi. **Optimizing Ph2 and Ph3 sample sizes.** There are situations when an indication is supplemental to existing indications. In this case, there is often a lower minimum requirement on exposure for safety assessment because the product has already been taken by many patients in the market place. In this case, a relevant question is how to plan Ph2 and Ph3 trials to optimize on the metric of choice. Figure 26.6 shows how this assessment could be done using ENPV as the basis for optimization assuming the Sigmoid Emax profile with maximum response of 1.1 NRS and the moderate tolerability profile. We include in Figure 26.6 results from both dose selection methods. For each curve the rightmost point plotted corresponds to the situation where the point with the requirement for 1500 observations mentioned in point 5 above was met. The curves suggest that a total sample size of approximately 135 (power=81.2%) for the Ph2 trial is the best under the target effect method. Under the maximum utility method, ENPV is maximized at a Ph2 sample size of 270 with Ph2 power = 97.5%. The optimal total sample size for Ph3 (combined over the two trials) is 1000 for the target efficacy method and 700 for the maximum utility method. The corresponding ENPV's are 1.42 and 2.79 ($Billion), respectively. The advantage of the maximum utility method over the target efficacy method is a 96% improvement in the ENPV.

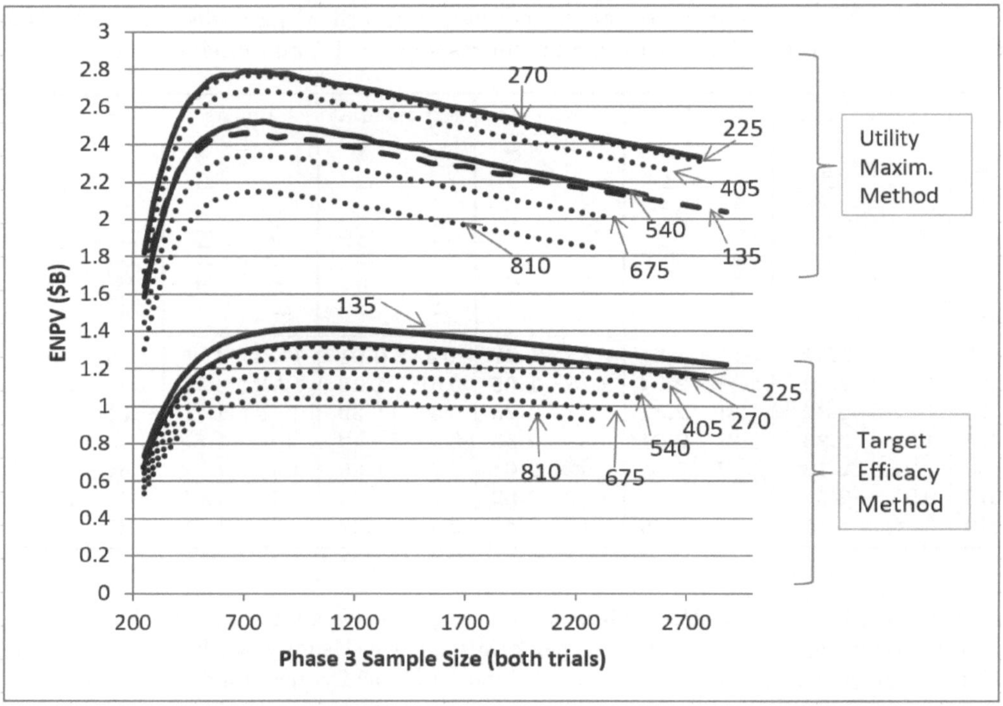

FIGURE 26.6: Optimum Ph2 and Ph3 trial sizes with no adjustment for ICH E1 safety database requirement.

The ENPV, being the mean of the NPV distribution, does not reflect downside financial risk associated with the program. To assess this it is important to consider the probability of making a loss or earning less than a hurdle value. It can also be sometimes more appropriate to maximize the probability of exceeding a threshold NPV value. In addition to ENPV and PoS, all these measures can be easily generated by the simulation approach outlined above.

26.4.3 Case study 3

Patel and Ankolekar (2015) have developed a model for dynamically optimizing budget allocation for Ph3 drug development portfolios that incorporates uncertainty in the pipeline. The objective of the model is to maximize ENPV of a portfolio over a planning horizon by determining the optimal designs of Ph3 trials for a given budget. The model is formulated as a Stochastic Integer Programming (SIP) model that incorporates uncertainty regarding availability of drugs in the pipeline. The SIP model provides an optimal policy that specifies the optimal design for each drug for every possible scenario of availability of future drugs for Ph3 trials. It optimizes the trade-off between committing budget to drugs available for Ph3 funding at any point in time and preserving budget for drugs in the development pipeline that will need funding in the future. Optimizing this trade-off is challenging because it is uncertain which drugs will need funding in the future as they may fail to progress to Ph3 (e.g. fail in Ph2 or safety studies). This important trade-off is not handled in a consistent, quantitative way in portfolio budgeting models used in practice today.

An advantage of the SIP mathematical structure is that it provides a flexible framework that can be modified to accommodate most practical situations. For example, one can easily impose constraints that may be important for practical implementation. Two such constraints are (1) upper and lower limits on budget usage for therapeutic areas, (2) a drug can become available for Ph3 trials only if another is drug is available. It can be applied to design options that are quite general. For example, group sequential and adaptive designs can be included, and outputs from program level models can be used as inputs to the model. The only requirement is that one has a range of design options with varying costs and revenues, and that success probabilities have been computed from the design parameters for each option. In contrast to the portfolio models developed by Chen and Beckman, the revenue and cost models can be quite general. For example, Ph3 trial costs often have large fixed cost components that do not vary with the number of subjects. Revenues can have time profiles that depend on factors such as time to patent expiry.

Patel and Ankolekar also develop a Monte Carlo simulation model to assess the technical, regulatory and commercial risk of the optimal budget allocation policy. If the risk (e.g. probability of making a loss or not meeting an important threshold ENPV) is considered to be too high the simulation model can be used to investigate proposed plans that reduce risk at an acceptable level of reduction of ENPV from its maximum value.

These models can be used to answer important what-if questions such as those that arise when in-licensing or out-licensing drugs or partnering with investors who share cost and risk of drug development in return for payments from revenues if the drug is approved for marketing.

An important advantage of the model is that it can be used for dynamic re-optimization of the portfolio when changes in the internal and external environment occur and as new information becomes available. This enables rapid, frequent and consistent realignment of the strategy to optimize future use of the budget available for re-allocation.

In an illustrative example they show how the optimization model can be used to decide on the best budget level to meet a target ROI. As a benchmark they first compute the maximum ENPV that is achievable if the design for each drug is calculated in isolation without regard to the budget. For Drug i this is $\max_j\{\text{ENPV}_{ij}\}$. The maximum ENPV that can be achieved for the portfolio is the sum of the maximum ENPV over all drugs. For the example, suppose this is \$11,197M and the corresponding budget required is \$293M. This gives an ROI of 38.3 (=11,197/293). The individual optimum sample sizes (and power) for drugs 1 to 7 are 674 (0.90), 852(0.90), 1176 (0.90), 1300 (0.95), 732(0.95), 1838(0.99), and 832(0.95).

We can use the SIP model to compute the maximum ENPV that can be achieved for different budget levels over a range below \$293. This shows us how the maximum ENPV for the portfolio varies with the size of the budget (B). For our example we display a plot of this relationship in Figure 26.7. The slope of the line joining the origin to a point on this curve for a given budget gives us the best ROI we can achieve at that budget.

Note that we need an efficient algorithm to find the best dynamic allocation for a given budget (one point on the curve). This is because with seven drugs and five designs, there are more than 280,000 possible allocations.

Notice that if we reduce the budget by about 50% to \$150M the maximum ENPV goes down by only 1%. We can increase ROI defined as ENPV/Budget from 38.2 to 73.8 (= 11,077/150) by using an optimal dynamic strategy to allocate Ph3 budget instead of a static strategy that maximizes portfolio ENPV by maximizing ENPV for each drug individually. The ROI has almost doubled!

The ROI increases to 100 by reducing the budget further to \$100M. However the maximum ENPV is \$10,295M, a reduction of 8% from the Maximum ENPV for a \$293 budget. Figure 26.7 shows the trade-off between ROI and Maximum ENPV in deciding on the level of budget to deploy for Ph3 trials. If one has a target ROI we can determine the budget required to maximize ENPV while meeting the target by using budget where the target

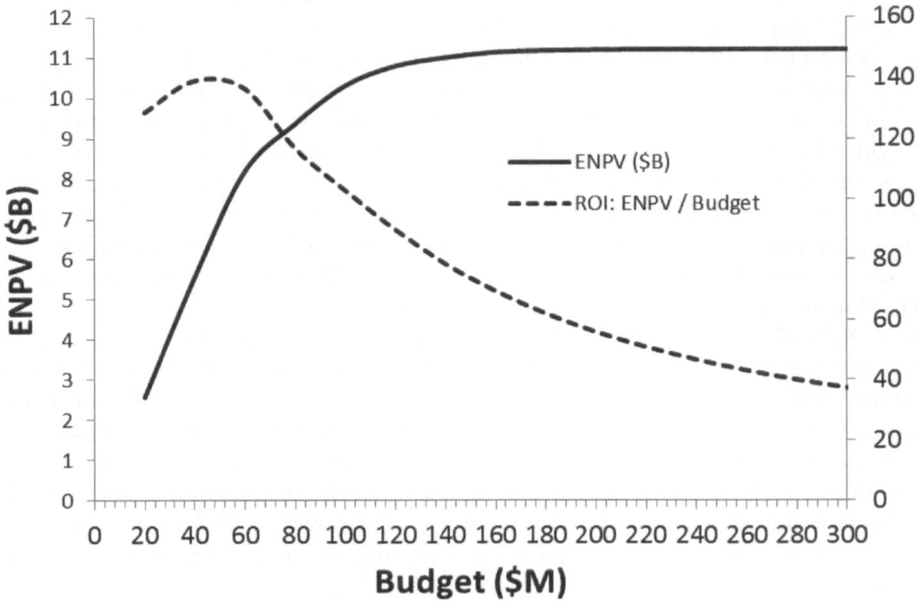

FIGURE 26.7: Portfolio ENPV and ROI for different budget levels.

ROI intersects the ROI curve. If, for instance, we have a target ROI of 90 we need a budget of \$120 to obtain the maximum possible ENPV of \$10,784M. The best budget allocation strategy for a budget of \$150M is shown in Table 26.4.

It is interesting to see that with a budget limited to \$150M, the optimal policy is to out-license Drugs 4 and 5 if Drug 3 is available; and also to out-license Drug 5 if Drug 4 becomes available. We have not considered the potential profit from out-licensing in calculating ENPV in Table 26.1. The chance of an out-licensing situation occurring is small here (about 1%) so it is unlikely to make a significant difference to the optimal dynamic policy. Out-licensing as well as in-licensing opportunities can be readily incorporated into the SIM model.

26.5 Research opportunities and potential for major impact in practice on program and portfolio strategy

In this chapter, our objective has been to provide clinical trial statisticians and decision analysts with an overview of the area of quantitative modeling to support drug development decisions at program and portfolio levels. Owing to space limitations, we have not touched on pioneering work in this area that has potential for expanding the scope of research in quantitative modeling beyond what we have covered. We describe some examples below.

1. More sophisticated models for regulatory decisions in late stage drugs: an example is the paper by Bolognese et al. (2017) that involves modeling of rules that regulators are likely to follow if there is interest in obtaining approval to market one or two doses of a

TABLE 26.4: Optimum allocation for budget = $150M.

Drug	Availability Scenario	Scenario Probability	Contribution to ENPV ($M)	Maximum Budget ($M)	Optimum Sample Size (Power)
1	-	1	2628	21	674 (0.90)
2	-	1	1364	28	852 (0.90)
3	-	0.1	822	43	832 (0.95)
4	D3 not available	0.09	311	47	898 (0.85)
	D3 available	0.01	Out-license / Partner		
5	D3, D4 not available	0.081	33	31	592 (0.90)
	Otherwise	0.019	Out-license / Partner		
6	D3, D4, D5 not available	0.6561	3858	55	1838 (0.99)
	Otherwise	0.2439	1428	39	1300 (0.95)
7	D3, D6 available	0.009	52	17	576 (0.85)
	D4, D6 available, D3 not	0.0081	43	15	504 (0.80)
	Otherwise	0.0829	538	24	832 (0.95)

drug. Another example is the area of progressive approval for different subpopulations, see e.g. Eichler et al. (2015).

2. Inclusion of payer responses to approved drugs in estimating revenues as would occur in the case of outcome dependent reimbursement, see e.g. Trusheim and Berndt (2015).

3. Assessment of the value of group sequential, adaptive, basket and umbrella trial designs at program and portfolio levels, see e.g. Antonijevic (2016).

4. Assessment of the value of biomarkers at program and portfolio levels, see e.g. Beckman et al. (2011, 2015).

5. Modeling the role of trial design in attracting external investments and partnerships to reduce risk by sharing post approval revenues at trial, program and portfolio levels see e.g. Fernandez et al. (2012); Huml (2015); Lo and Naraharisetti (2014); Sunesis (2014).

From a longer-term perspective, recent trends of increasing R&D expense and falling productivity levels have put pressure on pharmaceutical companies to manage drug development more efficiently and effectively to maximize returns. At the same time we are seeing a confluence of two rapidly expanding fields: life science and information technology. This confluence will lead to rapid growth in opportunities for research in quantitative models in program and portfolio optimization for novel systems for organizing drug discovery. For an example of a radically different system for drug development, see Trusheim et al. (2016). For quantitative models to play an important role to support decision making at program and portfolio levels in practice, we feel it is crucial that clinical statisticians and decision analysis experts work closely together to build sound data driven decision processes in pharmaceutical companies.

Bibliography

Antonijevic, Z. (2015). Need for optimal design of pharmaceutical programs and portfolios in modern medical product development. In Antonijevic, Z., editor, *Optimization of Pharmaceutical R&D Programs and Portfolios*, pages 3–16. Switzerland: Springer International Publishing.

Antonijevic, Z. (2016). The impact of adaptive design on portfolio optimization. *Therapeutic Innovation & Regulatory Science*, 50(5):615–619.

Antonijevic, Z., Kimber, M., Manner, D., Burman, C., Pinheiro, J., and Bergenheim, K. (2013). Optimizing drug development programs. *Therapeutic Innovation & Regulatory Science*, 47(3):363–374.

Beckman, R., Clark, J., and Chen, C. (2011). Integrating predictive biomarkers and classifiers into oncology clinical development programs: An adaptive, evidence-based approach. *Nature Reviews Drug Discovery*, 10:735–749.

Beckman, R., Clark, J., and Chen, C. (2015). Portfolio optimization of therapies and their predictive biomarkers. In Antonijevic, Z., editor, *Optimization of Pharmaceutical R&D Programs and Portfolios*, pages 155–180. Switzerland: Springer International Publishing.

Bode-Greuel, K. and Nickisch, K.J. (2008). Value-driven project and portfolio management in the pharmaceutical industry: Drug discovery versus drug development – Commonalities and differences in portfolio management practice. *Journal of Commercial Biotechnology*, 14(4):307–325.

Bolognese, J., Bhattacharyya, J., Assaid, C., and Patel, N. (2017). Methodological extensions of Phase 2 trial designs based on program-level considerations: Further development of a case study in neuropathic pain. *Therapeutic Innovation & Regulatory Science*, 51(1):100–110.

Bonabeau, E., Bodick, N., and Armstrong, R. (2008). A more rational approach to new-product development. *Harvard Business Review*, 86(3):96–102.

Brealey, R. A. (1983). *An Introduction to Risk and Return from Common Stock.* MIT Press, Cambridge, MA.

Chen, C., Beckman, R., and Sun, L. (2015). Maximizing return on investment in Phase II proof-of-concept trials. In Antonijevic, Z., editor, *Optimization of Pharmaceutical R&D Programs and Portfolios*, pages 141–154. Switzerland: Springer International Publishing.

Chen, C. and Beckman, R. (2009a). Optimal cost-effective designs of proof of concept trials and associated go-no go decisions. *Journal of Biopharmaceutical Statistics*, 19(2):424–436.

Chen, C. and Beckman, R. (2009b). Optimal cost-effective go-no go decisions in late-stage oncology drug development. *Statistics in Biopharmaceutical Research*, 1(2):159–169.

Chuang-Stein, C. and Kirby, S. (2014). The shrinking or disappearing observed treatment effect. *Pharmaceutical Statistics*, 13(5):277–280.

Chuang-Stein, C., Kirby, S., French, J., Kowalski, K., Marshall, S., Smith, M. K., Bycott, P., and Beltangady, M. (2011). A quantitative approach for making go/no-go decisions in drug development. *Drug Information Journal*, 45(2):187–202.

De Martini, D. (2013). *Success Probability Estimation with Applications to Clinical Trials.* New Jersey: Wiley.

De Martini, D. (2014). Allocating the sample size in Phase II and III trials to optimize success probability. *Epidemiology Biostatistics and Public Health*, 11(4):1–16.

De Martini, D. (2016). Profit evaluations when adaptation by design is applied. *Therapeutic Innovation & Regulatory Science*, 50(2):213–220.

DiMasi, J., Grabowski, H., and Hansen, R. (2016). Innovation in the pharmaceutical industry: New estimates of R&D costs. *Journal of Health Economics*, 47:20–33.

Eichler, H.-G., Baird, L., Barker, R., Bloechl-Daum, B., Børlum-Kristensen, F., Brown, J., Chua, R., Del Signore, S., Dugan, U., Ferguson, J., Garner, S., Goettsch, W., Haigh, J., Honig, P., Hoos, A., Huckle, P., Kondo, T., Le Cam, Y., Leufkens, H., Lim, R., Longson, C., Lumpkin, M., Maraganore, J., O'Rourke, B., Oye, K., Pezalla, E., Pignatti, F., Raine, J., Rasi, G., Salmonson, T., Samaha, D., Schneeweiss, S., Siviero, P., Skinner, M., Teagarden, J., Tominaga, T., Trusheim, M., Tunis, S., Unger, T., Vamvakas, S., and Hirsch, G. (2015). From adaptive licensing to adaptive pathways: Delivering a flexible life-span approach to bring new drugs to patients. *Clinical Pharmacology and Therapeutics*, 97:234–246.

Fernandez, J., Stein, R., and Lo, A. (2012). Commercializing biomedical research through securitization techniques. *Nature Biotechnology*, 30(10):964–975.

Frewer, P., Mitchell, P., C., W., and J., M. (2016). Decision-making in early clinical drug development. *Pharmaceutical Statistics*, 15(3):255–263.

Hee, S. and Stallard, N. (2012). Designing a series of decision-theoretic Phase II trials in a small population. *Statistics in Medicine*, 31(30):4337–4351.

Holmgren, E. B. (2013). *Theory of Drug Development.* CRC Press, Boca Raton, FL.

Huml, R. (2015). Investment considerations for pharmaceutical product portfolios. In Antonijevic, Z., editor, *Optimization of Pharmaceutical R&D Programs and Portfolios*, pages 49–69. Switzerland: Springer International Publishing.

Inoue, L., Thall, P., and Berry, D. (2002). Seamlessly expanding a randomized Phase II trial to Phase III. *Biometrics*, 58(4):823–831.

Julious, S. A. and Swank, D. J. (2005). Moving statistics beyond the individual clinical trial: Applying decision science to optimize a clinical development plan. *Biometrics*, 4:37–46.

Kirby, S., Burke, J., Chuang-Stein, C., and Sin, C. (2012). Discounting phase 2 results when planning phase 3 clinical trials. *Pharmaceutical Statistics*, 11:373–385.

Kloeber, J. and Kim, C. (2012). Portfolio Management Methods for Different Stages of Drug Development. KROMITE White paper. Accessed on 26 April 2017. `"http://www.kromite.com/dl/Kromite%20White%20Paper%20-%20Horses%20for%20Courses%20v1.pdf"`.

Levy, H. and Markowitz, H. (1979). Approximating expected utility by a function of mean and variance. *The American Economic Review*, 69(3):308–317.

Lindborg, S., Persinger, C., Sashegyi, A., Mallinckrodt, C., and Ruberg, S. (2014). Statistical refocusing in the design of Phase II trials offers promise of increased R&D productivity. *Nature Reviews Drug Discovery*, 13(8):638–640.

Lo, A. and Naraharisetti, S. (2014). New financing methods in the biopharma industry: A case study of royalty pharma, inc. *Journal of Investment Management*, 12(1):4–19.

Mallinckrodt, C., Molenberghs, G., Persinger, C., Ruberg, S., Sashegyi, A., and S., L. (2012). A portfolio-based approach to optimize proof-of-concept clinical trials. *Journal of Biopharmaceutical Statistics*, 22(3):596–607.

Marchenko, O., Miller, J., Parke, T., Perevozskaya, I., Qian, J., and Wang, Y. (2013). Improving oncology clinical programs by use of innovative designs and comparing them via simulations. *Therapeutic Innovation & Regulatory Science*, 47(5):602–612.

Nie, W., Zhou, Y., Simaria, A., and S.S., F. (2012). Biopharmaceutical Portfolio Management Optimization under Uncertainty, Proceedings of the 22nd European Symposium on Computer Aided Process Engineering, 17 - 20 June 2012, London. Accessed on 26 April 2017. "http://booksite.elsevier.com/9780444594310/downloads/ESC.445%20-%20Biopharmaceutical%20portfolio%20management%20optimisation%20under%20uncertainty.pdf".

O'Hagan, A., Stevens, J., and Campbell, M. (2005). Assurance in clinical trial design. *Pharmaceutical Statistics*, 4(3):187–201.

Parke, T., Marchenko, O., Anisimov, V., Ivanova, A., Jennison, C., Perevozskaya, I., and Song, G. (2017). Comparing oncology clinical programs by use of innovative designs and expected net present value optimization: Which adaptive approach leads to the best result? *Journal of Biopharmaceutical Statistics*, 27(3):457–476.

Patel, N. and Ankolekar, S. (2015). Dynamically optimizing budget allocation for Phase 3 drug development portfolios incorporating uncertainty in the pipeline. In Antonijevic, Z., editor, *Optimization of Pharmaceutical R&D Programs and Portfolios*, pages 181–200. Switzerland: Springer International Publishing.

Patel, N., Bolognese, J., Chuang-Stein, C., Hewitt, D., Gammaitoni, A., and Pinheiro, J. (2012). Designing Phase 2 trials based on program-level considerations. *Therapeutic Innovation & Regulatory Science*, 46(4):439–454.

Persinger, C. (2015). Challenges of portfolio management in pharmaceutical development. In Antonijevic, Z., editor, *Optimization of Pharmaceutical R&D Programs and Portfolios*, pages 71–80. Switzerland: Springer International Publishing.

Sharpe, P. and Keelin, T. (1998). How SmithKline Beecham makes better resource-allocation decisions. *Harvard Business Review*, 76(2):45–57.

Sharpe, W. (1981). Decentralized investment management. *Journal of the American Finance Association*, 36(2):217–234.

Spiegelhalter, D., Abrams, K., and Myles, J. (2004). *Bayesian Approaches to Clinical Trials and Health-Care Evaluation.* Wiley, New York, NY.

Sunesis (2014). "Using adaptive design to change an asset's risk profile" in Beyond Borders Biotechnology Industry Report 2014.

Trusheim, M., Shrier, A., Antonijevic, Z., Beckman, R., Campbell, R., Chen, C., Flaherty, K., Loewy, J., Lacombe, D., Madhavan, S., Selker, H., and Esserman, L. (2016). PIPELINEs: Creating comparable clinical knowledge efficiently by linking trial platforms. *Clinical Pharmacology and Therapeutics*, 100:713–729.

Trusheim, M. R. and Berndt, E. (2015). The clinical benefits, ethics, and economics of stratified medicine and companion diagnostics. *Drug Discovery Today*, 20:1439–1450.

Wang, S.-J., Hung, H., and O'Neill, R. (2006). Adapting the sample size planning of a Phase III trial based on Phase II data. *Pharmaceutical Statistics*, 5:85–97.

Whitehead, J. (1985). Designing Phase II studies in the context of a programme of clinical research. *Biometrics*, 41(2):373–383.

Index